COLLECTED PAPERS

Neuroscience Publications IV

Lazaros C. Triarhou

COLLECTED PAPERS

Neuroscience Publications IV, 2009–2013

Research conducted at the Department of Educational Policy, University of Macedonia School of Social Sciences, Humanities and Arts, Thessaloniki, Greece

Collected papers : neuroscience publications IV, 2009–2013.

Lazaros C. Triarhou, MD PhD
Professor of Neuroscience
Aristotelian University
Thessaloniki (Greece)

Copyright © 2023 by L. C. Triarhou
All rights reserved. No part of this book may be used or reproduced, in whole or in part, including illustrations, in any form by any electronic or mechanical means (beyond that copying permitted by Sections 107 and 108 of the U.S. Copyright Law and excerpt by reviewers for the public press), without permission in writing from the author.

Cataloging-in-Publication Data

Triarhou, Lazaros Constantinos
   Neuroscience Publications IV, 2009–2013 / Lazaros C. Triarhou.
   p. cm.
   Includes bibliographical references.
   ISBN: 979-8-865-09924-6
   Imprint: Independently published
   1. Neurosciences.   I. Title.   II. Series: Collected papers.

CONTENTS

Preface · Acknowledgments

2009

114. Triarhou LC: Alfons Maria Jakob (1884–1931), neuropathologist par excellence: Scientific endeavors in Europe and the Americas. *European Neurology 61:* 52–58, 2009

115. Triarhou LC, Vivas AB: Poetry and the brain: Cajal's conjectures on the psychology of writers. *Perspectives in Biology and Medicine 52:* 80–89, 2009

116. del Cerro M, Triarhou LC: Eduardo De Robertis (1913–1988). *Journal of Neurology 256:* 147–148, 2009

117. Triarhou LC: Exploring the mind with a microscope: Freud's beginnings in neurobiology. *Hellenic Journal of Psychology 6:* 1–13, 2009

118. Triarhou LC: Tripartite concepts of mind and brain, with special emphasis on the neuroevolutionary postulates of Christfried Jakob and Paul MacLean. In: Weingarten SP, Penat HO (eds) *Cognitive Psychology Research Developments.* Nova Science Publishers, Hauppauge, NY, 2009, p 183–208 [Reprinted in: Wilhelm CE (ed) *Encyclopedia of Cognitive Psychology.* Nova Science Publishers, Hauppauge, NY, 2012, vol. 2, p 489–513]

119. Théodoridou ZD, Triarhou LC: Fin-de-siècle advances in neuroeducation: Henry Herbert Donaldson and Reuben Post Halleck. *Mind Brain and Education 3:* 117–127, 2009

120. del Cerro M, Triarhou LC: Volume determination under the microscope, the simple way: The Delesse–Glagolev principle. *Micscape Magazine UK 161,* 2009

2010

121. Triarhou LC: Revisiting Christfried Jakob's concept of the dual onto–phylogenetic origin and ubiquitous function of the cerebral cortex: A century of progress. *Brain Structure and Function 214:* 319–338, 2010

122. Triarhou LC: Final publications of Christfried Jakob: On the frontal lobe and the limbic region. In: Flynn CE, Callaghan BR (eds) *Neuroanatomy Research Advances.* Nova Science Publishers, Hauppauge, NY, 2010, p 165–169

123. Triarhou LC: Bernhard Pollack (1865–1928). *Journal of Neurology 257:* 1585–1586, 2010

124. del Cerro M, Triarhou LC: The microscope of a shoeless doctor. *Micscape Magazine UK 171,* 2010

125. Koniari D, Triarhou LC: Otto Marburg's "On the question of amusia." *Functional Neurology 25:* 5–7, 2010

2011

126. Koniari D, Proios H, Tsapkini K, Triarhou LC: Singing but not speaking—A retrospect on music–language interrelationships in the human brain since Otto Marburg's *Zur Frage der Amusie* (1919). In: Columbus AM (ed) *Advances in Psychology Research, Volume 87.* Nova Science Publishers, Hauppauge, NY, 2011, p 239–248

127. Triarhou LC: A review of Edward Flatau's 1894 atlas of the human brain by the neurologist Sigmund Freud. *European Neurology 65:* 10–15, 2011

128. Hatzigiannakoglou PD, Triarhou LC: A review of Heinrich Obersteiner's 1888 textbook on the central nervous system by the neurologist Sigmund Freud. *Wiener Medizinische Wochenschrift 161:* 315–325, 2011

129. Théodoridou ZD, Triarhou LC: Christfried Jakob's 1921 theory of the gnoses and praxes as fundamental factors in cerebral cortical dynamics. *Integrative Psychological and Behavioral Science 45:* 247–262, 2011

2012

130. Théodoridou ZD, Triarhou LC: Challenging the supremacy of the frontal lobe: Early views (1906–1909) of Christfried Jakob on the human cerebral cortex. *Cortex 48:* 15–25, 2012

131. Théodoridou ZD, Triarhou LC: Christfried Jakob's late views (1930–1949) on the psychogenetic function of the cerebral cortex and its localization: Culmination of the neurophilosophical thought of a keen brain observer. *Brain and Cognition 78:* 179–188, 2012

132. Triarhou LC, del Cerro M: Ramón y Cajal erroneously identified as Camillo Golgi on a souvenir postage stamp. *Journal of the History of the Neurosciences 21:* 132–138, 2012

133. Triarhou LC: Cytoarchitectonics of the human cerebral cortex: The 1926 presentation by Georg N. Koskinas (1885–1975) to the Athens Medical Society. In: Bright P (ed) *Neuroimaging—Cognitive and Clinical Neuroscience.* InTech Publishers, Vienna, 2012, p 1–16

134. Triarhou LC: Alfred Fuchs (1870–1927). *Journal of Neurology 259:* 1764–1765, 2012

135. Triarhou LC: Erwin Stransky (1877–1962). *Journal of Neurology 259:* 2012–2013, 2012

136. Triarhou LC: Professor Bernhard Pollack (1865–1928) of Friedrich Wilhelm University, Berlin: Neurohistologist, ophthalmologist, pianist. *European Neurology 67:* 338–351, 2012

2013

137. Triarhou LC, del Cerro M: Ramón y Cajal as an analytical chemist of bottled water? Use (and misuse) of the great savant's repute by the industry. *Sage Open 3:* 1–12, 2013

138. Partsalis AM, Blazquez PM, Triarhou LC: The renaissance of the neuron doctrine: Cajal rebuts the Rector of Granada. *Translational Neuroscience 4:* 104–114, 2013

139. Triarhou LC: Anders Retzius (1796–1860). *Journal of Neurology 260:* 1445–1446, 2013

140. Théodoridou ZD, Triarhou LC: Evolution of Christfried Jakob's views on the frontal lobe, 1890–1949. In: Cavanna AE (ed) *Frontal Lobe: Anatomy, Function and Injury.* Nova Science Publishers, Hauppauge, NY, 2013, p 9–22

141. Théodoridou ZD, Koutsoklenis A, del Cerro M, Triarhou LC: An *avant-garde* professorship of neurobiology in education: Christofredo Jakob (1866–1956) and the 1920s lead of the National University of La Plata, Argentina. *Journal of the History of the Neurosciences 22:* 366–382, 2013

142. Triarhou LC: The cytoarchitectonic map of Constantin von Economo and Georg N. Koskinas. In: Geyer S, Turner R (eds) *Microstructural Parcellation of the Human Cerebral Cortex: From Brodmann's Post-Mortem Map to in Vivo Mapping of High-Field Magnetic Resonance Imaging.* Springer Verlag, Berlin, 2013, p 33–53

PREFACE

The present volume contains articles published from 2009 to 2013, while I was academically affiliated with the University of Macedonia in Greece. The papers revisit classical works by neuroscience pioneers Santiago Ramón y Cajal, Christfried Jakob, Alfons Maria Jakob, Eduardo De Robertis, Bernhard Pollack, Otto Marburg, Edward Flatau, Sigmund Freud, Heinrich Obersteiner, Georg N. Koskinas, Constantin von Economo, and Anders Retzius, among others. Topics range from the ontophylogeny of the cerebral cortex and the triune brain to music-language interrelationships in the human brain and neuroeducation.

I thank my colleagues and co-authors, the institutions that provided research support, and the editors and publishers of the journals or books which hosted the original versions.

Thessaloniki, October 2023

THE AUTHOR

Lazaros C. Triarhou holds an M.D. degree from the Aristotelian University School of Medicine (1981), E.C.F.M.G. Certification (1983), an M.Sc. in Neuroscience from the University of Rochester (1984), and a Ph.D. in Medical Neurobiology from Indiana–Purdue University (1987). He has served on the faculties of Indiana University School of Medicine (1988–2001), University of Macedonia School of Social Sciences, Humanities and Arts (2001–2021), and Aristotelian University Faculty of Philosophy (2021–2024). He has authored *Neural Transplantation in Cerebellar Ataxia* (Springer, 1997), *Dopaminergic Neuron Transplantation in the Weaver Mouse Model of Parkinson Disease* (Kluwer, 2002), *Neuromorphology* (Beta Medical Arts, 2017), *The Brain Masters of Vienna* (Springer, 2022), and *Life and Work of Georg N. Koskinas* (Beta Medical Arts, 2023); translated, revised and edited the first English edition of the *Economo–Koskinas Atlas of Cytoarchitectonics of the Adult Human Cerebral Cortex* (Karger, 2008) and a new English edition of von Economo's *Cellular Structure of the Human Cerebral Cortex* (Karger, 2009); and produced Greek translations of monographs by Nobel laureates Santiago Ramón y Cajal, Fridtjof Nansen, Albert Schweitzer, Christian de Duve, and Gerald M. Edelman. For his research in neural plasticity and regeneration he received the Honorable Weil Award from the American Association of Neuropathologists and the Science Prize in Medicine from the Bodossakis Foundation. He is acquisition editor of 'Pioneers in Neurology' for the *Journal of Neurology* and 'Cerebellar Classics' for the *Cerebellum*.

Historical Note

Eur Neurol 2009;61:52–58
DOI: 10.1159/000175123

Received: January 2, 2008
Accepted: February 18, 2008
Published online: November 25, 2008

Alfons Maria Jakob (1884–1931), Neuropathologist par Excellence

Scientific Endeavors in Europe and the Americas

Lazaros C. Triarhou

Economo-Koskinas Wing for Integrative and Evolutionary Neuroscience, Department of Educational and Social Policy, University of Macedonia, Thessaloniki, Greece

Key Words
Alfons Maria Jakob · Alpers disease · Creutzfeldt-Jakob disease · History of neuroscience · History of neuropathology

Abstract
The study briefly reviews the life and work of Alfons Maria Jakob (1884–1931), a notable representative of pre-war German neuropathology. Today Jakob is mainly remembered by neurologists for the spongiform encephalopathy with progressive dementia and spasticity that he, and Kiel neuropathologist Hans Gerhard Creutzfeldt (1885–1964), described independently. However, Jakob has left additional contributions to neuroanatomy, neuropathology and neuropsychiatry in the form of original articles and valuable monographs.

Copyright © 2008 S. Karger AG, Basel

A notable representative of German neuropathology [1–3], Bavarian neurologist Alfons Maria Jakob (fig. 1), was born on July 2, 1884 in Aschaffenburg am Main to a family of retailers. He studied medicine at the Universities of München, Berlin and Strassburg.

First Publications and Academic Career

The first scientific publication of Alfons Jakob dealt with the symptomatology, pathogenesis and pathological anatomy of the 'circular psychoses' [4]. Jakob completed his doctoral thesis on July 13, 1909 under the supervision of Robert Wollenberg (1862–1942), professor of psychiatry at Kaiser-Wilhelms-Universität Strassburg, on 'the pathogenesis of pseudobulbar palsy' [5] – a lower cranial nerve palsy resulting from supranuclear lesions, so named in 1877 by Lyon physiologist and Charcot student Jacques-Raphaël Lépine (1840–1919). Jakob reviewed 115 literature cases and clinicopathologically studied a 55-year-old male with cerebral atrophy, encephalomalacia multiplex, and circumscribed cerebellar hemorrhage.

On December 1, 1909 Jakob became an assistant physician at the psychiatric clinic directed by Emil Kraepelin (1856–1926) in München, where he trained in neuroanatomy with Alois Alzheimer (1864–1915) through May 1, 1911 [1].

Solicited by professor Wilhelm Weygandt (1870–1939), he moved in November 1911 to the psychiatric clinic of the Friedrichsberg State Hospital in Hamburg, where he eventually succeeded Theodor Kaes (1852–1913) as director *(Prosektor)* of the neuroanatomical laboratory. From the summer of 1915 until the end of World War I, Jakob served as a medical officer at the Belgian front. He was habilitated in neurology and psychiatry at Hamburg University in 1919 and became professor in 1924. He expanded the laboratory with serology, genetics, and experimental psychology sectors, and trained dozens of students from the United States, Russia, Japan, Turkey, Italy, Switzerland, Spain, Portugal and Uruguay [1]. He also kept a reputable medical practice. His brother Franz, also a physician, practiced in Nürnberg [6].

Creutzfeldt-Jakob Disease

At the 10th annual meeting of the Society of German Neurologists, held in Leipzig on September 18, 1920, O.B. Meyer presiding, von Weizsäcker read Jakob's report describing a clinicopathological syndrome in 3 patients (2 female, 51 and 34 years old, and 1 male, 43 years old) with spasticity and progressive dementia associated with cortical, striatal and spinal degeneration [7]. Jakob [8] expanded on those 3 cases in an additional paper. In 1920, Kiel neuropathologist Hans Gerhard Creutzfeldt (1885–1964) had independently published a similar case of a 22-year-old woman [9]. The text that follows gives an overview of what Jakob and additionally Creutzfeldt really described, compared to our current knowledge on spongiform encephalopathies. In-depth accounts have been given by Duckett and Stern [10], Poser and Bruyn [11], and Wolf and Foley [12].

'Creutzfeldt-Jakob disease' (CJD) was so named by Spielmeyer [13] and subsequently included amongst the organic psychoses in Bumke's 1928 *Handbook of Mental Diseases* [12]. The CJD concept is closer to a neuropathological syndrome rather than a single etiologic-nosological entity [10, 14]. Some 84 forms, 'types' or variants of CJD have been recorded on the basis of clinical and neuropathological criteria [15].

Today, CJD is classified as a prion disease ('prionosos') or transmissible spongiform encephalopathy (TSE), characterized by dementia, pyramidal, and extrapyramidal signs clinically, and by neuronal loss, spongiform changes, and astroglial reaction histologically [11, 12].

Scientific interest in CJD became renewed in 1957 with the description of kuru, a contagious disorder in natives of New Guinea [16] and its similarities to scrapie, a transmissible infectious disease in sheep [17, 18]; the concept of prion diseases was formulated 25 years later [19]. Animal forms of TSE, besides scrapie, include bovine spongiform encephalopathy ('mad cow disease') and mink encephalopathy [11].

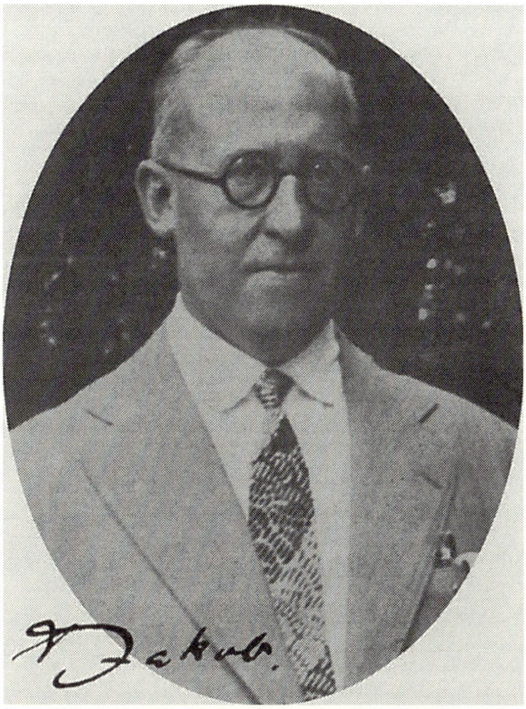

Fig. 1. Professor Alfons Maria Jakob (1884–1931). Photo from Brazilian textbook [36]; signature from an original offprint of his first article [4], hand-inscribed to Viennese neuropsychiatrist Erwin Stransky (1878–1962).

In all, Creutzfeldt studied 1 case [9, 20], and Jakob 7 cases, including the initial 3 cases [7, 8], case 4 [21], and case 5 described in his book on extrapyramidal disorders [22]. The brains of Jakob's patients 6 and 7 were further studied and published posthumously by his pupil Kirschbaum [23], who in his monograph reviewed 150 cases of CJD gathered over a 50-year period, including Creutzfeldt's and Jakob's original cases. English translations of Creutzfeldt's first paper [9] and of Jakob's report on case 4 [21] may be found in Rottenberg and Hochberg [24].

Creutzfeldt's case concerned a patient seen in 1913 at Alzheimer's clinic in Breslau. Because of World War I and Alzheimer's death, Creutzfeldt finalized his manuscript [9] after his 1919 move to Spielmeyer's department in Munich. Creutzfeldt published a sequel paper on the case [20].

Both articles were entitled 'On a particular focal illness of the central nervous system', conveying the possibility of having identified a new entity of unknown etiology [10].

The patient first presented with gait ataxia and developmental behavioral abnormalities when she was 16 [12]. The disease progressed irregularly, with remissions. The later clinical picture included pyramidal signs (paresis, spasticity and bilateral Babinski), hyperalgesia, intention tremor, facial hyperkinesia, nystagmus, myoclonus, dementia, mood changes and mutism [11]. Erythema multiforme bullosum, appearing as herpetiform small vesicles, made its appearance in the vicinity of the third ramus of the left trigeminal nerve. Stupor deepened, swallowing became impaired, and death ensued in status epilepticus [9, 10]. Two of the patient's five siblings had mental deficits and her mother had died of an unknown cause at the age of 56.

The neuropathological finds were focal neuron loss and neuronophagia in the postcentral and precentral gyri (particularly affecting the pyramidal cells of the third and deeper layers), bilateral degeneration of the corticospinal tracts, vascular reaction and astroglial hypertrophy also present in the basal ganglia, thalamus, cerebellum, brainstem and spinal cord [10]. Status spongiosus was not reported [11]. The diagnosis was an acquired polioencephalopathy. Creutzfeldt's case may actually be the first report of herpes zoster encephalopathy [10].

Jakob's first 5 cases [7, 8, 21, 22] and Creutzfeldt's case [9, 20] shared, in Jakob's opinion, a common neuropathological picture, a polioencephalopathy with lesions in the frontal lobe (deep cortical layers in particular) and changes in the rest of the cortex, striatum, thalamus (medioventral and lateral nuclei), substantia nigra, pontine tegmentum, cerebellum, brainstem and spinal cord. Jakob did not regard his first 4 cases as a homogenous group [10] and thought that the bulk of the pathological changes fell on the extrapyramidal system [25]. Diagnosis in cases 1 and 2 was syphilis, in case 3 malaria, and in case 4 chronic alcoholism [7, 8, 21]. In all likelihood, the diagnosis of CJD was correct in Jakob's case 3, the patient with progressive dementia, leg weakness and pain, ataxia, vertigo and diplopia [7, 8], and in case 5 [22], with diffuse vacuolation of the neuropil throughout cerebral cortical areas and the cerebellar molecular layer, typically seen in TSEs [11]. It is also interesting to note that the sister and maternal grandmother, along with 8 of her siblings, of Jakob's patient 6, a 44-year-old male, had died of an undeciphered nervous disorder; the brains of patient 6, his sister, and two of his children contained spongiform changes [11].

Jakob gave the disorder a neuropathological rather than a clinical name, 'spastic pseudosclerosis encephalopathy with disseminated foci of degeneration' [10]. He designated his subgroup of pseudosclerosis 'spastic', owing to the marked corticospinal degeneration [11, 12, 26]. Having access to Creutzfeldt's slides and the galleys of Creutzfeldt's chapter [20], Jakob considered Creutzfeldt's case as another example of spastic pseudosclerosis. However, Creutzfeldt objected to the term 'spastic pseudosclerosis' [11], preferring instead the general description 'progressive focal and diffuse degeneration of the gray matter' [10] and provisionally leaving the disorder without a specific clinical name [12].

The term 'pseudosclerosis' had been introduced in 1883 by the Berlin neuropsychiatrist Carl Westphal (1833–1890) [27] to describe what would later be identified as a juvenile form (Westphal variant) of Huntington chorea [28]. The eponym Westphal-Strümpell pseudosclerosis was also adopted in the German literature, based on additional cases reported by the Erlangen internist Adolf von Strümpell (1853–1925) in children [29].

A 'singular' case of pseudosclerosis with tonic rigidity and high-grade dementia, but without Babinski sign, sensory disturbances or thalamic lesions [30], marked histopathologically by interstitial hepatitis, gliosis in the striatum and globus pallidus, substantia innominata and cerebellar molecular layer, was reported by Economo and Schilder [31] in a 55-year-old man, before Creutzfeldt's first study [9] in the same journal. Although at some point considered to bear similarities with the classical descriptions of CJD [32], that case was probably Wilson disease [33]. Economo and Schilder [31] had inferred that their case affected the extrapyramidal system, with a distant relationship to paralysis agitans and olivopontocerebellar atrophy. Jakob [7] did observe interesting similarities between his first 3 cases and that of Economo and Schilder [31], but pinpointed that the latter was accompanied by liver damage, and thus found an agreement of his cases in all the substantial points only with the case of Creutzfeldt [9].

The question has been raised whether the disease that Creutzfeldt and Jakob independently described is the same, and the validity of Creutzfeldt's case report [9] as an instance of 'classical' CJD has been disputed [11, 12] on grounds of the patient's young age, the developmental symptoms, and the absence of extrapyramidal signs. Kirschbaum [23] and Katscher [34] favor 'Jakob-Creutzfeldt disease' (or 'Jakob's syndrome' [23]) over CJD, crediting Jakob as the major contributor to CJD, and a majority of authors currently consider Jakob's cases as the first true descriptions of CJD [10]. Proof that Jakob's later patients were true cases of CJD came with the identification of a *PRNP* gene mutation [35].

Thus, one may conceivably discern a connection between Jakob's 'syndrome' and the seeds for the eventual bestowal of two of the Swedish Academy's summa cum laude Prizes in Physiology or Medicine: to D. Carleton Gajdusek (and Baruch S. Blumberg) in 1976 'for their discoveries concerning new mechanisms for the origin and dissemination of infectious diseases', and to Stanley B. Prusiner in 1997 'for his discovery of prions, a new biological principle of infection'.

Travels to the Americas

On 27 March 1924, Jakob embarked on the maiden voyage of the Hamburg-American ocean liner *Deutschland* from Southampton, arriving in New York on April 6 [6]. He guest lectured at several institutions, including Columbia University [14].

Four years later, he journeyed to Latin America. In May through July 1928, he gave a 20-lecture course in Rio de Janeiro on nervous and mental pathology (fig. 2), with a theoretical and a practical part, using 4,000 microscopic preparations and transparencies [36]. He then travelled to São Paulo and Campinas, Brazil; Buenos Aires, where he met with physiologist Bernardo Alberto Houssay (1887–1971) and visited the neuroanatomical institute of his fellow countryman, Bavarian neuropathologist Christfried Jakob (1866–1956) [37, 38]; over the imposing Cordillera to Santiago de Chile and Valparaiso; and back, over the Andes, to Montevideo, Uruguay. Jakob gave a presentation of his South American impressions to the Hamburg Medical Association on December 11, 1928 [39].

Authored Works

Jakob published 80 articles on diverse topics [1–3], including cerebellar tumors (1910), trauma and secondary fiber degeneration (1912), cerebellar ataxia [40], multiple sclerosis (1913), epilepsy (1914), diffuse infiltrating encephalomyelitis (1914), spinal cord concussion (1919), endarteriitis syphilitica (1920), paralysis and tabes (1922), megalencephaly (1925), miliary gummata [41], and yellow fever [42], the latter co-authored with Amadeu Fialho and Eudoro Libanio Villela and presented at the 19th annual meeting of the Society of German Neurologists on 20 September 1929 in Würzburg, chaired by Otfrid Foerster (1873–1941). He published a review in Spanish on anatomo-psychiatric correlations [43] and one in Portuguese on multiple sclerosis [44]. Jakob was one of the proponents of the value of histopathology for elucidating the research problems of psychiatric diseases [25, 45].

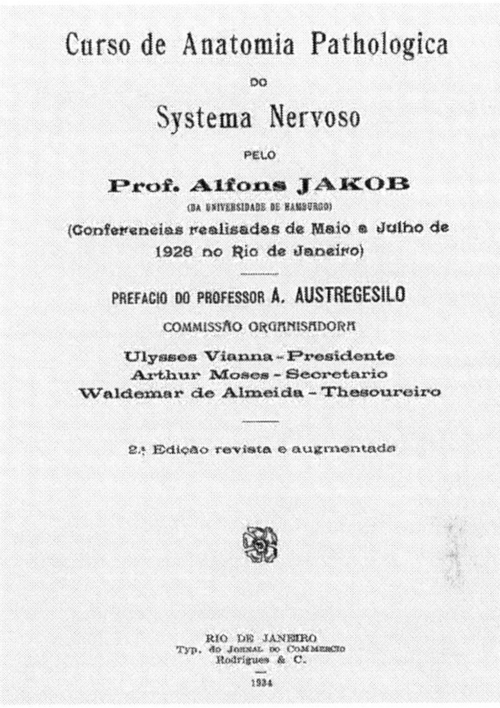
Curso de Anatomia Pathologica
DO
Systema Nervoso
PELO
Prof. Alfons JAKOB
(DA UNIVERSIDADE DE HAMBURGO)
(Conferencias realisadas de Maio a Julho de 1928 no Rio de Janeiro)
PREFACIO DO PROFESSOR A. AUSTREGESILO
COMMISSÃO ORGANISADORA
Ulysses Vianna - Presidente
Arthur Moses - Secretario
Waldemar de Almeida - Thesoureiro
2.ª Edição revista e augmentada
RIO DE JANEIRO
Typ. do Jornal do Commercio
Rodrigues & C.
1934

Fig. 2. Frontispiece of the second edition of Jakob's book containing his Brazilian lectures, published posthumously [36].

Jakob wrote the cerebellar chapter for Möllendorff's 1928 *Handbook of Microscopic Anatomy*, and the neurosyphilis chapter for Bumke's 1930 *Handbook of Mental Diseases* [2, 3]. He authored a monograph on extrapyramidal disorders [22], and contributed two scholarly volumes to Aschaffenburg's *Handbook of Psychiatry*, on normal and pathological neuroanatomy and neurohistology [46] and on special cerebral histopathology [47].

Jakob reviewed the *Cytoarchitectonics of the Adult Human Cerebral Cortex* of Economo and Koskinas [48] and the *Icones Neurologicae* of Strümpell and C. Jakob [49]. Strümpell and C. Jakob had produced the original epitome of *Icones Neurologicae* in 1897 [50]; the plates were re-edited by Müller and Spatz in 1926 with 13 folded plates, 11 of them 106 × 140 cm in size and two 140 × 212 cm [51].

Jakob called the Economo and Koskinas *Cytoarchitectonics* 'a masterpiece unique in the international medical literature', its 112 plates 'brilliant achievements in scientific microphotography', and its text a 'joy to the reader' [48]. Jakob found the nomenclature of Economo and Koskinas 'fully meaningful' in its departure from the methods of Vogt and Brodmann. In his own textbook on *Cerebral Anatomy and Histology,* Jakob [46] devoted two-thirds of the chapter on the architectonic organization of cortical fields to the findings of Economo and Koskinas and reproduced 23 of their original figures, arguing that 'at last we have acquired a perfect and complete map of the cerebral cortex by areas' [48].

Jakob is described as a 'private and disciplined individual, excellent and knowledgeable teacher and charismatic leader' [10]. Besides his own publications, Jakob conceived, and in part dictated, an estimated further 80 works by his students, in which he does not appear as a co-author [1].

Alpers Disease

At the third session of the 20th annual meeting of the Society of German Neurologists in Dresden on 20 September 1930, H. Curschmann presiding, Jakob presented a yet another new entity [52], studied in conjunction with his pupils Somoza, Freedom [53] and Alpers [54]. 'Alpers disease' or progressive infantile poliodystrophy (also called spongy glio-neuronal dystrophy [55]) is a mitochondrial disorder with autosomal recessive inheritance appearing in early infancy [56–58], leading to marked dementia, prominent seizures, spasticity and opisthotonus, and accompanied by liver failure [59, 60]. The histological hallmarks include almost total neuronal loss in the cortical gray matter with spongy changes and astrogliosis, and the molecular genetic defect is associated with mutations in the polymerase-γ *(POLG)* gene of the mitochondrial DNA (mtDNA) [61–63].

Postscript

Jakob gave his 'swan-song' presentation, on the nosology and localization of torsion dystonia with cinematographic and anatomical demonstrations, at the First International Neurological Congress in Berne [64], during the clinical-pathogenetic section of the afternoon of 3 September 1931, chaired by Gheorghe Marinescu (1863–1938).

Shortly after the Berne Congress, neurology lost two of its protagonists: Alfons Jakob on October 17, 1931 in Hamburg, at the age of 47, after an operation to contain complications of streptococcal osteomyelitis, from which he had been suffering for 7 years; and, within 4 days, Constantin von Economo in Vienna, at the age of 55. Three years later to the day, on October 17, 1934, the neuroscience world would lose yet another of its greatest, the venerated Santiago Ramón y Cajal.

Acknowledgements

The author gratefully acknowledges the courtesy of the Öffentliche Bibliothek der Universität Basel, Switzerland, for bibliographic assistance, and the Research Committee of the University of Macedonia, Greece, for subsidizing in part the publication costs.

References

1 Weygandt W: Zum Andenken an Professor Jakob. Dtsch Z Nervenheilk 1931;123:I–IV.
2 Lüthy F: Alfons Jakob. Schweizer Arch Neurol Psychiatr 1932;29:189–191.
3 Hassin GB: Alfons Maria Jakob (1884–1931); in Haymaker W (ed): The Founders of Neurology. Springfield, Thomas, 1953, pp 184–186.
4 Jakob A: Zur Symptomatologie, Pathogenese und pathologischen Anatomie der 'Kreislaufspsychosen'. J Psychol Neurol (Leipz) 1909;14:209–248, 1909;15:99–132.
5 Jakob A: Die Pathogenese der Pseudobulbärparalyse. Arch Psychiatr Nervenkrankh 1909;45:1097–1228.
6 Ancestry.com: New York Passenger Lists, 1820–1957. Provo, The Generations Network, Inc., 2006.
7 Jakob A: Über eigenartige Erkrankungen des Zentralnervensystems mit bemerkenswertem anatomischem Befunde (Spastische Pseudosklerose-Encephalomyelopathie mit disseminierten Degenerationsherden). Dtsch Z Nervenheilk 1921;70:132–146.
8 Jakob A: Über eigenartige Erkrankungen des Zentralnervensystems mit bemerkenswertem anatomischem Befunde (Spastische Pseudosklerose-Encephalomyelopathie mit disseminierten Degenerationsherden). Z Gesamte Neurol Psychiatr 1921;64:147–228.
9 Creutzfeldt HG: Über eine eigenartige herdförmige Erkrankung des Zentralnervensystems. Z Gesamte Neurol Psychiatr 1920;57:1–18.
10 Duckett S, Stern J: Origins of the Creutzfeldt and Jakob concept. J Hist Neurosci 1999;8:21–34.

11 Poser CM, Bruyn GW: Creutzfeldt-Jakob disease; in Koehler PJ, Bruyn GW, Pearce JMS (eds): Neurological Eponyms. New York, Oxford University Press, 2000, pp 283–290.
12 Wolf JH, Foley P: Hans Gerhard Creutzfeldt (1885–1964): a life in neuropathology. J Neural Transm 2005;112:I–XCVII.
13 Spielmeyer W: Die histopathologische Forschung in der Psychiatrie. Klin Wochenschr 1922;1:1817–1819.
14 Jakob A: The anatomy, clinical syndromes and physiology of the extrapyramidal system. Arch Neurol Psychiatry 1925;13:596–620.
15 Masters CL: Creutzfeldt-Jakob disease: its origins. Alzheimer Dis Assoc Disord 1989;3:46–51.
16 Gajdusek DC, Zigas V: Degenerative disease of the central nervous system in New Guinea; the endemic occurrence of kuru in the native population. N Engl J Med 1957;257:974–978.
17 Hadlow WJ: Scrapie and kuru. Lancet 1959;274:289–290.
18 Klatzo I, Gajdusek DC, Zigas V: Pathology of kuru. Lab Invest 1959;8:799–847.
19 Prusiner SB: Novel proteinaceous infectious particles cause scrapie. Science 1982;216:136–144.
20 Creutzfeldt HG: Über eine eigenartige herdförmige Erkrankung des Zentralnervensystems; in Nissl F, Alzheimer A (eds): Histologische und histopathologische Arbeiten über die Grosshirnrinde. Jena, Gustav Fischer, 1921, pp 1–48.
21 Jakob A: Über eine der multiplen Sklerose klinisch nahestehende Erkrankung des Zentralnervensystems (spastische Pseudosklerose) mit bemerkenswertem anatomischem Befunde. Mitteilung eines vierten Falles. Med Klin 1921;17:372–376.
22 Jakob A: Die extrapyramidalen Erkrankungen mit besonderer Berücksichtigung der pathologischen Anatomie und Histologie und der Pathophysiologie der Bewegungsstörungen. Berlin, Julius Springer, 1923.
23 Kirschbaum WR: Jakob-Creutzfeldt disease (Spastic Pseudosclerosis, A. Jakob; Heidenhain Syndrome; Subacute Spongiform Encephalopathy). New York, American Elsevier, 1968.
24 Rottenberg DA, Hochberg FH: Neurological Classics in Modern Translation. New York, Hafner, 1977.
25 Jakob A: Die Histopathologie im Dienste der psychiatrischen Krankheitsforschung. Arch Psychiatr Nervenkrankh 1927;81:68–98.
26 Jakob A: Über drei eigenartige Krankheitsfälle des mittleren Alters mit bemerkenswertem, gleichartigem anatomischem Befunde und ihre klinischen und anatomischen Beziehungen zur spastischen Pseudosklerose und zu metencephalitischen Prozessen. Dtsch Z Nervenheilk 1924;81:192–204.

27 Westphal C: Ueber eine dem Bilde der cerebrospinalen grauen Degeneration ähnliche Erkrankung des centralen Nervensystems ohne anatomischen Befund, nebst einigen Bemerkungen über paradoxe Contraction. Arch Psychiatr Nervenkrankh 1883;14:87–134, 767–769.
28 Holdorff B: Pioneers in Neurology: Carl Westphal (1833–1890). J Neurol 2005;252:1288–1289.
29 von Strümpell A: Ueber die Westphal'sche Pseudosklerose und über diffuse Hirnsklerose, insbesondere bei Kindern. Dtsch Z Nervenheilk 1898;12:115–149.
30 Jacob H, Pyrkosch W, Strube H: Die erbliche Form der Creutzfeldt-Jakobschen Krankheit (Familie Backer). Arch Psychiatr Z Neurol 1950;184:653–674.
31 Economo C, Schilder P: Eine der Pseudosklerose nahestehende Erkrankung im Praesenium. Z Gesamte Neurol Psychiatr 1920;55:1–26.
32 Liberski PP, Budka H: An overview of neuropathology of the slow unconventional virus infections; in Liberski PP (ed): Light and Electron Microscopic Neuropathology of Slow Virus Disorders. Boca Raton, CRC Press, 1993, pp 111–149.
33 Ransmayr G: Constantin von Economo's contribution to the understanding of movement disorders. Mov Disord 2007;22:469–475.
34 Katscher F: It's Jakob's disease, not Creutzfeldt's. Nature 1998;393:11.
35 Brown P, Cervenáková L, Boellaard JW, Stavrou D, Goldfarb LG, Gajdusek DC: Identification of a *PRNP* gene mutation in Jakob's original Creutzfeldt-Jakob disease family. Lancet 1994;344:130–131.
36 Jakob A: Curso de anatomia pathologica do systema nervoso, 2ª edição revista e augmentada. Rio de Janeiro, Rodrigues & Companhia, 1934.
37 Triarhou LC, del Cerro M: Semicentennial tribute to the ingenious neurobiologist Christfried Jakob (1866–1956). 1. Works from Germany and the first Argentina period, 1891–1913. Eur Neurol 2006;56:176–188.
38 Triarhou LC, del Cerro M: Semicentennial tribute to the ingenious neurobiologist Christfried Jakob (1866–1956). 2. Publications from the second Argentina period, 1913–1949. Eur Neurol 2006;56:189–198.
39 Jakob A: Reisebrief aus Südamerika. Dtsch Med Wochenschr 1929;55:281–282, 320–321, 365–368.
40 Jakob A: Zur Klinik und pathologischen Anatomie des chronischen Alkoholismus zugleich ein Beitrag zu die Erkrankungen des Kleinhirns. Z Gesamte Neurol Psychiatr 1912;13:132–152.
41 Jakob A: Über den Befund von miliaren Gummen bei der Paralyse. Z Gesamte Neurol Psychiatr 1926;102:313–319.

42 Jakob A, Fialho A, Villela EL: Über die Veränderungen im Zentralnervensystem bei Gelbfieber. Dtsch Z Nervenheilk 1929;111:111–116.
43 Jakob A: Investigaciones de anatomía cerebral y neuro-psiquiatria clínica. Rev Méd Germano-Ibero-Amer 1928;1:159–169.
44 Jakob A: Concepção actual da esclerose multipla. Brasil Med 1931;45:1101–1103.
45 Jakob A: Die Bedeutung der Histopathologie des Zentralnervensystems für die Erforschung der Geisteskrankheiten. Münch Med Wochenschr 1920;67:875–878.
46 Jakob A: Normale und pathologische Anatomie und Histologie des Grosshirns (mit besonderer Berücksichtigung der Histopathologie der Psychosen und extrapyramidalen Erkrankungen), erster Band: Normale Anatomie und Histologie und allgemeine Histopathologie des Grosshirns. Leipzig/Wien, Franz Deuticke, 1927.
47 Jakob A: Spezielle Histopathologie des Grosshirns, erster Teil. Leipzig/Wien, Franz Deuticke, 1929.
48 Jakob A: Referatenteil, Nerven- und Geisteskrankheiten: Die Cytoarchitektonik der Hirnrinde des erwachsenen Menschen. Von C. Freiherrn von Economo und G. N. Koskinas. Klin Wochenschr (Berl) 1926;5:37–38.
49 Jakob A: Bücherbesprechungen. Strümpell und Jakob, Icones neurologicae. Dtsch Z Nervenheilk 1927;98:154–157.
50 Strümpell A, Jakob C: Neurologische Wandtafeln zum Gebrauche beim klinischen, anatomischen und physiologischen Unterricht. München, Lehmann, 1897.
51 Strümpell A, Jakob C: Icones Neurologicae. Bilder zur makroskopischen Anatomie des Gehirns und zum Bahnenverlauf (Erläuterungen zur 2. Auflage von F. Müller und H. Spatz). München, Lehmann, 1926.
52 Jakob A: Über eigenartige frühinfantil einsetzende Erkrankungen des Großhirns mit besonderer Bevorzugung der grauen Substanz (Grosshirnrinde, Striatum, Pallidum und Thalamus). Dtsch Z Nervenheilk 1930;116:240–253.
53 Freedom L: Über einen eigenartigen Krankheitsfall des jugendlichen Alters unter dem Symptomenbilde einer Littleschen Starre mit Athetose und Idiotie. Dtsch Z Nervenheilk 1927;96:295–298.
54 Alpers BJ: Diffuse progressive degeneration of the gray matter of the cerebrum. Arch Neurol Psychiatry 1931;25:469–505.
55 Jellinger K, Seitelberger F: Spongy glio-neuronal dystrophy in infancy and childhood. Acta Neuropathol 1970;16:125–140.
56 Sandbank U, Lerman P: Progressive cerebral poliodystrophy – Alpers' disease: disorganized giant neuronal mitochondria on electron microscopy. J Neurol Neurosurg Psychiatry 1972;35:749–755.
57 Prick MJJ: Progressive Poliodystrophy: Association with Disturbances in Pyruvate Metabolism. Wijcken (Holland), Drukkerij Dukenburch, 1983.

58 Egger J, Pincott JR, Wilson J, Erdohazi M: Cortical subacute necrotizing encephalomyelopathy: a study of two patients with mitochondrial dysfunction. Neuropediatrics 1984;15:150–158.
59 Aicardi J: Diseases of the Nervous System in Childhood. London, MacKeith Press, 1992, pp 527–529.
60 Neville BGR, Collins JE, Surtees RAH: Paediatric neurology; in Walton J (ed): Brain's Diseases of the Nervous System, ed 10. Oxford, Oxford University Press, 1993, pp 453–477.
61 Nguyen KV, Østergaard E, Ravn SH, Balslev T, Danielsen ER, Vardag A, McKiernan PJ, Gray G, Naviaux RK: *POLG* mutations in Alpers syndrome. Neurology 2005;65:1493–1495.
62 Ferrari G, Lamantea E, Donati A, Filosto M, Briem E, Carrara F, Parini R, Simonati A, Santer R, Zeviani M: Infantile hepatocerebral syndromes associated with mutations in the mitochondrial DNA polymerase-γA. Brain 2005;128:723–731.
63 Davidzon G, Mancuso M, Ferraris S, Quinzii C, Hirano M, Peters HL, Kirby D, Thorburn DR, DiMauro S: *POLG* mutations and Alpers syndrome. Ann Neurol 2005;57:921–923.
64 Jakob A: Zur Frage der nosologischen und lokalisatorischen Auffassung der torsiondystonischen Krankheitserscheinungen; in Brouwer B, Sachs B, Riley HA, Dubois C, Fischer RF von, Schnyder P (eds): Comptes Rendus du 1er Congrès Neurologique International. Berne, Stämpfli, 1932, pp 255–256.

Poetry and the Brain

Cajal's conjectures on the psychology of writers

Lazaros C. Triarhou* and Ana B. Vivas†

ABSTRACT In 1902, Santiago Ramón y Cajal (1852–1934), the father of modern neuroscience and a 1906 Nobel laureate, contributed a preface to a book of poems by his fellow countryman, Spanish poet and dramatist Marcos Zapata (1844–1914). In that uncustomary—for his neuroscience followers—essay, Cajal unfolds his ideas on the literary genres of drama and comedy in relation to the workings of the human mind and sentiments. The same text was reissued almost half a century later in Spain and in Argentina under the title *The Psychology of Artists*. We present an English version of Cajal's essay, which may be of interest to both humanists and biologists, and which further denotes the celebrated neuroanatomist's attempt at understanding the mystery of the human mind.

A PASSING METEOR in the scientific and intellectual vault of the 20th century, Spanish histologist Santiago Ramón y Cajal (1852–1934) also probed the workings of the human brain from a behavioral perspective (Andres-Barquin 2002; Craigie and Gibson 1968; DeFelipe 2002; Garrison 1929; López-Muñoz, Boya, and Alamo 2006; Otis 2001; Williams 1954). Although Cajal was an ortho-

---

*Economo-Koskinas Wing for Integrative and Evolutionary Neuroscience, University of Macedonia, Thessaloniki.
†Department of Psychology, City Liberal Studies, Affiliated Institution of the University of Sheffield, Thessaloniki.
Correspondence: Lazaros C. Triarhou, M.D., Ph.D., University of Macedonia, 156 Egnatia Avenue, Bldg. Z–312, Thessaloniki, GR 54006, Greece.
E-mail: triarhou@yahoo.com.

Perspectives in Biology and Medicine, volume 52, number 1 (winter 2009):80–89
© 2009 by The Johns Hopkins University Press

POETRY AND THE BRAIN

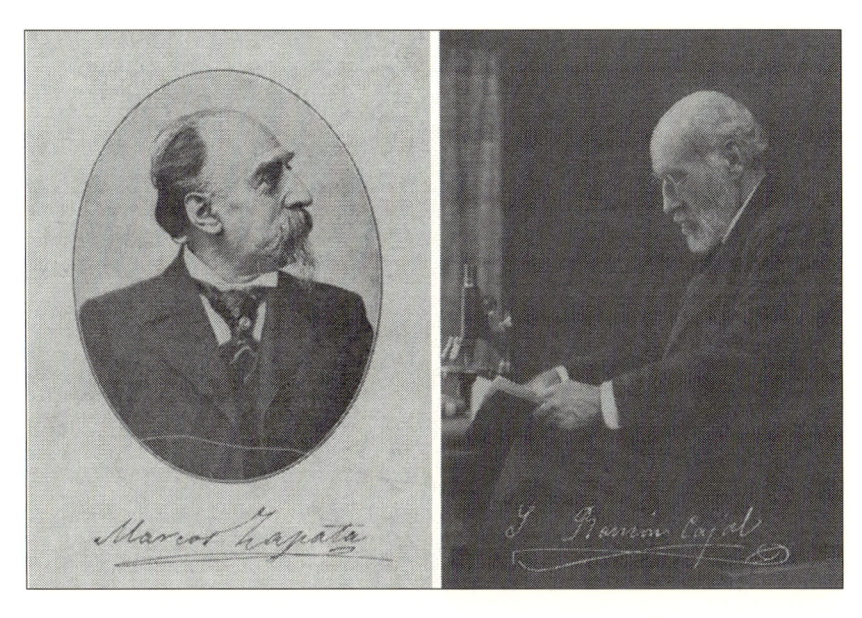

FIGURE 1

Spanish poet Marcos Zapata (left) at the age of 58 years. Santiago Ramón y Cajal (right) on his 70th birthday.

SOURCE: LEFT: ZAPATA 1902. RIGHT: PHOTO BY PADRÓ, MADRID.

dox anatomist, he constantly sought to understand the functional implications of his cytological findings. He briefly experimented with hypnotism, publishing a single case, his wife, and theorized on cognitive functions in "Conjectures on the anatomical mechanism of ideation, association and attention," placing special emphasis on the isolating properties of glia (Ramón Cajal 1889, 1895; Stefanidou et al. 2007).

In 1902, Cajal contributed a little-known preface to a book of poetry by his friend and compatriot, Spanish poet-dramatist Marcos Zapata (1844–1914) (Fig. 1; Ramón Cajal 1902). Zapata's *Poetry* is dedicated "to the excellency of the council of the forever heroic city of Zaragoza" and is structured into serious, satyrical, amorous, descriptive, dramatic, and chivalrous parts, and annals of Aragón.

Cajal's preface to *Poetry* is an essay on the hypothetical workings of the human mind and the expression of human sentiments in relation to drama and comedy; it was prompted by two key questions posed to him by Zapata. With some minor editing, the preface was reissued half a century later in a compilation of essays under the title *The Psychology of Artists* (Fig. 2; Ramón y Cajal 1945, 1954a). In a colorful style, Cajal combines scientific, philosophical, classical, even agricultural elements. Like any Cajal translation, the text poses the particular challenges stemming from his formal parlance, intricate syntax, and numerous regional idioms. The following translation, rendered from the original Spanish, attempts

winter 2009 • volume 52, number 1

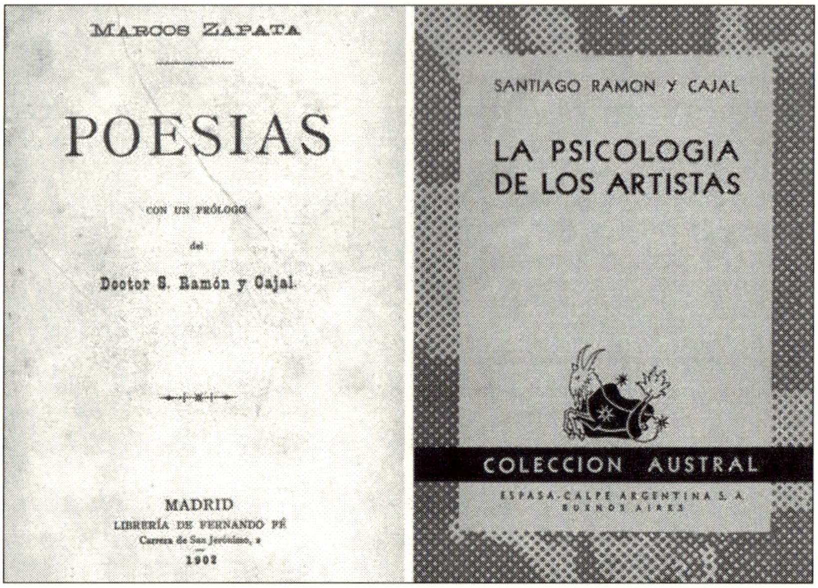

FIGURE 2

Frontispiece of Zapata's 1902 Poetry with a Preface by Doctor S. Ramón y Cajal (left) *and Cajal's 1954 edition of* The Psychology of Artists *(right).*

to maintain a balance between being faithful to the original and conforming to modern English usage.[1]

THE PSYCHOLOGY OF WRITERS

Señor don Marcos Zapata, my dear friend: You ask me, and you greatly honor me by seeking my advice, "What is the reason that I, like so many other scholars, live a comedy but write dramas, carry a happy conversation but have sad thoughts? Why do Andalusian people laugh when they speak, and cry when they sing?"

This is an excellent theme for a journal article on the psychology of writers; but it is of very doubtful use as the heading of a preface for a book of poetry. In such an uncommon request, I discern an element of the subtle humor that is so common to most serious writers and solemn dramatists; but whatever your intention is, and leaving you with all the responsibility of the strange incident, I go on, saying, plain and simply, the little that I can gather concerning these paradoxical contrasts.

I begin by admitting that the fact you allude to is very general, although it does not reach the proportions of a universal psychological law. This rhythm of bitter written and happy spoken words—and vice versa—corresponds to the

---

[1]First English version of Cajal's preface to Marcos Zapata's *Poetry* (Ramón Cajal 1902), translated from the original Spanish by the authors.

emotional order in the eternal alternation of pain and joy, weepiness and laughter. It is most common to our humorists, novelists, and dramatists.

In some writers, the dual manifestation of sentiment is accented to such a degree that it almost becomes a personality split. Two diametrically opposite subjects appear to exist in the minds of poets. They awake in turn, each featuring a particular mode for contemplating life and the world. Authors who lead a placid, serene, and tranquil life will write dramas, elegies, lamentations, novels, or melancholic stories. Those who live a true drama will search in fiction for a palliative and for the consolation of bitterness; they will write chronicles, happy verses, graceful and joyous stories, or spicy anecdotes. People assume what their needs are, based on an urge to complement what they already have. In this way, mental life can become integrated and full, and all brain systems can get their turn in the game.

What I say about writers equally applies to readers. The scientist, the philosopher, the statesman, being continuously immersed in serious and grave studies, devotes himself with avidity, in his hours of leisure, to pleasant literature, to spiritual and light conversations, even to the most innocent and childish games. Similarly, the humble craftsman, tired by the manual and boring work of monitoring, monotony that can be compared to the perpetual rotation of a wheel, tries to free his imagination in the golden domains of reveries; in passionate romance or in the horrendous drama of popular theater, he looks for a note of the picturesque, the beauteous, and the extraordinary, which are absent from his shady and routine existence.

Through a similar motive, the bourgeois, being idle and replete with commodities and pleasures, will find pleasure in horrifying novels and bloody dramas. The momentary vision of other people's pain becomes necessary to sting the numb nerves and to renovate and further sweeten the gratifying flavor of the cup of pleasure. It seems that, save exceptions, the people and the bourgeoisie form the inevitable public of dramatists. Conversely, authors of comedy must be contented with the timid class of intellectuals, those tired and sad beings whose overexcited nerves need sedatives instead of stimulants, pleasant emotions instead of passionate conflicts. Like the bolt that tears the cloud from which it is born, under deafening sounds, so thought wounds the brain, violently and painfully fraying its cells; the latter, as a remedy for their wounds, only request dreams without nightmares and distractions without emotions.

How might these facts be explained? I cannot pretend that I am guessing right; even less that I am exhausting all the various aspects of the problem. But I believe that the phenomenon in question fulfills two conditions: first, the sensation of cerebral weariness that continuously forces a change of mental disposition; and second, the physical necessity to engage the fallow or idle brain provinces into action. That necessity was wisely established by nature. It serves to prevent the forgetfulness and annihilation by disuse of those ideas, sentiments, and mental aptitudes which, due to the lack of a functional urgency and frequent use, and given the occasion, stop representing important elements of defense and prosperity for the individual and the species.

Just in case I have not made myself clear enough, I shall take the discussion a little further. In granting us ideas that become stabilized and improved by means of adaptation and progress, nature does not proceed capriciously. Instead, she offers them to us because they are useful—although not absolutely necessary—for the preservation of life. In any organism, the useless or the detrimental—whenever it appears—is short-lived. Primitive man was complete, albeit simple, because he exercised all his potentials equally. Modern man, on the other hand, belittled and polarized by the fragmentation of labor, cultivates intensely only one of his activities: the one that corresponds to his profession or social mission. For this reason, fallow brain cells, i.e. those responsible for functions not used every day, remind the self of their rights to an active life; they loudly demand a turn in the banquet, as soon as the occasion of a general recess arrives. Quite often, without waiting for permission from the faculties, they slyly increase their blood flow; moving from potential to action, they generate brilliant and conscious representations, which become combined, through imagination, into splashy and surprising constructions. Whenever the tension of nervous life reaches a maximum, during such a weaving and unweaving of the mind, the flow of ideas becomes molded into symbols; it surfaces either in the form of language and gesture or through pen and pencil.

Thus, the poet who through his writing or recitation evokes almost all his registers of solemn, painful, or emotive representations, feels, at the conclusion of the work and the restoration of his strength, that his mental retina is imperceptibly tinted in the complementary colors. As the poet complains of an unfair omission, opposite representations and emotions come to his mind. Unloaded in the motor apparatus through the law of cerebral dynamics, such representations and emotions aspire to live, at times with the ephemeral existence of unexpressed reveries, and then again with the most enduring existence borrowed from spoken word and the reminiscences of readers and listeners.

If we were to read through the lines of the problem, then the horror of death, which inactive or little evoked ideas seem to sense, may help clarify a fact that is well-known—but insufficiently understood—by physiologists. Everyone has noticed that when we dream, the special world of ideas and happenings that march before us usually becomes completely extraneous to the thoughts that preoccupy us and to the works that interest us or are demanded of us daily (there are exceptions that prove the rule). In analyzing dreams carefully, one sees that they reproduce scenes of our childhood or youth that we hardly remember, or fragmentary images, capriciously and absurdly combined, whose elements or sensory residues had not reached full revival for a long time nor, consequently, entered the field of consciousness.

In my experiments with hypnotism, I have often observed that ideas suppressed by suggestion tenaciously reappear in spontaneous dreams, sometimes provoking true obsessions. It is hence deduced that, in sleep, the subject does not rest fully. Only part of the brain rests: the part that became tired from the work during wakefulness. The fallow brain provinces—the cells on which unconscious images are recorded—watch and become excited, rejuvenating with exercise carried out surreptitiously of consciousness, in the same way that the veteran, weakened by life in the quarters, bolsters in maneuvers. With such gymnastics, these extraordinary contingents, a species of the reserve of ideas, become rapidly mobilized as soon as the exigencies of vigilant work and the unexpected eventful journeys of the struggle for life demand it. While many diurnal cerebral operations engage and wear out groups of cells scattered over the entire brain (particularly those involved in higher mental activities—in other words, the critical faculty, constantly ready to speak and listen), so do the majority of dreams constitute pieces of ideas that have not been spun, or that have been assembled in an extravagant manner. In that way, they somewhat resemble an absurd monster that has no proportions, harmony, or reason.

Nonetheless, what happens in dreams also happens in waking. It is only that in the latter situation, the critical faculty stays alert. Besides, none of the brain territories ever become fully asleep. Inhibited by consciousness, inactive cells quiesce. At the same time, they are always ready to enter into action at the minutest insinuation of the subject. Idle cells remain silent only while the laboring cells are engaged. In other words, during the break, mental forces already repaired, and deferred ideas, sentiments, and emotions, take their turn to compensate for the sterile rest. Then, the second human personality appears. In the man of science emerges the latent poet, drawing and embellishing the retort and the microscope. The dramatist throws away the tragic cothurnus and wears for some hours the suit of the harlequin and the buffoon. Heraclitus (the "dark philosopher") becomes Democritus (the "laughing philosopher"). Mechanical man, the shady helot who is worn out and grumbles, is succeeded by true man, who freely expands on all compressed activities of the spirit, and who feels in his heart the great, renewing, intense joy of living.

The cultivation of this second personality, which is complementary and harmonious to the other, is not imposed on us by nature out of a mere caprice, not even out of a pious goal of comforting the spirit for the hard task of the day that will follow. Nature's intentions in this, as in everything, are essentially utilitarian. Organs that are not used degenerate. The battle of life, in the end and after long struggles, will not be won by those whose one half of the brain becomes atrophic for the benefit of the other half. It will instead be won by those who selectively develop nervous territories consecrated to preferred professional activities, and who know how to maintain all mental forces intact in order to fully deploy them at the decisive strategic moment.

The preceding ideas can equally apply to your second question, "Why do Andalusian people laugh when they speak, and cry when they sing?"

It is clear that the unfolding and unrolling of personality, through the exhaustion of the antipodal mental phase, can also be observed in villages in the same way that it is observed in people. Like poets who write dramas but laugh when they speak, so unfortunate villages forget their griefs through the communicative joy of conversation, through the grace and charm of jokes, and through the arts of gallantry and beauty. Music shuffles the foundations of our dominant affects: despite the dissembled emotions while playing the guitar and singing the couplet, when people feel alone in their heart, the second personality will resonate (that is, with the sad and complementary note). The lips of the *cantaor*[2] modulate the melancholic lament that is exhaled by souls tired from endless work and sorrowed by irremediable poverty. What would happen to the Andalusian peasant, perhaps the most unfortunate in all of Spain, if the pious nature had not granted him—as a balsam for his present bitterness—the exquisite art of irony and grace, the easy inclination to laugh, and the profound preoccupation with love and gallantry?

Clearly, villages that are essentially individualistic, grave and semi-serious in their social setting, vary little in the emotional tone of their conversations and songs, their doings and sayings. Those villages, without being totally happy, are not so poor and unfortunate as to necessitate the cordial daily routine of joy evoked to passionately resume the interrupted furrow.

And that is enough for theories and annoying pseudoscientific considerations, for which I respectfully apologize to the readers.

On this occasion, such considerations do not even have the advantage of preparing the reader's palate (based on the law of contrasts). To be savored with delight, the virile, grand, and beautiful poetry of the author of *The Chapel of Lanuza*[3] does not need the bitter absinthe of my prose as an appetizer; even less so the poor praises of my critical incompetence in the literary field.

Your affectionate friend,

S. Ramón Cajal
July 5, 1902

COMMENT

It is only recently that Cajal's nonscientific writings have begun to be brought to the attention of modern readers. The preface to *Poetry* might appear unusual to the reader who is strictly accustomed to Cajal's scientific works. In speculating about the brain, Cajal addresses the lay audience that the book of poetry targeted. The text shows another, elegant side of the great neuroanatomist and a colorful style common in the early 1900s.

Cajal wrote his essay in the aftermath of Freud's *Traumdeutung* (1900). Cajal had copies of *The Interpretation of Dreams* and *The Psychopathology of Everyday Life*

---

[2] Flamenco singer.

[3] *La Capilla de Lanuza*, a heroic drama in one act, published by Zapata in 1871.

in his private library (Rusiñol Estragués and Ibarz Serrat 1999). Thus, Cajal's subjective narrative adopts a trend commonly used by psychologists at the time. Departing from lean neurological thought, he speculates on the nature of writing and its underlying emotions and purposes without employing the conventional methods of neurology or psychology; rather, his writing is based on apperception and intuition.

Cajal viewed his scientific life in a philosophical and artistic framework, and he epitomized it in his autobiography as a metaphor of poetry: "I have always aimed that my life should be lived as far as possible according to the counsel of the philosopher, that is, a living poem of intense action" (Jones 2006, p. 339). Metaphors from nature, art, technology, and farming abound in Cajal's maxims: "You complain about the censures from teachers, rivals, and adversaries, when instead you should welcome them: their hits don't hurt you, they sculpt you." Or, "The plant usually grows according to the dimensions of the pot. Talent confined to its corner will hardly blossom fully" (Ramón y Cajal 1936).

In his research, Cajal saw beyond morphology and inferred function from structure. One such example is his pinnacle discovery, the principle of dynamic polarization of neurons, extracted from the structural properties of dendrites and axons and their connectivity patterns. Cajal speculated amply about nervous tissue physiology, apart from conjecturing on the psychology of art: in many of his drawings, he denotes the flow of nervous impulses with the familial "arrows." Such examples can be seen in Figure 3, taken from his final manuscript, in which he reviews a life's work and reevaluates the evidence for the neuron theory (Ramón y Cajal 1954b).

Cajal's Preface to *Poetry* highlights an artistic side of his mind, an inextricable component of the same mental apparatus that achieved the better-known neuroscientific discoveries. Art—and poetry—do not follow the logic of science: their truth lies in perceiving and expressing beauty. In poetry, mountains can have a soul and birds can cry. By choosing to discourse upon the abstruse subject of emotive expression, Cajal deviated from the austere language of science: unorthodox as the essay may appear at first glance, it is not extraneous to the aesthetics of the tokens, steeped in the Quixotic locution of his cultivation and setting, that document Cajal's lifelong quest for verity through the science and art of histology.

References

Andres-Barquin, P. J. 2002. Santiago Ramón y Cajal and the Spanish school of neurology. *Lancet Neurol* 1(7):445–52.

Craigie, E. H., and W. C. Gibson. 1968. *The world of Ramón y Cajal with selections from his nonscientific writings*. Springfield, IL: Charles C. Thomas.

DeFelipe, J. 2002. Sesquicentenary of the birthday of Santiago Ramón y Cajal, the father of modern neuroscience. *Trends Neurosci* 25(9):481–84.

Freud, S. 1900. *Die Traumdeutung*. Leipzig: Franz Deuticke.

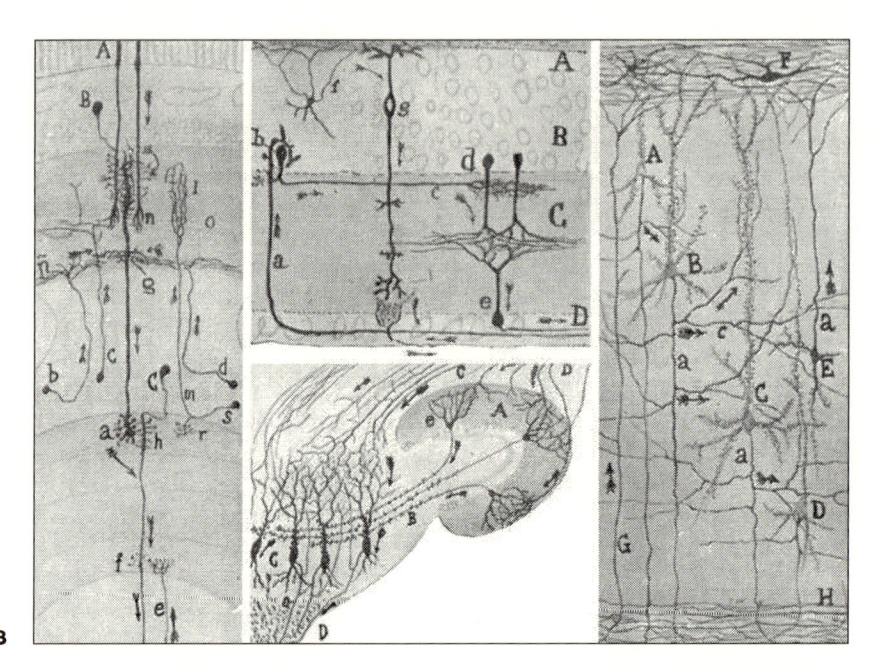

FIGURE 3

Drawings by Cajal of the neuronal circuits in the bee retina (left), avian retina (center top), mammalian fascia dentata and Ammon's horn (center bottom), and cerebral cortex (right). In his descriptors, Cajal uses phrases such as "schema of the course of the currents," "arrows indicate the direction of the currents," and "arrows mark the supposed direction of the nervous current."

SOURCE: FIGURES 40, 9, 39, AND 48, RESPECTIVELY, FROM CAJAL'S LAST MONOGRAPH, PUBLISHED POSTHUMOUSLY (RAMÓN Y CAJAL 1954B).

Garrison, F. H. 1929. Ramón y Cajal. *Bull NY Acad Med* 5(2):483–508.
Jones, E. G. 2006. The impossible interview with the man of the neuron doctrine. *J Hist Neurosci* 15(4):326–40.
López-Muñoz, F., J. Boya, and C. Alamo. 2006. Neuron theory, the cornerstone of neuroscience, on the centenary of the Nobel Prize award to Santiago Ramón y Cajal. *Brain Res Bull* 70(4–6):391–405.
Otis, L. 2001. Ramón y Cajal, a pioneer in science fiction. *Int Microbiol* 4(3):175–78.
Ramón Cajal, S. 1889. Dolores del parto considerablemente atenuados por la sugestión hipnótica. *Gaceta Méd Catal (Barcel)* 12(292):484–86.
Ramón Cajal, S. 1895. Algunas conjeturas sobre el mecanismo anatómico de la ideación, asociación y atención. *Rev Med Cirug Práct (Madrid)* 19(457):497–508.
Ramón Cajal, S. 1902. Prólogo. In M. Zapata, *Poesías*, 15–26. Madrid: Fernando Fé.
Ramón y Cajal, S. 1936. *Charlas de café: Pensamientos, anécdotas y confidencias*. Santiago de Chile: Lautaro.
Ramón y Cajal, S. 1945. *La Psicología de los artistas: Las estatuas en vida y otros ensayos inéditos o desconocidos*, 127–37. Vitoria: Industrias Gráficas Ortega.
Ramón y Cajal, S. 1954a. *La psicología de los artistas*, 118–25. Buenos Aires: Espasa-Calpe Argentina.

Ramón y Cajal, S. 1954b. *Neuron theory or reticular theory? Objective evidence of the anatomical unity of nerve cells*. Madrid: Consejo Superior de Investigaciones Científicas.

Rusiñol Estragués, J., and V. Ibarz Serrat. 1999. La recepción del pensamiento de Freud en la obra de Ramón y Cajal. Pontevedra: VII Congreso de la Sociedad Española de Historia de las Ciencias y de las Técnicas. http://www.unirioja.es/sehcyt/congr/pontevedra/resumenes.htm.

Stefanidou, M., et al. 2007. Cajal's brief experimentation with hypnotic suggestion. *J Hist Neurosci* 16(4):351–61.

Williams, H. 1954. *Don Quixote of the microscope: An interpretation of Santiago Ramón y Cajal (1852–1934)*. London: Jonathan Cape.

Zapata, M. 1902. *Poesías, con un prólogo del Doctor S. Ramón y Cajal*. Madrid: Fernando Fé.

PIONEERS IN NEUROLOGY

Manuel del Cerro
Lazaros C. Triarhou

Eduardo De Robertis (1913–1988)

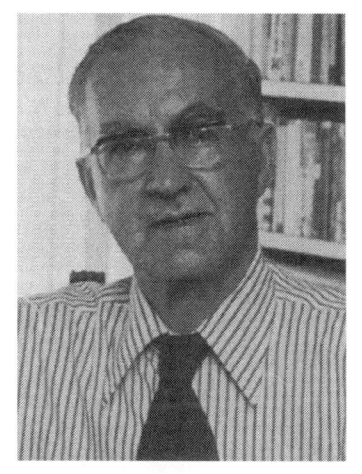

Eduardo De Robertis. © 1986 Plenum/Springer

Received: 31 May 2008
Accepted: 10 July 2008
Published online: 7 October 2008

Prof. M. del Cerro, MD
Depts. of Neurobiology and Anatomy,
and Ophthalmology
University of Rochester
Rochester, NY 14642, USA

Prof. L. C. Triarhou, MD, PhD (✉)
Economo-Koskinas Wing for Integrative
and Evolutionary Neuroscience
University of Macedonia
54006 Thessaloniki, Greece
Tel.: +30-2310/891-387
E-Mail: triarhou@uom.gr

Eduardo De Robertis, neurobiologist *par excellence*, was born on 11 December 1913 in Buenos Aires, to Italian immigrants. He graduated in medicine from the University of Buenos Aires in 1939 with gold medal [10]. As a student, he became interested in histology and worked with P. Rojas; in 1935 they discovered, with Sáez, that most amphibians have no morphologically distinguishable sex chromosomes [7].

Supported by B. Houssay, the later Nobel laureate, De Robertis secured fellowships to investigate parathyroid and thyroid function, with R. Bensley at the University of Chicago and with I. Gersh at Johns Hopkins (1939–1941). He continued that research in Buenos Aires, at the Department of Anatomy and Embryology (1941–1946), where he showed that gonadotrophin promotes gonadal maturation in toads.

In 1946, opposing the presidential candidacy of General Perón, he resigned his post and went on an 11-year self-imposed exile. At MIT in Boston, he studied axonal ultrastructure with F. Schmitt and described neurotubules (1946–1949). In 1949 De Robertis moved to the Biological Research Institute in Uruguay, headed by Cajal alumnus C. Estable. He organized the Cellular Ultrastructure Department, housing the first electron microscope in South America, and studied retinal ultrastructure, the separation of pre- and postsynaptic membranes as definitive proof of the neuron theory [6], and correlates of exocytosis in adrenal medullary cells [2].

In 1953 De Robertis went to Seattle to study with Bennett the ultrastructure of synapses in sympathetic ganglia of frogs and nervecord of earthworms (collected from Bennett's yard) [2]. In April 1954, the seminal discovery of synaptic vesicles in nerve terminals was separately announced by Palade and Palay at the American Association of Anatomists, and by De Robertis and Bennett at the Experimental Biology (FASEB) meeting. De Robertis and Bennett went further, associating synaptic vesicles with quantal acetylcholine and catecholamine release [4], a concept they supported with degeneration and stimulation experiments. Synaptosome isolation provided a direct approach to the study of synaptic function [5].

In 1957 De Robertis returned to Buenos Aires as professor and head of the Cell Biology Department and in August inaugurated the electron microscopic unit. In 1958 he was appointed director of the National Research Council.

His success (with Lasansky) to visualize for the first time protein-lipid bilayers in retinal photoreceptors and myelin-sheath membranes made was reported in the *New York Times* (29 April 1959). At the 1961 International Neuropathology Congress in Munich, De Robertis gave an update of synaptic ultrastructure, intersynaptic filaments, subsynaptic web and subcellular fractions [3]. Between 1962 and 1966, he reported the isolation of nerve terminal particles and characterized benzodiazepine receptors [1], formulated the unitary theory of neurohumoral secretion [8], and successfully blocked the effect of transmitters with antibodies against synaptosomes, three years before immunocytochemistry was introduced. He would say, "We all dissect, some with scalpel and forceps, others with the ultramicrotome or the ultracentrifuge, but it is the same, we all dissect". When the 1970 Nobel Prize in medicine was awarded to Katz, von Euler and Axelrod for discovering humoral transmitters in nerve terminals and their storage, release and inactivation mechanisms, many felt that De Robertis should have been included in the honour [1]. In the 1970s and 1980s he identified numerous receptors, investigated stress and anxiety, as well as hypothalamic and pineal function.

He published over 300 papers [9], translated Maximow and Bloom's *Textbook of Histology* (1944), and authored *General Cytology* (with Nowinski and Sáez, 1946; later *Cell Biology* and *Cell and Molecular Biology*, with Italian, Polish, French and Japanese translations); *Histophysiology of Synapses and Neurosecretion* (1964); *Biology of Neuroglia* (with Carrea, 1965); *New Atlas of Histology* (with di Fiore and Mancini, 1973); *Neurochemistry of Cholinergic Receptors* (with Schacht, 1974); *Synaptic Receptors* (1975); *Essentials of Cell and Molecular Biology* (with his son Eddy De Robertis, 1981).

De Robertis received multiple awards, national and international. He died in Buenos Aires on 31 May 1988. His place in the history of science rests on his fundamental discoveries on nervous tissue structure and function. His pupils include G. Rodríguez, A. Pellegrino, C. Cuello, J. Pecci-Saavedra, G. Jaim-Etcheverry, A. Solari, A. Lasansky, F. Wald, and one of us (MdC); they revere him as a gentleman of great dignity, who tried hard to hide a warm heart behind the façade of a stern, old-style professor. His department in Buenos Aires is now called "Eduardo De Robertis Institute of Cellular Biology and Neurosciences".

References

1. Barrios Medina A (1997) Eduardo De Robertis: un esbozo biográfico. www.houssay.org.ar/hh/bio/robertis.htm
2. Cuello AC (1989) Eduardo De Robertis (1913-1988). Brain Res 484:408-409
3. De Robertis E (1962) Fine structure of synapses in the CNS; Structure and chemical composition of isolated nerve endings. In: Jacob H (ed) IV.Internationaler Kongreß für Neuropathologie, Vol. II: Elektronenmikroskopie und Zellbiologie. Thieme, Stuttgart, pp 35-38, 54-57
4. De Robertis ED, Bennett HS (1955) Some features of the submicroscopic morphology of synapses in frog and earthworm. J Biophys Biochem Cytol 1:47-58
5. De Robertis EDP, Rodríguez de Lores Arnaiz G, Pellegrino de Iraldi A (1962) Isolation of synaptic vesicles from nerve endings of the rat brain. Nature 194:794-795
6. Estable C, Reissig M, De Robertis E (1954) Microscopic and submicroscopic structure of the synapsis in the ventral ganglion of the acoustic nerve. Exp Cell Res 6:255-262
7. Glick TF (1996) Science in twentieth-century Latin America. In: Bethell L (ed) Ideas and ideologies in twentieth-century Latin America. Cambridge University Press, New York, pp 287-359
8. Jaim-Etcheverry G (1984) Eduardo De Robertis at 70. Trends Neurosci 7:138-140
9. Mancini RE (1963) Eduardo De Robertis. Ediciones Culturales, Buenos Aires
10. Solari AJ (2006) Eduardo Diego Patricio De Robertis. Academia Nacional de Ciencias, Córdoba. http://acad.uncor.edu/academicos/resenia/robertis

EXPLORING THE MIND WITH A MICROSCOPE: FREUD'S BEGINNINGS IN NEUROBIOLOGY

Lazaros C. Triarhou
University of Macedonia, Thessaloniki, Greece

Abstract: Sigmund Freud (1856-1939), the acknowledged founder of psychoanalysis, started his research career as a promising neurobiologist. This article presents an overview of his early articles in neuroanatomy and a literature update regarding the awareness of Freud's origins in neurobiology. In all, Freud invested a decade studying animal histology, cell biology and basic neuroscience before turning to human neuropsychiatric disorders. Through his histological studies, Freud provided coherent evidence supporting the neuron doctrine and suggesting that the protoplasm consists of a contractile fibrillary network, the present-day cytoskeleton. Freud also documented movements of nucleoli in neurons, a phenomenon presently referred to as nuclear rotation. In certain instances, Freud's observations antedate later views by more than half a century and are important to our understanding of neuronal structure and intracellular motility.

Key words: Freud, History of neuroscience, Neurohistology, Neuron theory.

INTRODUCTION

Whether one may agree (Edelman, 1992; Gabbard, 2004; Kandel, 2002) or disagree (Eissler, 1995; McCrone, 2004; Tallis, 1996) with Sigmund Freud's propositions on the functioning of the mental apparatus, it is a common admission that psychoanalytic theory has had a considerable impact on twentieth century scientific, intellectual and cultural thought. Freud as a psychologist is viewed as one of the greatest explorers of the human mind that ever lived (Gay, 1988; Panek, 2004).

Acknowledgement: This article is based in part on an invited lecture given at the Conference on "Freud's legacy in contemporary science" that was organized by the School of Psychology of Aristotle University of Thessaloniki and the Psychological Society of Northern Greece, November 10th, 2006.
Address: Lazaros C. Triarhou, Department of Educational and Social Policy, School of Economic and Social Sciences, University of Macedonia, Egnatia 156, 540 06 Thessaloniki, Greece. E-mail: triarhou@uom.gr

On the occasion of celebrating the sesquicentennial anniversary of Freud's birth (May 6, 1856), the present study retraces his early research career in neurobiology. Freud's first skips in science happened during his medical school years at the University of Vienna. Beginning in 1875 as a sophomore medical student, until 1885, the year he went to Paris to study clinical neurology at *La salpêtrière* under the world-famous Jean-Martin Charcot (1825-1893), Freud explored the histological structure of nerve cells in fish and crustacea, subsequently focusing on human neuroanatomy and neuropathology.

Much of the neurohistological work took place in the Institute of Physiology at the University of Vienna headed by Ernst Wilhelm von Brücke (1819-1892), after whom the ciliary muscle in the eye, Brücke's muscle, is named. Carl Ludwig Brücke (1816-1895), Hermann von Helmholtz (1821-1894), and Emil du Bois-Reymond (1818-1896) dominate the history of physiology in the second half of the nineteenth century, finally delivering this science from all traces of speculation and mysterious forces ("vitalismus"); only physical concepts and the quantification of all processes count.

Freud had been exposed to Darwinian theory through the teachings of Solomon Stricker (1834-1898), his Professor of Histology (Stricker, 1872), and Carl Claus (1835-1899), his Professor of Zoology and Comparative Anatomy at the University of Vienna (Freud, Freud, & Grubrich-Simitis, 1978; Ritvo, 1990). He worked diligently at the Physiology Institute from 1876 to 1881 (the year of his graduation). Nevertheless, there was scant livelihood in it, and, as Brücke candidly informed him, no future[1]. Freud, who was contemplating marriage, reluctantly went into clinical medicine, specializing in what we could now call Neurology and Psychiatry (Freud et al., 1978). By then, based on his anatomical observations, Freud had published 14 original articles, some of them pioneering contributions to neuroscience, which gained him wide recognition among neurohistological, neuroanatomical and neuropathological circles.

Freud's contributions to neurobiology touch upon five cellular domains: (1) The emanation of nerve fibers from nerve cell somata (Freud, 1877b, 1878); (2) The emergence of the concept of cytoskeleton (Freud, 1882); (3) The movement of nucleoli in nerve cells (Freud, 1882; Henneguy, 1896); (4) The role of the nerve cell as a unit in the nervous system (Freud, 1884c), and (5) The existence of 'contact barriers' between nerve cells (Freud 1895/1966). These issues have been thoroughly covered in the literature (Bernfeld, 1949, 1951; Brito, 2002; Brun, 1936; Frixione, 2003; Gray, 1948, 1951; Jelliffe, 1937; Kandel, 1979, 1981, 2002; Pearce,

---

[1]. Brücke's two assistant professors were only ten years older than Freud, and unlike Freud, not Jewish.

1996, 2003; Solms, 1993, 1996, 1998, 2004; Sulloway, 1979; Triarhou & del Cerro, 1985, 1986, 1987a, 1987b).

FREUD'S WORKS IN BASIC NEUROSCIENCE

The first study carried out by Freud was, interestingly enough, on the microscopic structure of the eel testis, then known as Syrski's organ (Freud, 1877a). One should not attribute any "Freudian" connotation to the choice of topic, as it had been assigned to the young student by his mentor, Professor Carl Claus. Freud conducted his experiments on 400 specimens in two visits, during 1875 and 1876, to the Zoological Station in [then Austrian] Trieste, supported by travel grants from the Austrian Ministry of Education.

Original as his first study was, and important as his subsequent studies on cell motility were (Triarhou & del Cerro, 1987b), the basic science contributions of Freud that have better survived to our days were those on the structure of the nerve cells (Triarhou & del Cerro, 1985). Those contributions have been highly regarded by established researchers at the time and incorporated into the neuroscientific literature, including citations by Santiago Ramón y Cajal (1852-1934), the father of modern neurobiology[2], in his classic book *Textura del sistema nervioso del hombre y de los vertebrados* (Ramón y Cajal, 1897-1904) along with those of Nansen[3] (1861-1930) who apparently knew Freud (Fodstad, Kondziolka, & de Lotbiniere, 2000).

Freud conducted his histological studies on the nervous system of the lamprey (Petromyzon) (see Figure 1) and the river crayfish. In the legends of his histological drawings in the resulting publications in the Proceedings of the Imperial Academy of Sciences (Freud, 1877b, 1878, 1882), Freud gives technical information on the optical components used for his observations. Clearly, Freud, and Brücke's laboratory had a strong preference for the optics produced by Edmund Hartnack[4] (1826-1891).

---

2. Santiago Ramón y Cajal whose *Textura del sistema nervioso del hombre y de los vertebrados* (Ramón y Cajal, 1897-1904) is considered the cornerstone of modern neurobiology (Andres-Barquin, 2001; DeFelipe, 2002; Sotelo, 2003), and who shared the 1906 Nobel Prize in physiology or medicine with Camillo Golgi (1844-1926) for their investigations of the structure of the nervous system.

3. Fridtjof Nansen is another key protagonist who produced important groundwork supporting the individuality of nerve cells as structural and functional units of the nervous system. He was also an Arctic explorer, humanitarian, and winner of the 1922 Nobel Prize in peace.

4. This was a well-placed trust for Hartnack as an innovator (Bradbury, 1967) whose instruments are highly regarded by microscope historians (Moe, 2004). In 1857, Georges Oberhäuser (1798-1868), an uncle of Hartnack, went into partnership with his nephew in Paris to form the fine

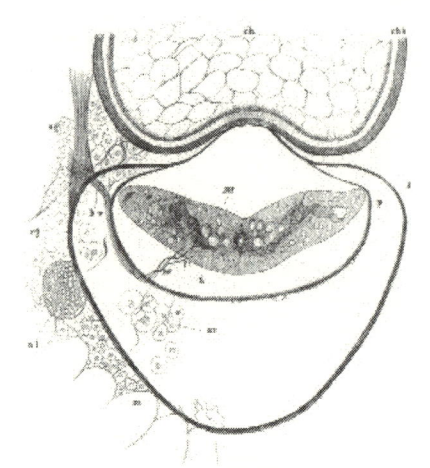

Figure 1. Freud's drawing of the lamprey spinal cord, from his first study on the petromyzon (Freud, 1877b).

Freud further worked out some new methods for dissecting and staining nervous tissue specimens (Freud, 1879, 1884a, 1884b), and summarized his histological findings in a review (Freud, 1884c) on the structural elements of the nervous system (Figure 2a and 2b).

Through his neurohistological studies, Freud became one of the early protagonists of the neuron doctrine (Koppe, 1983; Rueda Franco, 2001; Shepherd, 1991). Waldeyer (1891), working at the First Anatomical Institute in Berlin, coined the term "neuron" (first appearing in Homer, cf. Ochs, 2004) and popularized the neuron doctrine. Meanwhile, the subject had received substantial contributions from anatomists including Forel, Gowers, His, Kölliker, Nissl, and van Gehuchten (McHenry, 1969; Meyer, 1971; Ramón y Cajal, 1907; Shepherd, 1991).

---

instrument-making firm Oberhäuser & Hartnack. Hartnack assumed sole control of the firm in 1860. Ten years later, as a result of the Franco-Prussian war, Hartnack moved to Potsdam, leaving the Paris firm division Hartnack & Prazmowski to his partner Adam Prazmowski (1821-1888), a Polish professor of Mathematics and Astronomy who had previously worked at the Warsaw Observatory. Hartnack is credited with the first use of water-immersion lenses in the commercial production of microscopes and the adoption of the substage condenser in his later instruments. Microscopes by Hartnack, contemporary with the one that allowed Freud to observe nerve cells in the laboratory and to reach his fundamental histological conclusions, can be found in several microscope collections (Purtle, 1974; Turner, 1989).

Freud's beginnings in neurobiology

A NEW HISTOLOGICAL METHOD FOR THE STUDY OF NERVE-TRACTS IN THE BRAIN AND SPINAL CHORD.

BY DR. SIGM. FREUD,

Assistant Physician to the Vienna General Hospital.

In the course of my studies on the structure and development of the medulla oblongata I succeeded in working out the following method, which will be found a powerful aid in tracing the course of fibres in the central nervous system of the adult and the embryo.

Pieces of the organ are hardened in bichromate of potash, or in Erlicki's fluid (2½ parts of bichromate of potash and ½ of sulphate of copper to 100 parts of water), and the process of hardening is finished by placing the specimens in alcohol; thin sections are cut by means of a microtome and washed in distilled water. The washed sections are brought into an aqueous solution of chloride of gold (1 to 100) to which is added half or an equal volume of strong alcohol. This mixture is to

Figure 2a. Freud's technical paper in Brain *(Freud, 1884b).*

Die Structur der Elemente des Nervensystems.

Von

Dr. Sigm. Freud,

Sekundararzt im allgemeinen Krankenhause.

(Nach einem in psychiatrischen Vereine gehaltenen Vortrag.)

Sehr bald, nachdem Nervenzelle und Nervenfaser als die wesentlichen Bestandtheile des Nervensystems erkannt worden waren, begannen die Bemühungen, die feinere Structur dieser beiden Elemente aufzuklären, wobei die Hoffnung von Einfluss war, aus der erkannten Structur Schlüsse auf die physiologische Dignität derselben ziehen zu können. Es ist bekanntlich nicht gelungen, nach einer dieser beiden Richtungen befriedigenden Aufschluss und Einigung zu erzielen; dem einen Autor gilt die Nervenzelle als körnig, dem anderen als fibrillär; die Nervenfaser oder deren wesentlicher Bestandtheil, der Achsencylinder, dem einen als ein Fibrillenbundel, dem andern als eine Flüssigkeitssäule, und dem entsprechend wird die Nervenzelle hier als der eigentliche Herd der Nerventhätigkeit gewürdigt, dort zur Bedeutung eines Kernes der Schwann'schen Scheide degradirt.

Da ich nun glaube, dass in meiner Untersuchung „Ueber den Bau der Nervenfasern und Nervenzellen beim Flusskrebs"[1] eine wohl begründete Lösung des uns beschäftigenden Problems gegeben ist, will ich mir erlauben, den Inhalt derselben an dieser Stelle vorzubringen. Vorher muss ich es aber rechtfertigen, dass ich den Flusskrebs zum Object meiner Untersuchung gewählt, oder dass ich den

Figure 2b. Freud's review on the structural elements of the nervous system (Freud, 1884c).

FREUD'S WORKS IN CLINICAL NEUROSCIENCE

After his graduation from medical school, Freud worked in the Institute of Brain Anatomy headed by Theodor Meynert (1833-1892), his Professor of Psychiatry[5]. Freud published three works, based on the Weigert stain of incompletely myelinated human fetuses, on the connections of the superior olivary nuclei (Freud, 1885), on the origin and the course of the acoustic (eighth cranial) nerve (Freud, 1886), and on the anatomical relations of the restiform body in the medulla oblongata (Darkschewitz & Freud, 1886). These studies (Figure 3a and 3b), their precedence, and their caveats, have been discussed in detail by Wiest and Baloh (2002).

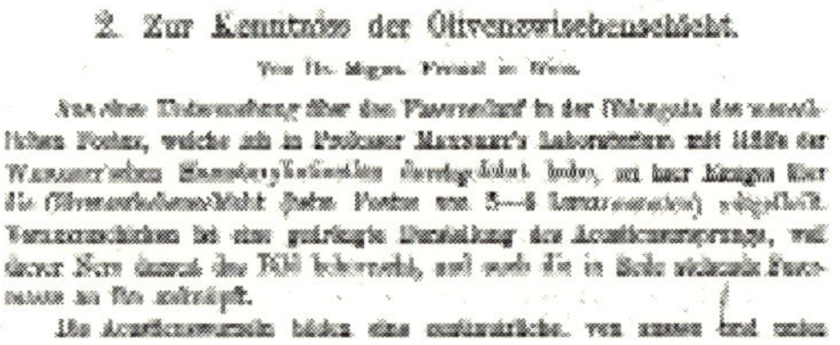
2. Zur Kenntniss der Olivenzwischenschicht.

Figure 3a. Freud's paper on the interolivary tract (Freud, 1885).

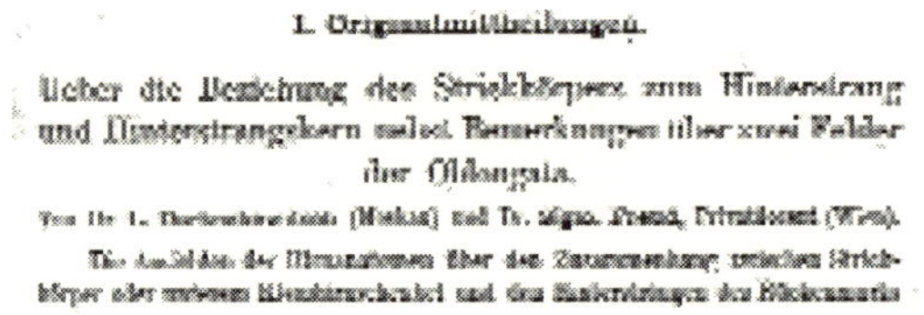
I. Originalmittheilungen.

Ueber die Beziehung des Strickkörpers zum Hinterstrang und Hinterstrangkern nebst Bemerkungen über zwei Felder der Oblongata.

Figure 3b. Freud's paper on the restiform body (Darkschewitsch & Freud, 1886).

Freud's subsequent endeavours in clinical neurology and aphasiology go beyond the scope of the present paper, as they are amply covered elsewhere (Delahanty, 1978; Fancher, 2000; Goldblatt, 1992; Greenberg, 1997; Jacyna, 2005; Jellinek, 1993; Kaplan, 1989; Mancia, 2004; Markowitsch, 1986; Miller, 1991a, 1991b; Miller & Katz, 1989), and eloquently dramatized in several novels (Morton, 1979, 1989; Spiel, 1987; Stone, 1971).

5. Meynert is generally credited with promoting a neuroanatomical basis for psychiatric diseases (Meynert, 1884/1968) and as setting the foundations for the cytoarchitectonic study of the human cerebral cortex (Meynert, 1872).

DISCUSSION

One of the first attempts at reconciling Freudian unconscious mental processes with neurophysiology was a speculative hypothesis put forth by Winson (1985), based on the evolution of the dreaming state in mammals. Two entries, on *Aphasia* and on the *Brain*, written by Freud in 1888 for the *Handwörterbuch der gesamte Medizin* (Handbook of General Medicine) that was compiled by Albert Villaret[6] (Solms & Saling, 1990), predate the renowned monograph on aphasia (Freud, 1891, 1891/1953, 1891/1983, 1891/1992) and shed light on historical aspects of the relationship between neurological science and psychoanalysis.

A meeting held at the New York Academy of Sciences in November 1995 (Bilder & LeFever, 1998) examined Freud's "Project" (Freud, 1895/1966) in a neuroscientific perspective. Freud's early scientific works from the "pre-analytic" period are further analyzed in a volume (Guttmann & Scholz-Strasser, 1998), the outcome of a conference organized in Spring 1997 by the Sigmund Freud Society and the Austrian Academy of Sciences. It is argued there that the new language Freud had to create for his system of psychotherapy, after departing from the territories of neurohistology and neurology, followed a similar epistemological approach, which allows current comparisons between his neuroscientific, and his later, psychoanalytic works.

Freud's ideas on hysteria, or sensory conversion disorder, seem to be validated by recent data from fMRI studies: selective alterations in primary sensorimotor cortical (S1) activity have been implicated in subjects with unexplained sensory loss (Ghaffar et al., 2006; Hurwitz & Pritchard, 2006).

Perhaps two other points concerning observations of Freud that pertain to contemporary neuroscience should be mentioned briefly. The first concerns the long-term potentiation of synaptic transmission, a reliable neurophysiological model of learning and memory that consists in the facilitation at the synapse in response to sustained activation. In his "Project", Freud theorized about representing memory at the contact barriers as "a permanent alteration following an event", thus anticipating several crucial physiological properties of long-term potentiation (Centonze et al., 2004; Kandel, 1981).

The other point concerns affective neuroscience (Peper & Markowitsch, 2001), and the pivotal role of Austrian physiologist Siegmund Exner (1846-1926), Freud, and French physician Israel Waynbaum (1862-uncertain), who might all be considered forerunners in that field, having had propounded a neural network theory of emotion that involved a stage of precortical processing, an idea compatible with

---

6. Published in Stuttgart by Ferdinand Enke (Volume I).

present-day views on the neural substrates and physiological characteristics of emotions.

The resonance of Freud's early scientific work in his later theorizing is striking, and the irruption of Newtonian concepts and causality to the exclusion of all others in physiology undoubtedly stood as a model for Freud's "dynamic" psychiatry (Triarhou, 1989). To quote du Bois-Reymond at the beginning of his career: «Brücke and I, we have sworn to each other to validate the basic truth that in an organism no other forces have any effect than the common physiochemical ones» (Jans Muller, M.D., personal communication, January 1989). Or, to go back all the way to Anaxagoras (500-428 B.C.), «The phenomena are a visible expression of that which is hidden» (Johansen, 1998, p. 73).

The neurobiological background in Freud's thought, and an avant-garde vision of the neurochemical correlates of mental disorders, becomes evident in the following fragment from *The question of lay analysis* (Freud, 1926/1978, p. 54, my translation[7]): «Considering the intimate relationship between the things that we distinguish as bodily and as mental, one may foresee that the day will come, when paths of knowledge and hopefully of influence will open up that will lead from the Biology of organs and from Chemistry to the field of the neuroses.»

REFERENCES

Andres-Barquin, P. J. (2001). Ramón y Cajal: A century after the publication of his masterpiece. *Endeavour, 25*, 13-17.

Bernfeld, S. (1949). Freud's scientific beginnings. *American Imago, 6*, 163-196.

Bernfeld, S. (1951). Sigmund Freud, M.D. 1882-1885. *International Journal of Psychoanalysis, 32*, 204-217.

Bilder, R. M., & LeFever, F. F. (1998). *Neuroscience of the mind on the centennial of Freud's project for a scientific psychology*. New York: The New York Academy of Sciences.

Bradbury, S. (1967). *The evolution of the microscope*. Oxford, UK: Pergamon.

Brito, G. N. O. (2002). Mind from genes and neurons: A neurobiological model of Freudian psychology. *Medical Hypotheses, 59*, 438-445.

Brun, B. (1936). Sigmund Freud's Leistungen auf dem Gebiete der organischen Neurologie [Sigmund Freud's achievements in the field of organic neurology]. *Schweizer Archiv für Neurologie und Psychiatrie, 37*, 200-207.

---

7. «Bei dem innigen Zusammenhang zwischen den Dingen, die wir als körperlich und als seelisch scheiden, darf man vorhersehen, daß der Tag kommen wird, an dem sich Wege der Erkenntnis und hoffentlich auch der Beeinflussung von der Biologie der Organe und von der Chemie zum dem Erscheinungsgebiet der Neurosen eröffnen werden».

Centonze, D., Siracusano, A., Calabresi, P., & Bernardi, G. (2004). The Project for a scientific psychology (1895): A Freudian anticipation of LTP-memory connection theory. *Brain Research Reviews, 46*, 310-314.

Darkschewitsch, L., & Freud, S. (1886). Über die Beziehung des Strickkörpers zum Hinterstrang und Hinterstrangskern nebst Bemerkungen über zwei Felder der Oblongata [On the relationship of the restiform body to the posterior column nucleus together with remarks on two fields of the medulla oblongata]. *Neurologisches Centralblatt, 6*, 121-129.

DeFelipe, J. (2002). Sesquicentenary of the birthday of Santiago Ramón y Cajal, the father of modern neuroscience. *Trends in Neurosciences, 25*, 481-484.

Delahanty, G. (1978). Freud y neurología [Freud and neurology]. *Neurología Neurocirugía y Psiquiatría, 19*, 18-26.

Edelman, G. M. (1992). *Bright air, brilliant fire: On the matter of the mind.* New York: Basic Books.

Eissler, K. R. (1995). The end of an illusion: Sigmund Freud and his 20th century. *Psyche, 49*, 1196-1210.

Fancher, R. E. (2000). Snapshots of Freud in America, 1899-1999. *American Psychologist, 55*, 1025-1028.

Fodstad, H., Kondziolka, D., & de Lotbiniere, A. (2000). The neuron doctrine, the mind, and the arctic. *Neurosurgery, 47*, 1381-1389.

Freud, E., Freud, L., & Grubrich-Simitis, I. (1978). *Sigmund Freud.* London: Deutsch.

Freud, S. (1877a). Beobachtungen über Gestaltung und feineren Bau der als Hoden beschriebenen Lappenorgane des Aals [Observations on the organization and finer structure of the lobe organ described as testes in the eel]. *Sitzungsberichte der kaiserliche Akademie der Wissenschaften, 75*, 419-431.

Freud, S. (1877b). Über den Ursprung der hinteren Nervenwurzeln im Rückenmark von Ammocoetes (*Petromyzon planeri*) [On the origin of the dorsal nerve roots in the spinal cord of Ammocoetes (*Petromyzon planeri*)]. *Sitzungsberichte der kaiserliche Akademie der Wissenschaften, 75*, 15-27.

Freud, S. (1878). Über Spinalganglien und Rückenmark des Petromyzon [On the spinal ganglia and the spinal cord of the Petromyzon]. *Sitzungsberichte der kaiserliche Akademie der Wissenschaften, 78*, 81-167.

Freud, S. (1879). Notiz über eine Methode zur anatomischen Präparation des Nervensystems [Note on a method for the anatomical preparation of the nervous system]. *Centralblatt für die Medicinischen Wissenschaften, 17*, 468-469.

Freud, S. (1882). Über den Bau der Nervenfasern und Nervenzellen beim Flußkrebs [On the structure of nerve fibers and nerve cells in the river crayfish]. *Sitzungsberichte der kaiserliche Akademie der Wissenschaften, 85*, 9-46.

Freud, S. (1884a). Eine neue Methode zum Studium des Faserverlaufs im Centralnervensystem [A new method to study the course of fibers in the central nervous system]. *Centralblatt für die Medicinischen Wissenschaften, 22*, 161-163.

Freud, S. (1884b). A new histological method for the study of nerve-tracts in the brain and spinal cord. *Brain, 7*, 86-88.

Freud, S. (1884c). Die Structur der Elemente des Nervensystems [The structure of the elements of the nervous system]. *Jahrbücher für Psychiatrie und Neurologie, 5,* 221-229.

Freud, S. (1885). Zur Kenntniss der Olivenzwischenschicht. *Neurologisches Centralblatt, 12,* 268-270.

Freud, S. (1886). Über den Ursprung des N. acusticus [On the origin of the acoustic nerve]. *Monatsschrift für Ohrenheilkunde, 20,* 245-251, 277-282.

Freud, S. (1891). *Zur Auffassung des Aphasien: Eine kritische Studie* [A view on the aphasias: A critical study]. Leipzig, Germany: Deuticke.

Freud, S. (1953). *On aphasia: A critical study* (E. Stengel, Trans.). London: Imago. (Original work published in 1891)

Freud, S. (1966). Project for a scientific psychology. In J. Strachey (Ed.), *The standard edition of the complete psychological works* of Sigmund Freud (Vol. 1, pp. 281-397). London: Hogarth. (Original work published in 1895)

Freud, S. (1978). Die Frage der Laienanalyse: Unterredungen mit einem Unparteiischen [The question of lay analysis: Conversations with an impartial person]. In A. Freud, & I. Grubrich-Simitis (Eds.), *Sigmund Freud Werkausgabe in zwei Bänden: Bd. 1. Elemente der Psychoanalyse* (pp. 17-69). Frankfurt am Main, Germany: Fischer. (Original work published in 1926)

Freud, S. (1983). *Contribution à la conception des aphasies: Une étude critique* (C. van Reeth, Trans.) [Contribution to the concept of the aphasias: A critical study]. Paris: Presses Universitaires de France. (Original work published in 1891)

Freud, S. (1992). *Zur Auffassung der Aphasien: Eine kritische Studie* [A view on the aphasias: A critical study]. Frankfurt am Main, Germany: Fischer. (Original work published in 1891)

Frixione, E. (2003). Sigmund Freud's contribution to the history of the neuronal cytoskeleton. *Journal of the History of the Neurosciences, 12,* 12-24.

Gabbard, G. O. (2004). Sigmund Freud, 1856-1939. *American Journal of Psychiatry, 161,* 2.

Gay, P. (1988). *Freud: A life for our times.* New York: Anchor Books Doubleday.

Ghaffar, O., Staines, W. R., & Feinstein, A. (2006). Unexplained neurologic symptoms: An fMRI study of sensory conversion disorder. *Neurology, 67,* 2036-2038.

Goldblatt, D. (1992). Freud and Sachs. *Seminars in Neurology, 12,* 147-150.

Gray, H. (1948). Bibliography of Freud's pre-analytic period. *Psychoanalytic Review, 35,* 403-410.

Greenberg, V. D. (1997). *Freud and his aphasia book: Language and the sources of psychoanalysis.* Ithaca, NY: Cornell University Press.

Guttman, G., & Scholz-Strasser, I. (1998). *Freud and the neurosciences: From brain research to the unconscious.* Vienna: Verlag der Österreichischen Academie der Wissenschaften.

Henneguy, L. F. (1896). *Leçons sur la cellule: Morphologie et reproduction* [Lessons on the cell: Morphology and reproduction]. Paris: Carré.

Hurwitz, T. A., & Prichard, J. W. (2006). Conversion disorder and fMRI. *Neurology, 67,* 1914-1915.

Jacyna, S. (2005). Freud's critical study. *Cortex, 41,* 101-102.

Jelliffe, S. E. (1937) Sigmund Freud as a neurologist: Some notes on his earlier neurobiological and clinical neurological studies. *Journal of Nervous and Mental Disease, 85,* 696-711.

Jellinek, E. H. (1993). Sigmund Freud: Neurologist. *Proceedings of the Royal College of Physicians of Edinburgh, 23,* 205-208.

Johansen, K. F. (1998). *A history of ancient philosophy: From the beginnings to Augustine* (H. Rosenmeier, Trans.). London, UK: Routledge.

Kandel, E. R. (1979). Psychotherapy and the single synapse: The impact of psychiatric thought on neurobiological research. *New England Journal of Medicine, 301*, 1028-1037.

Kandel, E. R. (1981). Calcium and the control of synaptic strength by learning. *Nature, 293*, 697-700.

Kandel, E. R. (2002). La biologie et le futur de la psychanalyse: Un nouveau cadre conceptuel de travail pour une psychiatrie revisitée [Biology and the future of psychoanalysis: A new conceptual framework for a revisited psychiatry]. *Évolution Psychiatrique, 67*, 40-82.

Kaplan, R. (1989). The neurological legacy of psychoanalysis: Freud as a neurologist. *Comprehensive Psychiatry, 30*, 567.

Koppe, S. (1983). The psychology of the neuron: Freud, Cajal and Golgi. *Scandinavian Journal of Psychology, 24*, 1-12.

Mancia, M. (2004). The dream between neuroscience and psychoanalysis. *Schweizer Archiv für Neurologie und Psychiatrie, 156*, 471-479.

Markowitsch, H. J. (1986). Physiological and comparative psychology: Current research interests. *American Psychologist, 41*, 1301-1305.

McCrone, J. (2004). Freud's neurology. *Lancet Neurology, 3*, 320.

McHenry, L. C. (1969). *Garrison's history of neurology*. Springfield, IL: Thomas.

Meyer, A. (1971). *Historical aspects of cerebral anatomy*. London: Oxford University Press.

Meynert, T. (1872). *Der Bau der Gross-Hirnrinde und seine örtlichen Verschiedenheiten* [The structure of the cerebral cortex and its regional variations]. Leipzig, Germany: Heuser.

Meynert, T. (1968). *Psychiatry: A clinical treatise on diseases of the fore-brain based upon a study of its structure, function, and nutrition* (B. Sachs, Trans.). New York: Haffner. (Original work published in 1884)

Miller, L. (1991a). *Freud's brain: Neuropsychodynamic foundations of psychoanalysis*. New York: Guilford.

Miller, L. (1991b). On aphasia at 100: The neuropsychodynamic legacy of Sigmund Freud. *Psychoanalytic Review, 78*, 365-378.

Miller, N. S., & Katz, J. L. (1989). The neurological legacy of psychoanalysis: Freud as a neurologist. *Comprehensive Psychiatry, 30*, 128-134.

Moe, H. (2004). *The story of the microscope*. Copenhagen: Rhodos.

Morton, F. (1979). *A nervous splendor: Vienna 1888-1889*. Boston: Little, Brown and Company.

Morton, F. (1989). *Thunder at twilight: Vienna 1913-1914*. New York: Macmillan.

Ochs, S. (2004). *A history of nerve functions: From animal spirits to molecular mechanisms*. Cambridge, UK: Cambridge University Press.

Panek, R. (2004). *The invisible universe: Einstein, Freud, and the search for hidden universes*. New York: Viking.

Pearce, J. M. S. (1996). Sigmund Freud. *Lancet, 347*, 1039-1041.

Pearce, J. M. S. (2003). *Fragments of neurological history*. London: Imperial College Press.

Peper, M., & Markowitsch, H. J. (2001). Pioneers of affective neuroscience and early concepts of the emotional brain. *Journal of the History of the Neurosciences, 10*, 58-66.

Purtle, H. R. (1974) *The Billings microscope collection*. Washington, DC: Armed Forces Institute of Pathology.

Ramón y Cajal, S. (1897-1904). *Textura del sistema nervioso del hombre y de los vertebrados* (Vol. I-III) [Textbook of the human and vertebrate nervous system]. Madrid: Moya.

Ramón y Cajal, S. (1907). Die histogenetischen Beweise der Neuronentheorie von His und Forel [The histogenetic proof of the neuron theory of His and Forel]. *Anatomischer Anzeiger, 30*, 113-144.

Ritvo, L. B. (1990). *Darwin's influence on Freud*. New Haven, CT: Yale University Press.

Rueda Franco, F. (2001). The neuron doctrine, the mind, and the Arctic. *Neurosurgery, 49*, 233-234.

Shepherd, G. M. (1991). *Foundations of the neuron doctrine*. New York: Oxford University Press.

Solms, M. (1993). Problems at the interface of psychoanalysis and neuroscience. *Contemporary Psychology, 38*, 719-720.

Solms, M. (1996). Towards an anatomy of the unconscious. *Journal of Clinical Psychoanalysis, 5*, 331-367.

Solms, M. (1998). An introduction to the neuroscientific works of Sigmund Freud. *Sartoniana, 11*, 283-304.

Solms, M. (2004). Freud returns. *Scientific American, 290*, 82-88.

Solms, M., & Saling, M. (1990). *A moment of transition: Two neuroscientific articles by Sigmund Freud*. London: The Institute of Psycho-Analysis & Karnac.

Sotelo, C. (2003). Viewing the brain through the master hand of Ramón y Cajal. *Nature Reviews Neuroscience, 4*, 71-77.

Spiel, H. (1987). *Vienna's golden autumn, 1866-1938*. London: Weidenfeld and Nicolson.

Stone, I. (1971). *The passions of the mind: A biographical novel of Sigmund Freud*. New York: Doubleday.

Stricker, S. (1872). *A manual of histology*. New York: Wood.

Sulloway, F. J. (1979). *Freud, biologist of the mind: Beyond the psychoanalytic legend*. New York: Basic Books.

Tallis, R. C. (1996). Burying Freud. *Lancet, 347*, 669-671.

Triarhou, L. C. (1989). *On the early neurohistological studies of Sigmund Freud: 50-year memorial lecture*. Indianapolis, IN: John Shaw Billings History of Medicine Society.

Triarhou, L. C., & del Cerro, M. (1985). Freud's contribution to neuroanatomy. *Archives of Neurology, 42*, 282-287.

Triarhou, L. C., & del Cerro, M. (1986). Sigmund Freud: A note on his neuroanatomic investigations. Thirty-eighth Annual Meeting of the American Academy of Neurology. *Neurology, 36*(Suppl. 1), 126.

Triarhou, L. C., & del Cerro, M. (1987a). The histologist Sigmund Freud, 1877-1884. Centennial Meeting of the American Association of Anatomists. *Anatomical Record, 218*, 140A.

Triarhou, L. C., & del Cerro, M. (1987b). The histologist Sigmund Freud and the biology of intracellular motility. *Biology of the Cell, 61*, 111-114.

Triarhou, L. C., & del Cerro, M. (2006). Sigmund Freud's microscope – On the 150th birthday anniversary of the histologist. *Micscape, 132*, http://www.microscopy-uk.org.uk/mag/artoct06/mc-freud.html

Turner, G. L' E. (1989). *The great age of the microscope: The collection of the Royal Microscopical Society through 150 years*. Bristol, UK: Hilger.

Waldeyer, H. W. G. (1891). Über einige neuere Forschungen im Gebiete der Anatomie des Centralnervensystems [On some newer researches in the area of the anatomy of the central nervous system]. *Deutsche Medizinisches Wochenschrift 17*, 1213-1218, 1244-1246, 1287-1289, 1331-1332, 1352-1356.

Wiest, G., & Baloh, R. W. (2002). Sigmund Freud and the VIIIth cranial nerve. *Otology and Neurotology, 23*, 228-232.

Winson, J. (1985). *Brain and psyche: The biology of the unconscious.* New York: Random House.

In: *Cognitive Psychology Research Developments*
Editors: Stella P. Weingarten and Helena O. Penat

ISBN 978–1–60692–197–5
© 2009 Nova Science Publishers, Inc.

Chapter 7

TRIPARTITE CONCEPTS OF MIND AND BRAIN, WITH SPECIAL EMPHASIS ON THE NEUROEVOLUTIONARY POSTULATES OF CHRISTFRIED JAKOB AND PAUL MACLEAN

Lazaros C. Triarhou[*]

Economo–Koskinas Wing for Integrative and Evolutionary Neuroscience,
University of Macedonia, Thessaloniki, Greece

ABSTRACT

The 'triune brain', conceived by Paul D. MacLean (1913–2007) in the late 1960s, has witnessed more attention and controversy than any other evolutionary model of brain and behavior in modern neuroscience. Decades earlier, in his book *Elements of Neurobiology* published in 1923 in La Plata, Argentina, neurobiologist Christfried (Christofredo) Jakob (1866–1956) had formulated a 'tripsychic' brain system, based on his deep understanding of biological and neural phylogeny. In a historical context, 1923 was also the year of publication of Sigmund Freud's *The Ego and the Id*, whereby the founder of psychoanalysis solidified his tripartite model of the mental apparatus. Tripartite systems of the human mind have been surmised since Plato and Aristotle; they continue to our era, an example being Robert J. Sternberg's triarchic theory of human intelligence. In view of the fact that both Jakob and MacLean invested a considerable part of their long and distinguished careers studying comparative, and particularly reptilian neurobiology, the present article revisits their neuroevolutionary models, underlining the convergence of their anatomical-functional propositions, in spite of a time distance of almost half a century.

---

[*] E-mail address: triarhou@uom.gr, phone +30 2310 891-387, fax +30 2310 891-388

INTRODUCTION

In the words of neurologist William E. DeMyer [1], "to understand the brain–thought–behavior triumvirate is the Holy Grail of neuroanatomy, as compelling to the researcher as a cyclonic vortex." Models to explain the mechanisms of operation of the human mental apparatus have been formulated since the era of classical Greece. The preponderance of such models appear to be 'tripartite,' without necessarily entailing that e.g. unipartite, bipartite or quintopartite models would be less meaningful.

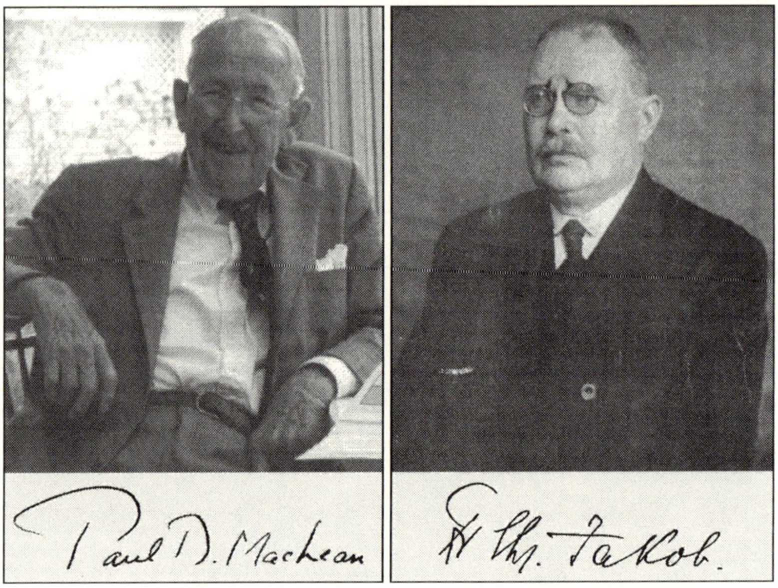

Figure 1. Left: Portrait of Paul D. MacLean (1913–2007), taken in 2001 by Kelly G. Lambert [81] © 2003 Elsevier Inc., reproduced with permission; signature from the author's private archive. Right: Portrait of Christofredo Jakob (1866–1956), from Orlando's book cover [15]; signature from Jakob's 1924 notes of pathological anatomy and physiology (full reference in [17]), courtesy of Staatsbibliothek Berlin.

The 'triune brain', conceived by neurobiologist-psychiatrist Paul D. MacLean (1913–2007) (Fig. 1), has been popularized way beyond the neurosciences. This becomes evident in the treatments by Arthur Koestler in chapter 16 ('The three brains') of his *Ghosts in the Machine* [2] – the concluding sequel of the trilogy which includes the 1959 *Sleepwalkers: A History of Man's Changing Vision of the Universe* and the 1964 *Act of Creation* –, and by Carl Sagan in chapter 3 ('The brain and the chariot') of his evolutionary saga *The Dragons of Eden* [3]. Further, the triune brain featured in a documentary produced by the National Film Board of Canada [4]. In recent years, the triune modular brain concept has been accommodated by the social sciences: Cory [5] suggested an extended dynamic model of neural social architecture, the 'conflict systems neurobehavioral' (CSN) model, placing more emphasis on behavioral than on neurological terms.

Concerning neuroanatomical terminology, Elliot Smith [6] coined the term *neopallium* in 1901 to denote a cortical organ that had the ability, based on progressive evolution, to learn with experience through a mechanism of sensory perception, associative memory, consciousness and response (Fig. 2). Elliot Smith [7 (pp. 31–38)] regarded the neopallium as fulfilling all the conditions of the Aristotelian *sensorium commune*.

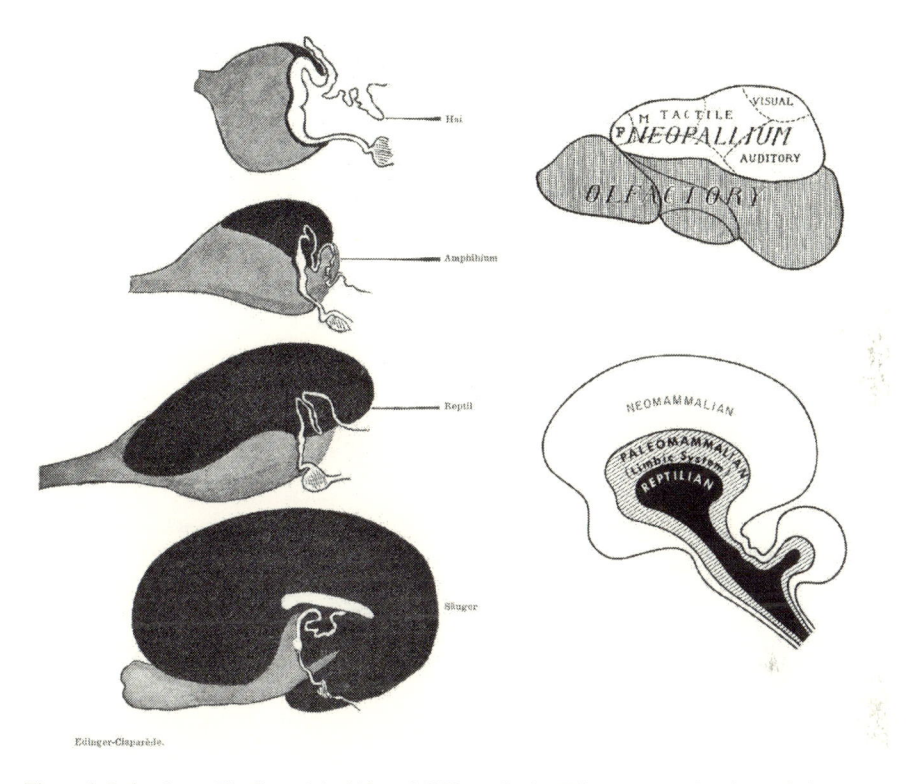

Figure 2. *Left column:* The first original idea of 1908, credited to Edinger, suggesting the evolutionary distinction of the brain into an 'old' *(gray)* and a 'new' part *(black)*. The drawing depicts, top to bottom, the brains of a shark, an amphibian, a reptile and a mammal. The *palaeëncephalon* exists from insects to man, and remains virtually unchanged from shark to elephant. The *neëncephalon* made its first appearance in fish and progressed all the way to humans, filling the entire skull. From figure 8 in Edinger [11 (p. 17)]. *Upper right:* Sir Grafton Elliot Smith introduced the term neopallium in 1901. The diagram shows the lateral aspect of the left cerebral hemisphere of a primitive mammal, the jumping shrew *(Macroscelides)*, and the relatively enormous extent of the primitive olfactory territories and small neopallium with its receptive areas for tactile, visual and auditory impressions. The anterior segment of the tactile area (from *M* back to the dotted line) represents the so-called 'motor area'. *F* represents the frontal area rudiment. From figure 7 in Elliot Smith [7 (p. 33)]. *Lower right:* Schematic representation of the theorized hierarchical organization in the triune brain concept of MacLean [73, 75]. The three basic components, in an ascending evolutionary order, are the *reptilian complex*, the *limbic system* (paleomammalian brain), and the *neocortex* (neomammalian brain), roughly subserving *instincts*, *emotions*, and *intellect*, respectively.

The designations *'paleo-'*, *'archi-'* and *'neo-'* for the cortex (pallium) on grounds of their sequential evolutionary appearance were introduced with a 1909 paper of Ariëns Kappers [8],[1] which subsequently led to similar designations for diverse brain regions, including the striatum, thalamus and cerebellum [10]. Kappers' mentor, Frankfurt anatomist Ludwig Edinger [11] had provided the fundamental intellectual stimulus the previous year, 1908, by systematizing the brain into *palaeëncephalon*, the highly conserved midbrain and hindbrain, and *neëncephalon*, the forebrain, which varies substantially among vertebrates, appearing for the first time in fish and increasing in size and complexity along the phylogenetic scale (Fig. 2). Edinger's core proposition, i.e. that the forebrain has evolved through a sequential addition of parts, is most likely the original idea from which MacLean's 'triune brain' concept derives [12 (p. 31)].

Tilney [13] used the term *archikinetic* to connote balance functions subserved by the medial group of the deep cerebellar nuclei (globose and fastigial), and *neokinetic* for the skilled movements of the face and limbs subserved by the lateral group (emboliform and dentate nucleus) in conjunction with the neopallium and the pyramidal system. According to Tilney [14], *neokinesis* is an extensive group of reactions comprising the externalized expression of the elaborate evolved coordination of eyes, head and hands.

Some of the most pertinent contributions to a neuroevolutionary approach of behavior have come from Christfried (Christofredo) Jakob (1866–1956) (Fig. 1), a German-born neuropathologist who spent most of his professional life in Argentina. Having studied under Friedrich Albert von Zenker (1825–1898) and Adolf von Strümpell (1853–1925) at Erlangen, Jakob subsequently became affiliated with the National Universities of La Plata and of Buenos Aires, where he established one of the most important neuropathological laboratories in South America. He is considered the father of Argentinian neurobiology and forensic histopathology and has left an invaluable legacy of 200 articles and 30 monographs in German and Spanish [15–17].

Jakob reached international renown through his early successful handbooks of clinical medicine [18] and neurology [19], as well as his atlases of human [20] and comparative neuroanatomy [21, 22] (Fig. 3 and 4). He later produced landmark works on evolutionary neurobiology, studying in detail dozens of species of the autochthonus Patagonian fauna, including the broad-snouted 'yacaré' (or *Caiman latirostris*), a reptile of the Alligatoridae family [23], and the 'pichiciego' (fairy armadillo or *Chlamyphorus truncatus*), a mammal of the Dasypodidae family [24].

---

1 In a footnote, Jakob [9 (p. 12)] argues that, to avoid confusion by various authors, the correct chronological order of the three terms on etymological grounds should be archi-, paleo- and neo-, since ἀρχή means origin or beginning, and should therefore precede παλαιός, which means old or ancient.

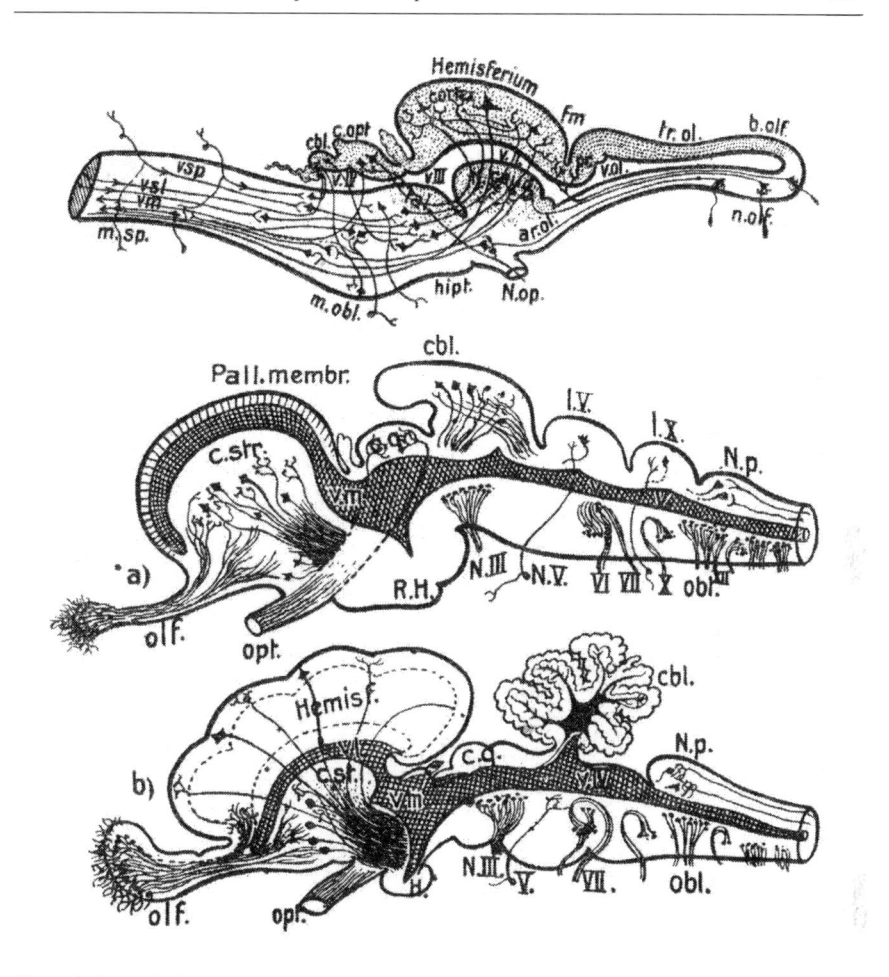

Figure 3. Sagittal schematic views of reflex and central nervous pathways in the brain of a reptile (top), a fish or 'lower vertebrate' (middle) and a mammal or 'higher vertebrate' (bottom). The atlases of comparative neuroanatomy by Jakob and Onelli [21, 22] are rare treasures of evolutionary information. In them, the anatomical properties and connections patterns of cortical (monostratified to polystratified), striatal, hypothalamic and mesencephalic structures, among others, are related from fish through reptiles to primates, as are the underlying functional correlations. Sources: top frame is from figure 7 on p. 8 in [21], also appearing on p. 13 in [22]; middle and bottom frames are from figure 1 on p. 6 in [21], also appearing on p. 11 in [22] and in figure 13 on p. 32 in [66]. Note that in the top frame the olfactory bulb is oriented to the right side; in the middle and bottom frames to the left.

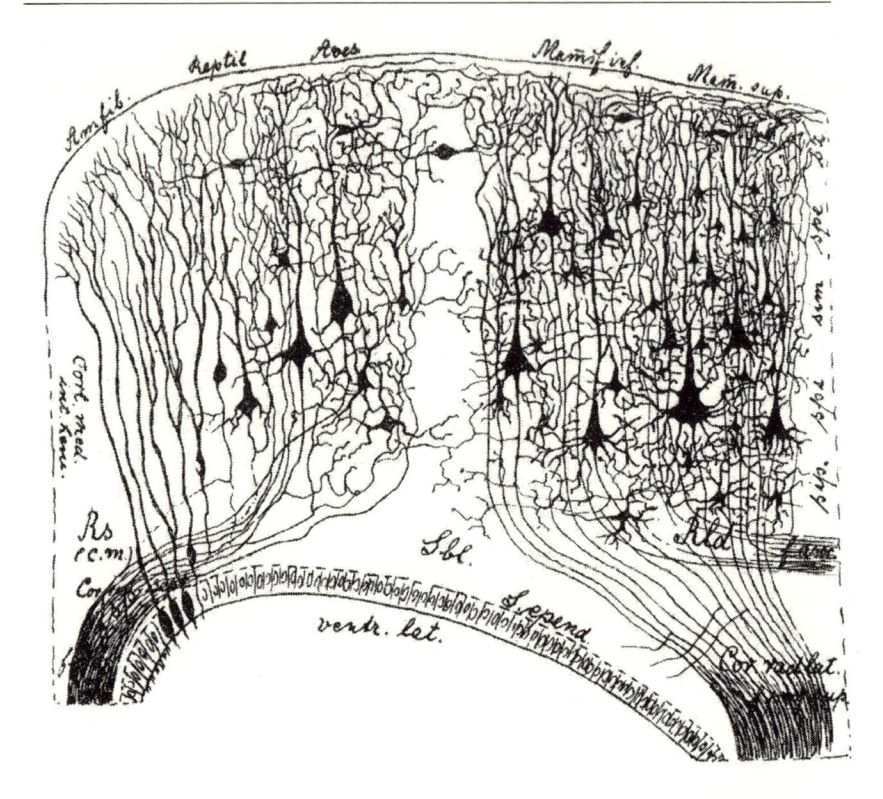

Figure 4. Phylogenetic evolution of the cerebral cortex from monostratified to polystratified. From left to right, amphibian, reptilian, avian, mammalian, and higher mammalian cortical layer structure. Source: from figure 32 on p. 23 in [21], also appearing on p. 16 in [22].

The aim of the present article is first, to revitalize an interest in the evolutionary concepts of Christofredo Jakob, a foremost neuroanatomist of the 20th century and perhaps one of the earliest pioneers in neurophilosophy; and second, to pinpoint the confluences between the anatomical-functional conceptions of Jakob and MacLean regarding their tripartite models of the human mind based on evolutionary criteria, despite a time distance of almost half a century. For a broader perspective, certain other tripartite models of the human mind from the classical antiquity through present are mentioned.

Both Jakob and MacLean invested a considerable part of their long and distinguished careers studying comparative neurobiology from reptiles (Fig. 5) to primates (Fig. 6), and both left their mark on scientific advances regarding the visceral and olfactory brain and the limbic system (Fig. 7). As a matter of fact, there is a whole line of evidence indicating that Jakob described the anatomical elements of the visceral brain some 30 years before the widely known 'circuit of Papez' came into being [25–31]. On the other hand, MacLean's contributions have been instrumental in both defining the limbic system and in sorting out some of its key emotional functions in normality and psychopathology [32–38].

Tripartite Concepts of Mind and Brain 189

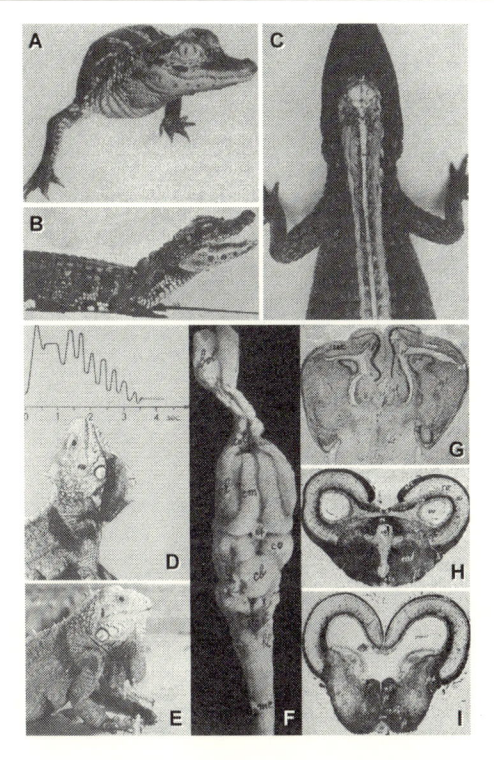

Figure 5. (**A**) A young alligator used for studies on temperature regulation and reproductive behavior at MacLean's Laboratory of Brain Evolution and Behavior at the National Institute of Mental Health [97]. (**B**) The yacaré *(Caiman latirostris)* displaying the innate 'terrorizing' reflex posture, an 'archineuronal brainstem reaction' [53 (p. 143)]. (**C**) Brain and spinal cord of a young yacaré ('alligator of Chaco') dissected in situ. One can discern the cerebral hemispheres, optic tectum, small cerebellum, and the dorsal medulla and spinal cord. From plate 37a in [9 (p. 97)]. (**D, E**) Onset and termination of a stereotypic 'head-nodding' behavior displayed by a male *Iguana iguana* lizard from South America; this type of fixed social signal may have evolved 150 million years ago. From work by MacLean's alumnus Detlev Ploog [100]. (**F**) Dorsal view of the iguana brain. The Ammonic zone or medial cortical *(cm)* and lateral cortical *(cl)* portion of the cerebral hemispheres can be seen, separated by the dorsal longitudinal lateral sulcus, which is the precursor of the hippocampal sulcus. *Abbreviations: bol,* olfactory bulb; *tol,* olfactory tubercle; *ep,* epiphysis (pineal); *co,* optic tectum; *cb,* cerebellum; X, vagus; *bl,* medulla oblongata; *mc,* spinal cord. From figure 86 in [9 (p. 136)]. (**G**) Coronal section of the anterior cerebrum of *Iguana iguana,* at the level of the basal commissure *(cb)* and its continuation towards the hypothalamus. Between the fascia dentata and Ammon's zone, the lateral sulcal depression is found. From figure 87 in [9 (p. 138)]. (**H**) The midbrain of *Iguana iguana.* Entry of the optic nerve *(II)* in the zonal layer *(stz)*; superior *(cs)* and inferior *(ci)* mesencephalic commissure in the tectum; at the bottom is the hypothalamic commissure *(cht).* Weigert stain, ×50. From figure 94 in [9 (p. 150)]. (**I**) Coronal section through the midbrain of *Iguana iguana,* showing the three layers of the optic body, the zonal *(sz),* the intermediate, and the deep *(stp),* as well as its commissure *(cc).* Laterally the optic bundle *(II)* enters into the zonal layer. From the deep layer derives the bulbar quadrigeminal descending fasciculus *(fcb)* also called by various authors tectospinal. In the ventral half one can distinguish the posterior longitudinal fasciculus *(fl),* the reticular formation and the basal (striodiencephalobulbar) fasciculus. Weigert stain, ×90. From plate XXXVIIa in [9 (p. 95)].

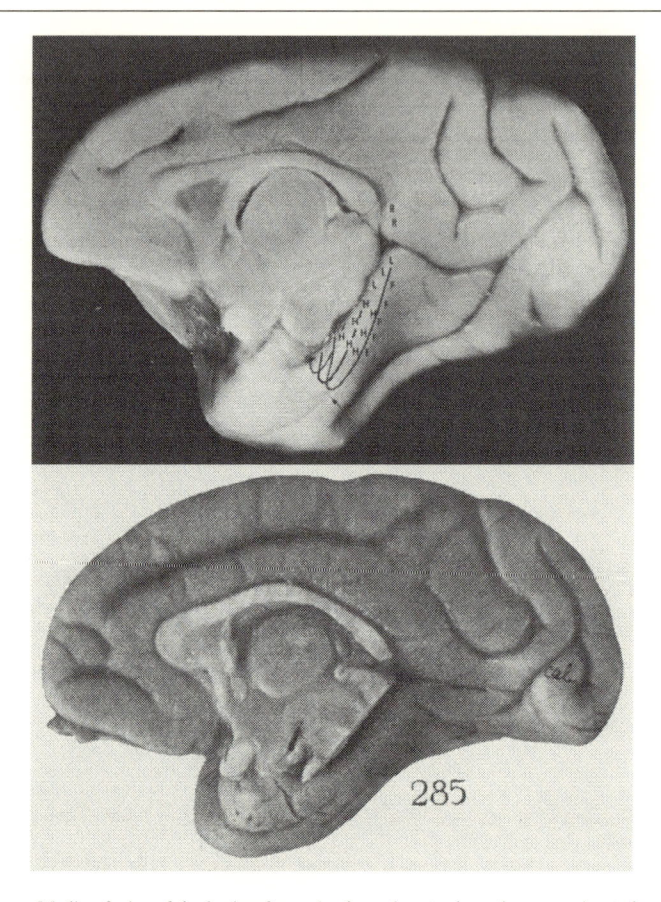

Figure 6. *Upper:* Median facies of the brain of a squirrel monkey to show the approximate location of light-responsive areas. *Abbreviations: H*, posterior hippocampal gyrus; *L*, parahippoampal portion of lingual gyrus; *R*, retrosplenial cortex; *F*, fusiform gyrus. Arrow shows the caudal extreme of rhinal sulcus at the caudal limit of the entorhinal area. From figure 5 in [75 (p. 343)]. *Lower:* Macroscopic brain specimen of a cebus monkey from Paraguay. From plate LXII in [22].

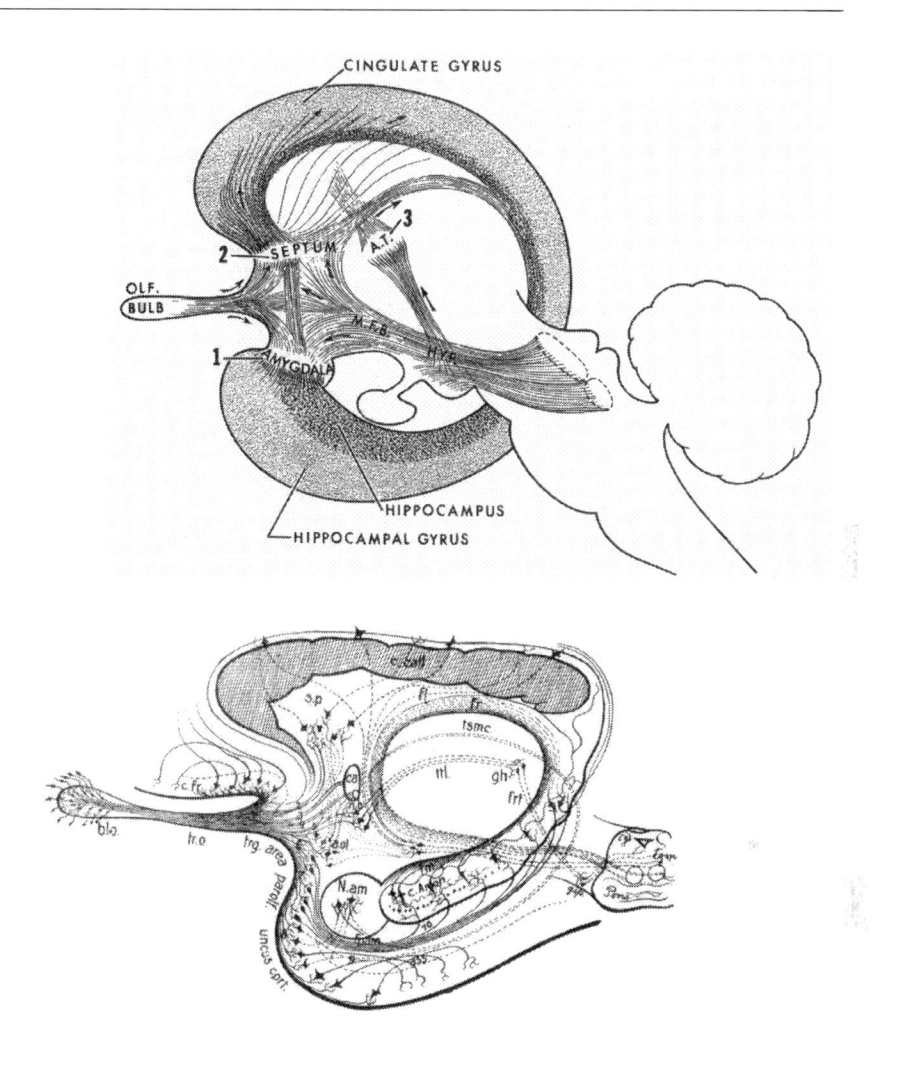

Figure. 7. Drawings of the limbic system and the rhinencephalon (olfactory brain) by MacLean [75] and Jakob [20]. *Upper:* Limbic cortex and its connections with brainstem structures. *Abbreviations: A.T.*, anterior thalamic nuclei; *HYP*, hypothalamus; *M.F.B.*, median forebrain bundle; *OLF*, olfactory [75 (figure 4 on p. 341)]. *Lower:* The rhinencephalon and the olfactory radiation, with the anatomical connections of the olfactory bulb, septum, anterior commissure and uncus hippocampi [20 (figure 15 on p. 19)].

PHILOSOPHICAL TRIPARTITE MODELS OF THE PSYCHE

Plato of Athens developed a tripartite concept of the human psyche in *Phaedrus* (370 B.C.) and in the *Republic* (360 B.C.). For him, the cerebrospinal marrow is the organic seat of the 'rational' or 'intelligent' (λογιστικόν), the 'temperamental' or 'courageous' (θυμοειδές), and the passionate or appetitive (ἐπιθυμητικόν), respectively occupying the cerebral, thoracic, and abdominal portion [39 (pp. 270–271), 40, 41]. Atomic philosopher Democritus of Abdera (c. 460–370 B.C.) may have anticipated Plato's tripartite division of the psyche [39 (pp. 254–255)], naming the brain the 'guard of the mind' (φύλαξ διανοίης), the heart the 'control of passion' (ὀργῆς τιθηνός), and the liver the 'cause of desire' (ἐπιθυμίης αἴτιον).

Burnet [42 (p. 149)] argues that the doctrine of the tripartite psyche was in reality Pythagorean. Among existing suggestions at the time, Plato adopted in *Timaeus* (360 B.C.) the landmark discovery made by Alcmaeon of Croton (500 B.C.) that the brain is the faculty of the mind [43]. Based on that thesis, Socrates speculates in *Phaedo* that the brain provides sensations (αἰσθήσεις); from these arise memory (μνήμη) and opinion (δόξα); and when stabilized, these become knowledge (ἐπιστήμη) [39 (p. 269)].

Cohen [44] surmises that, because the Bible makes God tripartite with the three persons of the Trinity and teaches that man is made in God's image, theologians have looked for a Biblical tripartite nomenclature for man: a unified totality, comprising the components of 'spirit' (πνεῦμα), 'psyche' (ψυχή), and 'body' (σῶμα), the only Biblical support for a doctrine of human tripartiteness found in the First Epistle to the Thessalonians (ε'23).

A noteworthy association from the domain of classical drama – not far from neuroscience in an essential way[2] – is a metaphorical tripartite model of the human psyche discerned in the Karamazov brothers of Fyodor Dostoyevsky's 1880 crowning success, Dmitri representing 'passion', Ivan 'intellect', and Alyosha 'contemplation' [46].

THE TRIPSYCHIC BRAIN SYSTEM OF JAKOB

In his 1923 *Elements of Neurobiology*, Jakob establishes three categories of 'neurodynamic' functions [47 (pp. 197–209)]:

(1) *plasmopsychisms* or *plasmodynamisms* (tropism, taxism, and pulsatile rhythms);
(2) *phylopsychisms* or *neurodynamisms* (simple serial or organized reflexes, otherwise instincts); and
(3) *ontopsychisms* or *psychodynamisms* ('gnosias', 'praxias' and 'symbolias').

Jakob [48] viewed motor and sensory elements and their connections as constituting a unit and a fundamental functional cortical arc that forms the basis of psychological phenomena. In the phylogenetic scale, *plasmopsychic* or *plasmodynamic* activities precede all other nervous functions [9].

---

[2] As highlighted by Steven Pinker [45], Dostoyevsky was not foreign to the nervous underpinnings of behavior. In his prison cell, prompted by a visit by the academician Rakitin, Dmitri Karamazov mulls over the fact that thinking results from quivering nerve tails and the chemistry inside the brain, rather than an immaterial soul.

The above three neurodynamic graduations are all primarily 'biophylactic', i.e. they serve to preserve life, respectively, at its fundamental, the species, and the organism levels [47]. They are found in varying distribution and combination among actual living beings: in the world of plants, as well as in protozoans and sponges one finds only *plasmopsychisms*; in metazoans with ganglionic nervous systems (e.g. hydropolyps, worms, molluscs and arthropods) through the inferior vertebrates (cyclostomes and fish) exist both *plasmopsychisms* and *phylopsychisms*; insects, having a cerebral ganglion, and fish, with their mesencephalon, might potentially exercise elemental *ontopsychic* functions; in amphibians through the higher vertebrates, including humans, one finds all three categories amalgamated and combined, with a predominance of the *ontopsychic dynamism*, which in humans has culminated into the symbolic psychisms (the elements of the intellectual world, of aesthetics and ethics), without though diminishing the concomitant existence of the more elemental levels.

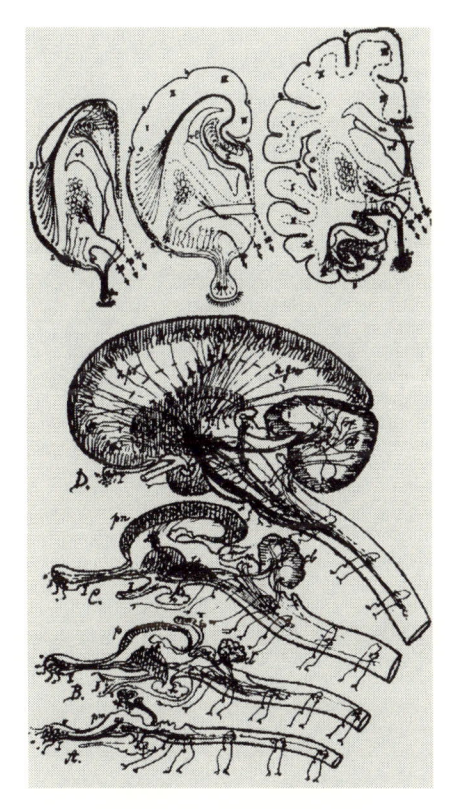

Figure 8. *Upper row:* Schematic drawing of the phylogeny of *archineuronal, paleoneuronal* and *neoneuronal* olfactory systems in a reptile *(left)*, a marsupial *(center)* and a primate *(right)*. From figure 110 in *El Yacaré* [23 (p. 100)]. *Lower group:* Schematic drawing of *primordial neural (A), archineural (B), paleoneural (C)* and *neoneural (D)* systems. From *The Neoencephalon, its Organization and Dynamism* [96 (plate 2)].

There are three underlying structural-functional hierarchical levels of the nervous system, designated as (*a*) *archineuronal*, (*b*) *paleoneuronal* and (*c*) *neoneuronal* (Fig. 8). *Archineuronal* and *paleoneuronal* levels are inherited[3] and constitute the substrate of *phylopsychic* or *neurodynamic* processes; the *neoneuronal* level subserves *ontopsychic* or *psychodynamic* processes, where individual experience becomes possible, and where the will resides [47, 50, 51 (pp. 18–30)].

The *archineuronal* system has a reflex function similar to the invertebrates, comprising simple visceral and somatic reflex arcs ('archikinesias') (Fig. 9, 10A). The *paleoneuronal* system hosts instinctive-automated reactions ('paleokinesias') and it becomes able to prolong the effects of stimuli over time, thus instigating a *chronotropic* ability (Fig. 9). Examples of paleokinetic systems [50, 52] can be found in the cerebellum and the corpus striatum (Fig. 10B, C).

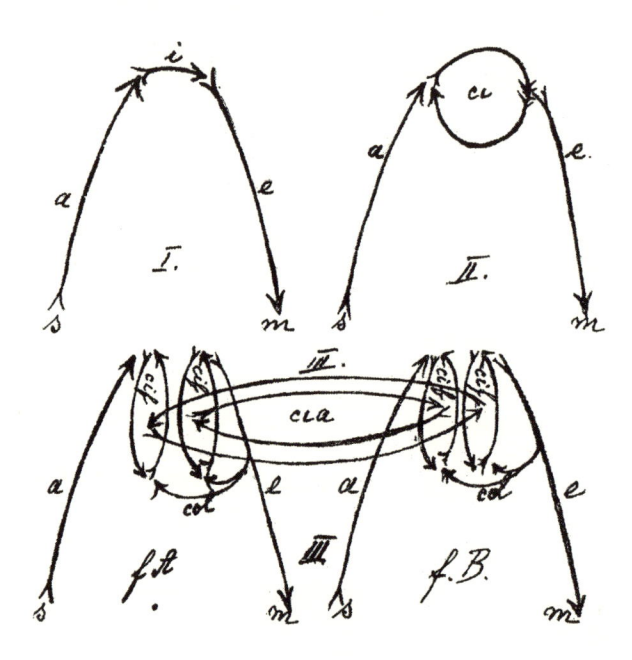

Figure 9. Diagrammatic scheme of *archikinesias (I), paleokinesias (II)* and *neokinesias (III)* according to Jakob [50 (p. 116)]. *Abbreviations: a, s*, sensory afferent system; *e, m*, motor efferent system; *i*, intercalated system; *ci*, intercalated microdynamism; *fA, fB*, cortical foci A and B; *cif*, focal intercalated microdynamism; *cia*, associative intercalated circuit; *col*, motor collateral

The higher *neoneuronal* system subserves conscious acts, individuality and consciousness ('neokinesias') (Fig. 9, 11); it comprises two sectors, the limbic cortex ('introyente' or endogenous sphere) and the lateral cortex ('ambiente' or external environment). Time responses vary approximately from 20–30 msec for the 'archikinesias'

---

[3] In his 1969 Hincks Memorial Lecture at Queen's University in Ontario, MacLean [49] begins his tripartite diatribe with 'Man's reptilian and limbic *inheritance*' (my italics).

and from 200–300 msec for the 'neokinesias' [53 (pp. 35–37)];[4] in the latter instance, the major distance can be established through a central or volitional neokinetic transformation in a reaction time of 110–120 msec (the "fourth dimension of thought").

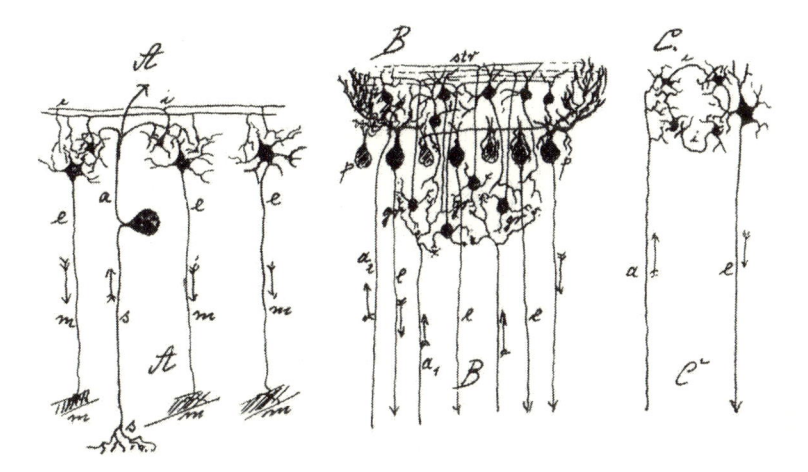

Figure 10. Histological organization of intercalated systems in (A) archikinesias, (B) cerebellar paleokinesias, and (C) striatal paleokinesias according to Jakob [50 (p. 119)]. *Abbreviations: a*, afferent; *e*, efferent; *m*, motor; *s*, sensory; a_1, mossy fiber; a_2, climbing fiber; *P*, Purkinje cells; *gr*, granule cells; *str*, stellate cells; *i*, intercalated element (interneuron).

Within the framework of the dynamic workings of the human cerebral cortex, the 'neokinesias' include (*i*) 'gnosias' (cognitive processes related to conscious orientation in one's environment), (*ii*) 'praxias' (individual active intervention) and (*iii*) 'symbolias' (ideative abstraction to facilitate interindividual communication, such as the sociogenetic processes on which human culture is based) [47, 50, 53 (pp. 41–66), 60; cf. also 29, 61, 62 (pp. 297–303), 63–65]. Jakob [66 (p. 16)] later elaborated on these three concepts in his *Documenta Biofilosófica*, commenting that 'gnosia' (attentive orientation), 'praxia' (active or passive intervention) and 'symbolia' (communicative verbal formulation) represent three intimately linked sensory-motor phases that together form the true psychogenetic trinity ('la verdadera trinidad psicocreadora'), from which "experience and thought are revealed as amalgamated neurodynamic realities."

Jakob treated the theme of the phylogeny of the *archicortex*, *paleocortex* and *neocortex* in greater detail in the second part of his 1945 monograph on the yacaré [23 (pp. 99–109)].

---

[4] These are remarkable calculations for having been written in the 1940s, if one considers that current views hold that consciousness arises from neurons in about 500 msec – the 'neural time factor' [54] – or less [55]; in other words, it takes a fraction of a second between the occurrence of a physiological stimulus in the parietal cortex and a subject becoming conscious of it [56], with the mind compensating for real time through a 'backward referral' experience [57]. On the efferent side, brain potentials fire a little over 300 msec before one has the conscious intention to act [58] and cerebral potentials may precede finger movement by up to 1 sec [59].

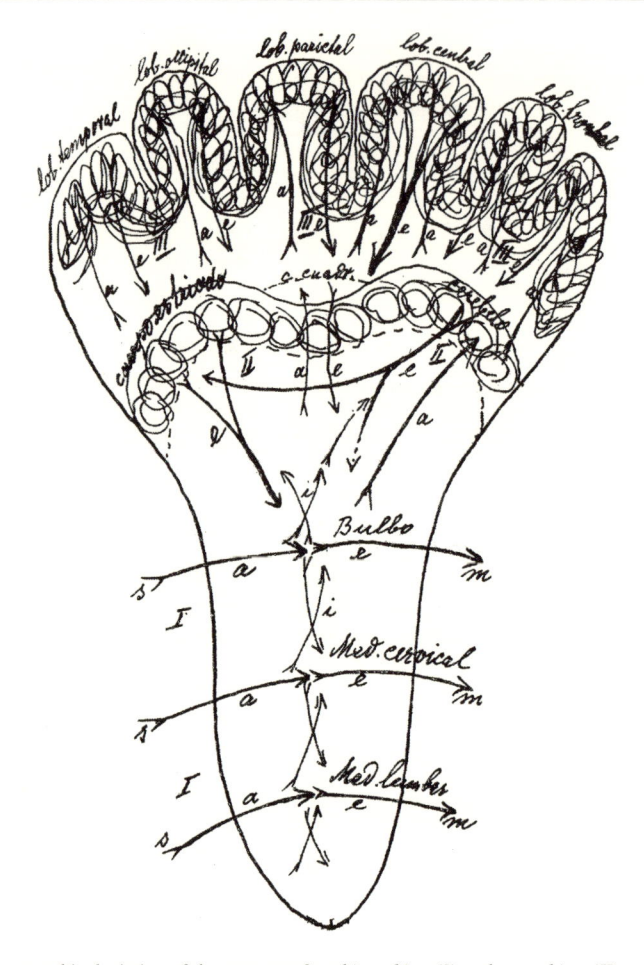

Figure. 11. Topographic depiction of the systems of *archipsychism (I)*, *paleopsychism (II)* and *neopsychism (III)* according to Jakob [50 (p. 127)].

THE TRIPARTITE MENTAL APPARATUS OF PSYCHOANALYSIS

Freud formally introduced the full scope of his infamous three-fold model of the mental apparatus – comprising the id ('das Es'), the ego ('das Ich'), and the super-ego or ego ideal ('das Über-Ich' oder 'Ich-Ideal') – in his 1923 book *Das Ich und das Es* [67], which was translated into English as *The Ego and the Id* [68]. Freud revisited and supplemented the theme a decade later (1933) in his *New Introductory Lectures* [69].

Jacobson [70] argues that Freud's contributions to the neuron doctrine may have been overestimated as part of "the blatant hero worship," which led to a reverberation of psychoanalytic thought in the new field of neuroscience. The theory of MacLean [71] on the processing of emotions by a network of deep brain structures seems to have found a general acceptance in the 1950s because of its conceptual correspondence to psychoanalytic theory [72]. As a matter of fact, MacLean [71] makes the point that "considered in the light of Freudian psychology, the visceral brain would have many of the attributes of the unconscious id." Regarding the assumed phylogenetic components of the 'triune brain,' MacLean [49, 73] does mention a correspondence to Freud's id, ego, and super-ego [74].

Sagan [3 (p. 79)] describes MacLean's triune brain model as being only in weak accord with the tripartite mind of psychoanalytic theory and stresses that, owing to the neuroanatomical connections between its three component parts, the triune brain must be useful, just like the metaphor for the human psyche found in Plato's *Phaedrus*. In that dialogue, Socrates likens the human soul to a chariot drawn by two horses, a black and a white, pulling in different directions and weakly controlled by the charioteer. Freud also described the *ego* as the rider of an unruly horse. Sagan [3] argues that an even better metaphor could be Freud's division of the mind into *conscious*, *preconscious* and *unconscious*.[5] A remarkable similarity can be seen between the metaphor of Plato's chariot and MacLean's neural substrates, the reptilian and paleomammalian brains corresponding to the two horses, and the neomammalian brain to the charioteer.

Freud's and Jakob's books, describing their respective landmark models of the tripartite mind and the tripsychic brain, were both published in the year 1923. Both investigators attribute a special emphasis to the body's projection pattern on the cerebral cortex: having a sound background and an early successful career in neuroanatomy, Freud [68] describes the ego as being "first and foremost a bodily ego, not merely a surface entity, but itself the projection of a surface." According to Freud, a neurological analogy for the ego is its identification with the "cortical homunculus of the anatomists." In a footnote first appearing in the authorized English translation of 1927 (absent from the German edition), this is further explained as the ego being "ultimately derived from bodily sensations, chiefly those springing from the surface of the body;" thus, it can be regarded as "a mental projection of the surface of the body, besides representing the superficies of the mental apparatus."

In his atlases of comparative and human neuroanatomy, Jakob [20–22] stresses in more detail the topographic dissociation of the body's projection pathways onto the lateral and medial surfaces of the cerebral hemispheres, depending on the perception of exogenous or endogenous signals, and introduces his pioneering concepts of the formation of sectors and pre-gyri, as well as the concept of a visceral brain with an anatomical correlate in the cingulate gyrus (reviewed in [31]).

---

5 In his paper on the phylogeny of the kinesias, Jakob [50] mentions a correspondence of plasmopsychic through archipsychic functions with the unconscious, of paleopsychic functions with the preconscious (which genetically precedes conscious phenomena, and thus is differentiated from the subconscious, which he considers part of the conscious), and of neopsychic functions with the conscious (Fig. 10).

THE TRIUNE BRAIN CONCEPT OF MACLEAN

Paul MacLean's conception of a 'triune' pattern and organization of the human brain includes three fundamental brain types or subsystems – each with its own subjectivity, intelligence, spacetime sense, memory, motor and other functions – intermeshing as one. Going phylogenetically and hierarchically from older to newer, over the past 200 million years, these are [49, 73, 75–78]:

(1) The *reptilian* brain at the base, the most ancient heritage, first evolved in primeval reptiles and the great lizards, forms the matrix of the upper brainstem and comprises most of the reticular formation, the midbrain, the hypothalamus, the basal ganglia (archipallium), and the cerebellum; it mediates biological and endocrine equilibrium, via stereotypic behaviors and vital functions, such as survival and self-preservation, sleep-wakefulness regulation, drinking and feeding, mating, territorial possession, imitation, aggression, flight and ritualized combat, and the establishment of social hierarchies. It assures an immediate response in the present and it is privileged concerning olfaction.

(2) The *paleomammalian* brain, the intermediate type that is distinguished by the presence of a primitive cortex, the limbic cortex; the limbic system is central in mediating feelings, emotions and affect – which necessitates a long-term memory and the motivation associated with it –, play, the sense of reality of oneself and the environment, the conviction of what is true or important, the recognition of offspring and parental care. It makes its appearance in the early mammals and it is based on the importance of vocalization and audition.

(3) The *neomammalian* brain, which 'mushroomed' late in evolution and is characterized by the more highly differentiated form of the neocortex (neopallium); it forms the basis of interpersonal communication via spoken and written language, arithmetic, rationality, creative abilities, and the intellect. Typical of humans, the neomammalian brain with its evolved frontal lobes, subserves (rather than 'understands', cf. [79]) reason and symbolic language; it is 'privileged' with regards to vision, abstraction, association, imagination and future anticipation.

According to the triune brain theory, the integrated human brain is a synthesis of the three successively evolved 'component' brains, which, while operating as a whole, retain their original attributes and functions. Limbic regions (e.g. anterior cingulate, medial frontal and insular), phylogenetically conserved to a higher degree than the neocortical regions which mediate cognitive capacities, are associated with emotional responses and their intrinsic affective attributes [73, 80]. The types of mental function for which the reptilian, limbic and neomammalian brain are responsible, are respectively assigned by MacLean [73] as 'protomentation', 'emotional mentation' and 'rational mentation'. In the relatively rapid human evolution, the three brain subsystems are imperfectly integrated, influencing individual and social behaviors that are under the commands of each individual or collective act.

MacLean chose the term 'triune' for his evolutionary brain theory because of the literal meaning of the word (three-in-one); the fact that his father was a Presbyterian minister may have something to do with such a choice, although MacLean reportedly regretted it [81], due to the potential confounding with the Christian doctrine.

FURTHER TRIPARTITE MODELS OF THE HUMAN MIND

In a temporal confluence, Knopp [82], studying patients with Gilles de la Tourette disease and acute schizophrenia, proposed – in the same year as MacLean [75] formally introduced the triune brain concept – a tripartite brain concept as well, whereby a balanced and continuous reconciliation among three components or at least two levels of central integration constitutes the 'rational brain'. According to Knopp's proposition, the limbic lobe, the hypothalamic network and the autonomic nervous system neurophysiologically subserve *visceral experience*, the nigrostriatal system and the limbic lobe *(conscious) emotional experience*, and the neocortex *social experience (effectuation)*.

In considering tripartite models of the mind, the synthetic neurophilosophical construct of Popper and Eccles [83] comes to mind, accounting for brain-mind interaction by means of their World 1 (liaison brain), World 2 (outer and inner sense and the self), and World 3 (cultural heritage).

In the cybernetic view, the nervous system operates as a tripartite system that involves *input* (sensory receptor), *integrating*, and *output* (muscle contraction) components [84]; this is based on a 19th century notion of anatomists and physiologists, and an ubiquitous principle of physiological psychology in the 20th century, of grouping brain structure and function into *sensory*, *association*, and *motor* systems [85]. Such properties accrete from the most fundamental properties of the nerve cell as a *receiving*, *conducting*, and *transmitting* functional unit, and the principle of dynamic polarization of neurons [86], which is at the core of neurobiology.

The triarchic model of the human mind propounded by Sternberg [87, 88] consists in *analytical*, *practical*, and *creative* sides of intelligence. Tigner and Tigner [89] argue that such a model may reflect the triptych developed by Aristotle of Stageira in his *Nicomachean Ethics* (350 B.C.). The Greek philosopher proposed a system of human intelligence comprising three virtues: 'theoretical' (διανόησις), 'practical' (φρόνησις), and 'productive' (ποίησις). The parallel conclusions of temporally disjoined inquiries by investigators working under disparate historical circumstances does not seem to be unusual in the historical evolution of psychological thought [89].

At the level of mind organization, Fodor [90] proposed a tripartite division of cognitive mechanisms, involving physical energy→symbol *transducers*, which record stimuli from the outside world and convert them into neural code, specialized modular *input systems*, which process raw data derived from the transducers, and a central *processor*, the site of higher cognitive processes that receives the outcome of input systems [91].

An established philosophical taxonomy, providing a tripartite structure of consciousness, divides it into *phenomenal*, *reflective*, and *access* consciousness [92, 93]. Phenomenal consciousness subserves the subjective feeling of mental content [94]; reflective consciousness is defined as the direct availability of the process of mental activities for access that allows one to access the steps of the reasoning process, whereas access consiousness is the direct availability of mental content that allows one to access the outcome of a reasoning process [93].

DISCUSSION

Based on the ideas exposed above, it becomes apparent that tripartite models abound in the attempt to shed light into the workings of the human brain and mind; they span over a spectrum from the philosophical to the biological. To attempt to draw parallels or pinpoint differences among various components in such a pleiad of systems forms a daunting task. Nonetheless, in considering the particular models in the evolutionary domain, Jakob's proposition of three hierarchically appearing 'psychisms' in the nervous system [47] seems to anticipate, by several decades, the 'triune brain' concept of MacLean [49, 75].

During his upbringing in Germany, Jakob acquired a strong background in philosophy [15] and throughout his career, Jakob [66, 95] maintained a philosophical perspective on biology in general and on neurobiology in particular (Fig. 12); he realized some of the earliest interpretations of the limbic or 'internal' brain as a viscero-emotional mechanism and the bidirectional communication between the internal organs and the splenial cortex, and the external environment and the lateral cortex [21, 22]. Although Jakob kept a distance from peripatetic metaphysics, he nevertheless adopted, in strictly biological terms, the Aristotelian notion of the psychic character (or 'psychism'): "That neurobiophylactic [neural life-protecting] complex of neuroenergetic reception, assimilation and reaction, which regulates the organism's vital necessities against variable factors in the external and inner environment, I call *psychism*" [96 (p. 8)]. In Jakob's synthesis, one can trace the influence of the precepts of his mentor von Strümpell, as well as of Italian positivism, particularly the views of philosopher Giovanni Marchesini (1868–1931) [30 (pp. 115–116)].

MacLean, on the other hand, planned to study philosophy before ending up studying medicine; he eventually proposed the creation of a new branch of knowledge ("epistemics") to look at things "from the inside out", combining neuroscience and psychology in an attempt to explain the subjective self and its relationship to the external and internal environment [97].

Jakob [47] attributed a life-preserving role ('biophylaxis') to phylopsychism – at the species – and ontopsychism – at the individual – level. MacLean highlighted the importance of the reptilian complex for integrating behaviors involved in self-preservation and in the preservation of the species [97].

Jakob [60] named 'praxias' the active individual intervention processes within the framework of the dynamic workings of the cerebral cortex, and treated 'tropism' within the spectrum of fundamental neurodynamic functions [47]; he further presented his ideas on life and mental experience relative to time at the basal, phylogenetic and ontogenetic levels in a paper under the encompassing title 'From tropism to the general theory of relativity' [98]. MacLean coined terms such as 'isopraxic' – to denote behaviors in which multiple members of a group perform the same thing – and 'tropistic' – to connote a behavior responding to partial representations of things, such as the marking on a prey [97].

In the 1990s, MacLean [99] placed special emphasis on the three cortical types that evolved in the forebrain of mammals, from mammalian-like reptiles (therapsids) through humans, to describe the idea of how resonance may contribute to the dynamic excitability of neural circuits by representing possible algorithms in the nervous system at the macroscopic, microscopic, molecular, and atomic level that underscore mental states and solutions for immediate or eventual actions. He suggested that the forebrain is particularly important as a 'central processor' for mental experience, including sensation, perception, drive, affect, thought, and the precise facts of science, and concluded that a refined picture of the structure and chemistry of the brain's circuitry accounting is needed, especially because of the central question of whether one may ever rely on the brain with its viscoelastic properties to reliably measure time and space and the general nature of things [99].

Over six decades earlier, in his classical exposé on the phylogeny of the kinesias, Jakob [50] employed the time spread of 'corollary discharge' – a mechanism proposed by Helmholtz, allowing a receiving system to either take into account or ignore self-generated sensory input during the monitoring of self-generated movements – in attempting to substitute *semovience* (the mind's capacity to generate new causal actions through experienced inner life). Jakob explained such a substitution with the mediation of axon collaterals, which upload neural activity into focal intercalated microcircuits, and an acquired 'associative system' [30 (pp. 121, 144)].

The ideas and propositions independently formulated by Jakob and by MacLean, despite their time distance and different environments, reflect a substantial convergence in their reasoning. Thus, studies attempting to penetrate human behavior by means of evolutionary hints, might benefit by taking a closer look at Jakob's contributions, which have largely remained unheeded in the English scientific literature and which contain information potentially pertinent to current problems in psychobiology.

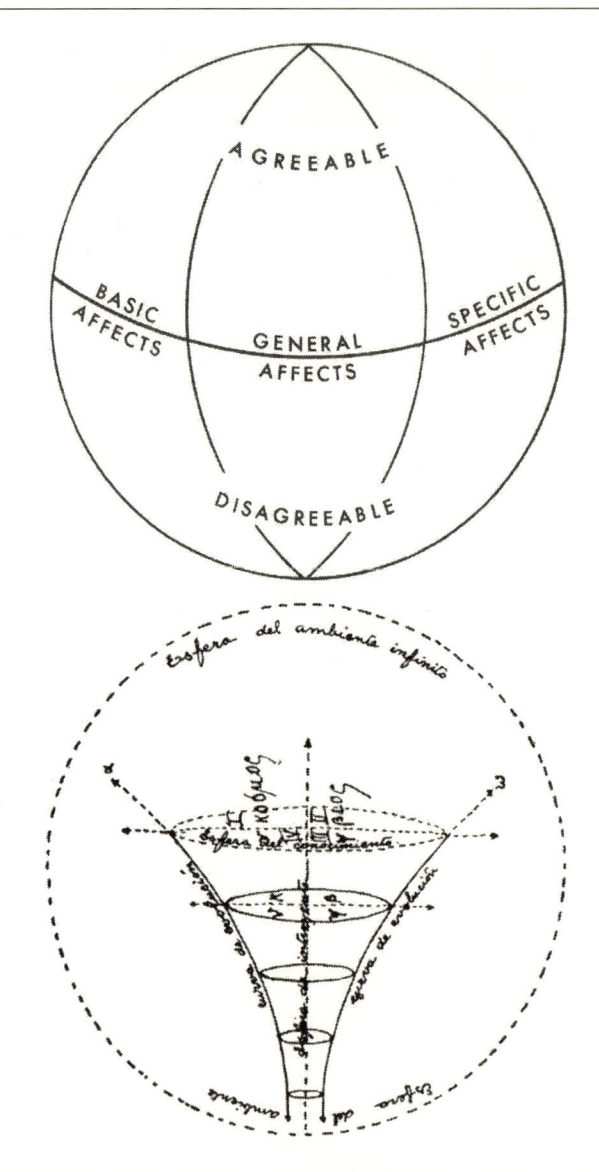

Figure 12. Upper: MacLean's [75 (p. 338)] scheme for viewing the world of affects, subjectively qualified into either agreeable or disagreeable. MacLean maintains that affects cannot be neutral, because "emotionally speaking, it is impossible to feel unemotional." He further subdivides affects into basic (informative about basic bodily needs), general (pertinent to situations, individuals or groups and the preservation of self or the species) and specific (occurring with activation of specific sensory systems). Lower: Jakob's [95] scheme of the empirical sphere with the four quadrants of the sciences: I. Cosmos (κόσμος), II. Life (βίος), III. Psyche (ψυχή) and IV. Order (νόμος). The sphere of the infinite environment is invaded by that of progressive knowledge, delimited by the curve of evolution.

CONCLUDING REMARKS

Born an ocean and five decades apart, Christofredo Jakob and Paul MacLean left their marks of productivity as interdisciplinary neuropsychiatrists, with special emphasis on comparative neurobiology and brain evolution. It is worth noting that the two investigators also died half a century apart, and published their tripartite models in 1923 and in 1970, respectively, when they both were 57 years of age. The fact that they never met, but formulated convergent propositions, can only lead one to recall the motto, "great minds think alike."

The extent to which the two neuroevolutionary constructs are empirically supported remains a controversial issue even today. Considering the recurring triune theories on the underpinnings of the mind, witnessed over twenty-five centuries of human inquiry, one may ponder over a putative tendency of the human brain itself to construct or understand tripartite models of reality. Perhaps the hypothesis of an evolutionary trend to develop tripartite models of existence could some day be put to rigorous experimental testing.

REFERENCES

[1] DeMyer, W. (1988). *Neuroanatomy*. Baltimore–Malvern: Williams & Wilkins/Harwal Publishing Co., p. 315.

[2] Koestler, A. (1967). *The Ghost in the Machine*. London: Hutchinson & Co. Ltd., pp. 267–296.

[3] Sagan, C. (1977). *The Dragons of Eden: Speculations on the Evolution of Human Intelligence*. New York: Random House, pp. 49–79.

[4] Thérien, G., Verrier, H., & Beaudet, M. (1984). *Les Trois Cerveaux*. Montréal: Office National du Film du Canada.

[5] Cory, G. A. Jr. (2003). MacLean's evolutionary neuroscience and the conflict systems neurobehavioral model: some clinical and social policy implications. In A. Somit, & S. A. Peterson (Eds.), *Human Nature and Public Policy: An Evolutionary Approach*. New York–Hampshire: Palgrave Macmillan, pp. 161–180.

[6] Elliot Smith, G. (1901). The natural subdivision of the cerebral hemisphere. *Journal of Anatomy and Physiology (London)*, 35, 431–454.

[7] Elliot Smith, G. (1927). *The Evolution of Man: Essays*, 2nd edn. London: Humphrey Milford–Oxford University Press.

[8] Ariëns Kappers, C. U. (1909). The phylogenesis of the paleocortex and archicortex compared with the evolution of the visual neocortex. *Archives of Neurology and Psychiatry (London)*, 4, 161–173.

[9] Jakob, C. (1941). *El Cerebro Humano: Su Ontogenía y Filogenía* (Folia Neurobiológica Argentina, Atlas III). Buenos Aires: Aniceto López.

[10] Swanson, L. W. (2000). What is the brain? *Trends in Neurosciences*, 23, 519–527.

[11] Edinger, L. (1909). Die Beziehungen der vergleichenden Anatomie zur vergleichenden Psychologie, Neue Aufgaben. In L. Edinger, & E. Claparède (Eds.), *Über Tierpsychologie: Zwei Vorträge* (aus dem Bericht über den III. Kongreß für Experimentelle Psychologie, 1908). Leipzig: J. A. Barth, pp. 1–30.

[12] Striedter, G. F. (2005). *Principles of Brain Evolution*. Sunderland, MA: Sinauer Associates, Inc.

[13] Tilney, F. (1927). The chief intracerebellar and precerebellar nuclei, with a demonstration with models and charts. *Brain*, 50, 275–276.

[14] Tilney, F. (1927). The brain stem of tarsius. A critical comparison with other primates. *Journal of Comparative Neurology*, 43, 371–432.

[15] Orlando, J. C. (1966). *Christofredo Jakob: Su Vida y Obra*. Buenos Aires: Editorial Mundi. http://electroneubio.secyt.gov.ar/Vida_y_obra_de_Christofredo_Jakob.htm

[16] Triarhou, L. C., & del Cerro, M. (2006). Semicentennial tribute to the ingenious neurobiologist Christfried Jakob (1866–1956). 1. Works from Germany and the first Argentina period, 1891–1913. *European Neurology*, 56, 176–188.

[17] Triarhou, L. C., & del Cerro, M. (2006). Semicentennial tribute to the ingenious neurobiologist Christfried Jakob (1866–1956). 2. Publications from the second Argentina period, 1913–1949. *European Neurology*, 56, 189–198.

[18] Jacob, C. (1898). *A Klinikai Vizsgálati Módszerek Atlasza a Belgyógyászati Diagnostica és a Különös Kór- és Gyógytan Alapvonalaival* (fordította Ritoók Zsigmond). Budapest: Singer és Wolfner Kiadása.

[19] Jakob, C. (1899). *Atlante del Sistema Nervoso nello Stato Sano e nel Patologico con un Sunto di Anatomia Patologica e Terapia del Medesimo*. Milano: Società Editrice Libreria.

[20] Jakob, C. (1911). *Das Menschenhirn: Eine Studie über den Aufbau und die Bedeutung seiner Grauen Kerne und Rinde*. München: J. F. Lehmann.

[21] Jakob, C., & Onelli, C. (1911). *Vom Tierhirn zum Menschenhirn: Vergleichend Morphologische, Histologische und Biologische Studien zur Entwicklung der Grosshirnhemisphären und ihrer Rinde. I. Teil. Tafelwerk nebst Einführung in die Geschichte der Hirnrinde*. München: J. F. Lehmann.

[22] Jakob, C., & Onelli, C. (1913). *Atlas del Cerebro de los Mamíferos de la República Argentina. Estudios Anatómicos, Histológicos y Biológicos Comparados sobre la Evolución de los Hemisferios y de la Corteza Cerebral*. Buenos Aires: Imprenta de Guillermo Kraft.

[23] Jakob, C. (1945). *El Yacaré (Caiman latirostris) y el Orígen del Neocortex: Estudios Neurobiológicos y Folklóricos del Reptil más Grande de la Argentina* (Folia Neurobiológica Argentina, Tomo IV). Buenos Aires: Aniceto López.

[24] Jakob, C. (1943). *El Pichiciego (Chlamydophorus Truncatus): Estudios Neurobiológicos de un Mamífero Misterioso de la Argentina* (Folia Neurobiológica Argentina, Tomo II). Buenos Aires: Instituto de Biología de la Facultad de Filosofía y Letras.

[25] Barraquer-Bordas, L. (1954). *Fisiología y Clínica del Sistema Límbico: Aportaciones Recientes al Conocimiento de las Bases Neurofisiológicas de la Personalidad*. Madrid: Paz Montalvo, pp. 136–137.

[26] Barraquer-Bordas, L. (1976). *Neurología Fundamental: Fisiopatología, Semiología, Síndromes, Exploración*, 3rd edn. Barcelona: Toray, p. 596.

[27] Orlando, J. C. (1964). Sobre el cerebro visceral. Documentación histórica de una prioridad científica. *Revista Argentina de Neurología y Psiquiatría*, 1, 197–201.

[28] Goldar, J. C. (1975). *Cerebro Límbico y Psiquiatría*. Buenos Aires: Salerno.

[29] Faccio, E. J. (1991). Christofredo Jakob y el origen del psiquismo. *Alcmeón – Revista Argentina de Clínica Neuropsiquiátrica*, 3, 331–348.

[30] Szirko, M. (1995). A la antropología ganglionar desde la kinesiología: un fallido ensayo de extrapolar lo orgánico (Noticia preliminar). *Electroneurobiología (Buenos Aires)*, 2, 104–169.

[31] Triarhou, L. C. (2008). Centenary of Christfried Jakob's discovery of the visceral brain: An unheeded precedence in affective neuroscience. *Neuroscience and Biobehavioral Reviews*, 32, 984–1000.

[32] MacLean, P. D. (1969). The hypothalamus and emotional behaviour. In W. Haymaker, E. Anderson, & W. J. H. Nauta (Eds.), *The Hypothalamus*. Springfield, IL: Charles C Thomas, pp. 659–678.

[33] Marino, R. Jr. (1975). *Fisiologia das Emoçoes: Introduçao à Neurologia do Comportamento, Anatomia e Funçoes do Sistema Limbico*. São Paulo, Brasil: Sarvier S.A. Editora do Livros Médicos.

[34] MacLean, P. D. (1985). Evolutionary psychiatry and the triune brain. *Psychological Medicine*, 15, 219–221.

[35] Lautin, A. (2001). *The Limbic Brain*. New York: Kluwer Academic–Plenum Publishers, pp. 69–98.

[36] Ploog, D. (2003). The place of the triune brain in psychiatry. *Physiology and Behavior*, 79, 487–493.

[37] Perna, G. (2005). *Las Emociones de la Mente: Biología del Cerebro Emotivo*. Madrid: Tutor.

[38] Reep, R. L., Finlay, B. L., & Darlington, R. B. (2007). The limbic system in mammalian brain evolution. *Brain Behavior and Evolution*, 70, 57–70.

[39] Beare, J. I. (1906). *Greek Theories of Elementary Cognition from Alcmaeon to Aristotle*. Oxford: Clarendon Press.

[40] Stocks, J. L. (1915). Plato and the tripartite soul. *Mind – A Quarterly Review of Philosophy*, 24, 207–221.

[41] Georgulis, K. D. (1957). Plato. *Helios Encyclopaedical Lexikon (Athens)*, 16, 7–81.

[42] Burnet, J. (1920). *Early Greek Philosophy*, 3rd edn. London: A. & C. Black, Ltd..

[43] Doty, R. W. (2007). Alkmaion's discovery that brain creates mind: A revolution in human knowledge comparable to that of Copernicus and of Darwin. *Neuroscience*, 147, 561–568.

[44] Cohen, E. D. (1988). *The Mind of the Bible-Believer*. Amherst, NY: Prometheus Books, p. 121.

[45] Pinker, S. (2002). *The Blank Slate: The Modern Denial of Human Nature*. London: Allen Lane, p. 85.

[46] Edgeworth, R. J. (1994). The tripartite soul in Plato, Dostoyevsky, and Aldiss. *Neophilologus*, 78, 343–350.

[47] Jakob, C. (1923). *Elementos de Neurobiología, volumen I: Parte Teórica* (Biblioteca Humanidades, Tomo III). La Plata, Argentina: Facultad de Humanidades y Ciencias de la Educación de la Universidad Nacional de La Plata.

[48] Jakob, C. (1914). La psicología orgánica y su relación con la biología cortical (Referat von R. Allers). *Zeitschrift für die Gesamte Neurologie und Psychiatrie*, 9, 804–805.

[49] MacLean, P. D. (1973). *A Triune Concept of the Brain and Behaviour* (The Clarence Hincks Memorial Lectures, Volume 2, edited by T. J. Boag and D. Campbell).

Toronto–Buffalo: Ontario Mental Health Foundation–University of Toronto Press, pp. 1–66.
[50] Jakob, C. (1935). La filogenia de las kinesias: Sobre su organización y dinamismo evolutivo. *Anales del Instituto de Psicología de la Facultad de Filosofía y Letras de la Universidad de Buenos Aires*, 1, 109–127.
[51] Jakob, C. (1940). *Ontogenia del Sistema Nervioso Humano*. La Plata–Buenos Aires: Universidad Nacional de La Plata, Facultad de Humanidades y Ciencias de la Educación–Imprenta López.
[52] Jakob, C. (1936). *La Organización Subcortical del Sistema Nervioso Central de los Vertebrados Superiores: El Paleoencéfalo y sus Funciones Instintivas*. La Plata–Buenos Aires: Facultad de Humanidades y Ciencias de la Educación, Universidad Nacional de La Plata–Imprenta y Casa Editora «Coni».
[53] Jakob, C. (1941). *Neurobiología General* (Folia Neurobiológica Argentina, Tomo I). Buenos Aires: Aniceto López.
[54] Libet, B. (1999). How does conscious experience arise? The neural time factor. *Brain Research Bulletin*, 50, 339–340.
[55] Gazzaniga, M. (1998). *The Mind's Past*. Berkeley–London: University of California Press, pp. 69–82.
[56] Libet, B., Alberts, W. W., Wright, E. W. Jr., Delattre, L., Levin, G., & Feinstein, B. (1964). Production of threshold levels of conscious sensation by electrical stimulation of human somatosensory cortex. *Journal of Neurophysiology*, 27, 546–578.
[57] Libet, B., Wright, E. W. Jr., Feinstein, B., & Pearl, D. K. (1979). Subjective referral of the timing for a conscious sensory experience: a functional role for the somatosensory specific projection system in man. *Brain*, 102, 193–224.
[58] Libet, B., Gleason, C. A., Wright, E. W. Jr., & Pearl, D. K. (1983). Time of conscious intention to act in relation to onset of cerebral activities (readiness potential): the unconscious initiation of a freely voluntary act. *Brain*, 106, 623–642.
[59] Kristeva, R., Keller, E., Deecke, L., & Kornhuber, H. H. (1979). Cerebral potentials preceding unilateral and simultaneous bilateral finger movements. *Electroencephalography and Clinical Neurophysiology*, 47, 229–238.
[60] Jakob, C. (1921). La teoría actual de las gnosias y praxias como factores fundamentales en el dinamismo de la corteza cerebral. *Crónica Médica (Lima)*, 38, 17–24.
[61] Szirko, M. (1991). Definición de psiquismo y de conocimiento sensible, retención de las memorias, evolución del sistema nervioso, y relaciones mente-cuerpo o nexo psicofísico, en la Escuela Neurobiológica Argentino-Germana. *Electroneurobiología (Buenos Aires)*, 1 [Supl. 2], I–XIV.
[62] Kurowski, M. (2001). *La Obra Psicológica de Juan Cuatrecasas Arumí (1899–1990)*. Madrid: Universidad Complutense, Facultad de Psicología.
[63] Crocco, M. (2004). ¡Alma e' reptil! Los contenidos mentales de los reptiles y su procedencia filética. *Electroneurobiología (Buenos Aires)*, 12, 1–72.
[64] Capizzano, A. A. (2006). Actualidad del pensamiento de Cristofredo Jakob. *Revista del Hospital Italiano de Buenos Aires*, 26, 71–73.
[65] Crocco, M. (2007). Christofredo Jakob. In *Wikipedia, la Enciclopedia Libre*. http://es.wikipedia.org/wiki/Christofredo_Jakob

[66] Jakob, C. (1946). *Documenta Biofilosófica. Folleto I. Biología y Filosofía. A: Aspectos de sus divergencias y concomitancias. B: Ensayo de Psicogenia orgánica* (Folia Neurobiológica Argentina, Tomo V). Buenos Aires: López y Etchegoyen.

[67] Freud, S. (1978). Das Ich und das Es [1923]. In A. Freud, & I. Grubrich-Simitis (Eds.), *Sigmund Freud Werkausgabe in zwei Bänden, Band 1: Elemente der Psychoanalyse*, 2. Aufl. Frankfurt a.M.: S. Fischer Verlag GmbH, pp. 369–401.

[68] Freud, S. (1974). *The Ego and the Id* [1923] (transl. by J. Riviere, ed. by J. Strachey). London: The Hogarth Press and the Institute of Psycho-Analysis, pp. 9–17.

[69] Freud, S. (1978). Neue Folge der Vorlesungen zur Einführung in die Psychoanalyse [1933]. In A. Freud, & I. Grubrich-Simitis (Eds.), *Sigmund Freud Werkausgabe in zwei Bänden, Band 1: Elemente der Psychoanalyse*, 2. Aufl. Frankfurt a.M.: S. Fischer Verlag GmbH, pp. 402–418.

[70] Jacobson, M. (1993). *Foundations of Neuroscience*. New York–London: Plenum Press, pp. 204–205.

[71] MacLean, P. D. (1949). Psychosomatic disease and the "visceral brain": Recent developments bearing on the Papez theory of emotion. *Psychosomatic Medicine*, 11, 338–353.

[72] Kolb, B., & Whishaw, I. Q. (1996). *Fundamentals of Human Neuropsychology*, 4th edn. New York: W. H. Freeman and Co., pp. 417–420.

[73] MacLean, P. D. (1990). *The Triune Brain in Evolution: Role in Paleocerebral Functions*. New York–London: Plenum Press.

[74] Peper, M., & Markowitsch, H. J. (2001). Pioneers of affective neuroscience and early concepts of the emotional brain. *Journal of the History of the Neurosciences*, 10, 58–66.

[75] MacLean, P. D. (1970). The triune brain, emotion, and scientific bias. In F. O. Schmitt (Ed.), *The Neurosciences: Second Study Program*. New York: Rockefeller University Press, pp. 336–349.

[76] MacLean, P. D. (1977). The triune brain in conflict. *Psychotherapy and Psychosomatics*, 28, 207–220.

[77] MacLean, P. D. (1990). *Les Trois Cerveaux de l'Homme: Textes Traduits de l'Américain, Notes et Commentaires de Roland Guyot* (Collection «La Fontaine des Sciences» dirigé par Gérard Klein). Paris: Éditions Robert Laffont, S.A..

[78] Schoffeniels, E., Schmerling, P., & MacLean, P. D. (1994). Journée Commemorative du Bicentenaire de Pierre Schmerling: Colloque: Théorie des trois cerveaux de Paul Donald MacLean et incidences en Psychiatrie: vendredi 15 novembre 1991, Hôpital Psychiatrique du Petit Bourgogne, Liège (*Acta Psychiatrica Belgica*, 94, fasc. 4–6). Bruxelles, Société de Médecine Mentale.

[79] Bennett, M. R., & Hacker, P. M. S. (2001). Perception and memory in neuroscience: a conceptual analysis. *Progress in Neurobiology*, 65, 499–543.

[80] Panksepp, J. (2002). The MacLean legacy and some modern trends in emotion research. In G. A. Cory, Jr., & R. Gardner, Jr. (Eds.), *The Evolutionary Neuroethology of Paul MacLean*. Westport, CT: Praeger, pp. ix–xxvii.

[81] Lambert, K. G. (2003). The life and career of Paul MacLean: A journey toward neurobiological and social harmony. *Physiology and Behavior*, 79, 343–349.

[82] Knopp, W. (1970). Man's tripartite brain and psychosomatic medicine. *Psychotherapy and Psychosomatics*, 18, 130–136.

[83] Popper, K. R., & Eccles, J. C. (1977). *The Self and its Brain.* Berlin–Heidelberg: Springer International, pp. 358–365.
[84] Hubel, D. H. (1979). The brain. *Scientific American,* 241, 44–53.
[85] Uttal, W. R. (2001). *The New Phrenology: The Limits of Localizing Cognitive Processes in the Brain.* Cambridge, MA: MIT Press, p. 25.
[86] Ramón y Cajal, S. (1954). *Neuron Theory or Reticular Theory? Objective Evidence of the Anatomical Unity of Nerve Cells* (transl. by M. Ubeda Purkiss, C.A. Fox). Madrid: Consejo Superior de Investigaciones Científicas/S. Aguirre Torre.
[87] Sternberg, R. J. (1984). Toward a triarchic theory of human intelligence. *Behavioral and Brain Sciences,* 7, 269–315.
[88] Sternberg, R. J. (1988). *The Triarchic Mind: A New Theory of Human Intelligence.* New York–London: Viking Press.
[89] Tigner, R. B., & Tigner, S. S. (2000). Triarchic theories of intelligence: Aristotle and Sternberg. *History of Psychology,* 3, 168–176.
[90] Fodor, J. A. (1983). *The Modularity of Mind.* Cambridge, MA: MIT Press.
[91] Sterelny, K. (1990). *The Representational Theory of Mind.* Oxford: Basil Blackwell Ltd., p. 75.
[92] Block, N. (1995). On a confusion about a function of consciousness. *Behavioral and Brain Sciences,* 18, 227–287.
[93] Sun, R. (2002). *Duality of the Mind: A Bottom Up Approach Toward Cognition.* Mahwah, NJ: Lawrence Erlbaum Associates Inc., pp. 176–190.
[94] Nagel, T. (1974). What is it like to be a bat? *Philosophical Reviews,* 4, 435–450.
[95] Jakob, C. (1945). El cerebro humano: Su significación filosófica. Ensayo de un programa psico-bio-metafísico, después de 50 años de dedicación neurobiológica. *Revista Neurológica de Buenos Aires,* 10, 89–110.
[96] Jakob, C. (1939). *El Neoencéfalo: Su Organización y Dinamismo.* La Plata–Buenos Aires: Universidad Nacional de La Plata, Facultad de Humanidades y Ciencias de la Educación–Imprenta López.
[97] Holden, C. (1979). Paul MacLean and the triune brain. *Science,* 204, 1066–1068.
[98] Jakob, C. (1922). Del tropismo a la teoría general de la relatividad: Un capítulo biopsicofiláctico. *Humanidades (La Plata),* 3, 45–58.
[99] MacLean, P. D. (1997). The brain and subjective experience: question of multilevel role of resonance. *Journal of Mind and Behavior,* 18, 247–268.
[100] Ploog, D. (1970). Social communication among animals. In F. O. Schmitt (Ed.), *The Neurosciences: Second Study Program.* New York: Rockefeller University Press, pp. 349–361.

Fin-de-Siècle Advances in Neuroeducation: Henry Herbert Donaldson and Reuben Post Halleck

Zoë D. Théodoridou[1] and Lazaros C. Triarhou[1]

ABSTRACT—This article focuses on two early attempts at bridging neuroscience and education, made by Henry Herbert Donaldson (1857-1938), a neurologist, and Reuben Post Halleck (1859-1936), an educator. Their works, respectively entitled *The Growth of the Brain: A Study of the Nervous System in Relation to Education* (1895) and *The Education of the Central Nervous System: A Study of Foundations, Especially of Sensory and Motor Training* (1896), witness early attempts at opening up paths for the application of neurobiological findings to education. We provide an exposé of select points from their monographs; published only 1 year apart, both texts constitute significant testimonies of that *Zeitgeist*. They shed light on contemporary discussions about gender, neuroplasticity, critical periods, nature and nurture, and sleep/awake rhythms and provide a much needed perspective on the difficulties of founding the new inter- and transdisciplinary field of neuroeducation.

"What we group under the name of the sciences is, as the application of the word in the plural shows, no single entity, but consists of many separate fields of knowledge, which often lie far apart. Through the increase of such knowledge, these fields increase, and their boundaries, originally far apart, approach each other more and more. The investigation of these border zones then becomes one of the most interesting problems in science and a new branch of

---

[1]Neuroscience Wing, Department of Educational and Social Policy, University of Macedonia, Thessaloniki, Greece

Address correspondence to Lazaros C. Triarhou, Neuroscience Wing, Department of Educational and Social Policy, University of Macedonia, 156 Egnatia Avenue, Building Z-312, Thessaloniki 54006, Greece; e-mail: triarhou@uom.gr

science itself, whereby the experience and methods of one speciality are applied to the other and entirely new points of view are reached that lead to fruitful work in both fields."

—Constantin von Economo (1876-1931)

Substantial progress in neuroeducation has taken place in the past dozen years, since Battro and Cardinali (1996) introduced the term. Diverse disciplines that investigate human learning and development have become integrated, bringing together education, biology, and cognitive science (Fischer et al., 2007). Additional terms used by authors in conjunction with this new branch of knowledge include "neurolearning" (cf. Petitto & Dunbar, 2004), "nurturing the brain" (Ito, 2004), "developing the brain" (Koizumi, 2004), "educational neuroscience" (Petitto & Dunbar, 2004), and "pedagogical neuroscience" (Fawcett & Nicolson, 2007).

In considering the fervent growth of the discipline, we note that the tradition of the attempt to bridge neuroscience with the humanities goes back more than a century. Henry Herbert Donaldson (1857-1938) and Reuben Post Halleck (1859-1936) are pioneers in that respect, perhaps belonging among the first scientists who tried, around the turn of the nineteenth century, to meet halfway between this "bridge too far" (Bruer, 1997). In 1895, Donaldson published *The Growth of the Brain* after thorough investigation. Within a year, Halleck (1896) followed suit with *The Education of the Central Nervous System*. Halleck (1895) had previously published a textbook of psychology entitled *Psychology and Psychic Culture*, which seems to be a prelude to his 1896 book, aimed at "giving the truths of psychology in an intelligible way to pupils under 20." In their studies, the two authors[1] emphasize major issues currently at the epicenter of neuroeducation. Their approaches bear the stamp of their times.

The present study examines select points from those works, including aspects of plasticity of the human brain and its implications for education, the "nature versus nurture" debate, the best teaching and learning strategies as they arise from brain research, and the role of nutrition, fatigue and sleep in learning outcomes. The bearing of the authors' differing backgrounds on their "neuroeducational" views are also discussed in the context of the challenges and difficulties one encounters in interdisciplinary integration.

HENRY HERBERT DONALDSON, PH.D., D.SC. H.C.

Donaldson (Figure 1) studied at Yale (B.A., 1879) and Johns Hopkins University (Ph.D. in biology, 1885) (Conklin, 1938; McMurrich & Jackson, 1938). His thesis was carried out under the supervision of G. Stanley Hall on the mapping of cutaneous temperature-sensitive areas (Norrsell, Finger, & Lajonchere, 1999). Donaldson was later awarded D.Sc. degrees *honoris causa* from Yale (1906) and Clark University (1937).

From early 1886 through the fall of 1887, Donaldson was trained in Europe under Forel in Zürich, von Gudden in Munich,[2] Meynert in Vienna, and Golgi in Pavia. Subsequently, Donaldson was appointed an associate in psychology at Hopkins (1887–1889), assistant professor of neurology at Clark (1889–1892),[3] professor of neurology at University of Chicago (1892–1906), where he also served as Dean (1892–1898), and finally, professor of neurology and director of research at the Wistar Institute of Anatomy and Biology in Philadelphia (1906–1938).

In 1889 Hall entrusted to Donaldson the brain of Laura D. Bridgman.[4] Bridgman was a woman who "had lost sight, hearing and to a great extent the senses of smell and taste from an attack of scarlet fever at the age of 26 months" (Hall, 1879). She died when she was 60 years old. Donaldson carried out some of the thoroughest quantitative studies of a single human brain until that time (Donaldson, 1890, 1891, 1892; McMurrich & Jackson, 1938); he pinpointed peculiarities in her brain, but was careful not to "phrenologize" the specimen (Burrell, 2004). Donaldson commissioned a plaster cast from a local artist, which is still kept in a display case at Perkins Institute (Burrell, 2004).

The special interest in Bridgman's brain was largely based on her unique achievements, considering her disabilities. She had been taught to speak, reaching a marked mental ability (Conklin, 1938) under the guidance of S. Gridley Howe. She was the first deaf-blind child to learn language (Freeberg, 2001) thanks to Howe's innovative educational practices.[5] His work was considered "so ingenious and successful" that it was described as "one of the greatest triumphs of pedagogic skills" (Hall, 1879).[6]

The results of Donaldson's studies, along with an exhaustive review of the available knowledge on the growth of the central nervous system until then, culminated in *The growth of the brain* (Donaldson, 1895), which went through several reprint editions.

The status of Donaldson as one of the most distinguished neuroscientists at the dawn of the 20th century is evidenced from his inclusion among 50 high-ranking scholars, the calibre of Obersteiner and von Lenhossék (Austro-Hungarian Empire), van Gehuchten (Belgium), Elliot Smith (Egypt), Déjerine and Raymond (France), Edinger, Flechsig, His and Weigert (Germany), Golgi and Mingazzini

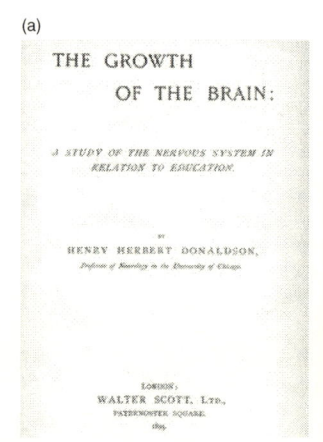

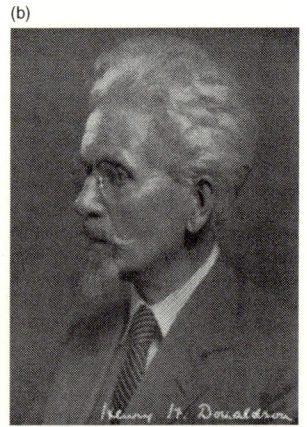

Fig. 1. Henry Herbert Donaldson (born May 12, 1857, Yonkers, NY; died January 23, 1938, Philadelphia, PA) and the frontispiece of his 1895 book *The growth of the brain*. Portrait © 1938 by the National Academy of Sciences of the United States of America; reproduced with permission from Conklin (1938).

(Italy), Ariëns Kappers (Netherlands), Bekhterev (Russia), Ramón y Cajal (Spain), Retzius (Sweden), von Monakow (Switzerland), Sherington (UK), and others, that made up the Brain Commission, the first international neuroscience organization, founded in 1903 in London (Richter, 2000). Berlin neuroanatomist Waldeyer—who in 1891 introduced the term *neuron* and "popularized" the neuron doctrine—served as its second president (Waldeyer, 1908a, b), from 1904 until the Commission's end of existence in 1914 at the outbreak of World War I.[7] Donaldson represented the only American Institute among 15 participating countries, and attended the Brain Commission's meetings in Vienna (1906) and Bologna (1909) (McMurrich & Jackson, 1938).

Donaldson was elected a member of the American Philosophical Society (1906) and the National Academy of Sciences (1914); he became President of the American Association of Anatomists (1916–1918) and American Neurological Association (1937), and was a member (1888–1938) and trustee (1912–1929) of the Marine Biological Laboratory in Woods Whole, MA (Conklin, 1938).

Donaldson studied cortical neuron number and weight and gray-white matter relationships (Donaldson, 1899), and developed methods of tissue processing (Donaldson, 1894). One of his most important contributions was establishing the Wistar albino rat as a standardized pure bred stock. Donaldson considered the 1:30 lifespan ratio between rat and human as reflecting a 30 times faster pace of growth of a nervous system with otherwise similar characteristics (Conklin, 1938; Donaldson, 1911; McMurrich & Jackson, 1938).

An ardent admirer of literature, music, and the arts, Donaldson was deeply concerned about social problems and welfare. His colleagues praised him as an investigator, leader, and counselor (Editorial, 1938). Following his will, his brain is part of the Wistar Institute's brain collection. During the last 40 years of his life, he published about 100 papers and monographs in developmental and comparative neuroanatomy without skipping a single year; his students and collaborators published an estimated 360 further works, in which he does not appear as a co-author (Conklin, 1938).

REUBEN POST HALLECK, M.A., LL.D. *H.C.*

The son of the Rev. Luther Calvin Halleck and Fannie Tuthill, a schoolteacher, Halleck (Figure 2) studied English at Yale (B.A., 1881; M.A., 1896). He was appointed principal of the Cherry Valley Academy, New York (1881), and subsequently instructor ("professor") in psychology, English literature and history at Louisville Male High School, Kentucky (1883), where he was promoted to vice president (1896) and principal (1897).

The Male High School was an unusual institution granted "all the rights and privileges of a university" (Smith & Phillips, 1996). Through 1913, students received a B.A. upon graduation (Kleber, Kinsman, Clark, Crews, & Yater, 2001).

In 1904 he was elected president of the Department of Secondary Education of the National Educational Association (Cattell, 1932; Kleber et al., 2001; Urofsky & Levy, 1972) and member of the council of the Southern Society for Philosophy and Psychology (Buchner, 1905). In 1907 Halleck became chairman of the National Educational Association Committee of Seventeen to discuss educational reforms (Kleber et al.,

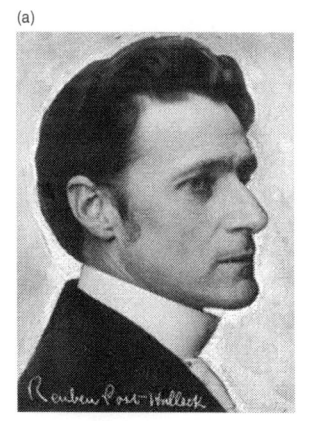

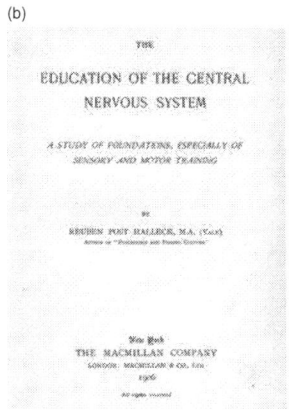

Fig. 2. Reuben Post Halleck (born February 8, 1859, Long Island, NY; died December 24, 1936, Louisville, KY) and the frontispiece of his 1896 book *The education of the central nervous system* (1906 reprint edition). Portrait credit: Courier-Journal Photograph of Professor "Rube" Halleck, famous Louisville Educator, Principal of Old Male High; courtesy of Filson Historical Society, Louisville, KY. Signature digitally etched onto photo from Halleck's 1930 book *Makers of our nation* with hand-inscribed dedication (private collection).

2001) and served as a Trustee of the American Printing House for the Blind (1918–1932) and President of the Society for the Study of Education (1906–1908) (Cattell, 1932).

Hallecks' works centered on educational psychology and pedagogical applications of physiological psychology (Cattell, 1932). He also wrote books on the history of the English and American literature, and patriotic studies (Smith & Phillips, 1996). His books include *Psychology and Psychic Culture* (1895), *History of English Literature* (1900), *History of American literature* (1911), *Halleck's New English Literature* (1913), *History of Our Country* (1923), *Our Nation's Heritage* (1925, with Juliette Frantz), *Founders of Our Nation* (1929), *Makers of Our Nation* (1930, with Frantz), *Our United States* (1935), and *The Story of English Literature* (1937).

Halleck retired in 1910 (Kleber et al., 2001) or 1912 (Cattell, 1932). For his services to education, the University of Kentucky granted him a LL.D. *honoris causa* (1912). He bequeathed part of his estate to educational institutions.

NEUROEDUCATIONAL IDEAS OF DONALDSON AND HALLECK

Both authors discuss factors related to environment (school, nutrition) and inner biological properties (gender, brain plasticity, and critical periods), that influence neurocognitive processes.

According to Donaldson (1895, pp. 5–6), *The Growth of the Brain* targets parents, teachers, and physicians. His book covers developmental and evolutionary aspects, on the basis of the importance of understanding growth changes as a fundamental factor for the welfare of all higher animals.

In discussing the factors that influence the growth of the nervous system and therefore learning, Donaldson (1895, pp. 342–344) considers formal education as "rather insignificant," insofar as it cannot overrun the limitations to cognitive development set by nature. Nevertheless, he claims that education can strengthen formed structures and awaken dormant abilities, and further supports the "modification" of education based on gender, due to physiologic sex differences.

Donaldson (1895) underscores the effect of biological factors—such as the inhibitory action of hunger and fatigue—on learning, implying that chronobiologic principles and dietary habits may affect performance. He attributes a special role to the timing of early experiences, arguing that the outcome of early deprivation of proper stimuli is irreversible, and tackles normative issues in his quest to provide a rational basis of pedagogic problems.

On the other hand, *The Education of the Central Nervous System* (Halleck, 1896) is an attempt to simplify complex neuropsychologic knowledge to provide teachers and parents with facts that would ensure a better nurture for their children. Halleck (1896) places special emphasis on early childhood and its importance in mental development. He argues that nutritive rhythms and periods of activity and rest should be taken into account in the educational process, since they directly affect cognitive abilities such as memory. He classifies memory in two ways: one based on particular modalities and their lobe localization (e.g. hearing and the temporal lobe), and a second differentiating conscious from unconscious memory.

Halleck acknowledges the power of the environment and its influence on the actualization of potential capacities, and addresses methodological issues such as (a) enriched environments as most helpful in the growing process, (b) the paramount role of imitation in cognitive, moral, and language development, and (c) sensory imagery as a means of brain modification.

Table 1 shows some examples of neuroeducational issues raised by Donaldson (1895) and Halleck (1896), juxtaposed to relevant ideas from the modern literature.

DISCUSSION

Some of the earliest attempts to couple neuroscience with education are recorded in the works of Forster (1815), Clarke (1874a, b), Crichton-Browne (1884), Halleck (1895), and Berry (1921). In particular, Clarke's *Sex in Education* (1874a) triggered one of "the most notorious controversies in the history of women's education" (Zschoche, 1989). Hall (1905) described it as a "holy war." Clarke argued that women have equal rights to men in education, but at the same time biologic constraints hamper intellectual performance, as maternity drains their energy (Clarke, 1874b). Clarke's arguments, deducted from biology, remind Social Darwinism, which became popular decades later. His ideas opposed feminists (Brubacher & Rudy, 1997) and especially Julia Ward Howe (1874), a social activist. The question whether gender differences have implications for education occupied Halleck (1906) as well. Donaldson and Halleck held that gender should be considered in educational practice. The adoption of single-sex schools has made a comeback, with support from neurobiological data (Sax, 2005).

It appears that the two authors tried to direct the attention to some of the most influential factors—as modern research indicates—at the interface of brain science and education. In his preface, Halleck (1896) characterizes the work of Donaldson (1895) as excellent but fatalistic. Period articles linked the two works (Wilder, 1897). Critics cordially recommended *The Growth of the Brain* for its "great pedagogical and psychological interest" (Trotter, 1896) despite the book's advanced level that conceivably rendered it more difficult for lay persons.

Table 1
Certain Issues Discussed by Donaldson (1895) and Halleck (1896), in Comparison with Pertaining Concepts from the Modern Neuroscience Literature

	Donaldson (1895)	Halleck (1896)	Current ideas
I. Environmental factors			
Formal education	"Education must fail to produce any fundamental changes in the nervous organisation" (p. 343). "No amount of education will cause enlargement or organisation where the rough materials, the cells, are wanting; and on the other hand, where these materials are present, they will, in some degree, become evident, whether purposely educated or not" (p. 355). "Education forms a more favorable environment [for the next generation]" (p. 361).	"We certainly have sound reasons for believing that we can by the proper training make our nervous systems more helpful machines" (p. 42).	"Education is a process of optimal adaptation such that learning is guided to ensure proper brain development and functionality" (Koizumi, 2004). "... extraordinary importance of environmental influences and education on the development of the functional architecture of the brain" (Singer, 2003). "Education plays a key role in cultural transformations: it allows members of a society, the young in particular, to efficiently acquire an ever-evolving body of knowledge and skills that took thousands of years to invent" (Fischer et al., 2007).
II. Innate factors			
Nature	"Nurture is of much less importance than nature" (p. 344).	"What make a genius are not the number of brain cells but the establishment of connections between them" (p. 59).	"... the nature-nurture controversy has not been put to rest, at least when it comes to education... genetic or heritable influences do not determine specific phenotypic outcomes; in the overwhelming majority of cases, they predispose for a number of phenotypes, each of which might or might not manifest in particular environments ..." (Grigorenko, 2007).
Gender differences	"In reactions ... the female [brain] has a more local responsiveness than the male, and back of all this is the matter of general physiology, which has its distinct modifications according to sex ... In women natural education is completed only with maternity, which we know to effect some slight changes in the sympathetic system and possibly the spinal cord ... Basing the inference on the size of the structural elements, we should infer that the typical central system in the female would be somewhat more easily fatigued, and also be slightly less complete in organisation" (p. 352).		"Sex differences in brain anatomy may explain some documented differences in behavior ... Sex difference in the percentage and asymmetry of the principal cranial tissue volumes may contribute to differences in cognitive functioning" (Gur et al., 1999).

Table 1
(Continued)

	Donaldson (1895)	Halleck (1896)	Current ideas
			"Logically, it would seem that given the different processing styles and strategies that members of each sex bring to the acquisition process and subsequent performance on a given cognitive task, educational interventions might be designed to capitalized on each of their predisposed styles of learning, ones that would in theory complement the brain activation patterns that characterize the prototypical male and female functional organization" (O'Boyle & Gill, 1998).
Diurnal rhythms	"In general there is a tendency to run down towards the middle of the afternoon, with a return of vigour later in the day ... After recuperative sleep ... there are general sensations of vigour and well-being" (p. 322).	"At certain times of the day both nervous and muscular energy are naturally at their maximum" (p. 64).	"... the impact of sleep/awake cycles in learning and health, a discipline we call *chronoeducation*" (Battro, 2005).
		"After a period of very fatiguing mental work, youthful brain cells will rise from a night's sound sleep with all the freshness of a spring morning" (p. 98). "Nutritive rhythms associated with the periods of activity and rest are established, with the result of economizing the bodily energy, and rendering its expenditure more effective" (p. 344).	"The concepts of time and timing—deeply controlled by the brain—need to be incorporated into any general view of educational processes" (Golombek & Cardinali, 2008).
Plasticity and critical periods	"The intensity with which any form of exercise is carried on during the growing period leaves its trace, and the absence of it at the proper time is for the most part irremediable. We should hardly expect much appreciation of colour in a person brought up in the dark, however good his natural endowments in this direction. Thus any lack of early experience may leave a spot permanently undeveloped in the central system a condition of much significance, for each locality in the cerebrum is not only a place at which reactions, using the word in a narrow sense, may occur, but by way of it pass fibres having more distant connections, and its lack of development probably reduces the associative value of these also" (p. 348).	"If the requisite means for training and developing the nervous system are not forthcoming early in life, even the possible genius may never develop a fraction of his earlier possibilities" (p. x).	"... in the cat, within the critical period between the fourth and eighth weeks, a deprivation as brief as a few days can have marked effects. This implies that for normal development normal environmental conditions must prevail throughout the critical period and not just during some small part of it" (Hubel & Wiesel, 1970).

Table 1
(Continued)

Donaldson (1895)	Halleck (1896)	Current ideas
	"Roughly speaking, the plasticity of nerve cells is inversely proportional to their age ... It is highly probable that such exercise tends to prolong the period of nerve plasticity ... Youthful human cells speedily repair many minor injuries from bruises, cuts, and burns..." (pp. 95–98).	"The onset of speech after left hemispherectomy in a nine-year-old boy ... appears to challenge the widely held view that early childhood is a particularly critical period for acquisition of speech and language ..." (Vargha-Khadem et al., 1997).
III. Contribution of the neurosciences to education		
"The aim at the moment, therefore, is to determine what limitations anatomy places to the educational process, and thus to obtain a rational basis from which to attack many of the pedagogical problems" (p. 342).		"Neuroscience data can be used to generate novel educational theories" (Byrnes & Fox, 1998).
		"... educators' perspectives include encouraging results regarding the levels of enthusiasm for the role of the brain in education ... those involved in bringing neuroscience and education together still have some work to do in establishing and communicating ideas and initiatives that can both become popular with teachers and meet scientific criteria for their basis" (Pickering & Howard-Jones, 2007).

Halleck (1896), on the other hand, was criticized for lack of original research; critics commented that the book should not be taken as serious scientific work (Editorial, 1897). The book was tagged incomplete, owing to the inadequate treatment of brain structure and function and the disproportional discussion of sensation and memory, while leaving out ideas such as the neuron theory (Editorial, 1896; Herrick, 1897). He was further criticized for lack of correct scientific thinking, and for making deductions based on inadequate data (Editorial, 1896). Thus, one of the most serious shortcomings of Halleck (1896) seems to parallel a common fault in modern neuroeducation: the over-literal interpretation of brain facts, risking a misapplication of neurobiology to education (Goswami, 2006).

In *The Education of the Central Nervous System* (Halleck, 1896), one may discern some of the currently held views and practices at the interface of neurology, psychology, and education. For example, the discovery of the "mirror neuron system" (Rizzolatti, 1996) and its functional implications reiterates the value of imitation in learning (Vogt et al., 2007). More than a century ago, Halleck stressed the primal role of impulsive imitation in human language acquisition, a point that can be viewed as a harbinger of modern linguistic theorizing (Chomsky, 1975; Pinker, 1994). Such a link is further supported by neuroimaging studies that suggest the involvement of Broca's area in both language and imitation functions (Kühn & Brass, 2008).

Halleck's emphasis on an environment enriched in sensory "material" is in line with experimental neurobiologic studies (cf. Cobayashi, Ohasi, & Ando, 2002), although caution should be exercised in jumping from animal research to human educational applications.

On the contrary, Donaldson (1895) is cautious, avoiding suggestions on educational practice(s). His is a primarily neurologic contribution, without immediate guidelines for those interested in the role of the brain in education. A substantial part of the work gives detailed information on the weight increase of the body, brain and spinal cord, comparative neuroanatomic points, and cytoarchitectonic and physiologic elements. Nevertheless, Donaldson can be credited as a pioneer of the interdisciplinary field of neuroeducation, having explicitly described its aims.

What adds special value to the works of Donaldson (1895) and Halleck (1896) is their clear focus on the relationship between brain and education, at a time when the latter field was chiefly dominated by psychologic theories. They both emphasized the influence of nutritive and diurnal rhythms and habits on intellectual work, arguments supported by current research, as dietary habits appear to directly affect cognitive performance (Bellisle, 2004; Spencer, 2008); the function of sleep is particularly addressed by the emerging field of chronoeducation (Cardinali, 2008).

Learning and memory occupied their thought as well. The types of organic memory described by Halleck are not foreign to the modern concepts of implicit and explicit memory (Schacter, 1987) or to modality-specific memory models (Baddeley, 1997).

A strong point in those works is the plasticity of the nervous system in conjunction with the concept of critical periods. Donaldson emphasizes the crucial role of early experience through an example (Table 1) that might be viewed as heralding the classic experiments of Hubel and Wiesel (1970) on the visual system.

In Halleck (1896), one encounters early uses of the terms "critical" and "plastic,"[8] pertaining to the modern concepts of the sensitive periods and the ability of the nervous system to improve itself through training. Halleck goes as far as mentioning the effects of timing on pronunciation in late second-language learners, a central argument in behavioral plasticity (Mayberry & Lock, 2003; Yeni-Komshian, Flege, & Liu, 2000).

Donaldson and Halleck share a common criterion about which brain facts may inform education; on the other hand, their views diverge with regard to the nature versus nurture debate. Differences between the neurologist and the educator become evident even in their writing style—Donaldson's balancing more on the punctilious, while Halleck's on the assimilable. Their (complementary) ideas could form—in conjunction—a rounded framework for planning educational interventions. Furthermore, in their theoretical constructs, the two pioneers of neuroeducation formulated concepts that, with the advent of technical innovations such as fMRI, would eventually be subjected to the verdict of the experimental test. Even the points of disagreement between the two authors touch upon long-debated issues.

Problems of communication can occur at the interface or borders of traditionally defined sciences, due to their differing and sometimes contradictory starting points and methods. Along that line, certain authors have discussed difficulties, inherent in any attempt of synthesis (Blake & Gardner, 2007; Fischer et al., 2007; Goswami, 2006). Accordingly, Goswami (2006) suggests a new dual role in interdisciplinarity through first, "interpreting neuroscience from the perspective of and in the language of educators" and second, through "feeding back research questions and ideas from educators to neuroscientists."

The two historic works that form the core of the present article witness the "basic human desire to improve our brains and minds" (Blakemore & Frith, 2005); now spanning over three centuries, they pinpoint the early development of ideas in the relation between education and neuroscience.

Acknowledgements—We thank Professor Manuel del Cerro of the University of Rochester, NY, for his generosity in presenting his personal copy of Donaldson's *The Growth of the Brain* to one of us (L.C.T.); Robin L. Wallace of Special Collections, Photographs and Prints at Filson Historical Society, Louisville, KY, for kindly providing the portrait of R. P. Halleck; and the anonymous reviewers for their constructive criticism that has led to an improved manuscript. Part of this work was presented at the 13th Annual Meeting of the International Society for the History of the Neurosciences, Berlin, Germany, June 18–22, 2008.

NOTES

1 They both were Yale graduates who must have overlapped in 1877–1879, Halleck as freshman/sophomore and Donaldson as junior/senior.
2 The respected neuroanatomist–psychiatrist and personal physician to King Ludwig II of Bavaria; the two men were found dead in the evening of June 13, 1886 in Lake Starnberg, mysteriously drowned or possibly murdered.
3 Solicited by his former mentor G. Stanley Hall, at the time president of the newly founded institution in Worcester, MA.
4 Following Hall's death, Donaldson also studied the brain of his mentor (Donaldson & Canavan, 1928).
5 In this sense Bridgman was Helen Keller's predecessor. The latter's education was based on Bridgman's example. Bridgman's fame was such at her times that even Charles Dickens (1842) visited her at the Perkins Institute for the Blind in Boston, where she used to live, and later wrote about her in his *American Notes*.
6 The instructional model provided by Laura Bridgman—the "greatest achievement in education yet made" in the words of Mary Tyler Peabody Mann (Mann, Sarmiento, & Velleman, 2005, pp. 130–132)—also inspired Domingo F. Sarmiento (1811–1888), the outstanding educator and President of Argentina (Ingenieros, 1928), to elaborate more "scientific" tools for special education in South America. Mary Mann, wife of the great American educator Horace Mann, had a long friendship with Sarmiento. In one of her many letters, she commented on the famous Seventh Annual Report of the Board of Education (1844) regarding the instruction of the "deaf-mutes" that inspired Sarmiento, then in England, to visit H. Mann in Boston. In a letter dated March 13, 1867, M. Mann told Sarmiento about the incredible feats of Bridgman (Mann et al., 2005). Sarmiento clearly recognized the impact of scientific research in education in his many interventions in public schools.
7 The two successive key events that reunited the world neuroscience community after the two world wars were the First International Neurological Congress of 1931 in Berne (Brouwer et al., 1932), and the founding in 1961 of the International Brain Research Organization (Richter, 2000).
8 William James (1891, p. 105) had already defined plasticity as "the possession of a structure weak enough to yield to an influence, but strong enough not to yield all at once"; in the neurobiology domain, Ramón y Cajal credits J. Minea, a pupil of the Romanian neurologist Georghe Marinescu, for defining plasticity in his 1909 doctoral thesis as representing "the totality of the metamorphic phenomena of the sensory neurone, provoked by the compression and transplantation of ganglia" (DeFelipe & Jones, 1991, p. 430).

REFERENCES

Baddeley, A. (1997). *Human memory: Theory and practice*. Exeter, UK: Psychology Press.
Battro, A. (2005). *New concepts in neuroeducation*. International School of Science Teaching—European Summer School for Primary Science Trainers. Retrieved June 28, 2008, from http://scienceduc.cienciaviva.pt/teachertraining/plenaries/S4_A_Battro.pdf
Battro, A. M., & Cardinali, D. P. (1996). Más cerebro en la educación [More brain in education] [Electronic version]. La Nación. Retrieved June 9, 2008 from http://www.byd.com.ar/cereln.pdf
Bellisle, F. (2004). Effects of diet on behaviour and cognition in children. *British Journal of Nutrition*, 92, S227–S232.
Berry, R. J. A. (1921). *Modern psychology*. Melbourne, Australia: Robertson & Mullens.
Blake, P. R., & Gardner, H. (2007). A first course in mind, brain, and education. *Mind, Brain, and Education*, 1, 61–65.
Blakemore, S. J., & Frith, U. (2005). The learning brain: Lessons for education: A précis. *Developmental Science*, 8, 459–471.
Brouwer, B., Sachs, B., Riley, H. A., Dubois, C., Fischer, R. F. von, & Schnyder, P. (Eds.). (1932). *Proceedings of the First International Neurological Congress*. Berne, Switzerland: Stämpfli & Cie.
Brubacher, J. S., & Rudy, W. (1997). *Higher education in transition: A history of American colleges and universities* (4th ed.). New Brunswick, NJ: Transaction Publishers.
Bruer, J. T. (1997). Education and the brain: A bridge too far. *Educational Researcher*, 26, 4–16.
Buchner, E. F. (1905). Proceedings of the first annual meeting of the Southern Society for Philosophy and Psychology, Baltimore, MD., and Philadelphia, PA., December 27 and 28, 1904. *Psychological Bulletin*, 2, 72–80.
Burrell, B. (2004). *Postcards from the brain museum: The impossible search for meaning in the matter of famous minds*. New York: Broadway Books.
Byrnes, J. P., & Fox, N. A. (1998). The educational relevance of research in cognitive neuroscience. *Educational Psychology Review*, 10, 297–342.
Cardinali, D. P. (2008). Chronoeducation: How the biological clock influences the learning process. In A. M. Battro, K. W. Fischer, & P. J. Léna (Eds.), *The educated brain: Essays in neuroeducation* (pp. 110–126). New York: Cambridge University Press.
Cattell, J. M. (1932). Halleck, Prof. Reuben Post. In *Leaders in education: A biographical directory* (1st ed.; pp. 390–391). New York and Lancaster, PA: The Science Press Printing.

Chomsky, N. (1975). *Reflections on language.* New York: Pantheon Books.
Clarke, E. D. (1874a). *Sex in education; or, a fair chance for girls.* Boston: James R. Osgood.
Clarke, E. D. (1874b). *The building of a brain.* Boston: James R. Osgood.
Cobayashi, S., Ohasi, Y., & Ando, S. (2002). Effects of enriched environments with different durations and starting times on learning capacity during aging in rats assessed by a refined procedure of the Hebb-Williams maze task. *Journal of Neuroscience Research, 70,* 340–346.
Conklin, E. G. (1938). Biographical memoir of Henry Herbert Donaldson, 1857-1938. *Biographical Memoirs of the National Academy of Sciences of the United States of America, 20,* 227–243.
Crichton-Browne, J. (1884). Education and the nervous system. In M. Morris (Ed.), *The book of health* (pp. 269–380). London–Paris–New York: Cassell.
DeFelipe, J., & Jones, E. G. (1991). *Cajal's degeneration and regeneration of the nervous system.* New York: Oxford University Press.
Dickens, C. (1842). *American notes for general circulation* (Vol. 1). London: Chapman & Hall.
Donaldson, H. H. (1890). Anatomical observations on the brain and several sense-organs of the blind deaf-mute, Laura Dewey Bridgman. I. *American Journal of Psychology, 3,* 293–342.
Donaldson, H. H. (1891). Anatomical observations on the brain and several sense-organs of the blind deaf-mute, Laura Dewey Bridgman. II. *American Journal of Psychology, 4,* 248–294.
Donaldson, H. H. (1892). The extent of the visual area of the cortex in man, as deduced from the study of Laura Bridgman's brain. *American Journal of Psychology, 4,* 503–513.
Donaldson, H. H. (1894). Preliminary observations on some changes caused in the nervous tissues by reagents, commonly employed to harden them. *Journal of Morphology, 9,* 123–166.
Donaldson, H. H. (1895). *The growth of the brain: A study of the nervous system in relation to education. The Contemporary Science Series.* Havelock Ellis (Ed.). London: Walter Scott. [Book available for download at: http://www.archive.org/details/growthofbrainstu00donauoft].
Donaldson, H. H. (1899). A note on the significance of the small volume of the nerve cell bodies in the cerebral cortex in man. *Journal of Comparative Neurology, 9,* 141–149.
Donaldson, H. H. (1911). On the influence of exercise on the weight of the central nervous system of the albino rat. *Journal of Comparative Neurology, 21,* 129–137.
Donaldson, H. H., & Canavan, M. M. (1928). A study of the brains of three scholars: Granville Stanley Hall, Sir William Osler, Edward Sylvester Morse. *Journal of Comparative Neurology, 46,* 1–95.
Editorial. (1896). The education of the central nervous system by R. P. Halleck [book review by H. C. W.]. *American Naturalist, 30,* 1032–1033.
Editorial. (1897). The education of the central nervous system: A study of foundations, especially of sensory and motor training by Reuben Post Halleck [book review]. *American Anthropologist, 10,* 121.
Editorial. (1938). Henry Herbert Donaldson. *Journal of Comparative Neurology, 68,* 4.
Fawcett, A. J., & Nicolson, R. I. (2007). Dyslexia, learning, and pedagogical neuroscience. *Developmental Medicine and Child Neurology, 49,* 306–311.
Fischer, K. W., Daniel, D. B., Immordino-Yang, M. H., Stern, E., Battro, A., & Koizumi, H. (2007). Why mind, brain, and education? Why now? *Mind, Brain, and Education, 1,* 1–2.

Forster, T. I. M. (1815). *Essay on the application of the organology of the brain to education.* London: The Pamphleteer.
Freeberg, E. (2001). The education of Laura Bridgman and the epistemological debates of the 19th century. *American Educator, 25,* 36–47.
Golombek, D. A., & Cardinali, D. P. (2008). Mind, brain, education, and biological timing. *Mind, Brain, and Education, 2,* 1–6.
Goswami, U. (2006). Neuroscience and education: From research to practice? *Nature Reviews Neuroscience, 7,* 406–411.
Grigorenko, E. L. (2007). How can genomics inform education? *Mind, Brain, and Education, 1,* 20–27.
Gur, R. C., Turetsky, B. I., Matsui, M., Yan, M., Bilker, W., & Hughett, P. (1999). Sex differences in brain gray and white matter in healthy young adults: Correlations with cognitive performance. *Journal of Neuroscience, 19,* 4065–4072.
Hall, G. S. (1879). Laura Bridgman. *Mind—A Quarterly Review of Psychology and Philosophy, 14,* 149–172.
Hall, G. S. (1905). *Adolescence: Its psychology and its relations to physiology, anthropology, sociology, sex, crime, religion, and education* (Vol. 2). New York: Appleton and Co., pp. 561–647.
Halleck, R. P. (1895). *Psychology and psychic culture.* New York–Cincinnati–Chicago: American Book Company.
Halleck, R. P. (1896). *The education of the central nervous system: A study of foundations, especially of sensory and motor training.* New York: Macmillan. [Book available for download at: http://www.archive.org/details/educationofcentr00halluoft].
Halleck, R. B. (1906). What kind of education is best suited in boys? *The School Review, 14,* 512–521.
Herrick, C. J. (1897). Halleck's education of the central nervous system (Literary Notices). *Journal of Comparative Neurology, 7,* 4–5.
Hubel, D. H., & Wiesel T. N. (1970). The period of susceptibility to the physiological effects of unilateral eye closure in kittens. *Journal of Physiology, 206,* 419–436.
Ingenieros, J. (1928). *Sarmiento, Alberdi y Echeverría: Los iniciadores de la Sociología Argentina* [Sarmiento, Alberdi and Echeverría: The founders of Argentinian sociology]. Buenos Aires: Editorial Pablo Ingegnieros.
Ito, M. (2004). 'Nurturing the brain' as an emerging research field involving child neurology. *Brain and Development, 26,* 429–433.
James, W. (1891). *The principles of psychology.* London: Macmillan.
Kleber, J. E., Kinsman, M. J., Clark, T. D., Crews, C. F., & Yater, G. H. (2001). Halleck, Reuben Post. In *The encyclopedia of Louisville* (pp. 366–367). Lexington, KY: University Press of Kentucky.
Koizumi, H. (2004). The concept of 'developing the brain': A new natural science for learning and education. *Brain and Development, 26,* 434–441.
Kühn, S., & Brass, M. (2008). Testing the connection of the mirror system and speech: How articulation affects imitation in a simple response task. *Neuropsychologia, 46,* 1513–1521.
Mann, M. T. P., Sarmiento, D. F., & Velleman, B. L. (2005). *"Mi estimado señor": Cartas de Mary Mann a Sarmiento (1865–1881)* ["My dear Sir": Letters of Mary Mann to Sarmiento (1865–1881)]. Buenos Aires, Argentina: Instituto Cultural Argentino Norteamericano (ICANA).
Mayberry, R. I., & Lock, E. (2003). Age constraints on first versus second language acquisition: Evidence for linguistic plasticity and epigenesis. *Brain and Language, 87,* 369–384.
McMurrich, J. P., & Jackson, C. M. (1938). Henry Herbert Donaldson, 1857-1938. *Journal of Comparative Neurology, 69,* 173–179.

Norrsell, U., Finger, S., & Lajonchere, C. (1999). Cutaneous sensory spots and the "law of specific nerve energies": History and development of ideas. *Brain Research Bulletin, 48*, 457–465.

O'Boyle, M. W., & Gill, H. S. (1998). On the relevance of research findings in cognitive neuroscience to educational practice. *Educational Psychology Review, 10*, 397–409.

Petitto, L. A., & Dunbar, K. (2004, October). New findings from educational neuroscience on bilingual brains, scientific brains, and the educated mind. Paper presented at conference on 'Building Usable Knowledge in Mind, Brain, and Education.' Cambridge, MA: Harvard Graduate School of Education.

Pickering, S. J., & Howard-Jones, P. (2007). Educators' views on the role of neuroscience in education: Findings from a study of U.K. and international perspectives. *Mind, Brain, and Education, 1*, 109–113.

Pinker, S. (1994). *The language instinct: How the mind creates language*. New York: Harper Collins.

Richter, J. (2000). The Brain Commission of the International Association of Academies: The first international society of neurosciences. *Brain Research Bulletin, 52*, 445–457.

Rizzolatti, G. (1996). Premotor cortex and the recognition of motor actions. *Cognitive Brain Research, 3*, 131–141.

Sax, L. (2005). *Why gender matters? What parents and teachers need to know about the emerging science of sex differences*. New York: Doubleday.

Schacter, D. L. (1987). Implicit memory: History and current status. *Journal of Experimental Psychology: Learning, Memory, and Cognition, 13*, 501–518.

Singer, W. J. (2003, November). *Brain development and education* [Electronic version]. Paper presented at 'Working Group on Mind, Brain, and Education.' Vatican City: Pontifical Academy of Sciences. Retrieved June 28, 2008 from http://www.vatican.va/roman_curia/pontifical_academies/acdscien/400_ann/cartella_a4_3nov_qxd.pdf

Smith, A. J., & Phillips, C. (1996). Reuben Post Halleck. In *The critical heritage* (Vol. 2; p. 186). London: Routledge.

Spencer, J. P. (2008). Food for thought: The role of dietary flavonoids in enhancing human memory, learning and neuro-cognitive performance. *Proceedings of the Nutrition Society, 67*, 238–252.

Trotter, W. F. (1896). The growth of the brain: A study of the nervous system in relation to education [book review]. *Mind: New Series, 5*, 421–422.

Urofsky, M. I., & Levy, D. W. (1972). *Letters of Louis D. Brandeis (Vol. 2) (1907–1912): People's attorney* (p. 176). Albany, NY: State University of New York Press.

Vargha-Khadem, F., Carr, L. J., Isaacs, E., Brett, E., Adams, C., & Mishkin, M. (1997). Onset of speech after left hemispherectomy in a nine-year-old boy. *Brain, 120*, 159–182.

Vogt, S., Buccino, G., Wohlschläger, A. M., Canessa, N., Shah, N. J., Zilles, K., et al. (2007). Prefrontal involvement in imitation learning of hand actions: Effects of practice and expertise. *NeuroImage, 37*, 1371–1383.

Waldeyer, W. (1908a). Document I of the report of the President of the Brain Commission [translated from the German by H. H. Donaldson]. *Journal of Comparative Neurology and Psychology, 18*, 87–90.

Waldeyer, W. (1908b). Report on the present status of the Academic Institutes for Brain Study, together with a report of the meetings of the Executive Committee of the Brain Commission, held at Berlin, March 14, 1908 [translated from the German by H. H. Donaldson]. *Anatomical Record, 2*, 428–431.

Ward Howe, J. (Ed.). (1874). *Sex and education: A reply to Dr. E. H. Clarke's 'Sex in education.'* Boston: Roberts Brothers.

Wilder, B. G. (1897). The desirability and the feasibility of the acquisition of some real and accurate knowledge of the brain by pre-collegiate scholars. *Science, 6*, 902–908.

Yeni-Komshian, G. H., Flege, J. E., & Liu, S. (2000). Pronunciation proficiency in the first and second languages of Korean-English bilinguals. *Bilingualism: Language and Cognition, 3*, 131–149.

Zschoche, S. (1989). Dr. Clarke revisited: Science, true womanhood, and female collegiate education. *History of Education Quarterly, 29*, 545–569.

VOLUME DETERMINATION UNDER THE MICROSCOPE, THE SIMPLE WAY: THE DELESSE PRINCIPLE

Manuel del Cerro (Pittsford, NY, USA) and Lazaros C. Triarhou (Thessaloniki, Greece)

OVERVIEW

Counting is a very intuitive activity, thus one would assume that estimating the number of particles within a solid mass by looking at microscopic slides would be simple. It is not so.

Volume estimation is not intuitive, thus one would assume that it should be difficult to achieve under the microscope. It is not so. It is something the amateur microscopist can easily do and that gives answers to a variety of interesting questions. This is the subject that we discuss below.

THE WHAT, THE WHY, AND THE HOW
Particle counting under the microscope

Determining the number of particles in a sample by counting them in a microscopic section is far more of an involved proposition that it may appear. The questions driving these counts are such as: "How many nerve cells are there in a cubic cm of brain cortex?" or "How many fungal particles are there in a parasitized fish (or ameba)?" or infinite variations of the same theme. Since we are going to use the term "particle(s)" often, a definition is in order. In 1940 R.M. Allen put it very simply: "This term, in a general sense, includes anything requiring counting." This definition of particle may appear overly inclusive but it serves the microscopist very well as we shall see later.

In practice, the validity of microscopic counting can be affected by the shape and size of the particles, their thickness relative to the thickness of the section, possible particle overlap within the section, and other factors (Abercrombie, 1946). Computer-assisted particle counting diminishes the effort but, surprisingly, it has only a modest effect on the validity of the final results. Many chapters in many books deal with the issue of particle counting. An entire new branch of morphometry dealing with it, the so-called "unbiased morphometry," has developed in the last quarter of a century particularly through the work of the group of H.J. Gundersen, at Aarhus, Denmark (Gundersen & Jensen, 1985; Gundersen, 1986; Pakkenberg & Gundersen, 1988). In view of the extensive bibliography available for particle counting, some of it highly specialized, we will not discuss it further. We should just note Haug's (1986) highly readable article on the history of morphometry. For those interested in the subject key references are given at the end of this article. Now that the background is dealt with, we shall discuss exclusively the estimation of *volume* using microscopic sections.

Volume estimates under the microscope

Here the questions are: "What is the relative volume of the red particles embedded in the yellow mass? (figure 1), or "What is the relative volume of nuclei in a sample?" or "What is the relative volume of fungal parasites within the body of a parasitized fish (or cell)?" Or infinite variations of the same theme (later we shall explore some practical examples). Answers to these questions can be very meaningful and can be obtained by an amateur microscopist working with very simple and very inexpensive tools. Now that we have discussed the "what" aspect of the problem we shall proceed to discuss "the why" and "the how."

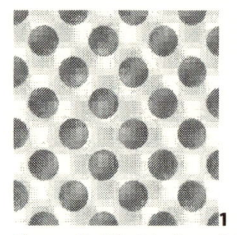

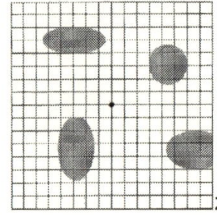

Figure 1. What is the relative volume of the red particles embedded in the yellow mass?

Figure 2. This diagram illustrates the application of the Delesse principle to a hypothetical random section. A grid is used as a testing probe and the number of hits on the whole field and on the particles is counted (details in the text).

In 1847 a French geologist and mines engineer, Auguste Delesse, proposed that: "in a rock, composed of a number of minerals, the area occupied by any given mineral on a surface of a section of the rock is proportional to the volume of the mineral in the rock."

The proposition was tested countless times and found valid, even if applied to surfaces other than those of rocks. It did not take long for microscopists to realize that "the Delesse principle" could be applied to tissue sections. Now we shall see how it is done.

The Delesse principle, flexible in application as it is, does have a few requirements. The first that the section in the mass that is to be tested be placed at random. The second that the particles whose volume will be estimated have well defined boundaries separating them from the background.

The first requirement is satisfied by sectioning the mass of material at any arbitrarily chosen plane. Fulfillment of the second has to be in the nature of the material tested (figures 1–4).

Once the basic requirements are fulfilled, the next step is to measure the area [a] of the particles ($ap_1...ap_n$) seen in the section and relate it to the total area (A) of the section. Delesse did this by first tracing the outline of the section on paper and also the outlines of each particle. Next, using scissors he cut out all the particles and weighed them. The relation between the weight of the combined cut-outs to the total weight gave him the relative volume of the particles contained in the sample. Delesse's procedure represents a tremendous simplification on any previously existing method of volume evaluation in rocks. Still, cutting with scissors each and all profiles drawn on a paper is a tedious approach to the problem. Alternatives were soon proposed, such as overlapping lines [l] on the drawing and determining the total length of line overlapping the particles, then determining the total length of lines overlapping the entire section, and finally determining the relationship between the two (Rosival, 1898). To do this with a computer program is simplicity itself; to do this manually is still laborious.

Other options were tried but the one that has gained popularity, and in the experience of one of us (MdC) is by far the best for the amateur, is manual point [p] counting (Glagolev, 1933). Here a sheath of paper or transparent material, having a number of clearly visible dots, is set under the drawing or picture and both are placed over an illuminated source. Next, the number of dots hitting the particles is counted, and so is the total number of points hitting the section outline. Instead of single points, a grid drawn on transparent material can be used in which case the line intersections (called "hits" from here on) are used for the purpose of the test (we shall illustrate all this in the examples given below). The relationship between the hits on the particles [a] and those on the entire surface of the section [A], is the same as the relationship between the volume of all the particles and the total volume ($V_v=P_p$). This relationship is usually expressed as a percentage: (hits on v/total hits) × 100 = %v.

Basically that is all. There are minor technical details that we shall review later. The procedure is easier to perform than to describe. We shall put it in action using a few examples.

Example 1

What percentage of volume is occupied in a hypothetical mass by the blue particles embedded in it?

Results and Comments. In this example there were a total of 289 hits; 42 corresponding to particles. As 42/289 = 0.145, and 0.145 × 100 = 14.5 the conclusion is that 14.5% of the total mass is occupied by the particulate material.

The grid used in this example is our favorite. It is a copy of the Amsler grid (also called Amsler chart). This is a most useful device for persons to test the condition of the maculae in their own eyes. Complimentary copies of it can be obtained at ophthalmologists or optometrists offices, or downloaded from the web. Including the intersections, the sites where the lines touch the borders, and the corners, the Amsler grid offers 289 test points. Obviously, the image of the grid may be reduced or enlarged to suit the sample to be tested.

One question often asked is: how many hits should be used to obtain reliable results? Experience has shown that a test point density that provides at least one hit per particle is acceptable. More than one hit/particle increases accuracy at the price of more time and effort. The same is true of the repetition of the testing changing the orientation of the grid each time. Statistical analysis of the results can determine the optimal strategy to achieve a chosen level of reliability. This is necessary for scientific research but seldom for amateur work.

Example 2

An oocyte, the cell that symbolizes life more than any other, is close to spherical and so is its nucleus. The question here is: what percentage of the total cell volume is occupied by the nucleus?

Results and Comments. A copy of the Amsler grid was placed under a copy of the image and both were placed on a light box. The number of hits falling on the entire cell were counted. A note was also made of hits on the cell nucleus. The total count was 293 hits, with 15 of them falling on the nucleus. Applying the Delesse principle we calculate that (15/293) × 100 = 5.1%, is the volume of the nucleus relative to the total volume of this cell.

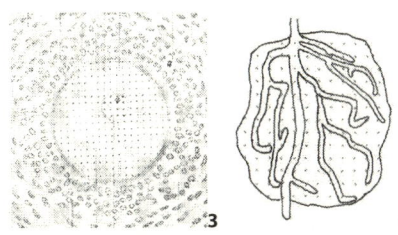

Figure 3. A sixty year old rendition of an oocyte and its surrounding cells by an artist who was working directly from the microscope. Test dots were marked on the entire oocyte and on its nucleus. See text for results and comments.

Figure 4. A copy of the Amsler's grid was set behind an old camera lucida drawing of the ameba. Using a light box for transillumination (a window pane is a workable alternative), the hits on the cell body were recorded as blue points and those on the invading fungus on red.

Example 3

An ameba still alive, is heavily infected by a parasitic fungus (figure 4). How much of the cell is occupied by the parasite?

Results and Comments. There were 139 total hits; 39 of them were on the fungal hyphae. As 39/139 = 0.28, and 0.145 × 100 = 28.0 the conclusion is that 28% of the cell mass is occupied by the fungus. Incidentally, this would be the equivalent of having 56 pounds of fungus infecting the body of a 200 pound human!

Comparison of the samples offered as example 1 and 3 shows some of the features that make of the Delesse principle such a useful and flexible tool. (1) It operates equally well with the smooth geometric particles of example 1, as with the highly irregular object in example 3. Provided that the borders of the particles are clearly defined, their shape is of no consequence. (2) One particle in example 1, the one to the right and down, illustrates another property of the Delesse principle: it operates as well with incomplete as with complete profiles. (3) Example 3 shows how the principle can in some instances, give information that is more meaningful than that of numerical estimation. For example, it would be quite meaningless to count as one particle the fungus branching profusely within the cell in example 3.

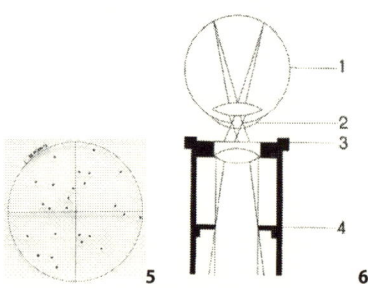

Figure 5. An enlarged view of the Zeiss 25 points ocular insert for volume determination according to the Delesse-Glagolev principle.
Figure 6. The line labeled "4" points to the ocular diaphragm. The this is the point where to place the insert shown on figure 5.

VARIATIONS OF A THEME

Point counts for applying the Delesse principle need not be limited to the use of pictures or drawings; they can be done while directly looking at the specimen through the microscope ocular. Zeiss representatives used to offer, somewhere in the 1970s or 1980s, an ocular grid with 25 randomly distributed dots (figure 5). If the original Zeiss insert is not available a similar one can be made by any amateur using a circular cover glass and a fine point marker. This grid is placed on the internal diaphragm of the ocular, just as it is done with ocular micrometers, for example (figure 6). This through-the-microscope approach has advantages and disadvantages when compared with the counting of points on a picture. It is faster of course, since no picture(s) need to be made; thus, it encourages the measuring of more fields from the same sample. The main disadvantage is that no permanent record of the counting is produced. Additionally, most observers find that point counting through an ocular is more demanding and tiring than simply doing it on a print placed on a desk top. It is however, a useful alternative to know and to use when appropriate.

CONCLUSION

The few examples of the application of Delesse's principle given above derive mostly from our interest in biomedical microscopy. They are by no means representative of the limits of application of the principle. On the contrary, there is practically no limit to the variety of samples to which the principle can be applied, including suitable electron micrographs. Research of recent date finds the principle applicable to the analysis of important medical questions (Schwartz and Recker, 2006).

We encourage every amateur microscopist to give the Delesse Priciple a try; it is informative and it is fun to do. We would much appreciate readers' feedback.

REFERENCES

Abercrombie, M. (1946) Estimation of nuclear population from microtome sections. *Anatomical Record* 94, 239–247.
Aherne, W.A., Dunhill, M.S. (1982) *Morphometry*. Edward Arnold, London, England, p. 205.
Allen, R.M. (1940) *The Microscope*. D. Van Nostrand Company, Inc., New York, USA, p. 159.
Bradbury, S. (1991) *Basic Measurement Techniques for Light Microscopy*. Oxford University Press, Oxford, England, p. 97.
Braendgaard, H., Gundersen, H.J.G. (1986) The impact of recent stereological advances on quantitative studies of the nervous system. *Journal of Neuroscience Methods* 18, 39–78.
Delesse, A. (1847) *Comptes Rendus Hebdomadaires des Sciences de L'Academie de Sciences* 25, 544–545.
Elias, H., Hyde, D.M. (1983) *A Guide to Practical Stereology*. Karger, Basel, Switzerland, p. 305.
Gundersen, H.J.G. (1986) Stereology of arbitrary particles. *Journal of Microscopy* 143, 3–45.
Mouton, P.R. (2002) *Principles and Practices of Unbiased Stereology: An Introduction For Bioscientists*. Johns Hopkins University Press, Baltimore, USA, p. 232.
Pakkenberg, B., Gundersen, H.J. (1988) Total number of neurons and glial cells in human brain nuclei estimated by the disector and the fractionator. *Journal of Microscopy* 150, 1–20.

REVIEW

Revisiting Christfried Jakob's concept of the dual onto-phylogenetic origin and ubiquitous function of the cerebral cortex: a century of progress

Lazaros C. Triarhou

Received: 22 November 2009 / Accepted: 20 January 2010 / Published online: 11 February 2010
© Springer-Verlag 2010

Abstract This paper revisits a concept combining the evolution, ontogeny and histophysiology of the cerebral cortex, presented, in a quest to explain cognition and behavior, by the neurobiologist Christfried Jakob (1866–1956) at the Second Annual Meeting of the International Society for Medical Psychology and Psychotherapy, organized by Oskar Vogt (1870–1959) in Munich in 1911. Jakob suggested a dual onto-phylogenetic origin and a ubiquitous cortical function, claiming that most receptive pathways end up in an 'outer fundamental layer', which derives from the rhinencephalic apparatus, whereas the 'inner fundamental layer' contains effector elements and derives from the striatum. With advancing evolution, the two fundamental layers become intermingled. By attributing a functional homogeneity to the cortex, Jakob contradicted the theories of Flechsig and Cajal on 'association' and 'mnemonic' areas. The merit of Jakob's concept rests, a century later, with the current resurgence of biological research at the evolutionary–developmental interface and the broadening anticipated from the re-integration of these two fields, especially by adding a functional dimension to the morphological traits.

Keywords Brain development · Brain evolution · Cerebral cortex · Cytoarchitectonics · Dorsal ventricular ridge · History of neuroscience · Pallium · Subventricular zone

Introduction

An understanding of neural development and evolution is inevitable for deciphering brain structure and function. The puzzle of the cerebral cortex in particular may become clarified by studying its evolutionary origins (Shimizu and Karten 1991) and the problem of neuronal homologies (Nauta and Karten 1970). As in general biology, so in neurobiology, research on phylogenetic accounts of ontogeny has been gaining momentum (Rakic and Kornack 2001).

Crucial studies on brain evolution and brain development came out from major laboratories between the 1870s and the 1930s (cf. Edinger 1896; Flatau and Jacobsohn 1899; Unger 1906; Brodmann 1909; Obersteiner 1913; Johnston 1915; Vogt and Vogt 1919; Ariëns Kappers et al. 1936). They contain a wealth of knowledge, not fully exploited by modern investigators, as they had been published in languages other than English.

This article revisits a theory proposed by Christfried Jakob (1866–1956), a Bavarian neuropathologist and the founder of Argentinian neurobiology, affiliated with the Universities of Buenos Aires and La Plata. Besides extensive research in comparative and human neuroscience, and numerous publications on cortical ontogeny, phylogeny and neuropathology, Jakob integrated such diversities as general biology, anthropology, paleontology, biogeography, philosophy and music. Half-way through his life, Jakob published in Munich two classic Atlases, called *The human brain* and *From animal brain to human brain* (Triarhou 2008c), and made a key presentation at the

Parts of this work were presented at the 3rd International Conference on Cortical Development, Crete, 22–25 May 2008, and the 38th Annual Meeting of the Society for Neuroscience, Washington, DC, 15–19 November 2008.

L. C. Triarhou (✉)
Economo-Koskinas Wing for Integrative and Evolutionary Neuroscience, University of Macedonia, 156 Egnatia Ave., 540 06 Thessaloniki, Greece
e-mail: triarhou@uom.gr

Second Annual Meeting of the International Society for Medical Psychology and Psychotherapy, organized also in Munich by Oskar Vogt on 25–26 September 1911. Jakob's communication was published the following year in two variants (Jakob 1912a, b); he maintained a constant interest in that concept (Jakob 1910b, 1913), and in 1916 published a Spanish version, with minor emendations and an added concluding paragraph (Jakob 1916).

Jakob suggested a dual evolutionary and developmental origin and an ubiquitous function of the cerebral cortex, based on data gathered during his 'first tenure' in Argentina, between 1899 and 1910 (Triarhou and del Cerro 2006a, b; Triarhou 2008b). He conducted hundreds of human neuropathological examinations and carried out comparative studies on over 100 species of the Patagonian fauna, including primates, the legless amphibian *Caecilia lumbricoides*, which resembles a giant earthworm but belongs to the order of the Gymnophiona, and the squamate reptile *Amphisbaena darwini* (blind viper).

Jakob claimed that all cortical regions contain receptive elements and that most sensory pathways end up in the 'outer fundamental cortical layer' (small and medium-size pyramidal cells), which onto-phylogenetically derives from the rhinencephalic apparatus. The 'inner fundamental layer' contains effector elements and derives from the striatum. With advancing evolution, the two fundamental layers become intermingled. Jakob attributes homogeneity to the cortex and contradicts Flechsig (1896, 1898) and Ramón y Cajal (1895, 1899, 1904, 1906) on the existence of dedicated association and memory areas.

The 'triple-synthesis' (evolutionary, developmental and physiological) has been viewed as one of Jakob's prime contributions to science (Moyano 1957; López Pasquali 1965; Orlando 1966; Meyer 1981; Fontana et al. 2002; Lores Arnaiz et al. 2002). Diego Outes, a pupil of Braulio Moyano (Jakob's successor at the Pathology Laboratory of the National Neuropsychiatric Hospital in Buenos Aires), revisited the topic of the dual cortex (*Doppelrinde*) twice (Outes and Benítez 1976; Outes 2006).

The current resurgence of research at the evolutionary–developmental interface of biology witnesses the promising re-integration of these two fields, after almost a century (Raff et al. 1999). With his larger Atlases, Jakob (1911; Jakob and Onelli 1911, 1913) pioneered evolutionary–developmental neurobiology. A cognoscente of 'cortical history' (*Die Geschichte der Hirnrinde*), Jakob promptly applied phylogenetic observations to the ontogeny of the human brain (Moyano 1957; López Pasquali 1965). The originality of his ideas is witnessed by the writings of his contemporaries (Ranke 1911; Siemerling 1911; von Economo and Koskinas 1925; Seldon and Szirko 2005).

Jakob has been compared in caliber to Ramón y Cajal. In their *Cytoarchitectonics*, von Economo and Koskinas (1925) express the view that future research on the cerebral cortex must be based on the fundamental work of Kaes (1907), Sammet (2006), Ramón y Cajal (1906), and Jakob (1911), Jakob and Onelli (1911). von Economo and Koskinas (1925) stress Jakob's *geniale Ansicht* (ingenious idea) regarding cortical phylo-ontogeny, Cajal's *ganz glänzend* (totally brilliant) use of the Golgi method, and Meynert's *geniale Intuition* (ingenious intuition) in associating the granularity in the area striata of the calcarine sulcus with sensory function (Meynert 1872).

Today, powerful cytochemical and molecular biological methods are available to neurobiologists for studying gene expression, the cascade of molecular pathways, cell–cell interactions, and the phylogeny of embryonic cortical development (Rakic 2007). A century ago, tools at hand were confined to the Nissl and Weigert stains and light microscopy, having to be compensated by the observer's acuity and imagination.

The present study makes Jakob's essay available in English. The discussion that follows re-examines Jakob's concept and the progress made since. The translation of Jakob's communication was rendered from the papers published in *Journal für Psychologie und Neurologie* (vol. 19, no. 1, pp. 379–382, 1912) and *Münchener Medizinische Wochenschrift* (vol. 59, no. 9, pp. 466–468, 1912). The sections added by Jakob in the Spanish version (*La Prensa Médica Argentina*, vol. 2, no. 23, pp. 305–307, 1916) appear in brackets. Figures were supplemented from sources explained in the captions.

Jakob (1918) mentions that he began studying the brains of Argentina's batrachians and reptiles in 1905, reporting his initial findings in an article (Jakob 1910a) and later in his books (Jakob 1911; Jakob and Onelli 1911, 1913). Originally, Jakob (1911; Jakob and Onelli 1911, 1913) wrote that the drawing on the relation of cortical layers depicted the brain of *Caecilia*, an amphibian belonging to the family of Gymnophiona, one of the three orders of modern amphibians (Zardoya and Meyer 2001). As Outes (2006) explains, Jakob (1918) subsequently clarified that the particular specimen had actually been an apod reptile, the *Amphisbaena darwini* (blind viper). The two species looked alike enough in external morphology and shared common habitats; the flaky epidermis and the more advanced brain form eventually led to the distinction of the Amphisbaena from the Gymnophion, whose vesicular brain reminded that of the urodela. The erratum has been remedied in the current translation. A systematic revisionary work on South American amphisbaenids did not appear until well into the 1960s (Gans 1966). Cytoarchitectonic studies have shown that the brain of *Caecilia* markedly differs from other amphibians in having a highly differentiated accessory olfactory bulb and a large overall extension of this brain region (Zilles et al. 1981).

On the ubiquity of the dual receptive–effector function of the cerebral cortex as the basis for a new biological conception of the cortical apparatus of mind

by Dr. Chr. Jakob (Buenos Aires) currently in Krailling by Munich

The historical development of our views on the origin and biological bases of mental forces can be divided into the following four phases:

1. The speculative period of antiquity and the middle ages, dominated by the theories of pneuma and ventricular localization.
2. The anatomical period of Vesalius and Varolio (inventor of the fiber teasing method), over to de le Boë Sylvius (1641, first essay on cortical localization) and Gall, characterized by diverse theories attempting to localize mental processes in the cerebral matter.
3. The physiological period of the nineteenth century that led us, experimentally and clinically, from Bouillaud and Flourens to Broca, Fritsch and Hitzig, Wernicke, and finally to Flechsig's theory on the varying importance of the cortex (projection and association centers), which came to a dead end with Ramón y Cajal's theory of 'mnemonic centers'.
4. The current biological–eclectic period, characterized by the systematic application and comparison of all methods, and by its biological trend.

In a systematic series of studies, I examined the regional structure and cortical layers (cyto-, myelo-, fiber-architecture), as well as the comparative histology, histogenesis and histopathogenesis, and their relation to normal and disturbed function. The most important questions toward a synthetic conception of the mental apparatus, which thus far remain unanswered, are:

a. Are there sectors in the human and animal cerebral cortex of an exclusively *receptive* nature and others of a purely *effector* nature or such of a purely *neutral* nature, and how are their components differentiated?
b. What is the evolutionary course of such sectors and what *fundamental differences* characterize the *human cortex*? Are there principal differences compared to animals or is it all about *gradual differentiation*?
c. Is the *origin of the cortex* mono- or poly-phyletic?

I have been addressing these questions for the past decade in collaboration with my students at the Institutes I head at the University of Buenos Aires (Laboratory of Hospital de Las Mercedes, Neurobiological Laboratory of National Women's Psychiatric Hospital, and Neurology Clinic of San Roque Hospital), using a vast collection of human brains, histopathologically (degeneration methods), experimentally in apes (*Cebus* from Paraguay), and comparatively anatomically in species of the South American fauna (Figs. 1, 2).

The results can be summarized as follows:

(I) *All regions of the human and animal cortex, with no exception, are receptive (the only peculiarity being the status of Ammon's formation, the phylogenetically oldest cortical region).*

This does not have to be discussed for cortical territories (visual, auditory, etc.) classified as 'projection centers'—von Monakow and Déjerine determined the fundamentals of anatomical fiber relations—but it becomes necessary for the remaining parts, i.e. frontal cortex, cingulate gyrus, precuneus, posterior parietal and temporal, temporopolar, and occipito-temporal regions. We systematically examined over 300 cortical areas (mostly softening processes) in serial sections for retrograde thalamic cellular changes with the Nissl–Lenhossék thionin stain. A preliminary study of the human thalamic nuclei was necessary (Jakob 1910a, 1911). We could discern that lesions of areas in all parts of the frontal cortex result in cell loss in most parts of the anterior lateral thalamic nucleus (the only exception being the small fronto-olfactory sector of the frontal base); in a similar manner, degenerative foci in the cingulate gyrus result in retrograde cell loss in the anterior and dorsal nucleus of the thalamus; degenerative foci in the precuneus and posterior parietal cortex result in retrograde cell loss in the dorsal rostral pulvinar (posterior nucleus, dorsal–anterior portion) and posterior lateral nucleus; degeneration of the anterior occipital area results in retrograde cell loss in the dorsal caudal pulvinar; degeneration of the posterior temporal area results in retrograde cell loss in the basal pulvinar (posterior nucleus, basal portion); and degeneration of the anterior temporal cortex in cell loss in the internal basal nucleus of the thalamus.

These data prove that the entire cortical surface has fiber systems receiving sensory stimuli that emanate from distinct thalamic regions, also on directed and descending pathways at the sensory mesencephalon and diencephalon; thus, the cortical surface is completely separated into sectorial receptive fields, each equipped with a specific modality. We obtained similar results in the ape brain. Degeneration areas must have a minimum size to lead to recognizable cell losses.

[One can verify, by translating the anatomical data into physiological facts that the entire cortical surface receives, from each distinct region of the thalamus, pathways which conduct the stimuli toward the cortex (centripetal paths or thalamocortical radiations). It is precisely the cells of origin of those pathways that degenerate secondarily as a consequence of cortical foci. As these pathways are further associated with the lower afferent sensory pathways of the midbrain and the diencephalon, it follows that the pallium

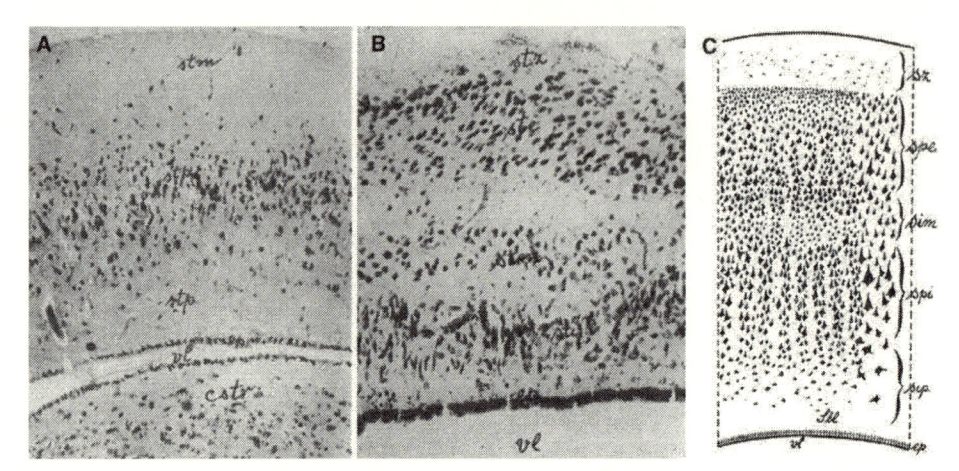

Fig. 1 a Ammon's cortex in the adult *Caiman latirostris* ('yacaré'). *stp* pyramidal cell layer, *stm* molecular layer, *vl* lateral ventricle, *ep* ependyma, *cstr* corpus striatum. Nissl stain ×150. From Jakob (1941, p. 168). **b** Lateral cortex of *Iguana iguana* with the molecular (*stz*), external (*ste*) and internal (*sti*) cortical layers, and an intermediate layer (*stm*). From Jakob (1941, p. 148). **c** Polystratified cortex of a higher mammal; *sz* molecular layer, *spe* external pyramidal layer, *sim* intermediate layer, *spi* internal pyramidal layer, *sip* interpyramidal layer, *sbl* basal layer (Jakob and Onelli 1913, p. 16)

is divided in its entire extent into zones that affect the form of sectors, each with distinct sensory modalities.

Moreover, if one takes into account the relations known to exist between the centers of projection and their respective thalamic nuclei, we conclude that for each sensory modality there are at least two adjacent cortical territories, one of which is *directly* connected with the basal thalamus, and the other *indirectly* connected via afferent pathways with the diencephalon (with the intercalation of the dorsal thalamic nuclei).

Thus, we arrive at the notion that the old 'projection centers' are identical to our direct primary cortical territories; secondary indirect territories (which phylogenetically mature later than primary) occupy parts of the old 'association centers'. The fact that lesions of the latter frequently develop in a latent form can be explained by the intervention of intact primary territories, whereas destruction of primary territories, of consequence to a secondary involvement of the baso-thalamic nuclei, must always disturb the conduction to secondary territories.

I obtained similar results in primates, whose structural plan completely agrees with the human brain. Such foci must always have a certain extent to produce secondary alterations that can be safely discerned.]

(II) *The principal part of these sensory radiations terminates at the external cortical layer.* [Outer layer = molecular layer, small, middle, larger outer pyramids + granular layer (intermediate layer).]

This trend can be proven with the Weigert method only at individual areas (degeneration of Gennari's strip in the calcarine sulcus) connected with the corresponding thalamic areas; on the other hand, with the Marchi method it is also confirmed in all other areas of both humans and apes, as well as in lower animals. Histological finds (myelination, impregnation) support this view as well. Further, for this purpose, indications are provided by the fact that the outer layer strongly increases always at the expense of the inner layer where ever radiations occur (visual, auditory, tactile cortex). This applies to the entire animal line.

[Studying the engravings of Ramón y Cajal, one can see that he invariably terminates the fibers in what I call the external layer, although he does stress that fact.]

(III) *The inner layer of the cortex has an effector function and exists everywhere.* (Inner layer = deep, large and middle pyramids, deep smaller and polymorphous cellular elements.)

That finding is first a logical result of the previous one, in the sense of a general structural plan of the central nervous system. It is further supported by the fact that everywhere in the cortex, where motor pathways emanate that project to lower centers (pyramidal pathway, bulbar pathways, hypothalamic bundles, pontine pathways, fornix system) this takes place without any exception in the inner layer; and anywhere that an overall effector character stands out, it is accompanied by an increase of the inner layer at the expense of the outer; this happens consistently in the entire animal line (Fig. 3). Definite proof must be furnished not by degeneration studies, but from the phylogeny of the two fundamental layers.

[It has been verified that the cerebral cortex does not in principle depart from the structural plan of lower spinal

Fig. 2 Evolution of the pallium and cortical mantle in five vertebrate species, from fish to human. From Jakob (1911, p. 34); Jakob and Onelli (1913, p. 12)

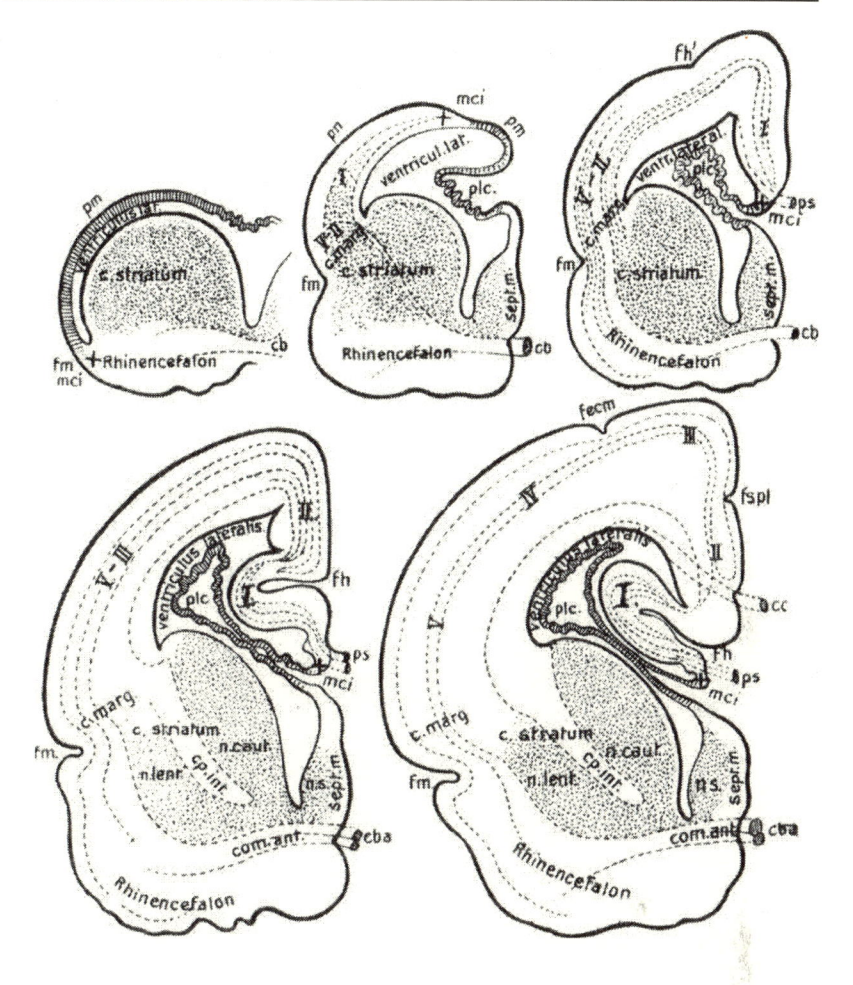

systems, since in them as well, through their entire extent, including the spinal cord, medulla and midbrain, the separate sensory and motor columns are arranged in parallel. The same happens in the cortex, where both fundamental layers run parallel. Similar to these regions, one or the other column may occasionally become overgrown or diminished, according to peripheral exigencies. This fact is repeated in the central apparatus in accordance with homologous laws. I attribute to the concept of such a sensory–motor disposition, for the entire corticality, the same importance for the future, that has been attributed in the history of neurology to the discovery of Bell and Magendie concerning the distinct functional nature of the ventral and dorsal roots.]

(IV) *Both fundamental layers have a uniform dual origin in mammals up to humans (monophyletic evolution) and something similar can be stated for various classes of lower vertebrates (reptiles in particular).* On the contrary, amphibians do not belong here. According to my studies, the *Amphisbaena* actually represents the fundamental type of evolution of the higher cortical apparatus up to humans (Figs. 4, 5). My comparative histological studies suggest that the two fundamental cortical layers have distinct origins: the receptive outer layer stems from the rhinencephalon (an old sensory part of the brain), whereas the effector inner layer from the corpus striatum (an old motor central nucleus) (Fig. 6). Despite its dual origin, with advancing evolution, the entire cortex reaches a correspondingly more internal intermingling of the two layers. In mammals, this proceeds as a consequence of the augmentation of cellular elements with a highly ramified protoplasm through the formation of axon collaterals, the occurrence of numerous intermediate and intercalated, and the secondary structural fusion of the fundamental cortical layers, which were initially separated in the anlage (Fig. 7); a principle that especially distinguishes the primate and human cerebral cortex.

Fig. 3 Cortical evolution from mono- to poly-stratified. *Left to right* amphibian, reptilian, avian, mammalian, and higher mammalian laminar structure. From Jakob and Onelli (1911, p. 23), (1913, p. 16)

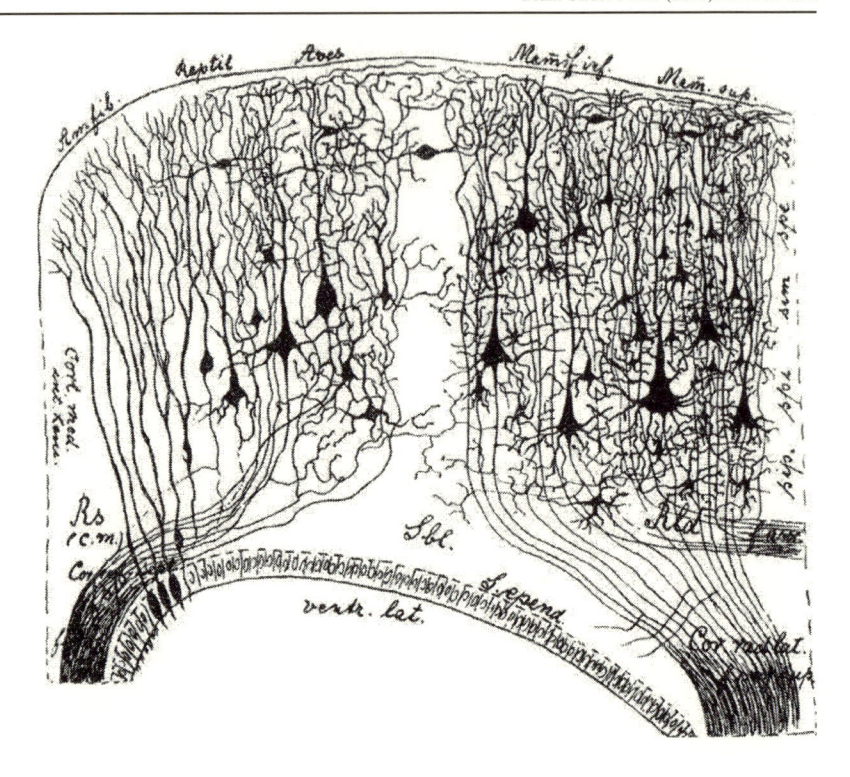

[The bilaminar cortical type can be seen in the brain of *Tapirus terrestris* (Fig. 8), and the union of both outer and inner cortical layers can be demonstrated in the brain of *Erinaceus europaeus* (Fig. 9).]

(V) *A cortex that is neither receptive nor effector (='association cortex') does not exist.*

The thorough study of the cortical surface yields consistent results. The dual-location fundamental layer type only knows one exception: in the entire animal line, the unistriate structure of Ammon's formation (the oldest olfactory cortical portion), which always exhibits only the lower, effector layer. Thus, the entire cortical mantle (pallium) is either sensorimotorily or motor-sensorily active (depending on the dominance of one or the other component). There is no part of the cortex that functions and acts solely as receptive or as effector, as far as the histological and experimental proof is concerned. A cortex that could exclusively claim the descriptor 'association cortex' or 'mnemonic center' does not exist. Such processes are functions of a dynamic nature of both fundamental layers at all localities. Accordingly, I proclaim, against the views of Flechsig and Ramón y Cajal, the equivalence of all cortical zones; with differences being only in gradation.

I thus arrive at the following conclusions:

The cerebral cortex develops monophyletically in the entire mammalian and human spectrum from two originally separate and also functionally different fundamental layers. Both components appear in the cortex in an ascending order into a more intrinsic contact than the case is in lower spinal, bulbar, and other systems. As a result of its structure, the cortex is reckoned as both receptive and effector throughout, the only change being functional qualities and their topographic relationships with lower centers.

As a consequence of the mutual penetration of both layers in mammals, and especially in humans, a process purely effector or exclusively receptive is not plausible at any cortical zone; each state of excitation has to momentarily release the corresponding other phase (receptive or effector). Thus, all cortical acts must a priori be defined as having a 'mixed' nature; an arbitrary separation into the two components seems irreconcilable with the cortical texture. Such a trend is fundamental for the understanding of cortical functions.

Therefore, each fundamental process in the domain of will or perception must carry a similar 'mixed' character; it is erroneous to speak of such processes as distinct (what actually happens is that, in each case, one component prevails over the other). They differ in tendency, not in essence. We thus arrive, from the past 'dualist' views of cortical mental processes, at a concept of 'cortical monism' for the entire functional repertoire. The outcome of those

I intend to revisit these new views on the nature and function of our mind apparatus. I would like to point out that these results, which derive from modern biological brain research, closely match in certain points the views of the newer philosophy (cf. Wundt's apperception theory, the doctrines of the subconscious, etc.). Thus, regarding the future of cortical biology, I would particularly emphasize the important point that the findings of mental research no more contradict those of brain research, as has been the case until now.

Discussion

Jakob (1895, 1898) had laid out a plan to study the brain in the early Atlases, which constituted a testimony to his versatility in neurohistology (Meyer 1981). The approaches considered meaningful to better understand the nervous system were (1) histological staining and serial section reconstruction of the adult human brain; (2) neuropathological changes and their sequels; (3) comparative neuroanatomy and neuroembryology; (4) human brain development and myelination; and (5) experimentally induced lesions in animals.

Within a dozen years of working in Buenos Aires, Jakob collected the tissues and was able to materialize his original plan of integrating data gathered from clinico-pathological correlations (e.g. focal cortical degeneration in neurosyphilis), lesion-induced retrograde degeneration (to track thalamocortical projections in monkeys), and comparative neurohistological studies (in diverse species of the Patagonian fauna). As Moyano (1957) relates, five decades later and a continent apart, Jakob had materialized his plans in the lavishly illustrated Atlas volumes of *Folia Neurobiológica Argentina*, which, in 1,200 pages, 1,000 figures and 650 macrophotographic plates, covered (I) human topographic neuroanatomy, (II) human neuropathology, and (III) cerebral ontogeny and phylogeny (Jakob 1939a, b, 1941).

Jakob and Onelli (1911, 1913) intended to establish a biological basis of mental phenomena, convinced that the comparative study of central nervous system structure and function would yield psychological clues, otherwise psychology is doomed to the limitations of its descriptive methods (Papini 1988). Jakob viewed the 'cortical apparatus of mind' as a mere quantitative evolution from animals to humans (Jakob 1914, 1945): 'Motivated by a study of animal language, I probed the varying production of affective language by galliformes: although humans surpass all animals through the free and extensive use of symbols, which only they know how to separate from the ensuing emotions, thus being able to intellectually rise to higher ideative constructions. Such an economy of thought facilitates a mental life freed from momentary emotional

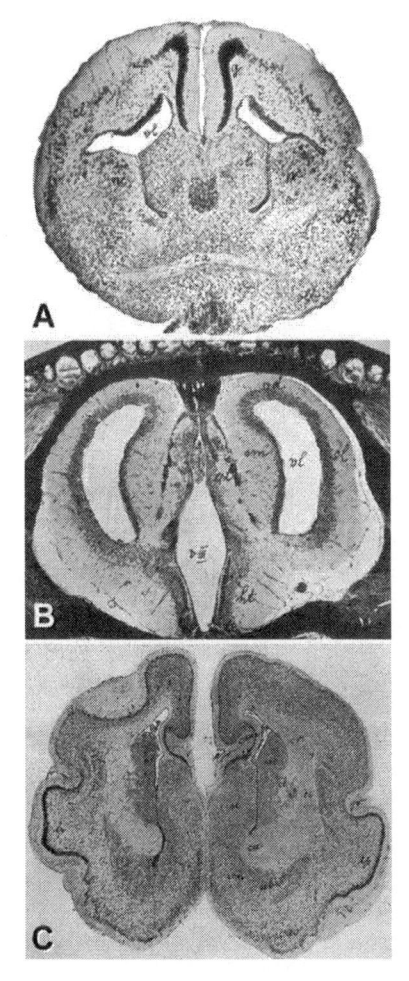

Fig. 4 Coronal sections in typical vertebrates of the Argentinian fauna. **a** *Amphisbaena darwini* initially thought to be *Caecilia lumbricoides*, but later corrected by Jakob (1918), cf. also Outes (2006). *g* Ammon's formation containing the fascia dentata and Ammon's cortex, *cl* lateral cortex, *sl* lateral septum, *olf* olfactory area, *vl* lateral ventricle, *nc* caudate nucleus, *ca* anterior commissure. Nissl stain. From Jakob and Onelli (1913, Plate 2.12). **b** Coronal section of the hemispheres and diencephalon in an amphibian (*Gymnophion* or *Chthonherpeton*). *cl*, *cd*, *cm*, lateral, dorsal, medial cortex; *vl*, *vIII*, lateral and third ventricle; *ht*, hypothalamus; *ept*, habenula or epithalamus. From Jakob (1941, p. 122). **c** Anterior coronal section in a marsupial ('comadreja' or *Didelphis paraguayensis*), Nissl stain. Gray paleoneuronal (Ammonic) and neoneuronal (dorsolateral) cortical formations. *fr* rhinal sulcus, *ao* olfactory area, *lp* piriform lobe, *sl* septum, *nc* caudate nucleus, *nl* lenticular nucleus. From Jakob (1941, p. 113)

views, which represent a new important biological basis for clinical, psychological (Jakob 1913) and physiological studies, contribute to bridging the gap between biological and mental phenomena.

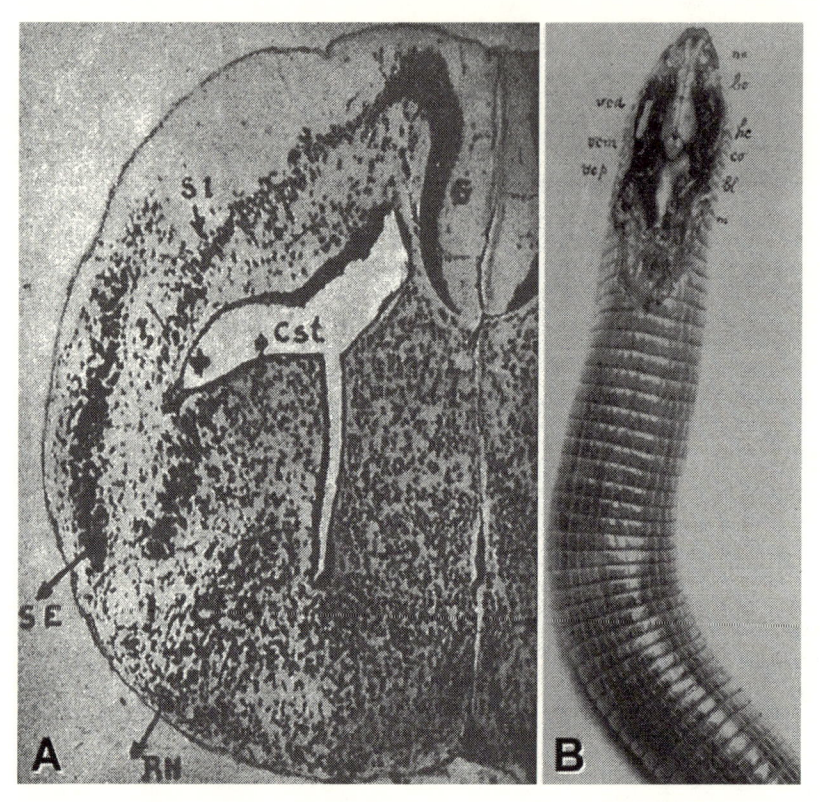

Fig. 5 a Photomicrograph of *Amphisbaena darwini* (Jakob 1918). The inner layer (*si*) of the lateral cortex continues dorsally toward Ammon's horn and ventrally toward the striatum (*Cst*). Jakob emphasized the ventral continuity, since the striatum is associated with motor function, although in this particular photomicrograph, the continuity with Ammon's horn is more conspicuous than that with the striatum. *se* outer layer, *Rh* rhinencephalon. From Outes (2006). **b** The brain of *Amphisbaena darwini* ('víbora ciega') dissected in situ, showing the olfactory bulb (*bo*), cerebral hemisphere (*hc*), rudimentary optic body (*co*), cerebellum, medulla oblongata (*bl*) and beginning of spinal cord (*m*). Magnification ×2. From Jakob (1941, p. 65)

responses, to which the animal psyche remains bound, but deep inside the psychogenetic vocabulary, numbering 8–10 in the hens, 500 in primitive man, and 50,000 or more in civilized peoples, lies an essentially quantitative question of intensity grade and extent, and not of qualitative differences concerning its biological basis.'

The originality of Jakob's ideas is reiterated by contemporary authors (Ranke 1911; Siemerling 1911). The lifelong interest of Jakob in fetal development is echoed in the fact that his first publication from Argentina was on cortical ontogeny during the first trimester of gestation (Jakob 1899), and one of his last books (Jakob et al. 1945) dealt with human embryology.

Flechsig (1896, 1898) had argued that 'illness of association areas is what, above all, produces mental diseases and thus forms the true object of psychiatry', agreeing with an earlier theoretical conjecture by Wernicke that mental diseases constitute alterations of association systems (Keegan 2003). Ramón y Cajal (1904, 1906, 1995) describes, following the groundwork by von Monakow, Déjerine, Siemerling, Vogt and others, that all the areas claimed by Flechsig to be association are connected with lower centers by way of projection fibers, a fact later acknowledged by Flechsig as well. Cajal hypothesizes the existence of three varieties of cortical areas (bilateral *perception*, and unilateral *primary* and *secondary mnemonic* areas), all of which issue centrifugal fibers: perception areas receive afferents from the thalamus, and mnemonic areas receive input from cortical perception areas. Cajal stands by Vogt's stance that the association area theory cannot adequately explain psychological mechanisms, and emphasizes that attempts to localize cognitive phenomena at 'privileged areas' amount to pursuing a chimera. In Cajal's view, intellectual operations result from the combined activity of multiple primary and secondary mnemonic areas (Ramón y Cajal 1904, 1906, 1995).

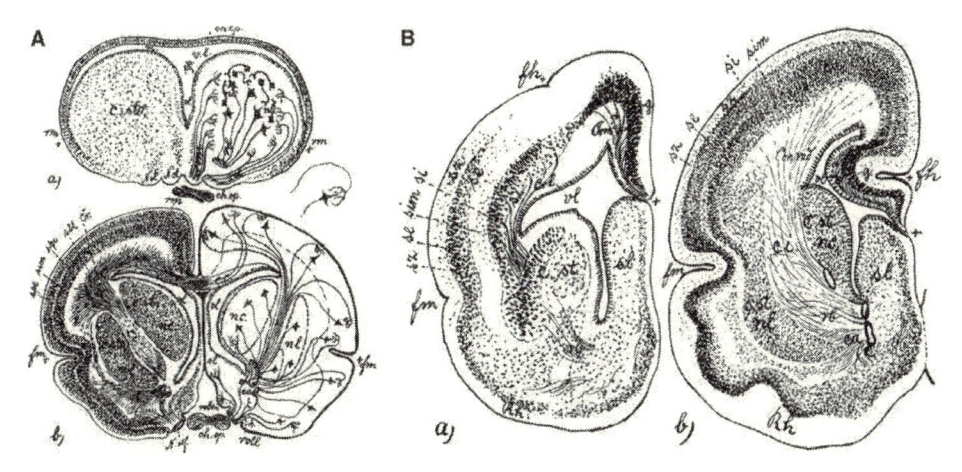

Fig. 6 a Coronal sections in a fish (*a*) and a mammal (*b*). The corpus striatum (*c str*) is robust, whereas the hemispheric mantle (pallium) appears as a thin ependymal membrane (*mep*) over the lateral ventricles (*vl*). From Jakob and Onelli (1911, p. 6), (1913, p. 15); field (A)/(*a*) also used by von Economo and Koskinas (1925). **b** Coronal sections of the cerebral hemispheres in the apod reptile *Amphisbaena darwini* (*a*) and the marsupial *Didelphis azarae* (*b*). The striatum (*c st*) appears robust. The thin pallium encloses the lateral ventricles (*vl*) dorsally; neurons are seen in the archipallium (*g*). These cells originate in the lateral band of the striatum and form the inner fundamental layer (*si*). The outer fundamental layer (*se*) grows over *si*. Therefore, *se* derives from the rhinencephalon (*Rh*) and later merges with *si*, which is derived from the striatum. *fm* marginal sulcus, *sz* molecular layer, *sim* intermediate layer, *fh* hippocampal sulcus, *g* fascia dentata, *ci* internal capsule, *sl* septum pellucidum, *nc* caudate nucleus, *nl* lenticular nucleus, *cor rad* corona radiata, *rb* radiatio basalis. From Jakob (1911, p. 38), (1911, p. 12), (1913, p. 14); also used by von Economo and Koskinas (1925)

In discoursing his evolutionary postulate of *progressive cerebration*, von Economo (1929) credits Jakob [and Onelli (1911)] for rightfully pointing out that the human organism 'is freed from the primitive and coarse law of the simple reflex; external stimuli no longer lead to a simple reflex, but, depending on past experiences, a different ingredient is obtained, whereby that simple reflex is finally converted to a process bearing the individual characters of the personality.'

A perspective from Jakob's intellectual progeny

Outes (2006) notes that Luys (1876), Nissl (1908) and Ariëns Kappers (1909) were forerunners of the idea that individual cortical layers may have discrete functions: Luys (1876) could be the first anatomist to think that each cortical layer has an individual and specific function. Thalamocortical connections were studied with the method of retrograde degeneration for the first time by Nissl (1908), who reflected on the meaning of each layer rather than cytoarchitectonics. Nissl (1908) suggested the existence of two parallel and superimposed cortical layers and attributed a distinct function to each one, the lower layer being concomitantly effector and receptive, and the upper fundamental psychic.

Jakob claimed that the entire cortex was receptive, against the views of Flechsig (1896, 1898), who, on the basis of his myelogenetic studies, had concluded that the primary association areas of the cortex did not project or receive any fibers.

Studying phylogeny, Ariëns Kappers (1909) suggested that the cortex is divided into an upper layer, with a receptive–psychic function, and a lower layer, with effector function, based on the finds that (1) the reptilian archicortex contains massive granule cells, almost double in number than pyramidal cells; (2) the forebrain of lower mammals shows a substantial increase of pyramidal cells in the hippocampus (archicortex), an area assuming projection and association functions; (3) the formation of an olfactory-mental field (subicular zone) in the mammalian hippocampus coincides with the appearance of a large number of pyramidal cells in the supragranular layer.

Ariëns Kappers (1909) further cited neuropathological data, such as those of Siebenmann and Bing (1907) who had reported reduced thickness of the lower layers in the auditory cortex of a deaf patient, and von Monakow (1905), who had made a similar observation in a case of deafness with lesions of the internal capsule. Thus, Ariëns Kappers (1909) concludes that 'the subgranular layers depend on the local subcortical system, whereas supragranular layers mostly depend on interregional associations with neighboring and distant cortical zones.' Supragranular pyramidal cells are the last to appear ontogenetically (Mott 1907) and would have association functions of a higher order (Ariëns Kappers 1909). That idea was later

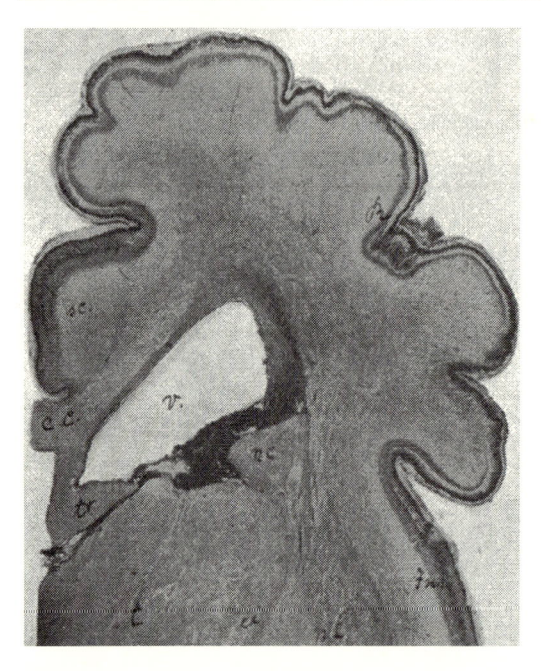

Fig. 7 Cerebral anlage of a human embryo at the beginning of the fifth month of gestation. von Economo and Koskinas (1925) discuss the cortical cell arrangement in a double layer, explaining that the 'fetal bilaminar type' corresponds to the two 'fundamental layers' of Jakob (1911), a trend seen in the human fetal brain and in the animal line, whereby the mixed 'sensorimotor function' of the entire human cortex is rooted. *cc* corpus callosum, *sc* supracallosal gyrus, *R* central sulcus, *ci* internal capsule, *nc* caudate nucleus, *nl* lentiform nucleus, *t* thalamus, *v* lateral ventricle. From Jakob (1911, p. 38)

developed by Kleist (1926, 1934), for whom the robust growth of layer III is typical of 'psychic' centers.

In a later schematic depiction of the cortex of *Lacerta* by Kuhlenbeck (1922), the neocortex or lateral cortex does not appear as bilaminar, and its lower parts seem to be in continuation with the corpus striatum (epistriatum); the lateral part of Ammon's horn is placed beneath the neocortex, at a position that could correspond to Jakob's inner layer (Outes and Benítez 1976; Outes 2006). Bilamination of the lateral cortex or primitive neocortex is more marked in the Amphisbaena (Jakob 1918) (Fig. 5).

Neuroanatomical and morphofunctional considerations

von Economo and Koskinas (1923) discovered that cortical areas known to be involved in sensory functions exhibit a homogeneous layering and a robust layer IV. The idea that sensory areas can be structurally distinguished from motor and association areas by the 'dusty' appearance of *koniocortex* is considered as one of Economo's major contributions to neuroscience (Marburg 1932). von Economo and Koskinas (1925) relied on Jakob's views, who had defined the inner cortical layers as effector and the outer as receptive (Marburg 1932). von Economo (1926) further showed that receptive areas only occupy the wall and sulcus floor of a gyrus and not the dome, a notion he subsequently used to explain the pattern formation of gyri.

von Economo and Koskinas (1925) devote a segment of their *Textband* to discussing the ideas of Jakob (1911; Jakob and Onelli 1911) and conclude that 'the future will show whether Jakob's novel and basic ideas on the fundamental layers and sector development will prove correct' (Figs. 6, 10, 11). An English translation of the corresponding section can be found in Seldon and Szirko (2005).

According to Meyer (1982), the concept of the 'sensorimotor' cortex, which has remained a problem for a century, is attributed to Munk (1881) by Mott (1894), with an early contribution by Bechterew (Bechterew and Meyer 1978). Flechsig (1896) understood that idea as an almost reflex-like unity between sensory and motor cortical function. Poliak (1932), Foerster (1936), Penfield and Boldrey (1937) and Penfield and Rasmussen (1950) resumed the idea of the sensorimotor cortex on the grounds of motor and somatosensory responses from both the postcentral and precentral gyrus. Another relevant point is that isolated giant cells of Betz, typically associated with motor function, spread over layer V from the giant pyramidal precentral area (FA_γ) to the giant pyramidal (PA) and intermediate (PC) postcentral areas, which are normally associated with sensorimotor function (von Economo and Koskinas 2008; von Economo 2009). The overwhelming majority of neurons that make up the brain and spinal cord, in fact all but motor neurons, cannot be classified as either sensory or motor in the strict sense (Nauta and Karten 1970).

A vindication of Jakob's views is echoed in *Gray's Anatomy* (Warwick et al. 1973): 'Even the simpler differentiation of the cortex into *sensory* areas receiving afferent projection fibres and *motor* areas projecting efferents—the remainder being regarded as 'silent' or *associational*—can no longer be considered appropriate, being itself an inaccurate over-simplification. Evidence has accumulated during the last three decades to show that the areas receiving or originating projection fibres are much more extensive than the initial classical studies indicated. Furthermore, the division into *receiving* and *originating* projection areas is by no means so distinct as first appeared… It is hence more appropriate to speak of the pre- and post-central areas as being *sensory–motor*; and since a mixture of afferent and efferent connections has been shown to exist also in respect to the projection fibres of the acoustic and visual *sensory* areas, they also are more accurately described as sensory–motor in character … It is this afferent–efferent character of most, and probably all, the sensory–motor areas which

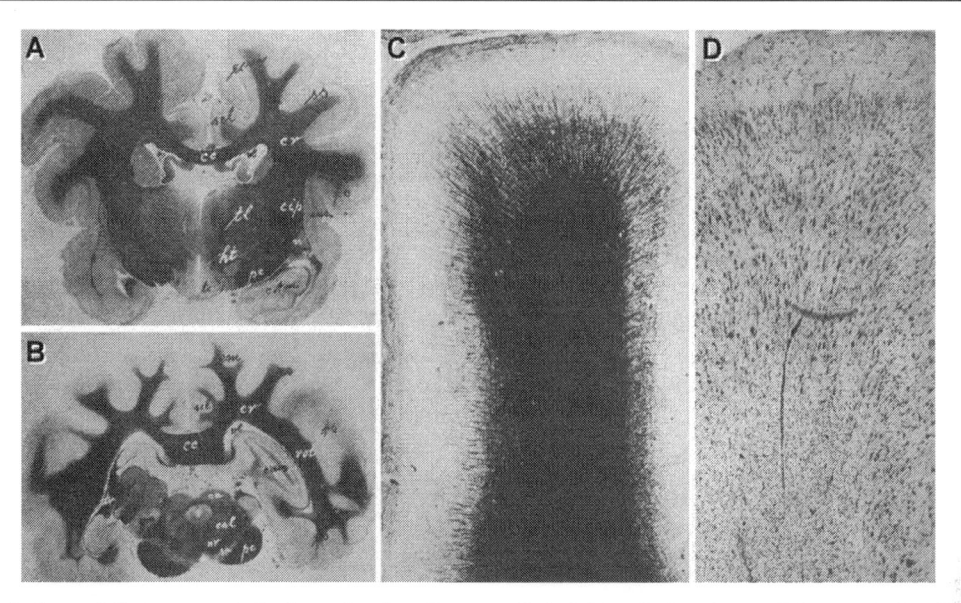

Fig. 8 Cerebrum of *Tapirus terrestris* ('tapir americano'). **a** Posterocapsular section of anterior cerebrum. Weigert method ×3/4. From Jakob (1941, p. 263). **b** Section through the knee of the corpus callosum. Weigert method ×2/3. From Jakob (1941, p. 263). **c** Cortical fibers. Prefrontal gyrus. Weigert method ×100. From Jakob and Onelli (1913, Plate 47.3). **d** Insular cortex. Nissl stain ×75. From Jakob and Onelli (1913, Plate 25.3)

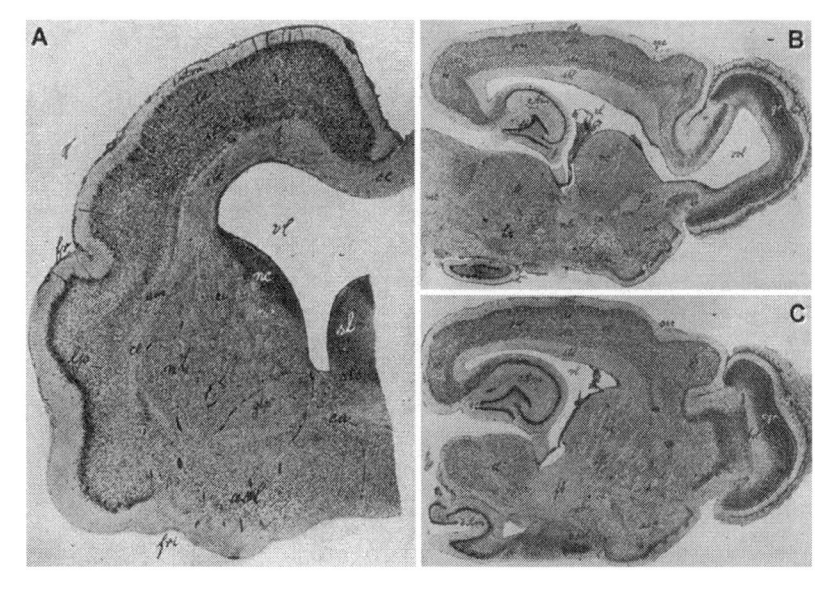

Fig. 9 Cerebrum of the hedgehog or *Erinaceus europaeus* ('erizo'). **a** Left hemisphere with neocortical divisions; the claustrum (*am*) continues upwards into the internal pyramidal layer. Nissl stain ×40. From Jakob (1941, p. 129). **b** Midsagittal section through the cerebral hemisphere, with the olfactory lobe. The neopallium continues toward Ammon's horn (*cAm*). At the base one distinguishes the olfactory (*aol*) and parolfactory (*apol*) areas, caudate nucleus (*nc*), fasciculus (*fb*) of nucleus basalis (*nb*), thalamus (*t*) and hypothalamus (*ht*). Nissl stain ×25. From Jakob (1941, p. 131). **c** A more lateral section. The capsular radiation (*rfb*) traverses the striatum in disseminated fascicles. The Ammonic zone (*zam*) is continuous with the inner cortical layer of Ammon's horn (*cAm*). Nissl stain ×25. From Jakob (1941, p. 131)

Fig. 10 Septal projection pathways (reptile) and lateral projection pathways (mammal) (Jakob and Onelli 1913, p. 26)

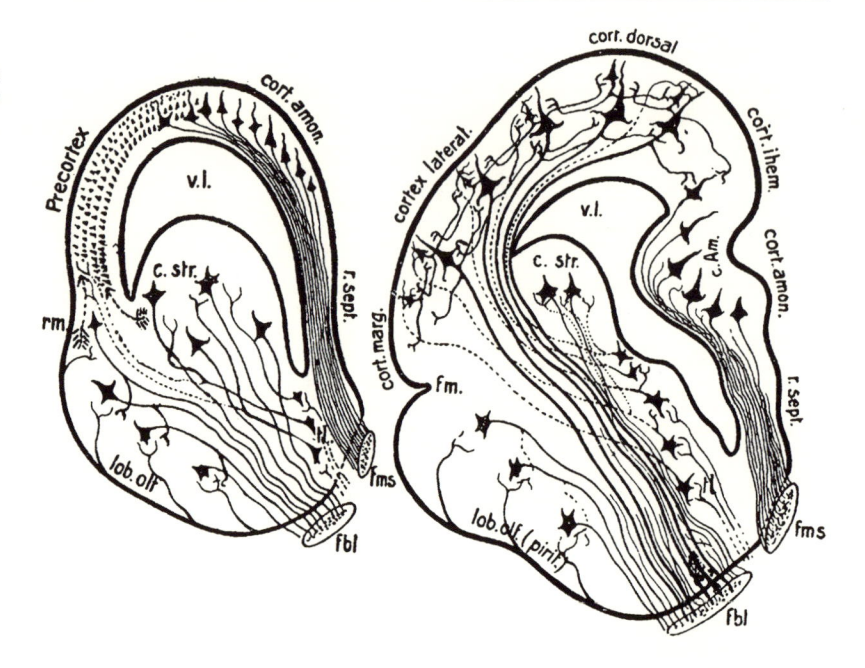

makes the concept of distinguishable motor and sensory parts of the cortex anatomically invalid and functionally misleading. It is clear from the above remarks that much less of the cerebral cortex remains to be dubbed as *associational*, in the vague but well-established meaning of the term.'

The term 'motor' is understood today as a function controlling movements via corticobulbar and corticospinal tracts, and it cannot be accepted, e.g. for the function of layer V neurons in V1 projecting to other cortical or subcortical areas (e.g., the lateral geniculate nucleus). The use of the term 'sensory–motor' by Jakob is more restricted and focused, otherwise all output systems are motoric and all input systems sensoric. Such an inflation of terminology might make the content of Jakob's idea cloudy in a modern context. Therefore, the terms 'effector' and 'receptive' are used to convey what he probably had in mind.

Tracing studies in mice indicate an overlap of neuron populations with simultaneous projections to both somatosensory and frontal association cortical areas, suggesting a widespread pattern of sensory–motor and premotor integration (Mitchell and Macklis 2005). The transcription factor *COUP-TFI* (or *Nr2f1*) appears to be necessary for balancing neocortical patterning, through a repression of motor (frontal) area identities and a specification of sensory (parietal and occipital) area identities (Armentano et al. 2007).

Kaas (1999) suggests that complex brains evolved from simpler brains not by adding vast amounts of general-purpose association cortex, but by expanding hierarchies to include additional areas for sensory processing and motor control; he bases his reasoning on the detection of multiple sensory and motor areas in what was once thought to be 'association cortex' territory in the cat, and the finding that sensory and motor representations occupy most of the neocortex in small-brain mammals.

Mounting evidence on the neural underpinnings of cognition supports the notion that neocortical operations are essentially multisensory at all levels of cortical processing, against an older view that senses operate independently (Ghazanfar and Schroeder 2006). Traditionally, it has been assumed that the integration of different kinds of sensory information in the cortical parenchyma was the task of specialized, higher-order association areas to produce a unified, coherent representation of the outside world. In contrast to such an assumption, recent data (reviewed by Ghazanfar and Schroeder 2006) suggest that much, if not all, of the neocortex is multisensory, which deviates us from the validity of probing the brain unimodally in addressing cognitive aspects, from development to social cognition.

The modern synthesis of functional evolution–development

The disciplines of evolutionary and developmental biology have operated separately for most of the twentieth century;

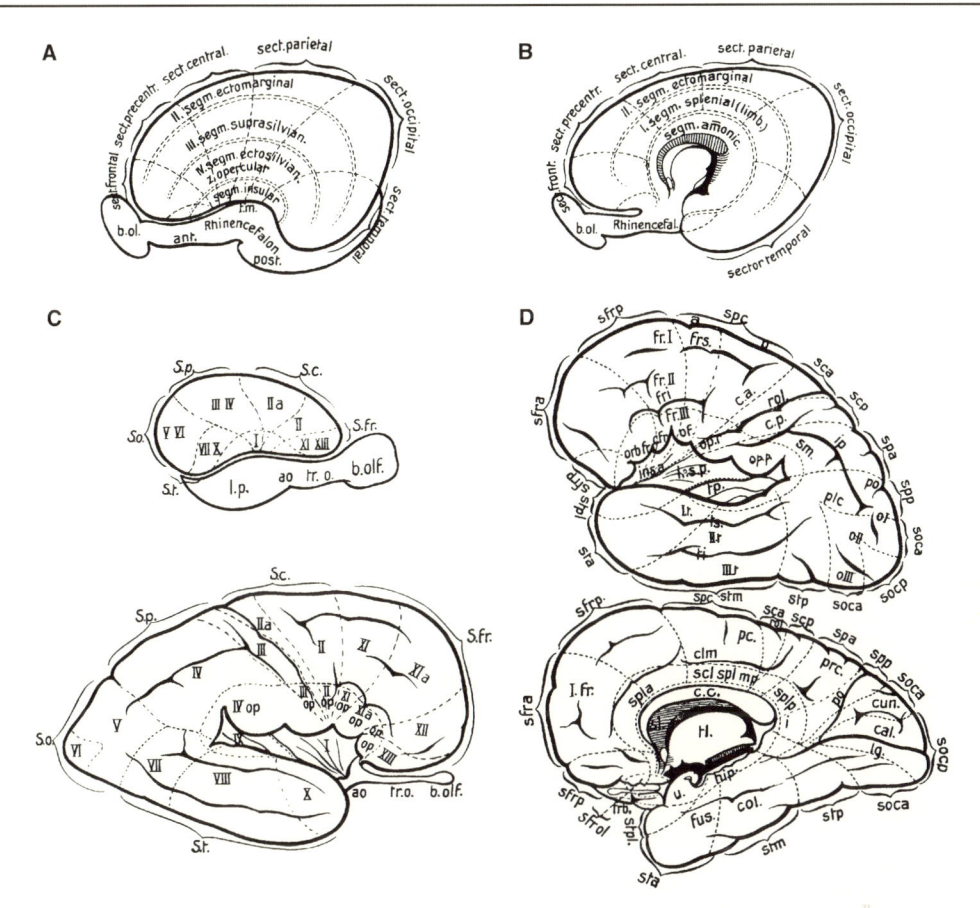

Fig. 11 a Lateral and **b** midsagittal facies depicting the hemispheric sector formation in the cerebral surface of a lissencephalic animal. The fan-shaped development of sectors and segments is shown in an anteroposterior direction. The insula forms the rotation point of such a growth. Jakob suggested the development of four sagittal cortical 'pre-gyri', laterally to Ammon's formation. He designated them as (*I*) gyrus splenialis or limbicus, where he places the *visceral cortex*, (*II*) the *bodily axis–hindlimb zone* located between the splenial and ectomarginal sulci, (*III*) the *forelimb zone* between the ectomarginal and suprasylvian sulci, and (*IV*) the *facio-mandibulo-lingual zone* between the suprasylvian and marginal sulci. The formation of these 'segments' has its origin in the base of the marginal sulcus, the insular area of higher mammals. From Jakob (1911, p. 33); Jakob and Onelli (1911, p. 19), (1913, p. 18); field (A) also used by von Economo and Koskinas (1925). **c** Sector formation in the cerebral hemispheric surface of a lissencephalic mammal (*upper*) and the gyrencephalic human brain (*lower*). The temporal lobe is pushed downwards and forward with the fan-shaped growth, whereas the occipital lobe is displaced caudally. From Jakob (1911, p. 34); Jakob and Onelli (1911, p. 20); Jakob and Onelli (1913, p. 18); figures also used by von Economo and Koskinas (1925). **d** Jakob's concept of sector formation in the human cerebral hemispheres (lateral and midsagittal views) in greater detail. From Jakob and Onelli (1911, p. 9), (1913, p. 36). Jakob considered the 'development of sectors' as the most important principle in the organization of the cerebral cortex, already noted in the brains of lower vertebrates such as edentates. He thus explained regional variations in cortical cytoarchitectonics, which he ascribed to five 'pre-sectors' and their sector partitions—frontal (with five partitions), central (three), parietal (three), occipital (two), and temporal (five)—as well as a robust 'subsector conformation'. The entire cortical mantle was viewed as a system of similarly constructed radiating sectors in a fan-shaped form, with their tip oriented towards the insula, and their expansions towards the upper hemispheric edge. Based on the pattern of fiber growth, he reckoned that sectors possess centripetal virgate parts in their coronae, with centrifugal segments consistently appearing only in certain areas across species. Jakob suggested that all sectors are receptively active, serving simultaneously both projection and association functions, and rejected the separation of the cortex into independent projection and association areas. For detailed reviews of these concepts, see Triarhou and del Cerro (2006a, b) and Triarhou (2008a, 2009)

some visionaries recognized this fact, but lacked the means for a conceptual and experimental synthesis (Raff et al. 1999).

The role of development as an evolutionary factor is currently studied in the context of 'Evolutionary Developmental Biology', with the discovery of the conservation of genes with prominent roles in development, and with a focus on developmental mechanisms that generate new variation (Raff 1996; Carroll 2005). A main goal is to understand how developmental mechanisms influence evolution and how such mechanisms evolved (Butler 1999). A comprehensive understanding of crucial evolutionary modifications of development with features of complete ontogenies, as opposed to static adult morphogenesis, is necessary, whereby multiple fields must be brought together into an interdisciplinary synthesis, seeking an integrated science of biological form (Raff et al. 1999).

An understanding of adaptive evolution requires the use of the entire conceptual spectrum, particularly the fusion of functional aspects with evolution and development (Breuker et al. 2006). One argument is that in many instances, evolution–development has emphasized a structural and partly historical perspective, without systematically addressing function. Therefore, Breuker et al. (2006) argue that the link to function is essential in gaining an integrated view of the role of development in evolution.

Phylogenetic considerations

Brain organization has been studied more in mammalian than in non-mammalian species, one reason being the fact that neuroanatomy received an early impetus from the neuropsychiatric clinic (Nauta and Karten 1970).

Brodmann (1909, 2006) described the comparative anatomy and cytoarchitecture of the cerebral cortex in numerous mammalian orders, from the hedgehog—with its unusually large archipallium—up to non-human primate and human brains; he introduced terms such as *homogenetic* and *heterogenetic formations* to denote two different basic cortical patterns, which, respectively, are either derived from the basic six-layer type or do not demonstrate the six-layer stage. Brodmann was intrigued by the phylogenetic increase in the number of cytoarchitectonic cortical areas in primates, and was astute in pointing out the phenomenon of phylogenetic regression as well (Striedter 2005). Vogt and Vogt (1919) laid the foundations of fiber pathway architecture; they defined the structural features of allocortex, proisocortex, and isocortex, and extensively discussed the differences between paleo-, archi-, and neo-cortical regions (Vogt and Vogt 1919; Vogt 1927; Zilles 2006).

The growth of the cortex by intercalation has been considered fairly well established (von Bonin 1963), in line with the neocortical evolutionary idea of Dart (1934) on a dual origin from hippocampal and prepiriform regions and an intercalation of newer parts between phylogenetically older parts.

Combining cyto- and myelo-architectonics, Sanides (1962, 1964) placed emphasis on transition regions (*Gradationen*) that accompany 'streams' of neocortical regions coming from paleo- and archi-cortical sources (Pandya and Sanides 1973). [Vogt and Vogt (1919) had already spoken of 'areal gradations'.] The idea of a 'koniocortex core' and 'prokoniocortex belt areas' in the temporal operculum (Pandya and Sanides 1973) was modified by Kaas and Hackett (1998, 2000), who speak of histologically and functionally distinct 'core', 'belt' and 'parabelt' subdivisions in the monkey auditory cortex, with specified connections.

While there are still open questions regarding the evolutionary origin of the mammalian neocortex, comparative studies indicate that at least three pallial subdivisions—lateral (olfactory), dorsal and medial (hippocampal)—characterized the roof of the cerebral hemispheres of earliest vertebrates (Northcutt and Kaas 1995). The forebrain of early mammals was dominated by an olfactory bulb, and the olfactory (piriform) cortex appeared large relative to the small amount of neocortex; in reptiles, the dorsal cortex—homolog of the mammalian neocortex—is proportionally almost as large in surface as the neocortex of early mammals, but thinner, comprising mainly a single pyramidal layer (Kaas 2008).

To adequately explain the evolution of the mammalian neocortex, an understanding of correlative changes in surrounding areas of the telencephalic pallium and subpallium, close neighbors in a common morphogenetic field and postulated sources of certain cortical neuron subsets, is deemed necessary (Puelles 2001). The developmental evidence that cells originating in a compartment corresponding to the dorsal ventricular ridge (DVR) become included in structures generated in a compartment corresponding to isocortex could reconcile the proposed evolutionary homology between the reptilian/avian DVR and mammalian isocortex (Aboitiz 1999).

The evidence seems to favor a correspondence of isocortex with the dorsal cortex of reptiles (Fig. 12b): sensory projections that terminate in the ventral pallium of reptiles end in the dorsal pallium (isocortex) of mammals, possibly owing to their phylogenetic participation in associative networks between dorsal, olfactory, and hippocampal cortices subserving spatial or episodic memory in early mammals (Aboitiz et al. 2003).

The mammalian neocortex is characterized by an inside-out developmental neurogenetic gradient, with deep layer neurons being born earlier than superficial layer neurons, whereas the reptilian cortex originates in a reverse, outside-in gradient (Goffinet et al. 1986; Aboitiz 1993; Aboitiz et al. 2002). The older, inferior layers (V–VI) of the mammalian isocortex resemble reptilian cortical cells in morphology, neurotransmitter signatures and subcortical connections, while the younger superficial layers (II–IV) exhibit their own local and corticocortical connections (Aboitiz et al. 2002).

It was suggested that the neocortex has resulted from a translocation of large neuronal masses, which in ancestral forms occupied subcortical stations, in particular the region of the external striatum (Nauta and Karten 1970). The superior and temporal neocortices in particular appear to resemble, from a phylogenetic viewpoint, the dorsal cortex and the DVR in reptiles, and the Wulst (a territory at the transition between the dorsalmost zone of the external striatum, or hyperstriatum, and the pallial mantle, characterized by a clearly defined layer of granule cells) and the DVR in the avian forebrain, respectively (Nauta and Karten 1970; Shimizu and Karten 1991; Reiner 2000). The lateral pallium of amphibians, reptiles and birds may be homologous to the hexalaminar cortex of mammals (Northcutt 1981); its expansion has been viewed as associated with a displacement of the hippocampal formation (archicortex) and the piriform cortex (paleocortex) toward the medial telencephalic wall (Rakic and Kornack 2001). The cytoarchitectonically continuous cortical plate (with a medial/dorsomedial hippocampal portion and a more dorsal portion) and the subcortical DVR form two portions of the pallium that are relevant to neocortical evolution in modern turtles (Reiner 2000).

The term 'dorsal ventricular ridge' was originally introduced by Johnston (1915) as a descriptive label (Lohman and Smeets 1991). Half a century earlier, Hunter (1861) had described in the lateral ventricle of reptiles the prominent eminence that would eventually bear his name: Hunter's eminence was viewed by many neuroanatomists during the early part of the twentieth century, perhaps including Jakob, as homologous to the basal ganglia of the mammalian brain (Fig. 12), thence the general application of the term 'striatum' to this structure (Lohman and Smeets 1991). Elliot Smith (1919) divided it into hypopallium, paleostriatum and amygdaloid complex; Ariëns Kappers et al. (1936) into neostriatum, paleostriatum and archistriatum; in modern usage, it comprises the DVR, the striatum and the amygdaloid complex (Lohman and Smeets 1991).

On the other hand, the three longitudinal cortical zones comprised mediodorsal, dorsal and lateral cortex (Edinger 1896), *Ammonsrinde*, dorsal and lateral cortex (Unger 1906), hippocampal, dorsal and piriform cortex (Goldby

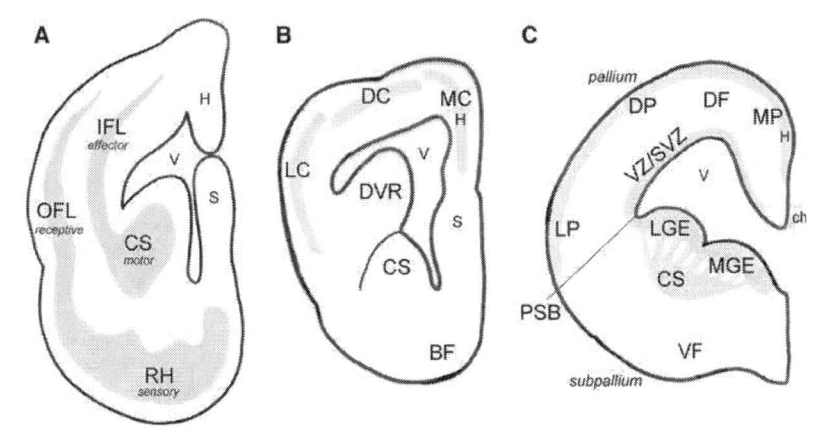

Fig. 12 **a** A summary of Jakob's idea on the dual onto-phylogenetic origin and ubiquitous function of the cerebral cortex, adapted from López Pasquali (1965, p. 30). Jakob mentions that the outer and inner cortical layers, respectively 'derive' from the rhinencephalon and the striatum (Jakob and Onelli 1911, p. 37); although the word 'migration' is not mentioned explicitly, the verb 'derive' logically implies that this is what he had in mind (Outes 2006). *CS* corpus striatum, *H* hippocampus (Ammon's horn), *IFL* inner fundamental layer, *OFL* outer fundamental layer, *RH* rhinencephalon, *S* septal nucleus, *V* lateral cerebral ventricle. **b** Modern view of forebrain phylogeny, shown in the reptilian cerebral hemisphere. The thin lateral cortex (*LC*) arises by radial migration from the lateral ependyma, whereas the dorsal ventricular ridge (*DVR*)—whose marked protrusion into the lateral ventricle led to being erroneously thought for a long time as homologous to the basal ganglia of the human brain—arises through the ventrolateral migration of neurons from the ependyma of the ventrolateral wall of the cerebral ventricle (Karten 1997). *BF* basal forebrain, *DC* dorsal cortex, *MC* medial cortex. Drawing based on Northcutt and Kaas (1995), Karten (1997), Tissir et al. (2002), and Aboitiz and Montiel (2007). **c** Modern view of mammalian forebrain ontogeny. The lateral ganglionic eminence (*LGE*) gives rise to the striatum (*CS*), and the medial ganglionic eminence to the globus pallidus; the medial pallium (*MP*) gives rise to the hippocampus, the lateral pallium (*LP*) to olfactory cortex, and the ventral pallium to the claustro-amygdaloid complex (Aboitiz and Montiel 2007). In the human forebrain, interneurons originate both in the ganglionic eminence and the ventricular (*VZ*) and subventricular (*SVZ*) zones. *ch* cortical hem, *DF* dorsal forebrain, *DP* dorsal pallium, *PSB* pallial-subpallial boundary, *VF* ventral forebrain. Drawings based on Northcutt and Kaas (1995), Karten (1997), Tissir et al. (2002), Aboitiz and Montiel (2007) and Rakic (2009)

1934), fascia dentata, Ammon's formation/general cortex and piriform cortex (Curwen 1937), and medial, dorsal and lateral cortex in modern usage (Lohman and Smeets 1991).

Although the consideration that the neocortex is elaborated from the rhinencephalon (Ariëns Kappers et al. 1936) is no longer tenable, it is conjectured that in primitive mammals the origin of the cerebral cortex was triggered, in a context of adaptation to nocturnal life, by the development of the olfactory system (Aboitiz 1992).

Herrick (1924), who acknowledges the contribution of Jakob and Onelli (1911) to the anatomy of the olfactory region in the opossum, emphasizes the large olfactory bulb that is connected with the remainder of the cerebral hemisphere by a distinct olfactory crus; in the latter, superficial cells assume a cortical cellular type, namely, piriform cortex laterally and anterior hippocampal cortex medially, which in turn extend forward in contact with the bulbar formation.

One puzzle was the striking discrepancy between the relatively small pallium and large striatum in sauropsids, and the apparent inverse ratios of large areas of pallium and only moderate amounts of striatum in mammals (Karten 1969). Nauta and Karten (1970) hypothesized that two distinct populations of founder cells contribute to cortical formation in mammals. One possibility is that DVR neuroblasts of ancient reptiles shifted into the lateral pallium and provided additional cells for the hexalaminar neocortex; the 'external striatum' of reptiles and birds is absent as such from mammals, which, conversely, feature a 'neocortex' in the pallial mantle (Nauta and Karten 1970; Rakic and Kornack 2001). Experiments in mouse chimeras support a dual origin, and further suggest that the two phylogenetically distinct populations stay segregated during development as the separate laminar and radial clones in the mammalian cerebral cortex (Kuan et al. 1997).

The resolution of the evolutionary origins of the neocortex, which has long puzzled anatomists, requires analyses of both developing and adult brains (Karten 1991). Studies in the mature reptilian and avian brain have clarified some basic questions on the origin of the neocortex, which can be viewed as consequent to two events: (1) The elaboration of constituent neuronal populations and their associated connections that are common to the telencephalon of non-mammalian and mammalian amniotes: such populations are found within the neocortex in mammals, whereas most of them are seen within the DVR and the dorsolateral ventricular ridge (DLVR) in reptiles and birds. (2) In mammals, the components of the DVR and DLVR are incorporated into the thin overlying pallium to form a laminated 'neocortex' (Karten 1991).

An onto-phylogenetic comparison of pallial organization indicates that the lateral cortex of reptiles is homologous to the avian and mammalian piriform cortex; the anterior DVR of reptiles is probably homologous to the neostriatum and ventral hyperstriatum of birds and to the endopiriform nucleus of mammals, whereas the posterior DVR of reptiles is most likely homologous to the archistriatum of birds and the mammalian amygdala; the dorsal cortex of reptiles is probably homologous to mammalian isocortex (Striedter 1997).

Multiple evolutionary origins of the neocortex have been proposed, based on its separation into the precursors of non-laminar and laminar regions; ancestral reptiles and proto-mammals have been thought of possessing discrete populations that were the precursors of cells of the SVZ of mammals and the DVR of non-mammalian amniotes (Shimizu and Karten 1991). Migratory routes may follow a mediolateral course from the DVR–SVZ in reptiles, and a lateral and dorsolateral course in mammals (Shimizu and Karten 1991).

In all, two major modern hypotheses have been proposed to explain the origin of the mammalian cortex (reviewed by Northcutt and Kaas 1995): the 'out-group hypothesis' holds that the DVR of living reptiles and birds and the isocortex of mammals are 'homoplastic' structures, representing independent transformations of the ancestral pallium. The 'recapitulation hypothesis' rejects the validity of the cerebral hemispheres of living amphibians as an appropriate out-group, and postulates that an additional pallial subdivision (the DVR) existed in the common ancestor of terrestrial vertebrates; thus, the presence of a DVR represents the primitive or ancestral condition, which has been retained in living reptiles and birds, while the mammalian isocortex arose by a dual differentiation of the dorsal cortex and a migration of the cells of the DVR. In that case, the DVR and the dorsal cortex of reptiles are viewed as homologous to the mammalian isocortex owing to the single transformation in one radiation.

Sauropsida (reptiles and birds) have a trilaminar dorsal cortex (corresponding to layers I, V and VI in mammals), whereas metatheria (marsupials) possess six-layer cortices; a SVZ—which appears to have emerged prior to the eutherian–metatherian split—may not be required for the generation of a hexalaminar cortex in all mammals, a clue supported by the absence of an organized SVZ in the South American gray short-tailed opossum (*Monodelphis domestica*) (Cheung et al. 2009).

Ontogenetic considerations

A dichotomy exists concerning the embryogenesis of the upper and the lower cortical layer in mammals (Fig. 12c), based on cytoarchitectonic and functional criteria, as well as axonal projections and gene expression.

Distinct neocortical neuron populations are generated within two spatially and molecularly segregated proliferative domains (Lai et al. 2008; Azim et al. 2009): progenitors of the dorsally located pallium positive for the transcription factor SOX6 give rise to excitatory projection neurons, whereas SOX5 positive progenitors of the ventrally located subpallium give rise to inhibitory interneurons (such an expression pattern becomes reversed in postmitotic neurons).

The deep cortical or infragranular layers (V–VI) are formed by early-generated neurons, born from dividing neuronal precursors at the ventricular zone (VZ). The upper cortical or supragranular layers (II–IV) derive from late-generated neurons, born through mitotic divisions of intermediate progenitor cells at the subventricular zone (SVZ) (Parnavelas et al. 2000; Molnár et al. 2006; Cheung et al. 2007; Noctor et al. 2007; Abdel-Mannan et al. 2008; Cubelos et al. 2008). Descending projection pathways to subcortical targets mainly arise from pyramidal neurons of the deep cortical layers, whereas projection neurons of the upper cortical layers do not extend long corticofugal axons (Kwan et al. 2008). Corticofugal axons (including corticothalamic and corticospinal fibers) that extend from neurons in the deep cortical layers are guided through the internal capsule, possibly through the specification of neurons expressing the transcription factors *Nfla* and *Nflb* (Plachez et al. 2008).

Specific genes, such as the homeodomain transcription factor *Cux-2*, selectively control the proliferation rates of SVZ precursors and therefore the number of upper cortical neurons (Cubelos et al. 2008). On the other hand, the nuclear factor I gene product NFIB is predominantly expressed in corticofugal projection neurons of the deep cortical layers, V and VI (Plachez et al. 2008).

Cells from the lateral/ventral pallium migrate to the lateral ganglionic eminence (LGE) and a number of cells cortically derived from the *Emx1* progenitor lineage persist in the adult striatum, thus being a putative source of neural diversity in the ventral telencephalon (Cocas and Corbin 2008).

Conclusion

It would be conjectural, even anachronistic, to attempt to guess to which structures, based on our current knowledge and nomenclature, correspond the areas construed by Jakob as the elements of his onto-phylogenetic and morpho-functional ideas (Fig. 12). Could what he described as 'striatum' in the reptilian forebrain be, at least in part, the dorsal ventricular ridge? Or could the ganglionic eminence of the embryonic human brain be included in what he viewed as striatal domains?

From the point of view of Outes (2006), it appears logical to think that the inner cell layer is the last migratory stream toward the pia, overlapping with the striatal mass insofar as this is also the last stream of a sector more inferior to the telencephalic vesicle; all this might indicate a kinship between these two sectors, both originating by the same secondary migratory wave.

The new foci of comparative neurobiology (Striedter 1998) comprise (1) the integration of comparative and developmental neurobiology and genetics to test phylogenetic hypotheses at a mechanistic level; (2) the comparative morphology of neural circuits and their relation to physiology and behavior; and (3) phylogenetic analyses of independently evolved similarities to discover general rules on how neural systems operate and become modified in the course of evolution. Jakob's functional evolutionary–developmental integration seems to endure, a century later. Concepts from the classical bibliography may thus complement the sophisticated modern means in deciphering the structural–functional workings of the brain and its mind.

Acknowledgments The author gratefully acknowledges Michael C. Triarhou, LL.M., for invaluable help with the German language, Professor Karl Zilles for constructive criticism, Noelia Fiorentino of *La Prensa Médica Argentina*, Buenos Aires, for a copy of Jakob's 1916 article, and Dr. Daniel S. Margulies for Jakob's biography by López Pasquali.

References

Abdel-Mannan O, Cheung AFP, Molnár Z (2008) Evolution of cortical neurogenesis. Brain Res Bull 75:398–404

Aboitiz F (1992) The evolutionary origin of the mammalian cerebral cortex. Biol Res 25:41–49

Aboitiz F (1993) Further comments on the evolutionary origin of the mammalian brain. Med Hypotheses 41:409–418

Aboitiz F (1999) Comparative development of the mammalian isocortex and the reptilian dorsal ventricular ridge: evolutionary considerations. Cereb Cortex 9:783–791

Aboitiz F, Montiel J (2007) Origin and evolution of the vertebrate telencephalon, with special reference to the mammalian neocortex. Adv Anat Embryol Cell Biol 193:1–112

Aboitiz F, Montiel J, Morales D, Concha M (2002) Evolutionary divergence of the reptilian and the mammalian brains: considerations on connectivity and development. Brain Res Rev 39:141–153

Aboitiz F, Morales D, Montiel J (2003) The evolutionary origin of the mammalian isocortex: towards an integrated developmental and functional approach. Behav Brain Sci 26:535–552

Ariëns Kappers CU (1909) The phylogenesis of the paleocortex and archicortex compared with the evolution of the visual neocortex. Arch Neurol Psychiatry (Lond) 4:161–173

Ariëns Kappers CU, Huber GC, Crosby EC (1936) The comparative anatomy of the nervous system of vertebrates, including man, 2 vols. Hafner, New York

Armentano M, Chou SJ, Tomassy GS, Leingärtner A, O'Leary DD, Studer M (2007) *COUP-TFI* regulates the balance of cortical patterning between frontal/motor and sensory areas. Nat Neurosci 10:1277–1286

Azim E, Jabaudon D, Fame RM, Macklis JD (2009) SOX6 controls dorsal progenitor identity and interneuron diversity during neocortical development. Nat Neurosci 12:1238–1247

Bechterew W, Meyer A (1978) The concept of a sensorimotor cortex: its early history, with especial emphasis on two early experimental contributions by W. Bechterew. Brain 101:673–685

Breuker CJ, Debat V, Klingenberg CP (2006) Functional evo-devo. Trends Ecol Evol 21:488–492

Brodmann K (1909) Vergleichende Lokalisationslehre der Großhirnrinde. J. A. Barth, Leipzig

Brodmann K (2006) Localisation in the cerebral cortex. Springer Science, New York (translated by L. J. Garey)

Butler AB (1999) Whence and whither cortex? Trends Neurosci 22:332–334

Carroll SB (2005) Endless forms most beautiful: the new science of evo devo. Norton, New York

Cheung AFP, Pollen AA, Tavare A, De Proto J, Molnár Z (2007) Comparative aspects of cortical neurogenesis in vertebrates. J Anat 211:164–176

Cheung AF, Kondo S, Abdel-Mannan O, Chodroff RA, Sirey TM, Bluy LE, Webber N, Deproto J, Karlen SJ, Krubitzer L, Stolp HB, Saunders NR, Molnár Z (2009) The subventricular zone is the developmental milestone of a 6-layered neocortex: comparisons in metatherian and eutherian mammals. Cereb Cortex Sep 2. (Epub ahead of print). doi:10.1093/cercor/bhp168

Cocas LA, Corbin JG (2008) Embryonic *Emx1+* progenitor cells generate diverse neural subtypes in the mature striatum. In: Fishell G, Kriegstein AR, Parnavelas JG (eds) Cortical development: stem cells, neurogenesis, migration, circuit formation, cortical disorders. Mediterranean Agronomic Institute, Crete, pp 43–44 (abstract)

Cubelos B, Sebastián-Serrano A, Kim S, Moreno-Ortiz C, Redondo JM, Walsh CA, Nieto M (2008) *Cux-2* controls the proliferation of neuronal intermediate precursors of the cortical subventricular zone. Cereb Cortex 18:1758–1770

Curwen AO (1937) The telencephalon of *Tupinambis nigropunctatus*. I. Medial and cortical areas. J Comp Neurol 66:375–404

Dart RA (1934) The dual structure of the *neopallium*: its history and its significance. Anat Rec 69:1–19

Edinger L (1896) Untersuchungen über die vergleichende Anatomie des Gehirns. III. Neue Studien über das Vorderhirn der Reptilien. Abh Senckenb Naturforsch Gesch 19:313–388

Elliot Smith G (1919) A preliminary note on the morphology of the corpus striatum and the origin of the neopallium. J Anat (Lond) 53:271–291

Flatau E, Jacobsohn L (1899) Handbuch der Anatomie und vergleichenden Anatomie des Centralnervensystems der Säugetiere. Karger, Berlin

Flechsig P (1896) Gehirn und Seele. Veit and Comp, Leipzig

Flechsig P (1898) Études sur le cerveau. Vigot Frères, Paris (trad. L. Levi)

Foerster O (1936) Motorische Felder und Bahnen: sensible corticale Felder. In: Bumke O, Foerster O (eds) Handbuch der Neurologie, vol 6. Springer, Berlin, pp 1–448

Fontana H, Belziti H, Requejo F (2002) El espacio perforado anterior y zonas aledañas. Consideraciones funcionales. Parte I. Rev Argent Neurocirug 16:1–11

Gans C (1966) Studies on amphisbaenids (Amphisbaenia, Reptilia). 3. The small species from Southern South America commonly identified as *Amphisbaena darwini*. Bull Am Mus Nat Hist 134:185–260

Ghazanfar AA, Schroeder CE (2006) Is neocortex essentially multisensory? Trends Cogn Sci 10:278–285

Goffinet AM, Daumerie C, Langerwerf B, Pieau C (1986) Neurogenesis in reptilian cortical structures: [^{3}H]-thymidine autoradiographic analysis. J Comp Neurol 243:106–116

Goldby F (1934) The cerebral hemispheres of *Lacerta viridis*. J Anat (Lond) 68:157–215

Herrick CJ (1924) The nucleus olfactorius anterior of the opossum. J Comp Neurol 37:317–359

Hunter J (1861) Essays and observations on natural history, anatomy, physiology, psychology and geology. van Voorst, London

Jakob C (1895) Atlas des gesunden und kranken Nervensystems nebst Grundriss der Anatomie, Pathologie und Therapie desselben. Lehmann, München

Jakob C (1898) An atlas of the normal and pathological nervous systems, together with a sketch of the anatomy, pathology, and therapy of the same. Baillière Tindall and Cox, London (translated by J. Collins)

Jakob C (1899) Sobre el desarrollo de la corteza cerebral. Rev Soc Méd Argent 7:397–403

Jakob C (1910a) La célula cortical en la locura (Estudios histopatológicos sobre las células piramidales en las enfermedades mentales). Anales de la Administración Sanitaria y Asistencia Pública: Ediciones de La Semana Médica. Imprenta de E. Spinelli, Buenos Aires, pp 263–267

Jakob C (1910b) La histoarquitectura comparada de la corteza cerebral y su significación para la psicología moderna. Argent Méd (B Aires) 8:437–438

Jakob C (1911) Das Menschenhirn: Eine Studie über den Aufbau und die Bedeutung seiner grauen Kerne und Rinde. Lehmann, München

Jakob C (1912a) Über die Ubiquität der senso-motorischen Doppelfunktion der Hirnrinde als Grundlage einer neuen, biologischen Auffassung des corticalen Seelenorgans. J Psychol Neurol (Leipz) 19:379–382

Jakob C (1912b) Ueber die Ubiquität der senso-motorischen Doppelfunktion der Hirnrinde als Grundlage einer neuen biologischen Auffassung des kortikalen Seelenorgans. Münch Med Wochenschr 59:466–468

Jakob C (1913) La psicología orgánica y su relación con la biología cortical. Arch Psiquiatr Criminol (B Aires) 12:680–698

Jakob C (1914) El lenguaje de los animales. Rev Jard Zool B Aires (Época II) 10:129–135

Jakob C (1916) Sobre la existencia simultánea de una doble función sensomotriz de la corteza cerebral come base de una nueva concepción biológica del órgano psíquico cortical. Prensa Méd Argent 2:305–307

Jakob C (1918) La filogenia cortical: sobre la corteza cerebral de gimnofiones y anfisbenas argentinas (abstract). Actas Trab 1er Congr Nacl Med (B Aires) 1:82

Jakob C (1939a) El cerebro humano: su anatomía sistemática y topográfica (Folia Neurobiológica Argentina, Atlas I). López, Buenos Aires

Jakob C (1939b) El cerebro humano: su anatomía patológica en relación a la clínica (Folia Neurobiológica Argentina, Atlas II). López, Buenos Aires

Jakob C (1941) El cerebro humano: su ontogenía y filogenía (Folia Neurobiológica Argentina, Atlas III). López, Buenos Aires

Jakob C (1945) El yacaré (*Caimán latirostris*) y el origén del neocortex: estudios neurobiológicos y folklóricos del reptil más grande de la Argentina (Folia Neurobiologica Argentina, Tomo IV). López, Buenos Aires

Jakob C, Onelli C (1911) Vom Tierhirn zum Menschenhirn: vergleichend morphologische, histologische und biologische Studien zur Entwicklung der Grosshirnhemisphären und ihrer Rinde. Lehmann, München

Jakob C, Onelli C (1913) Atlas del cerebro de los mamíferos de la República Argentina: estudios anatómicos, histológicos y biológicos comparados sobre la evolución de los hemisferios y de la corteza cerebral. Kraft, Buenos Aires

Jakob C, Jakob A, Pedace EA (1945) El embrión humano, folleto III: el proceso real de la gastrulación en un embrión con dos somitos. López, Buenos Aires

Johnston JB (1915) The cell masses in the forebrain of the turtle *Cistudo carolina*. J Comp Neurol 25:393–468
Kaas JH (1999) The transformation of association cortex into sensory cortex. Brain Res Bull 50:425
Kaas JH (2008) The evolution of the complex sensory and motor systems of the human brain. Brain Res Bull 75:384–390
Kaas JH, Hackett TA (1998) Subdivisions of auditory cortex and levels of processing in primates. Audiol Neurootol (Basel) 3:73–85
Kaas JH, Hackett TA (2000) Subdivisions of auditory cortex and processing streams in primates. Proc Natl Acad Sci USA 97:11793–11799
Kaes T (1907) Die Grosshirnrinde des Menschen in ihren Massen und in ihrem Fasergehalt: ein gehirnanatomischer Atlas mit erläuterndem Text und schematische Zeichnung. Fischer, Jena
Karten HJ (1969) The organization of the avian telencephalon and some speculations on the phylogeny of the amniote telencephalon. Ann NY Acad Sci 167:164–179
Karten HJ (1991) Homology and evolutionary origins of the 'neocortex'. Brain Behav Evol 38:264–272
Karten HJ (1997) Evolutionary developmental biology meets the brain: the origins of mammalian cortex. Proc Natl Acad Sci USA 94:2800–2804
Keegan E (2003) Flechsig and Freud: late 19th-century neurology and the emergence of psychoanalysis. Hist Psychol 6:52–69
Kleist K (1926) Die einzeläugigen Gesichtsfelder und ihre Vertretung in den beiden Lagen der verdoppelten inneren Körnerschicht der Sehrinde. Klin Wochenschr 5:3–10
Kleist K (1934) Gehirnpathologie. Barth, Leipzig
Kuan C, Elliott EA, Flavell RA, Rakic P (1997) Restrictive clonal allocation in the chimeric mouse brain. Proc Natl Acad Sci USA 94:3374–3379
Kuhlenbeck H (1922) Über den Ursprung der Großhirnrinde: eine phylogenetische und neurobiotaktische Studie. Anat Anz (Jena) 55:337–365
Kwan KY, Lam MM, Krsnik Ž, Kawasawa YI, Lefebvre V, Šestan N (2008) SOX5 postmitotically regulates migration, postmigratory differentiation, and projections of subplate and deep-layer neocortical neurons. Proc Natl Acad Sci USA 105:16021–16026
Lai T, Jabaudon D, Molyneaux BJ, Azim E, Arlotta P, Menezes JR, Macklis JD (2008) SOX5 controls the sequential generation of distinct corticofugal neuron subtypes. Neuron 57:232–247
Lohman AHM, Smeets WJA (1991) The dorsal ventricular ridge and cortex of reptiles in historical and phylogenetic perspective. In: Finlay BL, Innocenti G, Scheich H (eds) The neocortex: ontogeny and phylogeny. Plenum Press, New York, pp 59–74
López Pasquali L (1965) Christfried Jakob: su obra neurológica, su pensamiento psicológico y filosófico. López Libreros Editores S.R.L.–Talleres Gráficos de La Prensa Médica Argentina, Buenos Aires
Lores Arnaiz MR, Borrego Maturana F, Azzara S (2002) Las ideas de Christofredo Jakob sobre mapa cortical y functiones superiores. Rev Hist Psicol 23:9–36
Luys J-B (1876) Le cerveau et ses fonctions. Baillière, Paris
Marburg O (1932) Konstantin Economo Freiherr von San Serff. Dtsch Z Nervenheilk 123:219–229
Meyer L (1981) Cristofredo Jakob: a veinticinco años de su muerte. Acta Psiquiátr Psicol Amér Lat 27:13–14
Meyer A (1982) The concept of a sensorimotor cortex: its later history during the twentieth century. Neuropathol Appl Neurobiol 8:81–93
Meynert T (1872) Der Bau der Gross-Hirnrinde und seine örtlichen Verschiedenheiten, nebst einem pathologisch-anatomischen Corollarium. Heuser, Leipzig
Mitchell BD, Macklis JD (2005) Large-scale maintenance of dual projections by callosal and frontal cortical projection neurons in adult mice. J Comp Neurol 482:17–32
Molnár Z, Métin C, Stoykova A, Tarabykin V, Price DJ, Francis F, Meyer G, Dehay C, Kennedy H (2006) Comparative aspects of cerebral cortical development. Eur J Neurosci 23:921–934
Mott FW (1894) The sensory motor functions of the central convolutions of the cerebral cortex. J Physiol 15:464–487
Mott FW (1907) The progressive evolution of the structure and functions of the visual cortex in mammalia. Arch Neurol Pathol Lab Lond 3:1–48
Moyano BA (1957) Christfried Jakob (25/12/1866–6/5/1956). Acta Neuropsiquiátr Argent 3:109–123
Munk H (1881) Über die Funktionen der Großhirnrinde. Gesammelte Mitteilungen aus den Jahren 1877–1880, mit Einleitung und Anmerkungen. Hirschwald, Berlin
Nauta WJH, Karten HJ (1970) A general profile of the vertebrate brain, with sidelights on the ancestry of cerebral cortex. In: Schmidt FO (ed) The neurosciences second study program. Rockefeller University Press, New York, pp 7–26
Nissl F (1908) Experimentalergebnisse zur Frage der Hirnrindeschichtung (38. Versammlung der Südwestdeutschen Irrenärzte, Heidelberg, 2.–3. November 1907). Mschr Psychiatr Neurol 23:186–188
Noctor SC, Martínez-Cerdeño V, Kriegstein AR (2007) Contribution of intermediate progenitor cells to cortical histogenesis. Arch Neurol 64:639–642
Northcutt RG (1981) Evolution of the telencephalon in nonmammals. Annu Rev Neurosci 4:301–350
Northcutt RG, Kaas JH (1995) The emergence and evolution of the mammalian neocortex. Trends Neurosci 18:373–379
Obersteiner H (1913) Die Kleinhirnrinde vom Elephas und Balaenoptera. Arb Neurol Inst (Wien) 20:145–154
Orlando JC (1966) Christofredo Jakob: su vida y obra. Editorial Mundi, Buenos Aires
Outes DL (2006) A medio siglo de la muerte de Christofredo Jakob, 1956–2006: fuentes de la concepción biológica de la doble corteza. Electroneurobiología (B Aires) 14:3–28
Outes DL, Benítez I (1976) Sobre el origen de la concepción biológica de la doble corteza: a veinte años de la muerte de Christofredo Jakob, 1956–1976. Rev Neurol Argent 1:220–228
Pandya DN, Sanides F (1973) Architectonic parcellation of the temporal operculum in rhesus monkey and its projection pattern. Z Anat Entwicklungsgesch 139:127–161
Papini MR (1988) Influence of evolutionary biology in the early development of experimental psychology in Argentina (1891–1930). Int J Exp Psychol 2:131–138
Parnavelas JG, Anderson SA, Lavdas AA, Grigoriou M, Pachnis V, Rubenstein JL (2000) The contribution of the ganglionic eminence to the neuronal cell types of the cerebral cortex. In: Bock GR, Cardew G (eds) Evolutionary developmental biology of the cerebral cortex. Wiley and Sons, Chichester, pp 129–139
Penfield W, Boldrey E (1937) Somatic motor and sensory representation in the cerebral cortex of man as studied by electrical stimulation. Brain 60:389–443
Penfield W, Rasmussen TB (1950) The cerebral cortex of man: a clinical study of localization of function. MacMillan, New York
Plachez C, Lindwall C, Sunn N, Piper M, Moldrich RX, Campbell CE, Osinski JM, Gronostajski RM, Richards LJ (2008) Nuclear factor I gene expression in the developing forebrain. J Comp Neurol 508:385–401
Poliak SL (1932) The main afferent fiber systems of the cerebral cortex in primates. University of California Press, Berkeley, pp 107–207
Puelles L (2001) Thoughts on the development, structure and evolution of the mammalian and avian telencephalic pallium. Phil Trans R Soc Lond (Biol) 356:1583–1598
Raff RA (1996) The shape of life: genes, development, and the evolution of animal form. University of Chicago Press, Chicago

Raff RA, Arthur W, Carroll SB, Coates MI, Wray G (1999) Chronicling the birth of a discipline. Evol Dev 1:1–2

Rakic P (2007) The radial edifice of cortical architecture: from neuronal silhouettes to genetic engineering. Brain Res Rev 55:204–219

Rakic P (2009) Evolution of the neocortex: a perspective from developmental biology. Nat Rev Neurosci 10:724–735

Rakic P, Kornack DR (2001) Neocortical expansion and elaboration during primate evolution: a view from neuroembryology. In: Falk D, Gibson KR (eds) Evolutionary anatomy of the primate cerebral cortex. Cambridge University Press, Cambridge, pp 30–56

Ramón y Cajal S (1895) Algunas conjeturas sobre el mecanismo anatómico de la ideación, asociación y atención. Rev Med Cirug Práct (Madr) 19:497–508

Ramón y Cajal S (1899) The sensori-motor cortex. In: Story WE, Wilson LN (eds) Clark University 1889–1899 decennial celebration. Norwood Press, Norwood, MA, pp 311–382

Ramón y Cajal S (1904) Textura del sistema nervioso del hombre y de los vertebrados, tomo II, secunda parte. Moya, Madrid, pp 1121–1152

Ramón y Cajal S (1906) Studien über die Hirnrinde des Menschen, 5. Heft. Barth, Leipzig, pp 41–79 (übers. von J Bresler)

Ramón y Cajal S (1995) Histology of the nervous system of man and vertebrates, vol. II. Oxford University Press, New York, pp 707–729 (translated by N. Swanson and L.W. Swanson)

Ranke O (1911) Bücheranzeigen und Referate: Chr. Jakob und Cl. Onelli, Vom Tierhirn zum Menschenhirn; Chr. Jakob, Das Menschenhirn. Münch Med Wochenschr 58:2510–2512

Reiner AJ (2000) A hypothesis as to the organization of cerebral cortex in the common amniote ancestor of modern reptiles and mammals. In: Bock GR, Cardew G (eds) Evolutionary developmental biology of the cerebral cortex. Wiley and Sons, Chichester, pp 83–108

Sammet K (2006) Wilhelminian myelinated fibers—Theodor Kaes, myeloarchitectonics and the asylum Hamburg-Friedrichsberg 1890–1910. J Hist Neurosci 15:56–72

Sanides F (1962) Die Architektonik des menschlichen Stirnhirns. Springer, Berlin

Sanides F (1964) The cyto-myeloarchitecture of the human frontal lobe and its relation to phylogenetic differentiation of the cerebral cortex. J Hirnforsch 47:269–282

Seldon HL, Szirko M (2005) The comments on Professor Christfried Jakob's contributions made in *Die Cytoarchitektonik der Hirnrinde des erwachsenen Menschen* by Constantin von Economo and Georg N. Koskinas (1925). Electroneurobiología (B Aires) 13:46–73

Shimizu T, Karten HJ (1991) Multiple origins of neocortex: contributions of the dorsal ventricular ridge. In: Finlay BL, Innocenti G, Scheich H (eds) The neocortex: ontogeny and phylogeny. Plenum Press, New York, pp 75–86

Siebenmann F, Bing H (1907) Über den Labyrinth- und Hirnbefund bei einem an Retinitis pigmentosa erblindeten Angeboren-Taubstummen. Z Ohrenheilk (Wiesb) 54:265–280

Siemerling E (1911) Referat: Chr. Jakob und Cl. Onelli, Vom Tierhirn zum Menschenhirn; Chr. Jakob, Das Menschenhirn. Arch Psychiatr Nervenkrankh (Berl) 49:353–355

Striedter GF (1997) The telencephalon of tetrapods in evolution. Brain Behav Evol 49:179–213

Striedter GF (1998) Progress in the study of brain evolution: from speculative theories to testable hypotheses. Anat Rec (New Anat) 253:105–112

Striedter GF (2005) Principles of brain evolution. Sinauer Associates, Sunderland, MA

Tissir F, Lambert de Rouvroit C, Goffinet AM (2002) The role of reelin in the development and evolution of the cerebral cortex. Braz J Med Biol Res 35:1473–1484

Triarhou LC (2008a) Centenary of Christfried Jakob's discovery of the visceral brain: an unheeded precedence in affective neuroscience. Neurosci Biobehav Rev 32:984–1000

Triarhou LC (2008b) Christfried Jakob's 1911 proposition on the dual onto-phylogenetic origin and ubiquitous sensory-motor function of the cerebral cortex (abstract). In: Fishell G, Kriegstein AR, Parnavelas JG (eds) Cortical development: stem cells, neurogenesis, migration, circuit formation, cortical disorders. Mediterranean Agronomic Institute, Crete, pp 89–90

Triarhou LC (2008c) The books of Christofredo Jakob: lasting treasures of evolutionary neuroscience (abstract). Soc Neurosci Abstr 38:221.16

Triarhou LC (2009) Tripartite concepts of mind and brain, with special emphasis on the neuroevolutionary postulates of Christfried Jakob and Paul MacLean. In: Weingarten SP, Penat HO (eds) Cognitive psychology research developments. Nova Science Publishers, Hauppauge, NY, pp 183–208

Triarhou LC, del Cerro M (2006a) Semicentennial tribute to the ingenious neurobiologist Christfried Jakob (1866–1956). 1. Works from Germany and the first Argentina period, 1891–1913. Eur Neurol 56:176–188

Triarhou LC, del Cerro M (2006b) Semicentennial tribute to the ingenious neurobiologist Christfried Jakob (1866–1956). 2. Publications from the second Argentina period, 1913–1949. Eur Neurol 56:189–198

Unger L (1906) Untersuchungen über die Morphologie und Faserung des Reptiliengehirns. Anat Hefte 31:271–341

Vogt O (1927) Architektonik der menschlichen Hirnrinde. Zbl Gesamte Neurol Psychiatr 45:510–512

Vogt C, Vogt O (1919) Allgemeinere Ergebnisse unserer Hirnforschung. J Psychol Neurol (Leipz) 25:279–461

von Bonin G (1963) The evolution of the human brain. University of Chicago Press, Chicago

von Economo C (1926) Die Bedeutung der Hirnwindungen. Allg Z Psychiatr Psych-Gerichtl Med 84:123–132

von Economo C (1929) Der Zellaufbau der Grosshirnrinde und die progressive Cerebration. Ergebn Physiol 29:83–128

von Economo C (2009) Cellular structure of the human cerebral cortex. Karger, Basel (translated and edited by L. C. Triarhou)

von Economo C, Koskinas GN (1923) Die sensiblen Zonen des Großhirns. Klin Wochenschr 2:905

von Economo C, Koskinas GN (1925) Die Cytoarchitektonik der Hirnrinde des erwachsenen Menschen. Textband und Atlas. Springer, Wien

von Economo C, Koskinas GN (2008) Atlas of cytoarchitectonics of the adult human cerebral cortex. Karger, Basel (translated, revised and edited by L. C. Triarhou)

von Monakow C (1905) Gehirnpathologie, zweite Aufl. Hölder, Wien

Warwick R, Williams PL, Bannister LH (1973) Neurology. In: Warwick R, Williams PL (eds) Grays' Anatomy, 35th edn. Longman, Edinburgh, pp 745–1169

Zardoya R, Meyer A (2001) On the origin of and phylogenetic relationships among living amphibians. Proc Natl Acad Sci USA 98:7380–7383

Zilles K (2006) Architektonik und funktionelle Neuroanatomie der Hirnrinde des Menschen. In: Förstl H, Hautzinger M, Roth G (eds) Neurobiologie psychischer Störungen. Springer Medizin, Heidelberg, pp 75–140

Zilles K, Welsch U, Schleicher A (1981) The telencephalon of *Ichthyophis paucisulcus* (Amphibia, Gymnophiona [= *Caecilia*]): a quantitative cytoarchitectonic study. Z Mikrosk-Anat Forsch (Leipz) 95:943–962

In: *Neuroanatomy Research Advances*
Editors: C.E. Flynn and B.R. Callaghan

ISBN 978-1-60741-610-4
© 2010 Nova Science Publishers

Final Publications of Christfried Jakob: On the Frontal Lobe and the Limbic Region

Lazaros C. Triarhou[*]

Economo–Koskinas Wing for Integrative and Evolutionary Neuroscience,
University of Macedonia, Thessaloniki, Greece;

Abstract

One of the foremost neuroanatomists of the twentieth century, Christfried (Christofredo) Jakob (1866–1956) left a legacy of over 30 monographs and 200 papers, now becoming appreciated in the English biomedical literature. Born in Germany, he was summoned in 1899 to Buenos Aires by the Argentinian psychiatric academia. He spent the rest of his professional life (save for a brief return to Germany between 1910–1912) in affiliation with the National Universities of La Plata and Buenos Aires. The writings of Jakob cover a wide spectrum of topics, from the pathology of neuropsychiatric disorders to the phylogeny, ontogeny and dynamics of the cerebral cortex and their mental corollaries, and ultimately some of the most fundamental neurophilosophical questions. Although in many respects his innovative ideas opened up new ways of thinking in brain and behavior research, they still remain largely unheeded, most likely owing to their exclusive appearance in German or Spanish. The present study revisits Jakob's last two formal publications, dating to 1949. These are entitled 'The task of the frontal lobe in connection with a synthetic quantification of its constitutive elements' and 'The neuronal quantification of the limbic region in its relation to the endogenous affective sphere' (co-authored with his pupils Eduardo A. Pedace and Andrés R. Copello, respectively), and represent the culmination of Jakob's thought, integrating morphofunctional concepts in his quest for understanding the neuroanatomical fundamentals of the human mind. Cognitive function and emotional processing are at the core of current neurobiological research, and Jakob's pioneering concepts remain worthy of consideration six decades later.

[*] E-mail address: triarhou@uom.gr, phone +30 2310 891-387, fax +30 2310 891-388 (Corresponding author)

Introduction

Christfried (Christofredo) Jakob (1866–1956) was a German-born neuropathologist, neurobiologist and neurophilosopher, who spent most of his professional life in Argentina. Having worked under Friedrich Albert von Zenker (1825–1898) and Adolf von Strümpell (1853–1925) at Erlangen and Bamberg, Germany, Jakob subsequently became affiliated with the Universities of La Plata and Buenos Aires, and established one of the most important neuropathological laboratories in South America. Jakob is considered the father of Argentinian neurobiology [Orlando, 1966; Outes, 2006; Triarhou & del Cerro, 2006a, 2006b].

Brief Exposé of Jakob's Work

Jakob has left an invaluable treasure of over 30 monographs and 200 articles, written in German or Spanish, spanning over a wide range of diverse scientific topics [Orlando, 1966; Outes, 2006; Triarhou & del Cerro, 2006a, 2006b; Triarhou, 2007]. He had already reached international renown through early successful atlases of human [Jakob, 1911a] and comparative neuroanatomy [Jakob & Onelli, 1911, 1913]. He later produced landmark works on cortical and evolutionary neurobiology, studying in detail the normal and pathological human nervous system, as well as dozens of the autochthonous species – some extinct today – found in the Patagonian fauna, including the broad-snouted 'yacaré' (*Caiman latirostris*), a reptile of the Alligatoridae family [Jakob, 1945], and the 'pichiciego' or fairy armadillo (*Chlamyphorus truncatus*), a mammal of the Dasypodidae family [Jakob, 1943a].

On a coarse recounting, Jakob beginnings have a positivistic Virchowian view, mixed with Herbertian philosophy. His positivism is refined until 1912, when some general ideas of his mentor Theodor Ziehen are provisorily adopted; these, in turn, become gradually rejected around 1930, when a mystic, yet positivistic, *Weltanschaaung* from his travels gives him a less Kantian, more admirative stance in front of the cosmos. Such a dominant *leitmotiv* leads him to a more Pythagorean worldview, introducing even proportions such as the *section aurea* in neuronal counting, which becomes very clear in his articles of the late 1940s. From 1949 to 1953 Jakob sketched his interests in unpublished anthropological notes [Crocco, 2008].

Jakob's Final Publications

Among Jakob's strongest interests were the human frontal lobes [Pedace, 1949] and the limbic system, particularly the anatomical bases of emotion [Orlando, 1964; Triarhou, 2008a, 2008b].

The two articles that follow are the first English translations of Jakob's last two published papers [Jakob & Pedace, 1949; Jakob & Copello, 1949]. This endeavour forms part of an ongoing effort to make available select landmark works by Jakob not hitherto available in the English biomedical literature. Besides their historical interest, these documents contain valuable scientific information, especially in view of the current interest in the frontal lobe and the limbic region, as well their structure and function under normal and pathological circumstances.

Reflecting a life's culmination in the thought of the 83-year-old neurobiologist, the papers were presented at the Third South American Congress of Neurosurgery in Buenos Aires, on April 3–9, 1949, with Professor Ramón Carrillo (1906–1956), the great Argentinian neurosurgeon and social policy officer – and a Jakob alumnus [Crocco, 2006; Ordóñez, 2004] – as General Secretary of the Congress.

The two papers give a summary of mostly quantitative neuroanatomical data on the cellular and axonal components of the human frontal lobe, cingulate (supracallosal) and hippocampal (inferior limbic) gyrus. For the sake of numerical comparisons, it is herein reiterated that Economo & Koskinas [1925] had estimated the total number of neurons in the cerebral cortex of both hemispheres at about 14×10^9 (6×10^9 being the smaller granule cells and 8×10^9 all the remaining larger neurons); the current estimate of the number of nerve cells in the human cerebral cortex stands at 20×10^9 [Pakkenberg & Gundersen, 1997].

Conclusion

Jakob's views on frontal lobe function evolved over half a century, from his early anatomical and neuropsychological papers [Jakob, 1906a, 1906b, 1910, 1911b], through the 'middle period' [Jakob, 1913a, 1913b, 1921, 1923], all the way to the late neurobiological [Jakob, 1939a, 1939b, 1941a, 1941b, 1941c, 1943b] and neurophilosophical [Jakob, 1946] synthetic treatises.

A detailed discussion of the older views and the current state of affairs regarding the anatomical components of the 'visceral brain' has been given elsewhere [Triarhou, 2008a], as has the evolutionary context of Jakob's ideas [Triarhou, 2008b].

Acknowledgements

The author gratefully acknowledges the courtesy of the National Library of Medicine, Bethesda, MD, and Staatsbibliothek Berlin, Germany.

References

Crocco, M. (2006). Breve biografía de Ramón Carrillo (1906–1956). *Electroneurobiología (Buenos Aires),* **14**, 173–186.

Crocco, M. (2008). Personal communication, December 17, 2008.

Economo, C. von, & Koskinas, G.N. (1925). *Die Cytoarchitektonik der Hirnrinde des Erwachsenen Menschen.* Wien–Berlin: Julius Springer.

Jakob, C. (1906a). Estudios biológicos sobre los lóbulos frontales cerebrales. *La Semana Médica (Buenos Aires),* **13**, 1375–1381.

Jakob, C. (1906b). La leyenda de los lóbulos frontales cerebrales como centros supremos psíquicos del hombre. *Archivos de Psiquiatría y Criminología (Buenos Aires)*, **5**, 678–699.

Jakob, C. (1910). La significación de la histoarquitectura comparada para la psicología moderna. *Revista del Jardín Zoológico de Buenos Aires*, **6**, 159–162.

Jakob, C. (1911a). *Das Menschenhirn: Eine Studie über den Aufbau und die Bedeutung seiner Grauen Kerne und Rinde. I. Teil. Tafelwerk nebst Einführung in den Organisationsplan der Menschlichen Zentralnervensystems.* München: J. F. Lehmann's Verlag.

Jakob, C. (1911b). La histoarquitectura comparada de la corteza cerebral y su significación para la psicología moderna. *Archivos de Psiquiatría y Criminología (Buenos Aires)*, **10**, 385–387.

Jakob, C. (1913a). La biología en el sistema de las ciencias filosóficas y naturales. *Anales de la Academia de Filosofía y Letras*, **2**, 55–67.

Jakob, C. (1913b). La psicología orgánica y su relación con la biología cortical. *Archivos de Psiquiatría y Criminología (Buenos Aires)*, **12**, 680–698.

Jakob, C. (1921). La teoría actual de las gnosias y praxias como factores fundamentales en el dinamismo de la corteza cerebral. *Crónica Médica (Lima)*, **38**, 17–24.

Jakob, C. (1923). *Elementos de Neurobiología, vol. I: Parte Teórica.* La Plata, Argentina: Facultad de Humanidades y Ciencias de la Educación de la Universidad Nacional de La Plata.

Jakob, C. (1939a). *Folia Neurobiológica Argentina, Atlas I – El Cerebro Humano: Su Anatomía Sistemática y Topográfica.* Buenos Aires: Aniceto López.

Jakob, C. (1939b). *Folia Neurobiológica Argentina, Atlas II – El Cerebro Humano: Su Anatomía Patológica en Relación a la Clínica.* Buenos Aires: Aniceto López.

Jakob, C. (1941a). *Folia Neurobiológica Argentina, Atlas III – El Cerebro Humano: Su Ontogenía y Filogenía.* Buenos Aires: Aniceto López.

Jakob, C. (1941b). *Folia Neurobiológica Argentina, Tomo I. Neurobiología General.* Buenos Aires: Aniceto López.

Jakob, C. (1941c). La función psicogenética de la corteza cerebral y su posible localización. *Anales del Instituto de Psicología de la Facultad de Filosofía y Letras de la Universidad de Buenos Aires*, **3**, 63–80.

Jakob, C. (1943a). *Folia Neurobiológica Argentina, Tomo II. El Pichiciego (Chlamydophorus Truncatus): Estudios Neurobiológicos de un Mamífero Misterioso de la Argentina.* Buenos Aires: Aniceto López.

Jakob, C. (1943b). *Folia Neurobiológica Argentina, Tomo III. El Lóbulo Frontal: Un Estudio Monográfico Anatomoclínico sobre Base Neurobiológica.* Buenos Aires: Aniceto López.

Jakob, C. (1945). *Folia Neurobiológica Argentina, Tomo IV. El Yacaré (Caimán latirostris) y el Origen del Neocortex: Estudios Neurobiológicos y Folklóricos del Reptil más Grande de la Argentina.* Buenos Aires: Aniceto López.

Jakob, C. (1946). *Folia Neurobiológica Argentina, Tomo V. Documenta Biofilosófica, Folleto I. Biología y Filosofía.* Buenos Aires: López y Etchegoyen.

Jakob, C., & Copello, A.R. (1949). La cuantificación neuronal de la región limbica en su relación con la esfera introyental afectiva. *Archivos de Neurocirugía*, **6**, 475–481.

Jakob, C., & Onelli, C. (1911). *Vom Tierhirn zum Menschenhirn: Vergleichend Morphologische, Histologische und Biologische Studien zur Entwicklung der Grosshirnhemisphären und ihrer Rinde.* München: J. F. Lehmann's Verlag.

Jakob, C., & Onelli, C. (1913). *Atlas del Cerebro de los Mamíferos de la República Argentina: Estudios Anatómicos, Histológicos y Biológicos Comparados sobre la Evolución de los Hemisferios y de la Corteza Cerebral*. Buenos Aires: Guillermo Kraft.

Jakob, C., & Pedace, E.A. (1949). La misión del lóbulo frontal frente a una cuantificación sintética de sus elementos productores. *Archivos de Neurocirugía*, **6**, 467–474.

Ordóñez, M.A. (2004). Ramón Carrillo, el gran sanitarista Argentino. *Electroneurobiología (Buenos Aires)*, **12**, 144–147.

Orlando, J.C. (1964). Sobre el cerebro visceral. Documentación histórica de una prioridad científica. *Revista Argentina de Neurología y Psiquiatría*, **1**, 197–201.

Orlando, J.C. (1966). *Christofredo Jakob: Su Vida y Obra*. Buenos Aires: Editorial Mundi.

Outes, D.L. (2006). A medio siglo de la muerte de Christofredo Jakob, 1956–2006: Fuentes de la concepción biológica de la doble corteza. *Revista Electroneurobiología (Buenos Aires)*, **14**, 3–35.

Pakkenberg, B., & Gundersen, H.J.G. (1997). Neocortical neuron number in humans: effect of sex and age. *Journal of Comparative Neurology*, **384**, 312–320.

Pedace, E.A. (1949). Contribución de la Escuela Neurobiológica Argentina del Profesor Chr. Jakob en el estudio del lóbulo frontal. *Archivos de Neurocirugía*, **6**, 464–466.

Triarhou, L.C. (2007). Christofredo Jakob as a naturalist: the 1923 scientific voyage aboard HSDG *Cap Polonio* to La Tierra del Fuego. *Electroneurobiología (Buenos Aires)*, **15**, 61–116.

Triarhou, L.C. (2008a). Centenary of Christfried Jakob's discovery of the visceral brain: an unheeded precedence in affective neuroscience. *Neuroscience and Biobehavioral Reviews*, **32**, 984–1000.

Triarhou, L.C. (2008b). Tripartite concepts of mind and brain, with special emphasis on the neuroevolutionary postulates of Christfried Jakob and Paul MacLean. In: S. P. Weingarten, & H. O. Penat (Eds.), *Cognitive Psychology Research Developments*. Hauppauge, NY: Nova Science Publishers (in press).

Triarhou, L.C., & del Cerro, M. (2006a). Semicentennial tribute to the ingenious neurobiologist Christfried Jakob (1866–1956). 1. Works from Germany and the first Argentina period, 1891–1913. *European Neurology*, **56**, 176–188.

Triarhou, L.C., & del Cerro, M. (2006b). Semicentennial tribute to the ingenious neurobiologist Christfried Jakob (1866–1956). 2. Publications from the second Argentina period, 1913–1949. *European Neurology*, **56**, 189–198.

In: *Neuroanatomy Research Advances*
Editors: C.E. Flynn and B.R. Callaghan

ISBN 978-1-60741-610-4
© 2010 Nova Science Publishers

The Task of the Frontal Lobe in Connection with a Synthetic Quantification of its Constitutive Elements[1]

Christofredo Jakob and Eduardo A. Pedace
Service of Pathological Anatomy, Hospital Nacional de Alienadas, Buenos Aires

Introduction

The frontal lobes represent 25% of the human brain, i.e. about 350–370 g of cerebral mass, but reflect the latest acquisitions in the ascending neurophylogeny. These facts, solely considered from a quantitative standpoint, must alone testify to the higher task of their cortical functions. In them, contrary to the *cognitive orientation* of the experiences achieved by the individual and reserved for the other lobes of the cerebral hemispheres, we recognize the centers of experiential accumulation resulting from the personal *"intervention"*, progressively elaborated for the elemental and highest human skills, stimulated by the corresponding emotional manifestations.

Both zones, in close gnosio-praxic collaboration, execute the conscious activation of human mentality in its creative labor from the concrete to the abstract in an intimate synthesis between their endogenous and exogenous domains, i.e. from their affectivity and intellectuality, reciprocally.

It now becomes imperative, given the complexity of its structure, to extend in detail the radius of action of our quantitative knowledge directly towards the neuronal elements that intervene in its game of cortico-intercortical and subcortical focalization, projection and

---

[1] An English translation of 'La misión del lóbulo frontal frente a una cuantificación sintética de sus elementos productores,' originally published in *Actas del Tercer Congreso Sudamericano de Neurocirugía* (Buenos Aires, April 3–9, 1949), *Archivos de Neurocirugía*, vol. VI, no. 1–4, pp. 467–474 [Jakob & Pedace, 1949]; translated and edited from the Spanish text by L.C. Triarhou* with the help of A.B. Vivas.

* E-mail address: triarhou@uom.gr, phone +30 2310 891-387, fax +30 2310 891-388 (Corresponding author)

association (Figs. 1–5). Only in this way can we penetrate into the intimacy of its real psychogenetic dynamics. These data will speak clearer than what any graphic diagram or reproduction is capable of achieving: if vegetative vital phenomena rest on the principle of labor division among numerous collaborating units, this must be even more so in the case of cerebral operations, whose high degree of differentiation increasingly necessitates a greater affluence of cellular and axonal elements. The quantitative factor is the basis for every qualitative process resulting from the creations of such multiplying collaborations, since without capital of work there are no benefits, neither in the material nor in the ideal. Like all the other lobes, the frontal lobe has 'autochthonous' [intrinsic] focal elements (capital proper) as well; in addition, it requires the 'transfocal' [intermediary] systems of correlation (circulating capital), whose numerical capacity we will address in the following order:

(1) *Afferent and efferent axonal systems* of cortico-subcortical charge and discharge.

(2) *Cortico-pyramidal focal systems* of commemorative accumulation in its afferent and efferent layers.

(3) Short, semi-long, and long ipsilateral and contralateral *transcortical association systems*.

Afferent and Efferent Axonal Quantification

(a) The frontal afferent systems derive in their majority (more than 95%) from the thalamus, originating in its anterior one-third; the rest being of olfactory origin (medial frontobasal olfactory pathways), do not present any major interest, as they have been dealt with in various publications [Jakob, 1943].

The thalamofrontal systems pass through the genu and anterior segment, better to say the anterior radiation of the internal capsule, splitting up as the frontal corona radiata between the four frontal gyri: the superior limbic (supracallosal at the median facies), the superior, middle and inferior frontal gyri, at the dorsolateral hemispheric facies); a remaining segment of the radiation reaches the anterior insular pole.

In total these axons represent the considerable amount of 4 million among a total of 19 million axons in the capsula, as compared to the 15 million axons for the remaining cortico-retrofrontal; thus the ratio of the frontal contingent to the other centro-parieto-occipito-temporal lobes is of 4:15. (As can be seen, in our study on the frontal lobe we exclude the anterior Rolandic region and its axons, which belong functionally to the praxic centers as opposed to the remaining cognitive.)

The task of the frontal thalamic avalanche is distributed in two portions: a medial limbic of 400,000 axons, and a lateral of 3,600,000, in round numbers. (The counts were effected in magnified microphotographs of sections treated with the axon silver impregnation technique.)

The medial or limbic portion is formed with the continuation of the mamillothalamic system (bundle of Vicq d'Azyr) and carries according to our studies commenced over 30 years ago (that little by little appear to be confirmed) viscerosympathetic sensitivity from the respective thoracic organs until the pelvic, towards the supracallosal cortex, creating in this way the basis for the elemental notions, so variable physiologically, of the vegetative malaise and well-being.

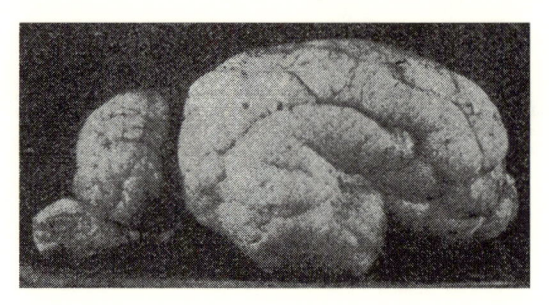

Fig. 1. Hemisphere of a sloth (*Bradypus tridactylus*, order *Edentata*) with its characteristic rotation and primordial segmentation system [Jakob & Pedace, 1949].

The lateral avalanche relays essentially the stimuli of the cerebello-rubro-thalamic radiation (superior hypothalamic radiation) and, with it, especially the cerebellar muscular sensitivity, further comprising other intercalated thalamic categories (its physiology represents still a very poor chapter in research).

The repartition of the afferent systems over the four frontal gyri is established approximately as follows (these numbers we consider nothing but an approximate orientation; their value is not absolute, but relative):

Superior limbic gyrus:	400,000 axons
Superior frontal gyrus:	1,600,000 axons
Middle frontal gyrus:	1,200,000 axons
Inferior frontal gyrus:	800,000 axons
Total:	4,000,000 axons

These afferent systems terminate as it is well known in the external pyramidal layer of the frontal cortex, a certain amount getting in through the tangential layer (possibly the phylogenetically oldest form according to the comparison with animal brains).

(b) The *frontal efferent* systems, corresponding to the first, can also be divided into two fascicles: medial and lateral. Both originate in the internal pyramidal layer, representing the medial portion, of superior limbic (supracallosal) origin via the limbic-tuberian tract with a total of 5,000 axons, that crossing through the corona radiata and its medial portion accompany the internal capsule, terminating little by little in the lateral paraependymal and tuberian sympathetic nuclei of the diencephalon (paleoneuronal sympathetic subcortical centers for the smooth-viscero-vascular musculature).

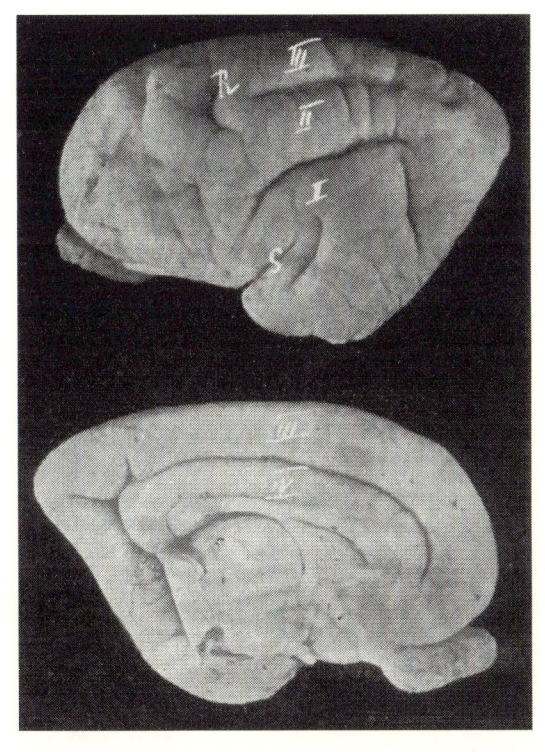

Fig. 2. Left hemisphere of a prosimian (*Cheiromys*) with its primordial gyral system [Jakob, 1943].

Along with them but coursing more laterally, emanate from the lateral frontal cortex 25,000 axons, which according to earlier studies formed the fronto-pontine tract; our own studies confirmed the concept of Meynert that part of them arrive at the substantia nigra (about 10,000 axons) and whose total represents, like the limbic-tuberian tract, the so-called *fronto-nigral* tract connected to the striated normokinesia and the frontal praxias.

The remaining 15,000 axons continue from the cerebral peduncle towards the dorsomedial pontine ganglia, forming the *fronto-pontine* tract, thus half of the frontal efferent pathways, together with the lateral thalamofrontal, close the dynamic afferent frontocerebellar loop, connected by the cerebellar pontine systems to the contralateral cerebellar hemisphere; thus result the two crossed pathways: the afferent cerebello-rubro-thalamic frontal system and the efferent cerebellar fronto-pontine system, i.e. the circuit of the neokinesic system superimposed on the paleokinesic (instinctive) and archikinesic (reflex).

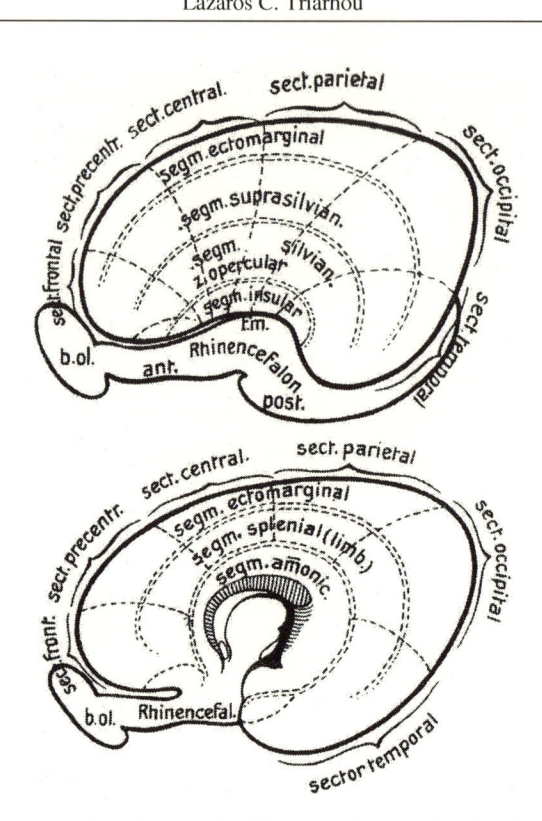

Fig. 3. Scheme of the segmentation and sectorization of the mammalian hemisphere [Jakob, 1911; Jakob & Onelli, 1911, 1913].

Its task connects evidently the frontal praxic dynamics to the cerebellar normokinesia for the appropriate execution of the volitive acts learned individually, from the most elemental skills to the mobilization of symbolic thought; such is the task of the lateral corticality, as opposed to the medial which is destined to contribute the vegetative affectivity oriented at the regulatory influence that the viscero-vasomotor endogenous functions, through the frontal limbic cortex, exercise in the reactive, biophylactic, neoneuronal phylogeny.

Then, by means of such medial afferent frontal radiations originates the notion of the *"anxiety"* of viscero-sympathetic origin in the frontal limbic cortex in pathological states; its elements represent, according to what has been exposed, only 10% of the thalamofrontal radiation.

The Frontal Pyramidal Elements

The frontal cortex presents as a site of contact between the afferent and efferent pathways, mentioned above, the system of transformation of the specific stimulations and reactions (endogenous-exogenous frontalization) and with it the final accumulation of its elaborations (frontalized commemorative function).

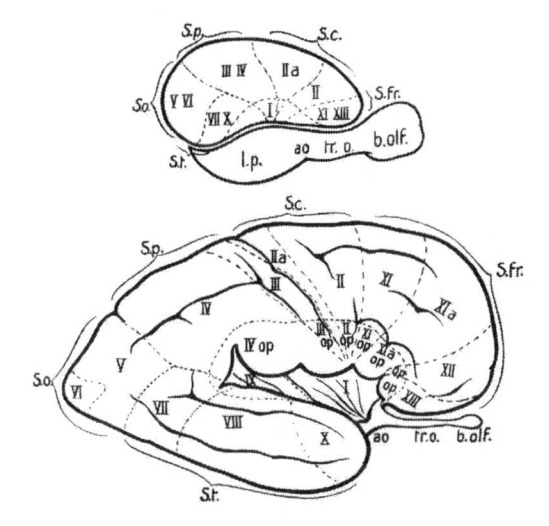

Fig. 4. Scheme of the cytoarchitectonic areas in the *Didelphis* (*upper*) and human brain (*lower*). Note the striking frontal phylogenetic development in the human [Jakob, 1911; Jakob & Onelli, 1911, 1913].

The first is effected by the neurodynamic exchanges of its receptive external pyramidal layer with the effector internal by the macrodynamic waves of charge and discharge. The focal accumulation, that constitutes the respective commemorative representation, is in charge of its minor elements (microdynamic waves); thus, from both layers this focal microdynamic charge is the one that encloses the outcomes of the personal praxic experience in the form of neurodynamic energy of the past, of increasing and available tension; for all acts of conscious intervention in the future (neokinesias) its latent game represents, consequently, the praxic capital of the individual in both domains: medial affective and lateral external environmental.

It is understood that the extension of possible interventions in humans requires an increased number of collaborative elements, without getting here into greater detail; in total we estimate for the frontal lobe (excluding always the anterior Rolandic) in the vicinity of 1,200 million pyramidal cells over a cell total of 5,000 million for each hemisphere (excluding the fusiform elements of the supra- and infrapyramidal layer). More than half (about 60%) belong to microdynamisms, the remaining part to systems of associative waves, as we shall see, and a small remnant to systems of discharge already studied (30,000).

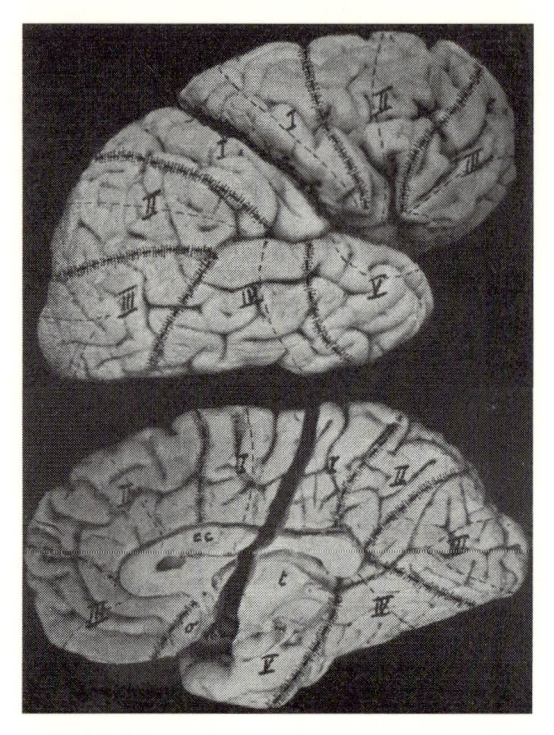

Fig. 5. The 'golden section' of the human cerebral hemisphere. External (*upper*) and midsagittal facies (*lower*). Note the importance of the frontal 'praxic' sectors [Jakob, 1943].

As far as the repartition of the pyramidal cells over the gyri are concerned, we only have an approximate orientation; taking into account the extent in surface, thickness and cell wealth, we calculate the following:

Cortex of the supracallosal (superior limbic) gyrus:	150 million
Cortex of the superior frontal gyrus:	450 million
Cortex of the middle frontal gyrus:	350 million
Cortex of the inferior frontal gyrus:	250 million
Total:	1,200 million

It will be interesting to establish next the coefficients between cells and projection axons; in general, to each afferent axonal element correspond about 300 pyramidal cells, whereas for an efferent neuron it is concentrated into the collaboration of more than 100 times (i.e. about 40,000 cells). Naturally, great regional differences exist in that respect.

Frontal Associative Systems

Although our histological knowledge offers sufficient information, one must confess that the functional relations are almost totally unknown; thus we will deal with them superficially, indicating only that the frontal lobe appears to possess the greater number of such special elements in its gyral association as much as contralaterally.

We know in the endogenous domain, as it was shown graphically by Burdach, the *cingulum* as an associative pathway composed of semi-long accumulated elements; their count has given us at different levels, from 25,000 to 35,000 axonal elements. In the lateral exogenous zone, in its dorsal portion, we have the arcuate fasciculus with 35,000 axons and in the base the uncinate gyrus with 12,000.

One should add an unknown but very high number of short intergyral systems (U-fibers), both in the limbic zone and the lateral gyri.

As far as the commissural system is concerned, we have in the genu of the corpus callosum a potent interfrontal pathway that we estimate at more than 1,500,000 axons split into afferent and efferent.

It is not possible to indicate a distribution of the corresponding gyri yet.

Conclusion

Having by this time finished our modest contribution to the numerical knowledge provisional of the frontal functions, we think that the presented numbers, without insisting on their absolute fidelity, will increase in the mind of our neurosurgeon colleagues somewhat more their medical responsibility when they cut so confidently axons and cells that will never be able to regenerate.

It is meaningful to note that our theory of the endogenous-exogenous cortical centers and systems, already conceived by one of us more than 30 years ago [Jakob & Onelli, 1913], anticipated a scientific basis accessible for the current psychosomatic clinical doctrines, confirming, through these cortical centers, the physio-psychological synthesis indispensable for the mutual collaboration and control between the human mind and body.

On the other hand, this short exposition in enough to understand the higher frontal task, both in its endogenous affective contribution and its exogenous praxic intervention; the real fact that the frontal lobe gathers so closely both domains of our conscious mentality, is a living indication for the current psychological concept, already established from the philosophy of Schopenhauer and Wundt, that in the volitive domain amalgamate intimately afferent affective intonations and efferent praxic skills as a creative frontal tribute, besides the postfrontal cognitive orientation for the total human mentality.

References

Jakob, C. (1911). *Das Menschenhirn: Eine Studie über den Aufbau und die Bedeutung seiner Grauen Kerne und Rinde. I. Teil. Tafelwerk nebst Einführung in den Organisationsplan der Menschlichen Zentralnervensystems.* München: J. F. Lehmann's Verlag.

Jakob, C. (1943). *Folia Neurobiológica Argentina, Tomo III. El Lóbulo Frontal: Un Estudio Monográfico Anatomoclínico sobre Base Neurobiológica.* Buenos Aires: Aniceto López.

Jakob, C. (1946). El trígono cerebral. Su significación neurobiológica. (Vía central eferente para la musculatura lisa víscero-vascular de la esfera gnósica-emotiva). *Revista Neurológica de Buenos Aires,* **11**, 2–36.

Jakob, C., & Onelli, C. (1911). *Vom Tierhirn zum Menschenhirn: Vergleichend Morphologische, Histologische und Biologische Studien zur Entwicklung der Grosshirnhemisphären und ihrer Rinde.* München: J. F. Lehmann's Verlag.

Jakob, C., & Onelli, C. (1913). *Atlas del Cerebro de los Mamíferos de la República Argentina: Estudios Anatómicos, Histológicos y Biológicos Comparados sobre la Evolución de los Hemisferios y de la Corteza Cerebral.* Buenos Aires: Guillermo Kraft.

Jakob, C., & Pedace, E.A. (1949). La misión del lóbulo frontal frente a una cuantificación sintética de sus elementos productores. *Archivos de Neurocirugía,* **6**, 467–474.

In: *Neuroanatomy Research Advances*
Editors: C.E. Flynn and B.R. Callaghan

ISBN 978-1-60741-610-4
© 2010 Nova Science Publishers

The Neuronal Quantification of the Limbic Region in its Relation to the Endogenous Affective Sphere[1]

Christofredo Jakob and Andrés R. Copello
Laboratory of Neuropathology, Hospital Nacional de Alienadas, Buenos Aires

Abstract

In the times of Broca one already separated the limbic gyrus from the rest of the hemisphere, an anatomical fact verified by phylogeny and ontogeny, and later by psychopathology, especially by the limbic form of Pick disease. This medial cortex is related to the periependymal tuberomamillary diencephalic paleoneuronal sympathetic centers (vasomotility and endocriny). Of the 5,000 million cortical pyramidal elements that a hemisphere has, 325 million correspond to the supracallosal gyrus and 75 million to the hippocampus; the former receives 600,000 axons from the anterior thalamic nucleus and emits the limbicotuberian pathway that is composed of 5,000 axons. The hippocampus, which is related to olfaction, hosts the central olfactory radiation (250,000 axons) and gives origin to the fornix (65,000 axons) to take stimuli to ipsilateral and contralateral periependymal and tuberian nuclei, to the peri-raphé nuclei of the mesencephalon and rhombencephalon from which it stimulates glands, vasomotility, etc. The supracallosal account as an associative path to the cingulum (25,000–35,000 axons) and U-fibers, and the hippocampus with only U-fibers and as an interhemispheric association to one-tenth of the genu of the corpus callosum, also to one-tenth of the anterior and interammonic commissures. In summary, the limbic gyrus maintains a functional independence from the rest of the hemisphere and is linked to viscero-vasomotor stimuli; as a phylogenetically older cortex, it provides us with the notion of well-being or vegetative malaise, getting to oscillate between euphoria and anxiety in a more pronounced manner. Thus, we deduce that here reside the bases for the affectively intoned feeling of endogenous ('introyental') mental life, as opposed to that which the lateral cortex carries out, toward the associative contribution for the total conscious mentality.

---

[1] An English translation of 'La cuantificación neuronal de la región límbica en su relación con la esfera introyental afectiva,' originally published in *Actas del Tercer Congreso Sudamericano de Neurocirugía* (Buenos Aires, April 3–9, 1949), *Archivos de Neurocirugía*, vol. VI, no. 1–4, pp. 475–481 [Jakob & Copello, 1949]; translated and edited from the Spanish text by L.C. Triarhou* with the help of A.B. Vivas.

* E-mail address: triarhou@uom.gr, phone +30 2310 891-387, fax +30 2310 891-388 (Corresponding author)

Introduction

Since the times of Broca, comparative neurobiology has separated the marginal cortical circle (supra and infracallosal) of the median hemispheric facies from the rest of the lateral hemispheric facies. Such a limbic zone essentially consisted of the supracallosal (superior limbic) and the hippocampal (inferior limbic) gyrus at the base. This purely anatomical concept has been confirmed in its phylogenetic existence and ontogeny, although its physiological study remained almost in darknesses, and it is just lately that psychopathology, especially the limbic form of Pick disease [Jakob, 1946b] opened up the possibility of elaborating clearer concepts with respect to its functions. In addition, normal and pathological histotopography have contributed to the clarification of certain limbic axonal relations with the periependymal and tuberomamillary diencephalic centers [Jakob, 1946a] that connect their cortical functions with those sympathetic paleoneuronal centers (vasomotility and endocriny). From it a fundamental concept emerges on the existence of distinct functions in two cortical spheres: the lateral cortex, represented by afferent and efferent pathways, is linked to the external environment; on the other hand, the internal ('introyental') medial limbic domain is related to sensitivity and viscerovascular motility. The former acts on striated musculature (pyramidal tract, etc.); the latter, on smooth musculature (fornix, etc.). As the latter is intimately associated with our emotive sphere (circulation, nutrition, inner secretions, etc.), it would represent our inner affective cortex; both together generate, intimately combined, the individual consciousness of the self (neopsychisms).

Anatomically, a large part of the limbic system belongs to the frontal lobe (supracallosal), and the remaining to the temporal lobe (hippocampus), but this one is also related to the frontal lobe through the intermediation of the olfactory area. Although altogether the limbic zone in humans only represents 10% of the cerebrum (in the descending phylogeny in animals it is inversed) one cannot speak in humans of a substantial and less functional reduction, without denying, of course, the superiority in lateral gain. It is for that reason of interest to know with greater detail, the quantity of functional elements that enter into its histoneuronal organization, because on the total of its elements evidently depends the efficacy of its impulses that dominate within the set of mental functions.

We divided its neuronal elements into the following three groups:

(1) Those corresponding to its cortical centers of neurodynamic accumulation (focalization of its commemorative work).

(2) Its elements of charge and discharge (afferent and efferent) in its projection toward subcortical regions.

(3) Those destined to its associative and commissural transcortical correlations with the rest of the corticality.

Pyramidal Cortical Elements

Of the total number of *pyramidal cortical elements* that in one hemisphere reach approximately 5,000 million [the count was obtained from magnified microphotographs of sections subjected to silver impregnation of cells and axons], correspond to the limbic zone around 400 million that we divide in the following manner: the superior limbic (supracallosal) cortex has 325 million, and the inferior limbic (hippocampus) 75 million. Each one represents the fundamental type of two superimposed layers. Thus, in the supracallosal gyrus, the receiving external layer of stimuli contains 225 million cells, and the effector internal layer 100 million cells. Between both layers the most numerous microdynamic elements form the stationary waves of sensory-motor consolidation. In the hippocampus, the receiving external layer is represented by the elements of the dentate gyrus (near 50 million) and the efferent external by the pyramidal cells of Ammon's horn (25 million). All these elements are the ones that store the acquired experience individually and transform it into volitional motor realizations, according to the mode of the received and transformed stimuli.

Afferent and Efferent Limbic Axons

To orient oneself really on the specific function of a cortical center, a knowledge of its pathways of charge and discharge is indispensable, because it is based on the category of those stimulations and reactions in its correlated projection that one must determine on the function of the focal center as it occurs with the two limbic zones, that in spite of being topographically and associatively reunited present essential differences.

(a) The *superior limbic gyrus* receives as afferent pathway (Fig. 1) to the *anterior dorsothalamic* radiation formed by a contingent of approximately 600,000 axons. Its anterior frontal portion, the greater of the two, participates with 65% (near 400,000 axons) and it is precisely about this portion that we have more precise functional information. In effect, the bundle of Vicq d'Azyr, which contains around 15,000 microaxons, terminates in the anterior thalamic nucleus; this bundle of very old phylogeny originates in the medial portion of the mamillary body and takes – according to confirmed personal observations a long time ago – viscerosympathetic stimuli of all thoraco-abdomino-pelvic organs, a fact so old in its phylogeny that it confirms in its relations to the individual and generic trophic functions (nutrition, sexuality) from the inferior mammals, although lacking to still penetrate into its special physiologic interpretation. In humans the observations of cases with tissue softening, such as progressive general paresis and Pick disease, confirm such facts.

In the same site of termination of the mamillothalamic fasciculus (Vicq d'Azyr) the frontal anterior radiation of the supracallosal gyrus originates precisely from the thalamic cells; the thalamus functions in general as an enormous multiplicator system, with an increase from the 15,000 axons of the bundle of Vicq d'Azyr to 500,000 of the thalamolimbic radiation, i.e. more than 30 times. These radiations extend in the form of a large fan in front of the genu of the internal capsule, from their dorsal portion to the base, entering the external pyramidal layer of the supracallosal cortex; their thicker fibers arrive at the tangential layer; they are reflected towards the external layer, a fact particularly demonstrative in mammals: the external tangential layer has nothing to do with association, as it was once considered, which is in fact evident in the inferior limbic gyrus. However, the pathway of discharge of the limbic is much more limited, also according to a general law that applies to all efferent radiations; it is represented by the *limbico-tuberian* pathway, formed by a contingent of around 5,000 axons and which, originating in the internal pyramidal layer of the cortex, continues crossing the radiation and genu of the internal capsule towards its base, where it occupies its more medial portion on the inside of the frontonigral and pontine systems [Jakob, 1947] to terminate in the lateral juxtaependymal and tuberian sympathetic nuclei of the diencephalon, and to conduct the stimuli from here by pathways little known towards the viscerovasomotor smooth musculature by means of the bulbospinal sympathetic reflex centers.

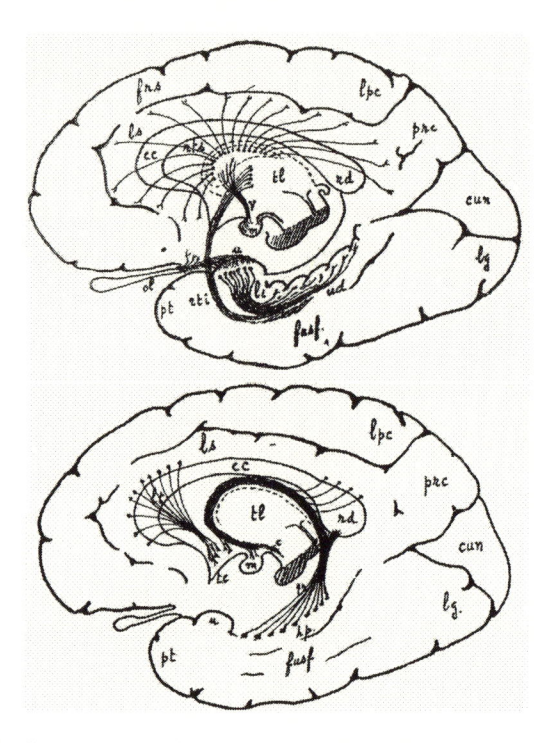

Fig. 1. Scheme of the afferent projection pathways to the superior and inferior limbic gyrus (*upper*) and of efferent projection systems (*lower*). Abbreviations: *c*, crus fornix; *hp*, hippocampus; *li*, inferior limbic; *ls*, superior limbic; *lt*, limbico-tuberian pahtway; *m*, mamillary body; *ol*, olfactory pathways; *rts*, superior thalamic radiation; *tc*, tuber cinereum; *tl*, thalamus; *tr*, fornical system; *u*, hippocampal uncus; *uc*, uncodentate system; *V*, bundle of Vicq d'Azyr [Jakob & Copello, 1949].

Thus closes the *limbic internal ('introyental')* functional circuit through which visceral affective states, from the euphoric to the anxious, are mediated, accumulated and discharging in the personal experience during normal individual life, biologically relating the limbic cortex to visceroendocrine functions. This is evidently a complex psychophysiological problem still not resolved, and common to the entire animal series, to which belong, among others, the care for personal hygiene and the young; cave and nest formation in animals; elimination of organic wastes via sphincters and regulation of nutritive and sexual functions.

The training for such functions begins in early childhood and never ceases; it is the evoked inner affect, which forms the biological basis of being, and which we connect foremost with cortical functions of the superior limbic gyrus. In these studies, human pathology has a most important part with its clinico-anatomical correlations.

(b) *Inferior limbic gyrus* (hippocampus). More has been known since earlier times about this gyrus, because comparative anatomy provided evidence as to the relation with the chemical sense of olfaction, a fact that already in itself links its cortical functions to the experience related to nutrition and sexuality, where the sense of olfaction dominates. The olfactory afferent central axons originate in the uncus of the hippocampus, where the lateral radiations also arrive from the olfactory area; that central radiation, that is the one of the hippocampus, integrated by near 250,000 axons (very approximately) crosses the subiculum (perforant fibers) and becomes distributed on a superficial surface; it arrives at the subicular external tangential layer, coursing soon, from that marginal zone to the hippocampal dentate gyrus, a pathway that Cajal called sphenodentate and which to our understanding is more appropriate to the dentate perforant radiation, a pathway that in animals originates in the piriform lobe (the uncus); so that topographically one should designate to it the name of *uncodentate* system. To this pathway become aggregated axons of the inferior thalamic sort/mode (gustative pathway?). We have therefore a second source of thalamo-temporal stimuli, whose true mission is in discussion; anyway, olfaction as a unique Ammonic function is debatable. Its pathway of discharge is far better known, originating in the Ammonic layer (effector layer of the hippocampus) integrated by an approximated contingent of 65,000 axons forming the well-known fornix (*cerebral trigonum*) that, as we have shown in a special work [Jakob & Copello, 1948] takes most of its axons towards the ipsilateral and contralateral periependymal and tuberian medial nuclei, and whose longer fibers arrive at the zone of the hypothalamic commissure, at the peri-raphé nuclei of the mesencephalon and the rhombencephalon. Again we have an efferent projection towards viscerosympathetic nuclei from which are stimulated the secretion and motility of the digestive and vascular systems.

Considering the mission of the superior limbic dynamic circuit associated here, we confirm its similar function in the visceral sympathetic inferior limbic circuit of the total internal environment ('introyente'). "Hunger and love emit from those cortices their categorical imperatives in the animal and human organism" [Jakob & Onelli, 1913].

It has functions already reflected and instinctively regulated by subcortical systems, but the evidence increasingly suggests the role of the limbic cortex as a neoneuronal superposed center individually dominant in relation to the lower archineuronal and paleoneuronal centers.

Associative Limbic Systems

Given the limited knowledge on the function of those systems that we know better from their histotopography, we shall only treat them briefly. In the area of the superior limbic gyrus is known in the first place for a long time the cingulum, a longitudinal system jointly formed by short and semi-long pathways that unite at distinct regions of the supracallosal gyrus. This path in front of the genu of the corpus callosum begin at the base, and taking a parallel course to the great interhemispheric commissure, it extends backwards, it reaches the splenium and following its curvature, the longer axons arrive all the way to the posterior parts of the hippocampus. In the entire trajectory, a part of its fibers irradiates to the supracallosal cortex, uniting in a double arc to its different portions. It is formed by a large amount of very fine axons (microaxons) which are disposed in a fascicular grouping; their count has given us as many as 25,000–35,000 axons, reaching the maximum in the frontal zone directly in front of the genu. In addition the supracallosal gyrus is connected by an appreciable amount with intergyral systems (U-fibers) to the entire medial facies of the hemisphere, being especially numerous in its anterior half (association with the superior frontal and paracentral lobules). The relations with the indusium griseum (*taenia tecta*) are doubtful.

In the inferior limbic gyrus, the associative existence is poorer; only some intergyral systems appear (U-fibers) that connect the hippocampus with the temporal internal facies. A quantification of these systems has not been possible for us until now. We shall not consider here the ancient occipitotemporal pathway, in the past interpreted as associative, since it belongs to the optic projection.

As far as the commissural interhemispheric association is concerned, it contributes by the anterior supracallosal gyrus a certain part of the genu of the corpus callosum, which we were able to calculate as one-tenth of its constitution; the larger amount of fibers is directed toward the frontolateral cortex. In the hippocampus we know the anterior and interammonic commissures; a count of the former has given us nearly 30,000 axons, but we must consider that part of it constitute crossed olfactory projection pathways, perhaps one-tenth as well.

Altogether we can affirm that the limbic endogenous zone is in ample associative contact with the ipsilateral and contralateral, especially as far as the superior limbic gyrus is concerned; in reality, numerous details still lack.

Conclusion

The following conclusion is drawn from the above exposition: the limbic gyrus maintains, as far as its afferent-efferent projections are concerned, a functional independence from the remaining gyri of the lateral neocortex, which are related to the outer environment. This important circuit is not fully understood yet; being phylogenetically older cortex, it provides us with viscerovasomotor signals and the feeling of well-being or of vegetative malaise, oscillating between euphoria and anxiety. Thus, we can deduce that here reside the bases for the affectively colored feelings of inner mental life, as opposed to those subserved by the lateral cortex, thus providing the association for integrated conscious mentality. In spite of these centers existing in lower vertebrates, it is in mammals that they successively become associated with the lateral outer effects, intensifying the intellectualization of states in higher consciousness in relation to the elementary nature of the others. Only in primates, and especially in humans with their verbal symbolization, one rises to a supreme mental degree, where the sphere of inner feelings of visceral origin becomes amalgamated with the environmental gnosio-praxic experience; in that superior synthesis arises the neopsychic sphere, from the concrete to the most abstract. But it consists, according to the most ideal reasoning that invariably accompanies it, although in a latent form, the affective endogenous stimulation forming the indispensable biophylactic individual-genetic basis, a priori, of all human existential life, as popular psychology already guesses when it says that the head needs the help of the heart if it wants to produce lasting values.

In this study on the limbic-endogenous cortical centers, we attempted to achieve a constructive synthesis for the creation of those inner affective mental phenomena in their relation to external cognitive phenomena. The associative process between both systems creates the conscious and total personality: affect and cognition, respectively located at the medial fornical-limbic and at the lateral pyramidal systems. The effects of the involuntary smooth musculature in combination with the voluntary striated muscles present an indisputable and fruitful basis for current doctrines in the psychosomatic sphere, because the internal-environmental interactions form the basis for this psychosomatic dynamic unity that represents the old concept of body and mind.

References

Jakob, C. (1946a). El trígono cerebral: su significación neurobiológica (vía central eferente para la musculatura lisa víscero-vascular de la esfera gnósica-emotiva). *Revista Neurológica de Buenos Aires*, **11**, 2–36.

Jakob, C. (1946b). La demencia progresiva: un análisis neurobiológico de la enfermedad de Pick. *Revista Neurológica de Buenos Aires*, **11**, 81–94.

Jakob, C. (1947). La significación neurobiológica y clínica de la cuantificación de los sistemas cerebrales. *Revista Neurológica de Buenos Aires*, **12**, 229–245.

Jakob, C., & Copello, A.R. (1948). La psicointegración introyento-ambiental orgánica y sus problemas para la neuropsiquiatría y psicología (primera parte: su filogenía constructiva). *Revista Neurológica de Buenos Aires*, **13**, 63–79.

Jakob, C., & Copello, A.R. (1949). La cuantificación neuronal de la región limbica en su relación con la esfera introyental afectiva. *Archivos de Neurocirugía*, **6**, 475–481.

Jakob, C., & Onelli, C. (1913). *Atlas del Cerebro de los Mamíferos de la República Argentina: Estudios Anatómicos, Histológicos y Biológicos Comparados sobre la Evolución de los Hemisferios y de la Corteza Cerebral*. Buenos Aires: Guillermo Kraft.

PIONEERS IN NEUROLOGY

Bernhard Pollack (1865–1928)

Lazaros C. Triarhou

Received: 12 March 2010 / Accepted: 30 March 2010 / Published online: 15 April 2010
© Springer-Verlag 2010

Bernhard Pollack wrote the first standard reference on histological staining methods for the nervous system [7]. He worked at Berlin's First Anatomical Institute, headed by Wilhelm Waldeyer [6], the Neuropsychiatric Institute of Emanuel Mendel [1], the Institute for Infectious Diseases directed by the later Nobel laureate Robert Koch [3], and at the research laboratory of the Eye Clinic with Paul Silex [4, 8, 10]. He collaborated with Max Bielschowsky [1] and Edward Flatau [9], who called Pollack "the man with the great work on the nervous system".

Born into a Prussian-Jewish family, Pollack was the youngest of five children [5]. He became fluent in German, French, Italian, English, Polish, Latin and Greek. His father Jakob was a tradesman who amassed a commanding fortune by being a supplier to the Prussian Army during the Austro-Prussian War of 1866; his mother's family (Ledermann) came from Silesia (Fig. 1).

Pollack became an *approbierter Arzt* (assistant physician) and completed his doctoral thesis in pathology (on metastatic lung tumors) in April 1893 at the Faculty of Medicine of Leipzig University, a leading institute at the time. Pollack's teachers were Waldeyer and Carl Weigert [7]. Cancer pathology had been a research interest of Waldeyer and his student Weigert during their early years in Breslau, prior to their seminal work on the nervous system.

Pollack joined the Berlin Medical Society in 1896 and practised in Silex's Policlinic as an *Oberarzt* (attending physician), attaining the reputation of a distinguished ophthalmologist. He attended the 15th Internal Medicine

L. C. Triarhou (✉)
Economo-Koskinas Wing for Integrative and Evolutionary Neuroscience, University of Macedonia, Thessaloniki, Greece
e-mail: triarhou@uom.gr

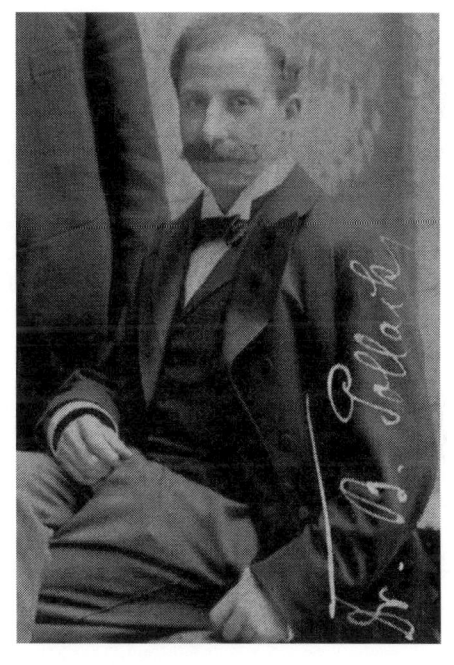

Fig. 1 Bernhard Pollack (1901). Credit: http://de.wikipedia.org/wiki/Siegfried_Kalischer; original at *Akademie der Künste*, Berlin [2]. Signature from a dedication copy of Flatau's 1894/1899 *Atlas of the Human Brain* (author's archive)

Congress (Berlin, June 1897), 12th International Internal Medicine Congress (Moscow, August 1897) [2], and 10th International Ophthalmology Congress (Lucerne, September 1904). Between 1899 and 1909, he reported cases to the Berlin Ophthalmological Society (ocular filariasis, metastatic choroidal carcinoma, spindle cell sarcoma of the frontal sinus, and Mikulicz disease or Sjögren syndrome), also compiling the Society's proceedings for the *Zeitschrift für Augenheilkunde*, in addition to the proceedings of the Berlin Physiological, Medical and Psychiatric-Neurological Societies.

Pollack published his compendium of staining methods for nerve tissue in 1897; it was dedicated to Waldeyer and Weigert. By 1905, the book had gone through three German editions and English, French, Russian and Italian translations. Specific instructions and a comprehensive bibliography covered most neurohistological stains known at the time. The chapters described dissection of the central and peripheral nervous system, macroscopic examination and conservation for museum purposes, hardening, embedding and sectioning, changes in brain weight depending on fixative, micrography, macro- and microphotography, stains for neurons, fibres and glia, and practical suggestions on choice of technique for normal or pathological neurohistology. He also discussed changes in brain weight according to gender, age, and hemispheric dominance. The methods of Ehrlich, Nissl, Weigert, Golgi, Cajal, Marchi, Flechsig, Freud, Nansen, Lenhossék, Frey, Roncoroni and Azoulay were described, as well as those of others; a separate chapter covered the retina, with reference to Cajal and Dogiel.

The book received favourable reviews from Theodor Ziehen and Alfred Walter Campbell, who called the author "a thoughtful, accomplished, and well-practised microscopist", highlighting the minute commentaries on each staining procedure and the distinction between important and unimportant methods. Its practical merits were thoroughly recommended by the *British Medical Journal*.

Pollack further wrote papers on neuroglia and its stains [6], the innervation of the mammalian eye [1], nerve cell damage from botulinum toxin [3], a primary tumour (suspected neurofibroma or myxosarcoma) of the optic disc [4], metachromasia of the sclera in tuberculous panophthalmitis [8], and optic nerve damage with mental signs following skull fracture [10]. His last publication, on the histology of an optic nerve gliosarcoma, appeared posthumously in the *Festschrift* for Flatau [9].

Pollack served on the editorial boards of *Jahresbericht über Neurologie und Psychiatrie* and *Centralblatt für Praktische Augenheilkunde*, reviewing literature on staining and anatomical methods in neurological research. Having been appointed Professor of Ophthalmology at the Friedrich-Wilhelms-Universität in 1919, his renown extended beyond continental Europe. Bernhard Pollack died in 1928 at the age of 63. He was twice married and is not known to have had children. His residence at Blumes Hof 15 would be expropriated in 1939–1941 by the Nazi regime as Jewish property, while his sister Betty Friedmann and her daughter would fall victim at Auschwitz.

Besides an acknowledged scientist and medical scholar, Pollack was a fine pianist, pupil of the composer Moritz Moszkowski. At the age of 25, Pollack had published a four-hand piano transcription of his master's *Second Suite for Orchestra*, op. 47 (Hainauer, 1890). He performed with the Austrian composer Fritz Kreisler in America and with the Hungarian violinist Joseph Szigeti in Berlin. Pollack's brother Joseph, who died young in a railway accident, was also musically gifted, having being accepted for a piano audition by Franz Liszt [5]. In 1911 Pollack founded the *Berliner Ärzte-Orchester*, an ensemble of musically talented physicians. Now, a century later, the orchestra is still active, performing a wide repertoire of symphonic works.

References

1. Bielschowsky M, Pollack B (1904) Zur Kenntniss der Innervation des Säugethierauges. Neurol Cbl 23:387–394
2. Eisenberg U (2005) Vom „Nervenplexus" zur „Seelenkraft"—Werk und Schicksal des Berliner Neurologen Louis Jacobsohn-Lask. Lang, Frankfurt
3. Kempner W, Pollack B (1897) Die Wirkung des Botulismustoxins (Fleischgiftes) und seines specifischen Antitoxins auf die Nervenzellen. Dtsch Med Wochenschr 23:505–507
4. Kurzezunge D, Pollack B (1903) Ein Fall von primärer Neubildung auf der Papille des Opticus. Z Augenheilk 10:302–308
5. Lichtheim R (1970) Rückkehr—Lebenserinnerungen aus der Frühzeit des Deutschen Zionismus. Deutsche Verlags-Anstalt, Stuttgart
6. Pollack B (1896) Einige Bemerkungen über die Neuroglia und Neurogliafärbung. Arch Mikrosk Anat 48:274–280
7. Pollack B (1897) Die Färbetechnik des Nervensystems. Karger, Berlin
8. Pollack B (1903) Ueber das Verhalten der Sclera bei Panophthalmie. Z Augenheilk 9:218–223
9. Pollack B (1929) Gliom des Nervus opticus. In: Bornsztajn M (ed) Recueil de travaux offert à Édouard Flatau. Gebethner-Wolff, Varsovie, pp 595–600
10. Waterman O, Pollack B (1904) Fracture of the basis cranii followed by atrophy of both optic nerves and peculiar psychic phenomena. J Nerv Ment Dis 31:250–257

Micscape Magazine UK • Issue 171 • January 2010
ISSN 1365–070X • http://www.microscopy-uk.org.uk

THE MICROSCOPE OF A SHOELESS DOCTOR

Manuel del Cerro (Pittsford, NY, USA) and Lazaros C. Triarhou (Thessaloniki, Greece)

INTRODUCTION

The political and social phenomenon known as the "Cultural Revolution" (officially: "The Great Proletarian Cultural Revolution," a creature of Mao Zedong), took place in China from 1966 to 1976. Today, the Cultural Revolution is considered both in China and abroad as a vastly destructive, tragic, and unnecessary event.

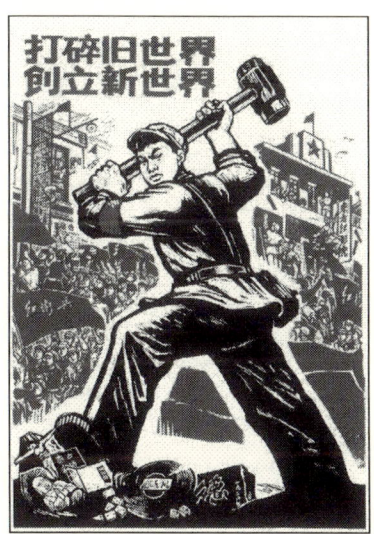

Figure 1. Fanaticized youngsters, the "Red Guard," were the enforcers of the Cultural Revolution. Here a Red Guard is about to smash a crucifix, a statuette of Buddha, books, a set of dice, and other objects. In the upper right a man is being thrown down from the upper floor of a building. (Courtesy University of Westminster Chinese Poster Collection.)

The tremendous social upheaval produced by the Cultural Revolution affected all sectors of the society (1–4). Physicians, particularly those with academic affiliations, were among the most prominent victims. Thousands of them were sent to practice in the countryside under dismal conditions. The guiding idea was they needed to be "re-educated" by the peasantry (3). In practice, they became the "Shoeless Doctors."

One of us had the privilege of meeting a survivor of that ordeal, and the honor of being presented with the microscope used by him during that time. Here is the story of the microscope of a Shoeless Doctor.

THE MICROSCOPE

Description. Microscope #095 MdC Collection—"Cultural Revolution" Chinese-made monocular microscope (figure 2). A 12.5 × 8 cm horseshoe base is continuous with a triangularly shaped metal pillar; the pillar is connected to the arm at the inclination joint. The pillar and the limb are made of flat metal pieces. There is a fork-mounted, concave mirror with a diameter of 3 cm. A wheel of diaphragms with five openings is located underneath the stage. The 7 × 7 cm stage has two stage clips. There is no fine focus; coarse focus is by rack and pinion controlled by a knob located on the right side. The tube moves up and down along two thin flanges that hold it on axis. The tube itself is made of plastic. The ocular screws at the top of the body tube; it is made of wood with a metal ring holding the field lens in place. The single, divisible objective has a non-standard screw thread (figure 3); it is 21 mm long with a barrel diameter of 12 mm. Two components form the objective; the upper one has an internal fix diaphragm with an unusually small opening. There are no visible inscriptions on the microscope. A sticker attached to the underneath the base reads in Chinese characters: "Qualification for production made by equipment manufactory of the National Science Association. Examiner: [difficult to read], 2 (?). Year 1961, month...day..." When set in the vertical position and focused using element 1 of the objective, the instrument stands 22.5 cm tall.

Optical Performance. Using element 1 of the objective the magnification is about 100×; the image is dim and uneven across the field. The field of view is 1,400 μm across. When both elements of the objective are used together the magnification is about 250×; the image is dimmer, as expected, but not worst. It is possible that the second element compensates in part for the severe flaws of element 1. The field of view is 400 μm across. This is an instrument resembling a toy microscope, but it is sturdier than a toy (it weights 1,042 g). The instrument however is usable only for rudimentary medical work.

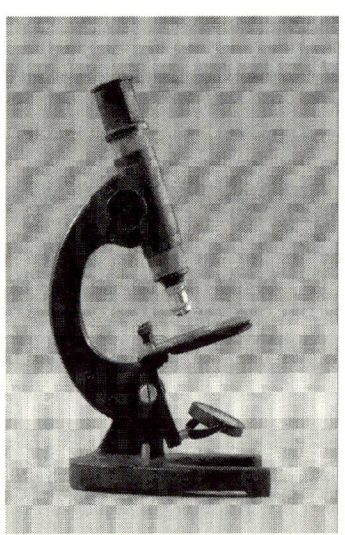

Figure 2. The cultural revolution microscope.

Provenance. This instrument was used by Huimin Zhou, M.D., while practicing in the Chinese countryside during the times of the "Cultural Revolution." The microscope came to the Collection in January 1987 as a gift to Manuel del Cerro, M.D. from Dr. Zhou. Dr. Zhou had become Professor and Director of the Center for Ultrastructure Research, Quingdao Medical College, Quingdao, China, and was internationally recognized for his work on the effects of leprosy on the eye.

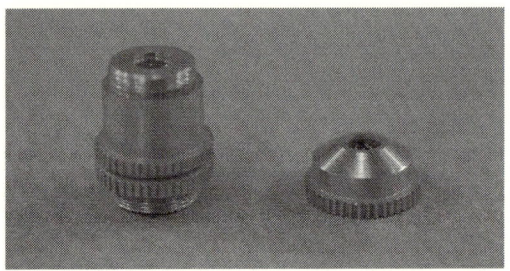

Figure 3. The two components of the divisible objective; the one to the left attaches to the microscope body.

COMMENTS

It is ironic that the Cultural Revolution that tried with so much ardor to destroy as much of the Chinese cultural heritage as possible, including priceless books and works of art, has left mementoes of its own. This rare example of a microscope of a Shoeless Doctor is one of them. Looking at it we honor the victims of that ordeal.

ACKNOWLEDGMENTS

We thank Dr. Harriet Evans and Dr. Katie Hill, University of Westminster, London, UK, for kindly allowing us to reproduce the image used as figure 1.

REFERENCES

1. Anonymous (2009) Cultural Revolution. http://en.wikipedia.org/wiki/Cultural_Revolution
2. Anonymous (2009) Cultural Revolution. http://encarta.msn.com/encyclopedia_761580637/cultural_revolution.html
3. Grenville, J.A.S. (1994) A History of the World in the Twentieth Century. Harvard University Press, Cambridge, MA, pp. 627–641.
4. Roberts, J.M. (1999) Twentieth Century. The History of the World, 1901 to 2000. Viking-Penguin, New York, pp. 719–721.

editorial

In 1919, Viennese neurologist Otto Marburg (1874–1948) reported the case of a patient with motor aphasia and preserved singing ability. He took the opportunity to discourse on the hemispheric lateralization of language and music functions, and also on the interaction of the two cerebral hemispheres in musical expression.
"Zur Frage der Amusie" (1919) was published in Arbeiten aus dem Neurologischen Institute an der Wiener Universität, *22, 106-112. In tribute to Marburg's neurological legacy and as an attempt to disseminate his neuroscientific ideas, Marburg's entire essay, in German is here translated into English by Dimitra Koniari MA and Lazaros C. Triarhou MD, PhD of the University of Macedonia, Greece.*

Otto Marburg's "On the question of amusia"

While linguistic expression is an ability enabled almost exclusively by the left cerebral hemisphere, increasing evidence shows that the right hemisphere ensures the ability of musical expression. Nevertheless, it is questionable whether such a clear independence exists for musical expression, that is, whether musical expression is completely detached from language and has its own centers. Previous authors, particularly Gowers (1) and Ballet (2), dealt intensively with this question of independence. Gowers (1) supported the view that singing, particularly singing with words, contrary to conscious, intellectual language, can be understood only as an automatic language process: one does not think in words when singing. This is a tenet that can hardly be taken for granted. However, if Gowers (1) is correct, then one can assume that the automatic language of singing comes from the right hemisphere, which takes us back to the earlier views of Hughlings Jackson (3).

Conversely, Ballet (2) places musical language between emotional and artificial language. The organization of musical images is less complex and occurs earlier [in life] than that of word images. When language is disrupted, artificial language, which is acquired later, is the first to be disturbed, and only then is musical and affect language [disturbed]. Such an opinion fits only those cases of aphasia in which musical expression is retained, despite the presence of otherwise full-blown aphasia; not those in which musical expression declines, while language remains intact. Therefore, Ballet (2) also accepts that there exist cases in which word and tone images are coordinated. Anyhow – and the credit for this goes to Edgren (4) – previous observations on disorders of musical ability (i.e. amusia) highlight the existence, in such cases, of independent anatomical localizations. For tone deafness (sensory amusia) he finds a center located left of that for word deafness in the superior and middle temporal gyrus. For motor amusia, in accordance with Ludwig Mann's standard case (5), the posterior segment of the right middle frontal gyrus and adjacent part of the anterior central gyrus is considered typical. However, the actual damage appears more severe in clinical case descriptions in which it corresponds to a cyst; conversely war cases in which the sensitivity disturbance is due to the anterior central gyrus do not correspond to the clinical descriptions by Mann (5). The described loss of sensitivity of thumb and index finger may be due only to a process in the parietal lobe. Kurt Mendel's case (6), even though it closely matches that of Mann (5), does not show perfect localization for several reasons: first of all because it is a gunshot wound, which often results in multiple foci, and, second, because the foci in this case also affect not only the middle frontal gyrus, but also a large part of the parietal lobe. Something similar probably applies to the less advanced case described by Max Mann (7). Moreover, the latter cases can be compared to one from the collection of Edgren (4), and specifically to Nadine Skwortzoff's case (8). Here, there is a patient with a large focal softening of the left hemisphere also affecting the foot of the middle and inferior frontal gyrus, who could sing despite a secondary, though small, focus in the right middle frontal gyrus.

Thus, the following question remains open to discussion: should we understand amusias in the sense of Ballet (2) or in the sense of Gowers (1)? In other words, are they something independent located in the right half of the brain, or are they part of the general field of the aphasias, in the left side?

However, it is open to question whether a definite resumé can be drawn from cases, like the one that I present next. It concerns a nonetheless frequently described case of aphasia with a preserved capacity to sing, like, for example, the one that Hugo Liepmann (9) presented recently.

My own observations concern a 23-year-old soldier, J.K., who was wounded by a tangential gunshot on October 16, 1915, at the Italian front. As far as could be ascertained despite his underlying aphasia, he remained unconscious for five days after the gunshot wound, repeatedly vomiting, until he was put on debridate [trimebutine maleate] at the beginning of November. Then, he came to von Eiselsberg's clinic on December 16. His status from December 17 was as follows: in the left parietal area, there was a triangular defect in the bone with the base at the midline; there was a tiny prolapse with marked granulations and pronounced secretion. The patient was hemiparetic on the right, such that the right lower extremities were completely paralyzed. There was also a right hypoesthesia including a disturbance of deep sensitivity, reduction of superficial reflexes, while the cord reflexes were clonic. Positive Babinski sign.

The most striking symptom was his motor aphasia. While he could understand everything that was said to him and could also recognize symbols without any problems, he was unable to say or repeat another person's words spontaneously. Furthermore, it could not be determined, for certain, whether he could read. He wrote his name correctly with his left hand, and drew letters and numbers laboriously. He could not count large numbers, despite several attempts to do small calculations with the fingers. The language disturbance changed little during the observation. He tried to pronounce individual words, getting no further than the syllable *geh*. Another time, it is reported that he uttered the phrase *geh weg, geh weiter*.

One day, a patient next to him began singing the song *Ich hatt' einen Kameraden*. The patient repeated the song like an echo [in echolalia] and, clearly and intelligibly articulating each word, finished the song along with his neighbor. Subsequent attempts with other folk songs always had the same effect, in which, naturally, the visual component was completely excluded. The patient had thus the ability to repeat a song with complete linguistic expression, while otherwise lacking language expression abilities, like spontaneous singing and word repetition.

In early January 1916, the patient began repeating the individual words *geben, geh weg*, while his repetition of singing continued invariably well. In the middle of January he presented with a raised temperature, became somewhat confused, and had a Jacksonian attack involving the right side of his body. There was an abscess in the prolapse, which was drained on January 20, 1916. He developed acute meningitis and died on January 21, 1916.

The autopsy on January 21, 1916 (performed by lecturer Wiesner[1]) showed: an old gunshot wound on the head, tangential shot, expanded defect within the region of the left temporal and parietal bone; incision and drainage of an old cerebral abscess at the parieto-frontal transition; expanded tissue softening from trauma and hemorrhage in the area of the operated field, bleeding in the left lateral ventricle; suppurative leptomeningitis particularly over the right cerebral hemisphere and the base of the brain; fibrous thickening of the dura at the bones at the edge of the lesion.

[Other findings were:] lobar pneumonia in both inferior lobes of the lungs; parenchymatous degeneration of liver and kidneys; acute spleen tumor; hyperplasia of the follicles in the tongue base, spleen and small intestinal mucous membrane; follicle-like formations of the esophagus; foramen caecum, appendix 10.5 [cm]; testes normal size; tuberculosis-negative.

The abscess can be localized quite precisely: it occupies anteriorly the superior frontal gyrus, posteriorly the upper parietal lobule, reaching medially the cortical edge, laterally the upper third of the two central gyri. It extends little in depth, and is in any case not deep enough to have damaged the language pathways at all. However, what seems most important, is that, macroscopically, apart from the fresh meningitis, the left language regions, enclosing the insula, seem to be completely clear, without the smallest indications of inflammation or hemorrhage. Certainly, the right hemisphere has been adequately studied and showed no deviation from normal and, in particular, no enlargement of the middle front gyrus. It is unlikely that the histological studies to be conducted later will plausibly reveal any substantial damage.

In summary, the 23-year-old patient had developed an abscess in the left fronto-parietal lobe, caused by a tangential gunshot, which led him to develop motor aphasia and right hemiplegia. The aphasia should be characterized as incomplete, since the patient, despite the absence of spontaneous language and word repetition, could write letters, count small numbers, and probably read, since he could copy. However, the most essential point is his capacity to sing with words, despite the loss of spontaneous singing ability.

Considering the localization of the abscess in relation to the symptoms of the defect, the loss of movement and sensitivity are undoubtedly related, as both central gyri are affected by the abscess. On the other hand, the aphasia is more difficult to explain satisfactorily, especially considering that, despite a similar extent of involvement of the motor and sensory language areas of the focus, only the former suffered. It was clear from the beginning that there could not have been major destruction of the language area, since the aphasia was not complete. Nevertheless, it is probable that the abscess affected the motor language area more readily than the sensory one, which is separated from the damaged area by the Sylvian fossa.

The most outstanding feature, the preservation of the ability to repeat songs with words, is more difficult to explain. If one agreed with Gowers (1), that singing works only through linguistic automatism, which is carried out by the right hemisphere, then the present case could be explained fully. However, it is highly unlikely that such a split of language exists, whereby words that fail to be expressed with the spoken voice can be elicited by a tone or rhythm other than the one of language. Musicians, on the basis of their experience, have completely rejected Gower's assumption anyway. It also seems here that the individuality of the singer plays a crucial role; the majority holds singing to be inspired by the meaning of the words. Ballet's view is easier to understand, according to which earlier acquisitions are better formed and remain more easily perceived than those acquired later, including therefore the less well established artificial language. Perhaps this remaining ability of musical expression represented a recovery of the aphasia, which might have been total only in the beginning. Indeed, the linguistic expression of my patient began to return.

However, how does this case fare in the light of the observations of Mendel (6) and Edgren (4)? According to Edgren (4), tone deafness is attributed to a left-sided focus, somewhere in front of the locus of sensory aphasia (although Edgren pays little attention to the fact that the right side was also affected, albeit not as completely as the left, but nevertheless noticeably). However, in the case of L. Mann (5) the focus was only on the right side, just as Mendel (6) presupposes in his case and M. Mann (7) as well. It should be consistently, and repeatedly, pointed out that previous cases do not allow a firm conclusion, but only confirm that the right hemisphere is important for the ability of musical expression. Certainly, [the right hemisphere] alone cannot be held responsible. We need only recall the aforementioned case of Skwortzoff (8) to realise that the opinion of Hermann Oppenheim (10), that we are far from having clarified this question further, holds good.

---

[1] The Viennese pathologist Richard von Wiesner (1875–1954) [translators' note].

These intricate processes could be easier to understand, if one supposed that both hemispheres intervene when dealing with musical expression, in such a way that damage of just one hemisphere generally does not induce major disturbances of musical expression. Also, cases with a unilateral lesion usually present incomplete disturbances, although even that is not absolutely necessary; for it might be assumed that in amusia, as with as in other forms of aphasia, individuality plays a large part. The more highly language is developed, the more it is represented in the left side. The less highly, or the more it approaches automatic and affect language, the more it becomes localized bilaterally. Such an explanatory attempt by no means deprives amusia of its independence; nevertheless, it brings amusia closer to aphasia of which it may be a subcategory.

Otto Marburg (1874-1948)
First Surgical Clinic, University of Vienna.

Essential references

1. Gowers WR. Vorlesungen über die Diagnostik der Gehirnkrankheiten (German translation by J. Mommsen). Freiburg; Mohr 1886
2. Ballet G. Le langage interieur et les diverses formes de l'aphasie, 2ème édn. Paris; Félix Alcan 1888
3. Hughlings Jackson J. Singing by speechless (aphasic) children. Lancet 1871;98:430-431
4. Edgren JG. Amusie (musikalische Aphasie). Dtsch Z Nervenheilk 1894;6:1-64
5. Mann L. Casuistische Beiträge zur Hirnchirurgie und Hirnlocalisation. III. Ein operierter Fall von traumatischer Herderkrangung des rechten Frontallappens mit Sectionsbefund (vocale motorische Amusie). Mschr Psychiatr Neurol 1898;4:369-378
6. Mendel K. Kriegsbeobachtungen: Motorische Amusie und Narkolepsie. Neurol Cbl 1916;35:354-361
7. Mann M. Ein Fall von motorischer Amusie. Neurol Cbl 1917;36:149-151
8. Skwortzoff N. De la cécité et de la surdité des mots dans l'aphasie (thèse de doctorat, faculté de médecine de Paris). Paris; Delahaye 1881
9. Liepmann HK. An der Berliner Gesellschaft für Psychiatrie und Nervenkrankheiten einen Aphasischen zeigen, bei dem eine sohon vor Jahrzehnten beschriebene Erscheinung besonders stark hervortritt. Neurol Cbl 1916;35:170-171
10. Oppenheim H. Frage an Herrn Liepmann, ob die Aphasie hier eine rein organisch bedingte ist oder ob neben dem materiellen Prozeß noch ein funktionelles Moment eine Rolle spielt. Neurol Cbl 1916;35:171

In: Advances in Psychology Research. Volume 87
Editor: Alexandra M. Columbus, pp. 239–248
ISBN 978-1-61470-171-2
© 2011 Nova Science Publishers, Inc.

Chapter 10

SINGING BUT NOT SPEAKING: A RETROSPECT ON MUSIC-LANGUAGE INTERRELATIONSHIPS IN THE HUMAN BRAIN SINCE OTTO MARBURG'S *ZUR FRAGE DER AMUSIE* (1919)

D. Koniari[1], H. Proios[2], K. Tsapkini[3] and L. C. Triarhou[1,*]

[1]Neuroscience Wing, University of Macedonia, Thessaloniki, Greece;
[2]Abteilung für Neuropsychologie, Neurologische Klinik, Universitätsspital Zürich, Switzerland;
[3]Department of Neurology, Johns Hopkins Medicine, Baltimore, MD, USA

ABSTRACT

This chapter reviews the relation between human neural systems for language and music as revealed by spoken and sung words, in light of a 1919 contribution by the eminent Viennese neurologist Otto Marburg (1874–1948), placing special emphasis on early neurological ideas in the European continent. Although the topic has been addressed for more than a century, there remain unresolved issues, especially in the light of the increasing evidence that music and language share common processing components. Marburg distanced himself from the holding suggestions at the time on the selective localization of music functions in the right or the left hemisphere; instead, he argued that the two cerebral hemispheres interact during music expression. Such a view might have verged on the heretic then, but is in line with the current neuropsychological evidence.

---

[*] E-mail address: triarhou@uom.gr, phone +30 2310 891-387, fax +30 2310 891-388 (Corresponding author)

INTRODUCTION

One of the eminent neurologists of the 20th century, Otto Marburg (1874–1948) headed Vienna's Neurological Institute as professor and successor to Heinrich Obersteiner (1847–1922), its founder. Marburg (Figure 1) belonged to the intellectual élite forced to leave Austria in the aftermath of the 1938 Nazi *Anschluss* [37,42].

In 1919, Marburg [20] published, in German, a case of motor aphasia and preserved singing ability in words (Figure 2), an English translation of which has been provided [18]. The patient was a soldier who had sustained a tangential gunshot wound at the Italian front; he had been hospitalized at the First Surgical Clinic of the University of Vienna, headed by Anton von Eiselsberg (1860–1939), who often consulted Marburg on neurological matters. The patient became hemiparetic on the right side. One day during his hospitalization, despite a persisting inability to speak, the patient joined another patient in singing a popular song,[1] articulating each word understandably. He remained unable to complete other language expressions, to repeat words or to sing alone spontaneously. With time, language expression began to improve.

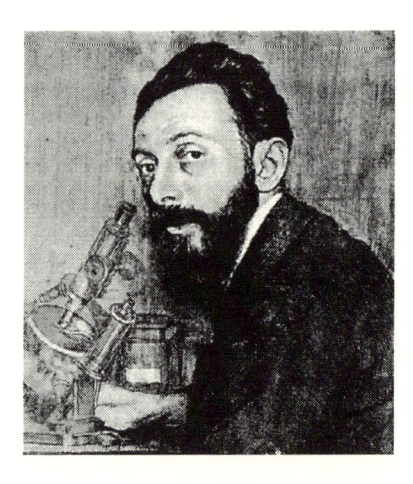

Figure 1. Sketch of Professor Otto Marburg during his years at Obersteiner's Neuropathology Institute in Vienna, appearing in a special Marburg anniversary issue of *Confinia Neurologica* (today *Stereotactic and Functional Neurosurgery*, published by S. Karger AG, Basel) on his 70th birthday, by his pupil Ernst A. Spiegel, who had founded the journal in 1938 [37].

The case gave Marburg an opportunity to discuss the ability of aphasic patients to verbalize words while singing familiar songs. Though Marburg entitled his article *On the question of amusia*, his patient was not truly amusic. In discussing the dissociation between speaking and singing with words, Marburg raised important questions on the representation

---

[1] The tune *Ich hatt' einen Kameraden* was popular among soldiers in World War I. The original lyrics, *Der gute Kamarad*, had been written by Ludwig Uhland of Tübingen in 1809, and set to music by Friedrich Silcher (1789–1860) in 1825, based on the old folk melody *Ein schwarzbraunes Mädchen hat ein'n Feldjäger lieb* (http://www.bdzv.de/kurt_oesterle.html).

and independence of music and language in the brain, and presented his own synthesis on the localization of musical abilities.

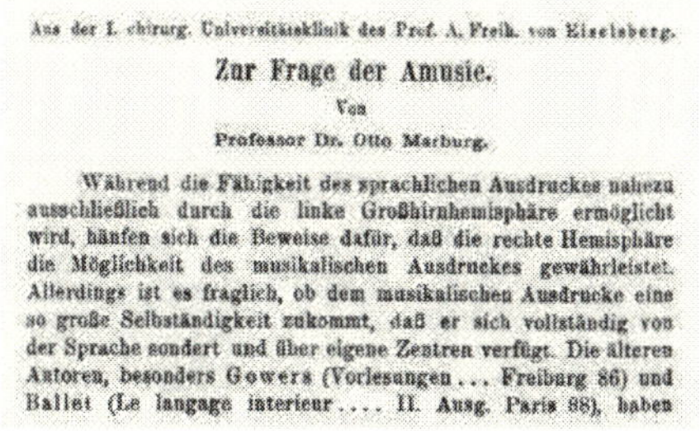
Aus der I. chirurg. Universitätsklinik des Prof. A. Freih. von Eiselsberg.

Zur Frage der Amusie.

Von

Professor Dr. Otto Marburg.

Während die Fähigkeit des sprachlichen Ausdruckes nahezu ausschließlich durch die linke Großhirnhemisphäre ermöglicht wird, häufen sich die Beweise dafür, daß die rechte Hemisphäre die Möglichkeit des musikalischen Ausdruckes gewährleistet. Allerdings ist es fraglich, ob dem musikalischen Ausdrucke eine so große Selbständigkeit zukommt, daß er sich vollständig von der Sprache sondert und über eigene Zentren verfügt. Die älteren Autoren, besonders Gowers (Vorlesungen ... Freiburg 86) und Ballet (Le langage interieur .... II. Ausg. Paris 88), haben

Figure 2. Title page of Otto Marburg's 1919 article on amusia in Obersteiner's *Arbeiten* [20]. Courtesy of the Niedersächsische Staats- und Universitätsbibliothek Göttingen, Germany.

Singing in Aphasia

The term *amusia* was coined in 1888 by the German anatomist August Knoblauch (1836–1919) to denote a 'disorder of the faculty of musical expression' [22]. Knoblauch [16] further presented a diagram of 'centers' and 'pathways' supporting music perception and its potential disorders, using the respective diagram for language of Ludwig Lichtheim (1845–1928) as a template [15].

The first known case of motor aphasia with preserved word articulation during singing was probably reported in 1745 by the Swedish historian Olof von Dalin (1708–1763), who described the case of a farmer's son who, after 'an attack of a violent illness', had lost the movement of his right limbs and could not speak except for saying 'yes'; however, he could recite prayers and sing hymns learned prior to the illness, with the help from persons singing along at the beginning of the hymn [4,30].

In 1895, Johan Gustaf Edgren (1849–1929) published a monograph on amusia and its relation to aphasia. He reported that Jean-Pierre Falret (1794–1870), in the entry on aphasia in the *Dictionnaire encyclopédique des sciences médicales*, underlined that aphasic patients could preserve the ability to sing familiar songs in two ways: either with single syllables, as in the case of a patient described by Béhir in 1836—who could sing *La Marseillaise* and *La Parisienne* using the syllable 'tan'—or with full words in the song [6]. Edgren [6] reviewed the previously published cases and commented that aphasia without a loss of singing with words is common, but the loss of singing alone without aphasia occurs rarely (a single case of a professional singer described by Brazier).

Patients with motor aphasia who could sing a song text, but at the same time unable to recite or verbalize the same words in spoken language, puzzled neurologists in the late 19th century. In the 'localizationist' spirit, speculations sprung to explain them. Marburg [18,20] revisits the ideas of the French neurologist Gilbert Ballet (1853–1916) and the English neurologist Sir William Richard Gowers (1845–1915).

Ballet was a student of Jean-Martin Charcot (1825–1893) and his views on aphasia were compatible with those of his mentor. In his thesis, Ballet [3] states that music and language are representations co-localized in the left hemisphere, the only difference being that the former occur earlier in life and are thus more robust. Accordingly, music representations are the last to be disturbed when there is a memory deficit of language. Knoblauch [16] also suggested that music was a function of the left hemisphere, and placed its centers and pathways in the proximity of the pertinent language areas [15].

The prevailing assumption, until the advent of modern neuropsychological methods, was a hemispheric independence of language and music abilities. With language localized in the left hemisphere, the right hemisphere was considered to mediate music functions. Such a view was supported by Gowers [9], who had suggested that the ability to articulate words while singing might be preserved in patients with motor aphasia due to a clear dissociation between language used in songs (musical language) and language used in conversational speech (propositional language). *Propositional language* expresses ideas ('divergent' in current terminology), whereas *musical language*, which is emotional and nonpropositional, expresses through simple and automatic modalities ('convergent' in current terminology). Gowers [9] was not the first to attribute an automatic, and therefore right hemispheric, nature to singing. John Hughlings Jackson (1835–1911) had already made a distinction between propositional and nonpropositional speech, by characterizing singing as a form of automatic nonpropositional speech, and suggested that each hemisphere was responsible for independent functions; in the event of left hemispheric damage affecting propositional speech, sensorimotor processes in the right hemisphere could still allow the expression of emotional automatic language, such as singing [12,13].

Marburg [18,20] appears puzzled by the discrepancy of previous clinical observations on disturbances of music functions and raises two objections to the earlier interpretations. First, cases of motor aphasia without loss of singing could hardly clarify the issue of independence of linguistic and musical functions: "It should only be consistently highlighted, again and again that previous cases do not make possible a firm decision, but only assure that the right hemisphere is important for the ability of musical expression."

Lesion studies may only reveal whether a region is involved in a function, but not whether such a region is necessarily the only one involved; they show the correspondence between localization and symptom, and not between localization and function. This view was supported by the neurologist Kurt Goldstein (1878–1965), among others [45]. Moreover, the idea that singing operates solely by linguistic automatism is not in accordance with the singers' personal approach toward singing, for "the majority seeks singing to be inspired by the meaning of the words." Thus, Marburg formulates his own hypothesis on the nature of music expression, with the involvement of both cerebral hemispheres.

Marburg [20] is an early voice of reservation on the duality of brain functions regarding language and music. He states that "it is questionable whether such a clear independence exists for musical expression, that is, whether musical expression is completely detached from language and has its own centers" and concludes that "both hemispheres intervene when dealing with musical expression, in that way that losses of a hemisphere generally not induce the same substantial disturbances."

The hypothesis, although novel at the time, is in line with current neuropsychological views suggesting that, contrary to language, there is no specific center for music functions in either cerebral hemisphere. Music processing is based on widely spread neural networks over the entire brain, which underlie the basic components of music, e.g. pitch, timbre, rhythm and meter [2] and can present anatomical and functional differences among subjects, depending on gender [17], musical education [34], and type of music-learning activities [10]. The exact neural networks mediating singing remain incompletely understood, as does the question why can aphasic patients sing.

NEUROBIOLOGY OF SINGING

Singing as a form of musical expression helps the individual interact and communicate from early infancy through late life [41]. Singing may integrate characteristics shared by music (i.e. pitch, melody, rhythm) and speech (i.e. phonological constraints, syntax, semantics) in a way that renders the separation of one from the other difficult. For instance, most studies dealing with singing are subscribed under the general quest of neural substrates of music-processing and rather highlight the musical characteristics of singing—such as pitch and rhythm accuracy—in the absence of a linguistic content (singing with the same syllable, e.g. 'la-la-la' or humming, and not with words). Further, the singing ability is heterogeneous among normal subjects, spanning over a spectrum from singing at a high standard to being 'out of tune'. Thus, it is meaningful for research on the function of singing to adopt repeated-measures designs with the same subject-singer serving as his/her own control [28], something not always possible, especially in clinical cases.

Lesion studies of motor aphasia without vocal amusia, as in Marburg's case report [20], suggested that singing with words might depend on the right cerebral hemisphere. In a modern study of 24 patients with motor aphasia resulting from a cerebrovascular accident in the left inferior frontal lobe [46], 21 of the subjects (or 88%) could preserve singing with words of familiar songs to some degree and 12 of the subjects (or 57%) very fluently, despite their hesitant and anarthric speech. Studies with sodium amylobarbital injection into the carotid artery (Wada test) were also consistent with the hypothesis of a right hemispheric dominance in singing. Singing with words was relatively spared after injection into the left carotid artery, despite the resulting aphasia; on the other hand, injection into the right carotid artery produced vocal amusia with loss of pitch control [8].

The importance of an intact right hemisphere for the ability of fluent singing is also supported by cases of vocal amusia without aphasia in musicians. Infarctions involving the superior temporal cortex of the right hemisphere [40] or the right planum temporale [19] led to serious singing deficits, particularly in pitch control. Right frontal lobe resection for intractable seizures [21] deprived a choir director from the ability to sing familiar melodies, while he could accurately identify them by hearing. On the other hand, aphasia due to a left cerebrovascular accident did not prevent a well known mezzo-soprano from singing; although she speaks with difficulty (her speech is aphasic and dysarthric), she can still sing opera (J. Kaplan and H. Proios, unpublished observations).

In non-musicians, infarct in both middle cerebral arteries [27] or in the right middle cerebral artery [24] produced serious singing deficits. Cases of vocal amusia without aphasia are more difficult to observe and to evaluate in non-musicians, mainly for two reasons. First, patients may not complain about the loss of their singing or music functions, which was not the case in the patient of Peretz et al. [27]. Second, there is limited information concerning the patients' previous musical abilities in order to detect differences, which was not the case in the patient of Murayama et al. [24].

Although in most clinical cases of selective amusia without aphasia a major conclusion is that they point to a possible dissociation between music and speech functions, there is a case of a non-aphasic patient, amateur musician, who, following a right hemisphere stroke, showed dissociation between recognition of instrumental and song melodies [38]. The patient could not anymore identify familiar instrumental melodies but could recognize and identify familiar song melodies presented without accompanying lyrics, including newly learned melodies. The authors suggested that this ability of their patient resided in an intact associated representation of the lyrics in the speech lexicon. Similar findings have been reported in patients with a sustained unilateral lobectomy for the relief of intractable epilepsy [33]. Left temporal lobectomy impaired text recognition, and right temporal lobectomy impaired recognition of melody in the absence of lyrics. However, following left or right temporal lobectomy, melody recognition was also impaired when the song was sung with new words. The authors suggested that there might be a dual code for songs in memory. According to the type of encoding involved in memory, verbal code is related to left temporal structures, whereas the melodic code might depend on either or both temporal lobe mechanisms.

While there is general agreement, from clinical and experimental studies, on right hemisphere involvement in singing, the localization of the responsible site in the brain has proven to be more difficult than the localization of the corresponding site for speech. Transcranial magnetic stimulation (TMS) produces speech arrest when applied over left frontal regions. However, when applied over homologous or other regions of the right frontal lobe, only a few subjects show abolishment of melody production while singing: two out of ten in Epstein et al. [7] and none out of five in Stewart et al. [39]. The latter authors speculate that possibly the neural networks underlying melody production through singing are more diffuse in the brain or that melody production may just be more robust than speech production and hence less susceptible to interference.

NEUROIMAGING OF MUSIC-LANGUAGE INTERACTIONS

The diffusion in the brain of the neural networks subserving singing can be studied with functional neuroimaging methods, which pose a challenge to classical views on the existence of distinct cerebral neural substrates for music and language processing, and show common activation patterns between singing and speaking with the possibility of a right hemispheric advantage for listening to and production of singing (with words or vocalizations) and a left hemispheric advantage for listening to and production of speech.

Singing a single vowel in a single pitch [29] appears to increase cerebral blood flow in cortical areas related to motor control related to speech, such as the supplementary motor area, anterior cingulate cortex, precentral gyri, anterior insula (and the adjacent inner face of the precentral operculum) and cerebellum, with some possible hemispheric asymmetries in both motor and auditory regions (an asymmetrical activation was noted in the right ventral precentral gyrus). A functional MRI study of overt singing a well-known instrumental (non-lyric) tune from Mozart's *Eine kleine Nachtmusik* showed cerebral activation predominantly in the right sensorimotor cortex, including the posterior inferior frontal gyrus, the right anterior insula, and the left cerebellar hemisphere, whereas opposite response patterns emerged during a speech task [32]. Similar activation patterns of singing (by improvising melodic phrases) and speaking (by improvising linguistic phrases), with striking overlap and differences in lateralization tendencies, were also observed in a PET study with amateur musicians [5], which found a much more bilateral pattern of activity. Both tasks activated the supplementary motor area bilaterally, the left primary motor cortex, the premotor cortex bilaterally, the left pars triangularis, the left primary auditory cortex, the secondary auditory cortex bilaterally, the anterior insula, the left anterior cingulate cortex, basal ganglia, ventral thalamus and posterior cerebellum, with the music generation task favoring activation in the dorsal part of the right temporal pole and right frontal operculum. In general, there appears to be a strong bilateral representation for music tasks across the spectrum of non-musicians, amateurs, and experts.

Shared neural substrates between overt singing and speaking, were also found in another functional MRI study [26], with singing provoking a much stronger activation on the right. That study used non-musicians and found a strong right hemispheric effect. The authors used the same words/phrases for both conditions in order to compare differences in hemodynamic responses. Common areas of activation to both tasks included the inferior precentral and postcentral gyri, the superior temporal gyrus, and the superior temporal sulcus bilaterally. The singing condition additionally revealed activation in the mid-portions of the right superior temporal gyrus, and the most inferior and middle portions of the primary sensorimotor cortex. It has been suggested that music and language share common neural resources of perception and production that appear to be also located in brain regions comprising the human mirror-neuron system [23].

Our current view of the interrelationship between singing and speaking functions is still incomplete. Nonetheless, the functional neuroimaging studies clearly show that singing and speaking share common bilateral neural networks, whereby singing activates more neural substrates than speaking. Perhaps those additional areas might offer some clues as to why singing abilities can be spared when speaking abilities become seriously damaged [5,14,26].

CONCLUSION

Cases of motor aphasia without loss of singing with words led to the classical hypothesis of laterality of function, i.e. that this phenomenon can occur because of left hemisphere involvement in propositional (generative or divergent) speech, whereas the right hemisphere is involved in automatic (convergent) speech, including the singing of familiar songs. Marburg [20] appears to be one of the first authors to voice reservations regarding a duality of brain functions involved in music and language, and to suggest that music functions are subserved by both cerebral hemispheres. His thesis is consistent with modern data that support the involvement of diffuse neural networks throughout the human brain in music functions. Considering the neural processes that underlie singing with words, several brain imaging studies have shown differences in neural activity for speech and singing, and mainly support a common neural activation pattern in the left hemisphere with additional right hemispheric involvement in singing.

Important evidence on singing vs. speaking in non-fluent aphasia indicates that verbral production, be it sung or spoken, results from the operation of similar mechanisms [11], and that singing in synchrony with an auditory model—choral singing—is more effective than choral speech in improving word intelligibility, in all likelihood because choral singing entrains more than one auditory-vocal interface [31]. In experiments with TMS it becomes apparent that both auditory and visual speech perception facilitate the excitability of the motor system involved in speech production [44].

Further, most aphasic patients are not professional musicians or highly musical. Thus, the ability to sing with words seems to reflect a rather general brain trait in motor aphasia. Such a finding has led investigators to suggest that, following damage to language areas of the left cerebral hemisphere, music may facilitate word production in aphasic patients by stimulating latent language capacities in homologous language areas of the right cerebral hemisphere [1]. 'Melodic intonation therapy' (MIT) is an aphasia treatment approach most effectively used with expressive aphasic patients; it uses intoned melodies and intonational contours as a means of improving verbal productions [25,43]. The rationale for MIT is that the intact right hemisphere is specialized for melodic functions, and that a facilitation of verbal responses can be achieved with four levels of programmed cued instructions beginning with drills using vocal melodic lines and hand-tapping in response to clinician cues [36]. The MIT's unique engagement of the right hemisphere, both through singing and tapping with the left hand to prime the sensorimotor and premotor cortices for articulation, appear to account for its effect over nonintoned speech therapy [35].

REFERENCES

[1] M.L. Albert, R.W. Sparks and N.A. Helm, Melodic intonation therapy of aphasia, *Arch Neurol* 29 (1973), 130–131.

[2] E. Baeck, The neural networks of music, *Eur. J. Neurol.* 9 (2002), 449–456.

[3] G. Ballet, *Le langage intérieur et les diverses formes de l'aphasie, éd 2*, Félix Alcan, Paris, 1888.

[4] A.L. Benton and R.J. Joynt, Early descriptions of aphasia, *Arch. Neurol.* 3 (1960), 205–222.

[5] S. Brown, M.J. Martínez and L.M. Parsons, Music and language side by side in the brain: a PET study of the generation of melodies and sentences, *Eur. J. Neurosci.* 23 (2006), 2791–2803.

[6] J.G. Edgren, Amusie (musikalische Aphasie), *Dtsch. Z. Nervenheilk.* 6 (1894), 1–64.

[7] C.M. Epstein, K.J. Meador, D.W. Loring, R.J. Wright, J.D. Weissmann, S. Sheppard, J.J. Lah, F. Puhalovich, L. Gaitan and K.R. Davey, Localization and characterization of speech arrest during transcranial magnetic stimulation, *Clin. Neurophysiol.* 110 (1999), 1073–1079.

[8] H. Gordon and J. Bogen, Hemispheric lateralization of singing after intracarotid sodium amylobarbitone, *J. Neurol. Neurosurg Psychiatry* 37 (1974), 727–738.

[9] W.R. Gowers, *Lectures on the Diagnosis of Diseases of the Brain*, J. and A. Churchill, London, 1885.

[10] W. Gruhn, Music learning: neurobiological foundations and educational implications, *Res. Stud. Music Educ.* 9 (1997), 36–47.

[11] S. Hébert, A. Racette, L. Gagnon and I. Peretz, Revisiting the dissociation between singing and speaking in expressive aphasia, *Brain* 126 (2003), 1838–1850.

[12] J. Hughlings Jackson, On a case of loss of power of expression; inability to talk, to write, and to read correctly after convulsive attacks, *Br. Med. J.* 2 (1866), 92–94, 326–330.
[13] J. Hughlings Jackson, Singing by speechless (aphasic) children. *Lancet* 98 (1871), 430–431.
[14] K.J. Jeffries, J.B. Fritz and A.R. Braun, Words in melody: An $H_2^{15}O$ PET study of brain activation during singing and speaking, *NeuroReport* 14 (2003), 749–754.
[15] J.K. Johnson and A.B. Graziano, August Knoblauch and amusia: a nineteenth-century cognitive model of music, *Brain Cogn* 51 (2003), 102–114.
[16] Knoblauch, Amusie, *Dtsch. Arch. Klin. Med.* 43 (1888), 343–344.
[17] S. Koelsch, B. Maes, T. Grossmann and A. Friederici, Electric brain responses reveal gender differences in music processing, *NeuroReport* 14 (2003), 709–713.
[18] D. Koniari and L.C. Triarhou, Otto Marburg's 'On the question of amusia', *Funct. Neurol.* 25 (2010), 5–7.
[19] B. Lechevalier, L. Rumbach, H. Platel, J. Lambert, C.H. Chouard and P. Tran Ba Huy, Amusie isolée révélatrice d'une lésion ischémique du planum temporal droit. Rôle du lobe temporal dans l'appréhension de la musique, *Bull Acad. Natl. Méd.* 190 (2006), 1697–1709.
[20] O. Marburg, Zur Frage der Amusie, *Arb Neurol Inst Wiener Univ* 22 (1919), 106–112.
[21] S. McChesney-Atkins, K.G. Davies, G.D. Montouris, J.T. Silver and D.L. Menkes, Amusia after right frontal resection for epilepsy with singing seizures: case report and review of the literature, *Epil. Behav.* 4 (2003), 343–347.
[22] Meyer, The frontal lobe syndrome, the aphasias and related conditions, *Brain* 97 (1974), 565–600.
[23] Molnar-Szakacs and K. Overy, Music and mirror neurons: from motion to 'e'motion, *Soc. Cogn. Affect. Neurosci.* 1 (2006), 235–241.
[24] J. Murayama, T. Kashiwagi, A. Kashiwagi and M. Mimura, Impaired pitch production and preserved rhythm production in a right brain-damaged patient with amusia, *Brain Cogn.* 56 (2004), 36–42.
[25] Norton, L. Zipse, S. Marchina and G. Schlaug, Melodic intonation therapy: shared insights on how it is done and why it may help, *Ann. NY Acad. Sci.* 1169 (2009), 431–436.
[26] E. Özdemir, A. Norton and G. Schlaug, Shared and distinct neural correlates of singing and speaking, *NeuroImage* 33 (2006), 628–635.
[27] Peretz, S. Belleville and S. Fontaine, Dissociations entre musique et langage après attente cérébrale: un nouveau cas d'amusie sans aphasie, *Rev. Can. Psychol. Exp.* 51 (1997), 354–367.
[28] Peretz, L. Gagnon, S. Hébert and J. Maçoir, Singing in the brain: insights from cognitive neuropsychology, *Music Perc.* 21 (2004), 373–390.
[29] D.W. Perry, R.J. Zatorre, M. Petrides, B. Alivisatos, E. Meyer and A.C. Evans, Localization of cerebral activity during simple singing, *NeuroReport* 10 (1999), 3979–3984.
[30] R. Prins and R. Bastiaanse, The early history of aphasiology: from the Egyptian surgeons (c. 1700 B.C.) to Broca (1861), *Aphasiology* 20 (2006), 762–791.
[31] Racette, C. Bard and I. Peretz, Making non-fluent aphasics speak: sing along! *Brain* 129 (2006), 2571–2584.

[32] Riecker, H., Ackermann, D. Wildgruber, G. Dogil and W. Grodd, Opposite hemispheric lateralization effects during speaking and singing at motor cortex, insula and cerebellum, *NeuroReport* 11 (2000), 1997–2000.

[33] S. Samson and R.J. Zatorre, Recognition memory for text and melody of songs after unilateral temporal lobe lesion: evidence for dual encoding, *J. Exp. Psychol.* 17 (1991), 793–804.

[34] G. Schlaug, The brain of musicians: a model for functional and structural adaptation, *Ann. NY Acad. Sci.* 930 (2001), 281–299.

[35] G. Schlaug, S. Marchina and A. Norton, From singing to speaking: why singing may lead to recovery of expressive language function in patients with Broca's aphasia, *Music Percept.* 25 (2008), 315–323.

[36] R. Sparks, N. Helm and M. Albert, Aphasia rehabilitation resulting from melodic intonation therapy. *Cortex* 10 (1974), 303–316.

[37] E.A. Spiegel, Professor Dr. Otto Marburg, *Confin Neurol.* 7 (1946), 1–2.

[38] W.R. Steinke, L.L. Cuddy and L.S. Jakobson, Dissociations among functional subsystems governing melody recognition after right-hemisphere damage, *Cogn. Neuropsychol.* 18 (2001), 411–437.

[39] L. Stewart, V. Walsh, U. Frith and J. Rothwell, Transcranial magnetic stimulation produces speech arrest but not song arrest, *Ann. NY Acad. Sci.* 930 (2001), 433–435.

[40] Y. Terao, T. Mizuno, M. Shindoh, Y. Sakurai, Y. Ugawa, S. Kobayashi, C. Nagai, T. Furubayashi, N. Arai, S. Okabe, H. Mochizuki, R. Hanajima and S. Tsuji, Vocal amusia in a professional tango singer due to a right superior temporal cortex infarction, *Neuropsychologia* 44 (2006), 479–488.

[41] S.E. Trehub, The developmental origins of musicality, *Nat. Neurosci.* 6 (2006), 669–673.

[42] L.C. Triarhou, Professor Otto Marburg—universal neurologist and the 'dean of teachers', *Wiener. Klin. Wschr.* 120 (2008), 622–630.

[43] B.W. Vines, A.C. Norton and G. Schlaug, Stimulating music: combining melodic intonation therapy with transcranial DC stimulation to facilitate speech recovery after stroke, in: *Transmitters and Modulators in Health and Disease: New Frontiers in Neuroscience*, S. Shioda, I. Homma and N. Kato, eds., Springer, Tokyo, 2009, pp. 103–114.

[44] K.E. Watkins, A.P. Strafella and T. Paus, Seeing and hearing speech excites the motor system involved in speech production, *Neuropsychologia* 41 (2003), 989–994.

[45] N. Wertheim, Is there an anatomical localization for musical faculties? in: *Music and the Brain*, M. Critchley and R.A. Henson, eds., William Heinemann, London, 1977, pp. 282–297.

[46] Yamadori, Y. Osumi, S. Masuhara and M. Okubo, Preservation of singing in Broca's aphasia, *J. Neurol. Neurosurg. Psychiatry* 40 (1977), 221–224.

History of Neurology

Eur Neurol 2011;65:10–15
DOI: 10.1159/000322500

Received: July 13, 2010
Accepted: November 2, 2010
Published online: November 29, 2010

A Review of Edward Flatau's 1894 Atlas of the Human Brain by the Neurologist Sigmund Freud

Lazaros C. Triarhou

University of Macedonia, Thessaloniki, Greece

Key Words
Human nervous system · Edward Flatau · Sigmund Freud · Gustaf Retzius · Brain atlas · History of neuroanatomy · Neuron theory

Abstract
In 1894, the Polish neurologist Edward Flatau (1868–1932), working in Berlin, published an exquisite photographic atlas of the unfixed human brain, preceding by 2 years *Das Menschenhirn*, the reference work of Gustaf Retzius (1842–1919) in Stockholm. In his early career as a neuroanatomist and neurologist, Sigmund Freud (1856–1939) wrote a review of Flatau's atlas for the *Internationale klinische Rundschau*, which has not been included in the 'Standard Edition of the Complete Psychological Works'. The aim of the present paper is twofold: to document Freud's review, and to revive the largely forgotten atlas of Flatau. The full text of Freud is presented in translation. Further, one element Flatau, Retzius and Freud had in common is discussed: their early role as protagonists and firm supporters of Ramón y Cajal's neuron theory, the cornerstone of modern neuroscience.

Copyright © 2010 S. Karger AG, Basel

Introduction

The paths of Edward Flatau (1868–1932), the founder of Polish neurology, and Sigmund Freud (1856–1939), the acknowledged father of psychoanalysis, crossed in 1897, while they were both serving on the editorial board of Karger's *Jahresbericht über die Leistungen und Fortschritte auf dem Gebiete von Neurologie und Psychiatrie* ('Annual Report on the Accomplishments and Progress in the Fields of Neurology and Psychiatry'). The general editor of that journal was Emanuel Mendel (1839–1907); the editorial board comprised such eminent brain researchers as Vladimir Bekhterev (1857–1927), Max Bielschowsky (1869–1940), Ludwig Jacobsohn (1863–1941), Siegfried Kalischer (1862–1954), Lazar Minor (1855–1942), Heinrich Obersteiner (1847–1922), Arnold Pick (1851–1924), Bernhard Pollack (1865–1928) and Theodor Ziehen (1862–1950) [1].

From his student years, in the late 1870s, through the 1890s, Freud occupied himself with the histology, anatomy and pathology of the nervous system, before permanently switching to psychology [2]. In 1891, he published his *Critical Study on Aphasia*, a neurology classic [3]. During those 'neurological' years, Freud regularly reviewed neuropsychiatric articles and books for medical journals. Two such reviews concern anatomical works,

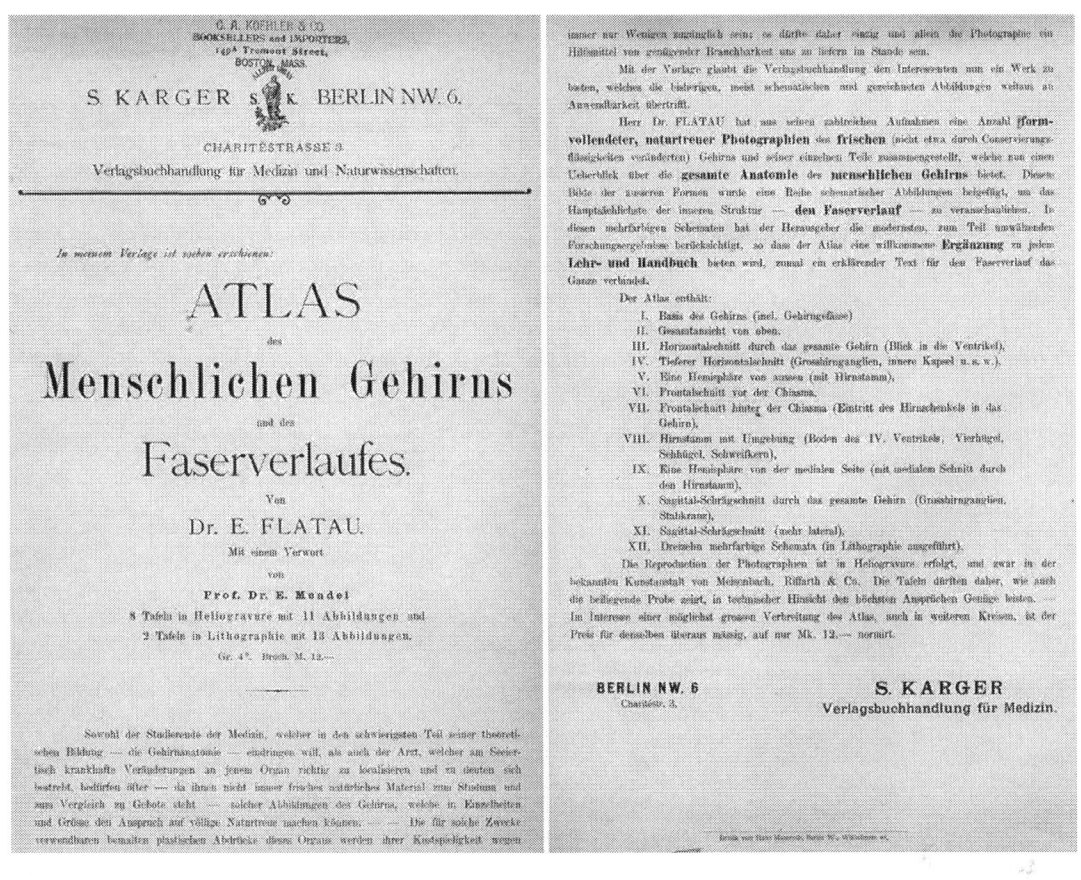

Fig. 1. A kit by the Samuel Karger Verlag in Berlin for the promotion of Flatau's 1894 *Atlas of the Human Brain* (author's archive).

namely, Obersteiner's textbook on the central nervous system [4], and Flatau's atlas of the human brain [5]. These two reviews have not been included in the *Standard Edition of the Complete Psychological Works* [6]. They are listed as works '1887e' and '1894b', respectively, in the *Ausgewählte Bibliographie* by the Freud Museum in Vienna (http://www.freud-museum.at/cms/online/freud/themen/biblio.htm).

Flatau was born in Płock, Poland. He graduated from Moscow University in 1892 and worked in Berlin between 1893 and 1899, the year he returned to Warsaw [7, 8]. In 1894, at the age of 26 years, Flatau published his *Atlas of the Human Brain and the Course of Nerve Fibres* [9]. That work (fig. 1), in large quarto (27×36 cm), most likely represents the first photographic atlas of the human brain in the German language. It appeared in print 2 years prior to the publication in Stockholm of the photographic atlas *Das Menschenhirn* by Gustaf Retzius (1842–1919), perhaps the most outstanding work in macroscopic neuroanatomy of the 19th century [10].

Flatau used whole and dissected human brains, unfixed and only rinsed in water. He applied small diaphragms to effect a better depth of field, and took long-exposure photographs, with exposure times of 20–30 min for uneven surfaces (ventral, dorsal, lateral and medial facies, plates I, II, V and VII), and up to 10 min for flat sections (horizontal, coronal and sagittal, plates III/IV, VI and VIII) [9, 11] (fig. 2). A schematic color chro-

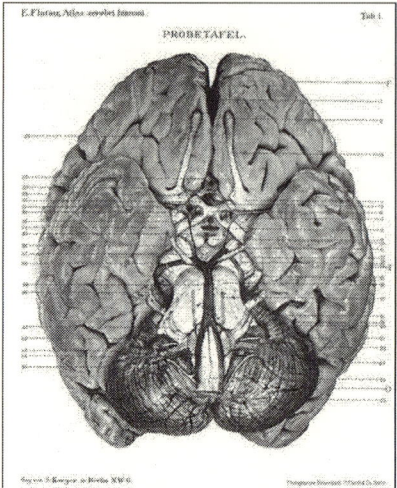

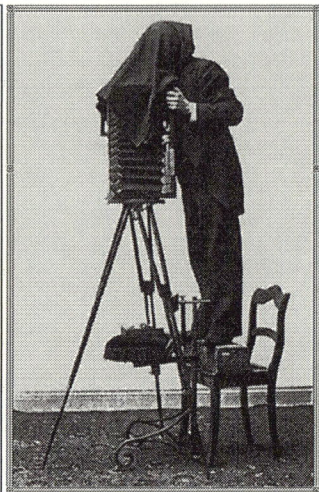

Fig. 2. A sample plate *(Probetafel)* from Flatau's *Atlas of the Human Brain* by Karger, Berlin, left, depicting the ventral cerebral facies (author's archive). Flatau demonstrating his method for macroscopically photographing fresh human brains, right; from a technical article [11] traced from a citation by Pollack [51] (courtesy: Universitätsbibliothek Hamburg).

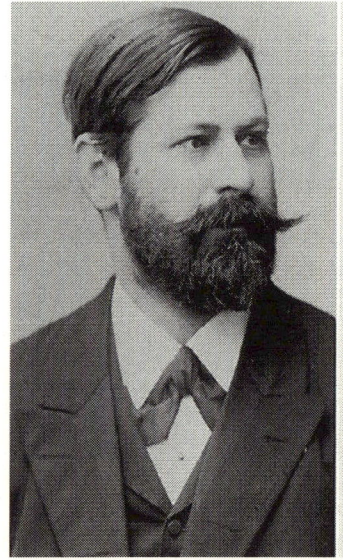

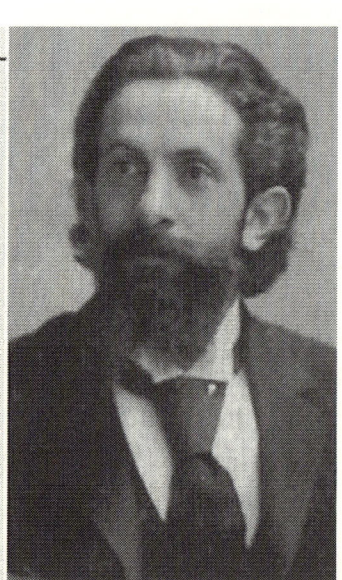

Fig. 3. The 35-year-old Sigmund Freud in Vienna, left (credit: Sigmund Freud Museum, London). Freud's review [5] of the Flatau atlas, middle (courtesy: Universitätsbibliothek der Medizinischen Universität Wien). The 33-year-old Edward Flatau in Berlin, right (credit: Wikimedia Commons, http://upload.wikimedia.org; original photograph traced by Eisenberg [18] in the Berta Lask Archive, Berlin Academy of Arts).

molithograph depicted central brain pathways and connections [9, 12].

The work had been carried out in the laboratory of the Neuropsychiatric Institute of Emanuel Mendel, who also contributed the preface. The atlas was simultaneously published in German, English, French, Polish and Russian [9, 12]. A supplement on microscopy [1] and an inclusive second, revised and enlarged edition [13] were issued 5 years later, including seven additional plates (IX–XV) depicting the cranial nerve nuclei, midbrain, pons, medulla, and spinal cord. Flatau incorporated his 1897 discovery – known as Flatau's law – that the greater the length of a fiber in the spinal cord, the more eccentrically it is located [14], as well as key findings from his degeneration studies [13]. The supplemental work for the second edition was carried out at the Anatomical Institute of Wilhelm Waldeyer (1836–1921).

With Jacobsohn, Flatau co-authored another classic, the *Handbook of Comparative Anatomy of the Mammalian Central Nervous System* [15]. With Minor, they co-edited a two-volume *Handbook of Neuropathology* [16, 17]. Both texts became indispensable references for their contemporaries and successors [18, 19].

An English translation of Freud's review [5] follows (fig. 3). The review of Obersteiner's textbook [4] forms the subject of a separate paper.

The Review by Freud

Dr. Flatau hereby offers physicians and students an atlas of the human brain, which depicts the various full views and some of the most important brain sections in eight plates (11 figures). These plates – from photographs of fresh brain – give an almost three-dimensional impression of the cerebral facies, in clear and characteristic sections, overall deserving to be designated as a superb teaching aid, suitable as a totally reliable reference for both self-study, in the case of not having access to fresh material, and for comparisons at autopsy and the like.

A leading 'schematic plate' in this atlas attempts to give an overview of our knowledge on the course of fiber pathways in the central nervous system in 13 multi-colored drawings, incorporating the known accounts of Mendel, Bekhterev and Edinger on this theme, and continuing with the opposing views of Golgi and Ramón [y Cajal] on the structure of the nervous tissue. The 27 text pages are devoted to the explanation of these schematic drawings. The price of the work (12 marks) is minimal if one considers its breadth and beauty. Author and publisher deserve the appreciation of the medical community for this valuable work.

Sigmund Freud

[Atlas of the Human Brain and the Course of Nerve Fibres. By Ed. Flatau. With a Foreword by Prof. E. Mendel. S. Karger Verlag, Berlin 1894. (Critical Reviews and Literary Notices.)]

Comment

Photographic versus Drawn Atlases of the Human Brain

The *Iconographie Photographique* [20] by the French neurologist Jules Bernard Luys (1828–1897) constitutes the first photographic atlas of the human brain. Prior to that artistic drawings were used to depict brain structure in standard atlases of the time [21–24]. The advent of the photographic technique, with its acclaimed precision, would eventually secure more impartial, impersonal and authentic reproductions of brain form, deemed by investigators to be more accurate than drawings and engravings [25]. In the words of Koskinas [26], '…the hitherto investigations of the brain depicted things schematically and therefore subjectively; if one aims at representing specimens accurately, one makes use of photography; photographic documentation constitutes the most truthful testimony of an exact depiction of nature, as it provides a truly objective image of things as these bear in natural form, size and arrangement.'

The industrious Luys ('subthalamic nucleus of Luys') developed an original view of the structural and functional organization of the brain, and contributed to our knowledge of the neuropathological aspects of mental illness [27]. The *Iconographie* [20] was illustrated with 70 plates containing 81 original albumen prints of brain sections (fixed in a chromate-glycerin solution), plus schematic drawings from his hand.

Édouard Brissaud (1852–1909; upturned 'sulcus of Brissaud' on the superolateral convexity of the superior parietal area) authored the *Anatomie du cerveau de l'homme* accompanied by a splendid atlas with 43 plates [22], drawn by himself in what appears to be a fine art; that prodigious work is still relevant today [28].

The pinnacle of photographic brain atlases of the late 19th century is considered to be the 167-page text volume and the 96-collotype plate volume in large quarto (30×39 cm) of Retzius [10]. The massive opus of scholarship was issued in a limited run of 500 sets. The text was organized in three parts, dealing with the development of the human brain, the morphology of the human brain, and the surface pattern of cortical sulci and gyri in 100 adult hemispheres (35 male right, 40 male left, 12 female right, and 13 female left). The plates comprised 486 drawings (by Sigrid Andersson, Hilma Bundsen, Gustaf Wennman and Ebba Flodman) and 327 directly reproduced photolithographs in natural size; about one third of the plates covered prenatal development (2–9 months of gestation), and the remaining two thirds depicted the adult macroscopic brain structure, with emphasis on individual variations. Specimens were fixed in chrome-osmium-acetic acid, potassium bichromate or formalin. Retzius clarified some of the more difficult problems of cerebral morphology. The wealth of the illustrations and their detailed description rendered *Das Menschenhirn* the best work ever offered until then [29], and also addressed age and gender differences. Retzius made some new discoveries, such as the saccular eminence on the tuber cinereum, the homologue of the saccus vasculosus of lower vertebrates, the relations of the amygdala, and new gyri in the rhinencephalon, the gyrus ambiens and semilunaris, and the fasciolar gyrus. He paid homage to his late father, anatomy professor Anders Retzius (1796–1860) of Karolinska Institutet, by dedicating *Das Menschenhirn* in commemoration of the latter's 100th birthday, and by naming the rudimentary intralimbic gyri after him ('gyri of Anders Retzius').

Freud, Neurology and the Neuron Doctrine

Freud made substantial contributions to basic neuroscience and clinical neurology [2, 30, 31]. He carried out pioneering neuroanatomical studies, using the Weigert method, on the connections of the superior olivary nuclei, on the origin and course of the eighth cranial nerve, and on the relations of the restiform body, as well as neuropathological studies on acute polyneuritis, aphasia, and infantile cerebral diplegia. He suggested, decades ahead of his time, that the trigeminal nucleus might be involved in migraine, also ascribing an important role to the meninges and the innervation of blood vessels [30]. With his histological studies on the spinal ganglia and spinal cord of the lamprey and the structure of nerve cells and fibers in the river crayfish, Freud became one of the early protagonists of the neuron theory [2, 32, 33]. He demonstrated the fibrillary structure of the protoplasm and documented the phenomenon of nuclear rotation in neurons [34]. Moreover, in his 1895 *Project for a Scientific Psychology* [6], Freud proposed the term *Contactschranke* ('contact barriers') to denote what Charles S. Sherrington (1857–1952) would term 'synapses' 2 years later at the suggestion of the Euripides scholar Arthur W. Verrall (1851–1912) of Trinity College [35]. The actual visualization of such 'barriers' and definite proof of the neuron theory would be established half a century later by means of the electron microscope [33, 36].

The value of Flatau's atlas reaches beyond gross morphology. It firmly supports Ramón y Cajal's *neuronismo*. Flatau had joined the Anatomical Institute only 2 years after Waldeyer, his director, had introduced the term *neuron* to denote the nerve or ganglion cell [37]. The word 'neuron' (Greek νεῦρον = nerve) first appears in Homer [38]. Waldeyer [37] adopted the term 'neuron' (Greek νευρών = nerve cell) and popularized the neuron theory, largely based on the landmark discoveries of Ramón y Cajal [39–41], and the substantial contributions of Forel, van Gehuchten, Gowers, His, Kölliker, von Lenhossék, Nansen, Nissl, and others [33, 36, 42–44]. Studying a wide variety of invertebrate and vertebrate species, Retzius had also provided evidence that helped establish the neuron theory [45, 46].

In the first paragraph of his atlas, Flatau states: 'The function of the dendrons is not as yet positively known, some authors (Ramón) being of the opinion that they are nervous; others (Golgi) believe them to have a trophic influence upon the cells. A nerve cell, with its nerve fiber process and the terminal branches of the latter, forms *a nerve unit or 'neuron' of Waldeyer*. The nervous system is made up of an immense number of those independent units, communicating with and influencing one another by contact' [9, 12].

Flatau took a clear stance for neuronism in a subsequent review [47]. He further provided experimental data for the unity of the neuron using the Nissl method, by cutting the oculomotor nerve and detecting secondary changes in the oculomotor nucleus [48]. Fully comprehending the technical basis of brain fixation procedures [49], staining methods [50, 51] and the caprices of silver impregnation [52], Flatau analyzed secondary degeneration after limb amputation in rodents, rabbits and dogs, as well as the effects of toxins, by using the Golgi and Marchi methods [16, 17, 53, 54].

References

1 Flatau E: Supplement zur ersten Auflage vom Atlas des menschlichen Gehirns und des Faserverlaufes. II. Mikroskopischer Theil. Berlin, Karger, 1899.
2 Triarhou LC, del Cerro M: Freud's contribution to neuroanatomy. Arch Neurol 1985;42:282–287.
3 Freud S: Zur Auffassung der Aphasien – Eine kritische Studie. Leipzig-Wien, Franz Deuticke, 1891.
4 Freud S: Literarische Anzeigen – Anleitung beim Studium des Baues der nervösen Centralorgane im gesunden und kranken Zustande. Von Dr H Obersteiner. Wiener Med Wochenschr 1887;37:1642–1644.
5 Freud S: Kritische Besprechungen und literarische Anzeigen – Atlas des menschlichen Gehirns und des Faserverlaufes. Von Ed Flatau. Int Klin Rundschau 1894;8:1131–1132.

6 Freud S: The Standard Edition of the Complete Psychological Works, vol I (1886–1899): Pre-Psycho-Analytic Publications and Unpublished Drafts (transl. by J Strachey and A Freud). London, Hogarth Press/Institute of Psycho-Analysis, 1966.
7 Simchowicz T: Edward Flatau. Schweiz Arch Neurol Psychiatr 1933;31:165–168.
8 Triarhou LC: Edward Flatau (1868–1932). J Neurol 2007;254:685–686.
9 Flatau E: Atlas des menschlichen Gehirns und des Faserverlaufes. Berlin, Karger, 1894.
10 Retzius G: Das Menschenhirn – Studien in der makroskopischen Morphologie. Stockholm, Königliche Buchdruckerei P Norstedt & Söner, 1896.
11 Flatau E: Über die photographischen Aufnahmen der frischen anatomischen Präparate, speziell des Gehirns. Int Med Photogr Monatsschr 1895;2:97–102.
12 Flatau E: Atlas of the Human Brain and the Course of the Nerve-Fibres (transl. by W Nathan and JH Carslaw). Berlin, Karger/Glasgow, Bauermeister, 1894.
13 Flatau E: Atlas des menschlichen Gehirns und des Faserverlaufes, zweite wesentlich vermehrte und verbesserte Auflage. Berlin, Karger, 1899.
14 Flatau E: Das Gesetz der excentrischen Lagerung der langen Bahnen im Rückenmark. Z Klin Med (Berl) 1897;33:55–152.
15 Flatau E, Jacobsohn L: Handbuch der Anatomie und Vergleichenden Anatomie des Centralnervensystems der Säugetiere. Berlin, Karger, 1899.
16 Flatau E: Degenerazioni secondarie del midollo spinale; in Flatau E, Jacobsohn L, Minor L (eds): Manuale di Anatomia Patologica del Sistema Nervoso, vol 2 (trad. del E Morandi). Torino, Unione Tipografico-Editrice Torinese, 1909, pp 885–920.
17 Flatau E: Anatomia patologica del tetano; in Flatau E, Jacobsohn L, Minor L (eds): Manuale di Anatomia Patologica del Sistema Nervoso, vol 2 (trad. del E Morandi). Torino, Unione Tipografico-Editrice Torinese, 1909, pp 1205–1217.
18 Eisenberg U: Vom 'Nervenplexus' zur 'Seelenkraft' – Werk und Schicksal des Berliner Neurologen Louis Jacobsohn-Lask (1863–1940). Frankfurt am Main, Peter Lang, 2005.
19 Richter J: Ulrike Eisenberg – Vom 'Nervenplexus' zur 'Seelenkraft' (book review). J Hist Neurosci 2007;16:225–227.
20 Luys J: Iconographie photographique des centres nerveux: atlas de soixante-dix photographies avec soixante-cinq chémas lithographiés. Paris, Baillière, 1873.
21 Luys J: Recherches sur le système nerveux cérébro-spinal: sa structure, ses fonctions et ses maladies; accompagné d'un atlas de 40 planches. Paris, Baillière, 1865.
22 Brissaud É: Anatomie du cerveau de l'homme: morphologie des hémisphères cérébraux, ou cerveau proprement dit; atlas et texte. Paris, Masson, 1893.
23 Jakob C: Atlas des gesunden und kranken Nervensystems nebst Grundriss der Anatomie, Pathologie und Therapie desselben. München, Lehmann, 1895.
24 Strümpell A, Jakob C: Neurologische Wandtafeln (Icones Neurologicae) zum Gebrauche beim klinischen, anatomischen und physiologischen Unterricht. München, Lehmann, 1897.
25 de Rijcke S: Light tries the expert eye: the introduction of photography in nineteenth-century macroscopic neuroanatomy. J Hist Neurosci 2008;17:349–366.
26 Koskinas GN: Cytoarchitectonics of the human cerebral cortex. Proc Athens Med Soc 1926;92:44–48.
27 Parent A, Parent M, Leroux-Hugon V: Jules Bernard Luys: a singular figure of 19th century neurology. Can J Neurol Sci 2002;29:282–288.
28 Walusinski O: Jacques Poirier – Édouard Brissaud, un neurologue d'exception dans und famille d'artistes (book review). Eur Neurol 2010;64:192.
29 von Waldeyer-Hartz W: Nachruf Gustaf Retzius, mit einem Bildnis. Anat Anz 1920;52:261–268.
30 Pearce JMS: Fragments of Neurological History. London, Imperial College Press, 2003.
31 Triarhou LC: Exploring the mind with a microscope: Freud's beginnings in neurobiology. Hellenic J Psychol 2009;6:1–13.
32 Køppe S: The psychology of the neuron: Freud, Cajal and Golgi. Scand J Psychol 1983;24:1–12.
33 Shepherd GM: Foundations of the Neuron Doctrine. New York, Oxford University Press, 1991.
34 Triarhou LC, del Cerro M: The histologist Sigmund Freud and the biology of intracellular motility. Biol Cell 1987;61:111–114.
35 Shepherd GM, Erulkar SD: Centenary of the synapse: from Sherrington to the molecular biology of the synapse and beyond. Trends Neurosci 1997;20:385–392.
36 Van der Loos H: The history of the neuron; in Hydén H (ed): The Neuron. Amsterdam, Elsevier, 1967, pp 1–47.
37 Waldeyer HWG: Über einige neuere Forschungen im Gebiete der Anatomie des Centralnervensystems. Dtsch Med Wochenschr 1891; 17: 1213–1218,1244–1246,1287–1289,1331–1332,1352–1356.
38 Ochs S: A History of Nerve Functions – From Animal Spirits to Molecular Mechanisms. Cambridge, Cambridge University Press, 2004.
39 Ramón y Cajal S: Die histogenetischen Beweise der Neuronentheorie von His und Forel. Anat Anz (Jena) 1907;30:113–144.
40 Ramón y Cajal S: Neuron Theory or Reticular Theory? Objective Evidence of the Anatomical Unity of Nerve Cells (transl. by M Ubeda Purkiss and CA Fox). Madrid, Consejo Superior de Investigaciones Científicas – Instituto Ramón y Cajal, 1954.
41 Ramón y Cajal S: The Neuron and the Glial Cell (transl. and ed. by J de la Torre and WC Gibson). Springfield, Thomas, 1984.
42 von Lenhossék M: Der Feinere Bau des Nervensystems im Lichte Neuester Forschungen. Berlin, Fischer's Medicinische Buchhandlung H Kornfeld, 1893.
43 McHenry LC: Garrison's History of Neurology. Springfield, Thomas, 1969.
44 Meyer A: Historical Aspects of Cerebral Anatomy. London, Oxford University Press, 1971.
45 Retzius G: Punktsubstanz, 'nervöses Grau' und Neuronenlehre. Biol Untersuch N Folge (Stockholm-Jena) 1905;12:1–19.
46 Larsell O: Gustaf Magnus Retzius (1842–1919); in Haymaker W, Baer KA (eds): The Founders of Neurology. Springfield, Thomas, 1953, pp 83–86.
47 Flatau E: Ueber die Neuronenlehre. Z Klin Med (Berl) 1895;28:51–65.
48 Flatau E: Einige Betrachtungen über die Neuronenlehre im Anschluss an frühzeitige, experimentell erzeugte Veränderungen der Zellen des Oculomotoriuskerns. Fortschr Med (Berl) 1896;16:210–225.
49 Flatau E: Beitrag zur technischen Bearbeitung des Centralnervensystems. Anat Anz (Jena) 1897;13:323–329.
50 Flatau E: Ueber die Färbung von Nervenpräparaten. Dtsch Med Wochenschr 1895; 21:212–214.
51 Pollack B: Die Färbetechnik des Nervensystems, zweite, vermehrte und verbesserte Auflage. Berlin, Karger, 1898.
52 Flatau E: Ueber die zweckmässige Anwendung der Golgi'schen Sublimatmethode für die Untersuchung des Gehirns des erwachsenen Menschen. Arch Mikrosk Anat (Bonn) 1895;45:158–162.
53 Goldscheider A, Flatau E: Ueber die Pathologie der Nervenzellen. Arch Psychiatr Nervenkrankh 1897;30:309–312.
54 Goldscheider A, Flatau E: Normale und pathologische Anatomie der Nervenzellen auf Grund der neueren Forschungen. Berlin, Fischer's Medicinische Buchhandlung H. Kornfeld, 1898.

A review of Heinrich Obersteiner's 1888 textbook on the central nervous system by the neurologist Sigmund Freud

Paul D. Hatzigiannakoglou and **Lazaros C. Triarhou**

Economo-Koskinas Wing for Integrative and Evolutionary Neuroscience, University of Macedonia, Thessaloniki, Greece

Received December 8, 2010, accepted (after revision) April 12, 2011

Eine kritische Besprechung des Neurologen Sigmund Freud über die „Anleitung beim Studium des Baues der nervösen Centralorgane" (1888) von Heinrich Obersteiner

Zusammenfassung. Im Jahre 1888 fasste der österreichische Neuroanatom Heinrich Obersteiner, Gründer des Wiener Neurologischen Institutes, die damals aktuellsten Kenntnisse zusammen und bezog seine eigenen Forschungsergebnisse über die normale und pathologische Anatomie des menschlichen Nervensystems ein, indem er seine „Anleitung beim Studium des Baues der nervösen Centralorgane im gesunden und kranken Zustande" veröffentlichte. Das Buch wurde weltweit zur „Bibel für Generationen von angehenden Neurologen" und übte einen entscheidenden Einfluss auf die folgende Entwicklung der Neurologie als eigenständige medizinische Wissenschaft. In seiner frühen Karriere als Neuroanatom erstellte Sigmund Freud eine literarische Anzeige über das Obersteiner'sche Lehrbuch, die in der *Wiener Medizinischen Wochenschrift* erschien. Jene Anzeige wurde jedoch nicht in der „*Standard Edition of the Complete Psychological Works*" eingeschlossen. Durch die vorliegende Arbeit wird nun eine englische Übersetzung der Freud'schen Besprechung zur Verfügung gestellt; dazu wird der historische Rahmen vorgeführt, vor allem hinsichtlich des Einflusses von Theodor Meynert auf seine hervorragenden Studenten Freud und Obersteiner.

Schlüsselwörter: Menschliches Zentralnervensystem, Heinrich Obersteiner (1847-1922), Sigmund Freud (1856-1939), Theodor Meynert (1833-1892), Geschichte der Neurowissenschaften

Summary. In 1888, the Austrian neuroanatomist Heinrich Obersteiner, founder of Vienna's Neurological Institute, published his "*Introduction to the Study of the Structure of the Central Nervous Organs in Health and Disease*", a fundamental textbook in which he summarised the state-of-the-art knowledge available then on the normal and pathological anatomy of the human nervous system, incorporating many of his original research findings. The book became "the Bible for generations of budding neurologists" worldwide and was crucial for the eventual development of neurology as an independent medical discipline. In his early career as a neuroanatomist, Sigmund Freud wrote a review of Obersteiner's book for the *Wiener Medizinische Wochenschrift*. That review was not included in the "*Standard Edition of the Complete Psychological Works*". The present article provides an English translation of Freud's review and further discusses its historical context, especially regarding the influence of Theodor Meynert on his two illustrious students, Freud and Obersteiner.

Key words: Human brain structure, Heinrich Obersteiner (1847-1922), Sigmund Freud (1856-1939), Theodor Meynert (1833-1892), history of neuroscience

Introduction

Heinrich Obersteiner (1847-1922), the founder of Vienna's Neurological Institute, and Sigmund Freud (1856-1939), the acknowledged father of psychoanalysis, both began their research careers as medical students in the neurohistology laboratory of Vienna University's Physiological Institute, headed by Ernst Wilhelm von Brücke (1819-1892). Obersteiner entered university in 1865 and graduated in 1870; Freud entered in 1873 and graduated in 1881. In 1897, both Obersteiner and Freud served on the editorial board of Karger's *Jahresbericht über die Leistungen und Fortschritte auf dem Gebiete vom Neurologie und Psychiatrie* ("Annual Report on the Accomplishments and Progress in the Fields of Neurology and Psychiatry") under the general

---

Correspondence: *Prof. Lazaros C. Triarhou, MD, PhD*, Economo-Koskinas Wing for Integrative and Evolutionary Neuroscience, University of Macedonia, Egnatia 156, Bldg. Z-312, 54006 Thessaloniki, Greece.
Fax: ++30-2310891388, E-mail: triarhou@uom.gr

editorship of the Berlin neuropsychiatrist Emanuel Mendel (1839–1907) [1].

Obersteiner was born in Vienna into a family of physicians on 13 November 1847; he died in Vienna on 19 November 1922. His first publication, as a 20-year-old medical student, was "On the development and growth of the tendon" [2]. (Ten years later, Freud's first publication appeared, "On the origin of the dorsal spinal roots in the Petromyzon" [3], written as a 21-year-old medical student.) Obersteiner became *Dozent* in 1873, *Extraordinarius* in 1880, *Ordinarius* in 1898 and *Hofrat* in 1906; he was also awarded an honorary doctorate from Oxford University [4, 5]. In 1882, with a generous personal donation of half a million crowns accepted by the Austrian Ministry of Culture, he founded the "University Institute for the Anatomy and Physiology of the CNS" (renamed the "Neurological Institute" in 1900), the world's first interdisciplinary brain research centre and served as its first director until his retirement in 1919 [4, 6]. He was succeeded by Otto Marburg (1874–1948) [7]. His contributions to neurology are diverse and include studies on progressive paresis, epilepsy, allochiria, intoxication psychoses and spinal anatomy, as well as comparative studies of the anatomy of the elephant, whale and human cerebellum. A true *Künstlerarzt*, Obersteiner was a gifted musician, exceedingly fond of the classical repertoire, and conducted the *Wiener Ärzte-Orchester* [8, 9].

In 1888, Obersteiner published the first edition of his "*Introduction to the Study of the Structure of the Central Nervous Organs in Health and Disease*" in German [10]. This book went through four further German editions over the following 25 years; it was twice translated into English (Fig. 1) and Russian, as well as into French and Italian [11–13]. Obersteiner largely relied on his own research findings for the book, integrating many original observations into the subject matter with a remarkable modesty, and his characteristic tendency for "objectification" and anonymity [5, 14]. Otto Marburg remarked that "it is always the disadvantage of a textbook, whereby the author's own research can become lost, and one might hardly appreciate how many of his own new findings that book contains" [5], "that it would be difficult to list singly" [4].

This textbook [10] represents one of the first comprehensive works on the normal and pathological

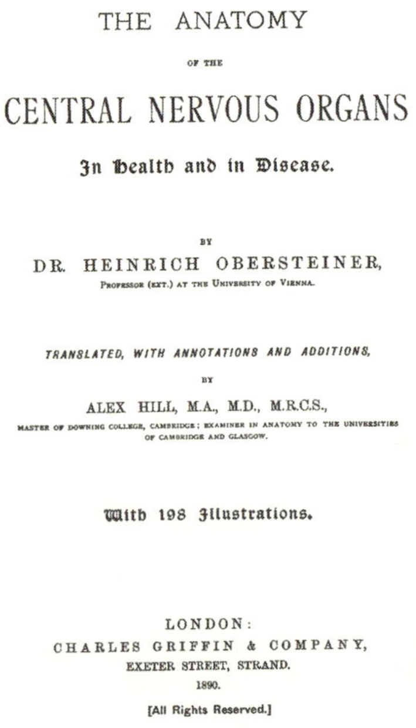
THE ANATOMY

OF THE

CENTRAL NERVOUS ORGANS

In Health and in Disease.

BY

DR. HEINRICH OBERSTEINER,

PROFESSOR (EXT.) AT THE UNIVERSITY OF VIENNA.

TRANSLATED, WITH ANNOTATIONS AND ADDITIONS,

BY

ALEX HILL, M.A., M.D., M.R.C.S.,

MASTER OF DOWNING COLLEGE, CAMBRIDGE; EXAMINER IN ANATOMY TO THE UNIVERSITIES OF CAMBRIDGE AND GLASGOW.

With 198 Illustrations.

LONDON:
CHARLES GRIFFIN & COMPANY,
EXETER STREET, STRAND.
1890.

[All Rights Reserved.]

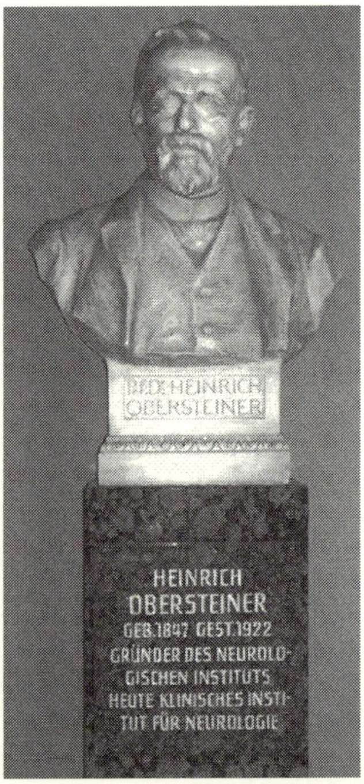

Fig. 1: Title page of the 1890 English version of Obersteiner's textbook [12], left (author's archive). Heinrich Obersteiner's marble bust, right, decorating the *Arkadenhof* at the University of Vienna (photo by one of the authors, July 2006). The bust was initially located at the Neurological Institute on Schwarzspanierstrasse, having been unveiled on 23 November 1907 during the silver anniversary celebrations for the Institute's creation in 1882 [15]

anatomy of the nervous system with functional correlations, which established the new field of basic and clinical neuromorphology [14]. It was a systematically presented syllabus of all the organic knowledge on the subject. It was the first time that an attempt was made to sum up all the state-of-the-art knowledge at the time that was necessary to logically study the brain and spinal cord, including techniques, cells, individual brain provinces, macroscopic and microscopic aspects and a review of pathways. He managed to present, with clarity and simplicity, material on each theme that had been considered unapproachable until then [6]. For the first time, brain research was treated as a branch of medicine, a fact of crucial importance for the eventual development of neurology as a medical discipline. Its tremendous educational and publishing success was so appreciated that it truly became, according to Marburg, "the textbook of the entire neurological world" [5, 15].

Obersteiner was a most influential neurologist. He was called the "unequalled master of theoretical neurology" by Otto Marburg [4], the "grand master of neuroanatomy and neuropathology" by Erwin Stransky [16], the "patriarch of neurology" by Franz Seitelberger [5] and *"magister magistrorum"* by Alfred Schick [9]. Numerous important neurologists from the European North and South and Asia and the Americas, of diverse nationalities and faiths, who shared a common interest in scientific and cultural exploration, were trained at the Obersteiner Institute. They include Ariëns Kappers, Bailey, Campbell, von Economo, von Frankl-Hochwart, Hunt, Karplus, Koskinas, Marburg, Neuburger, Pollak, Redlich, Spiegel, Stengel, Stransky and Tsiminakis [5, 17]. The students were cognisant of their mentor's impact: "He has given us more than life; he has given us a world of the spirit that nourishes life" [4].

In 1903, 50 high-ranking scholars, including Ariëns Kappers, Bekhterev, Cajal, Déjerine, Edinger, Flechsig, van Gehuchten, Golgi, His, von Lenhossék, Mingazzini, von Monakow, Obersteiner, Raymond, Retzius, Sherrington, Waldeyer and Weigert, banded together to found the Brain Commission, the first international neuroscience organisation and forerunner of IBRO, the International Brain Research Organisation [18]. Waldeyer served as president from 1904 until the end of the Commission's existence in 1914 with the outbreak of World War I [19, 20], while Obersteiner served as the Commission's first vice president [14, 21].

In his early career in neuroanatomy, neuropathology and clinical neurology [22, 23], Freud regularly reviewed neuropsychiatric articles and books for medical journals. Between 1887 and 1893, he published over a dozen such reviews of neurological and

1887. Wiener Medizinische Wochenschrift Nr. 50. 1642

Literarische Anzeigen.

Anleitung beim Studium des Baues der nervösen Centralorgane im gesunden und kranken Zustande. Von Dr. H. Obersteiner. 406 pp. Leipzig und Wien, Toeplitz und Deuticke, 1888.

Besprochen vom Dozenten Dr. Sigm. Freud.

Die letzten drei Jahre haben uns mit drei Darstellungen der Lehre vom Gehirnbaue beschenkt, in welchen die didaktische Absicht in den Vordergrund tritt. Die erste derselben Edinger's „Zehn Vorlesungen über den Bau der nervösen Centralorgane, 1885" ist ein kurzer, aber vortrefflich gelungener Versuch, welcher aus der Anatomie des Centralorgans alles dasjenige hervorhebt, was derzeit physiologisch oder pathologisch verwerthbar erscheint, und sich dabei wesentlich auf die Resultate stützt, die man der Anwendung der Flechsig'schen Methode (Studium des Faserverlaufes am frontalen Centralorgane) verdankt. Das zweite Werk, der Traité élémentaire d'Anatomie médicale du système nerveux von Féré (dem Adjunkten der Salpêtrière), ist schätzenswerth, wo es die klinischen und pathologisch-anatomischen Ermittlungen der Charcot'schen Schule zusammengestellt, aber unselbständig und selbst armselig, sobald es den feineren Bau des Centralorgans und den Faserverlauf in demselben behandelt.

Das hier vorliegende neue Buch von Obersteiner ist hingegen als die — soweit sie reicht — zuverlässigste und vollstän-

2

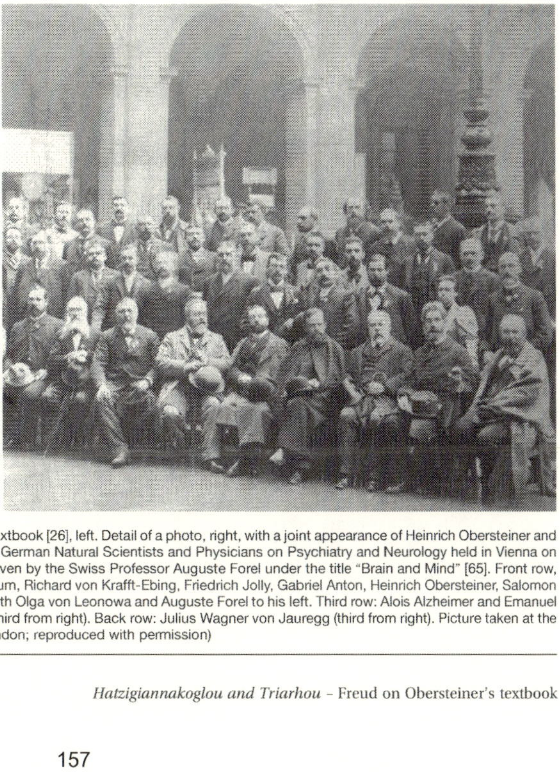

Fig. 2: Freud's review of the first German edition of Obersteiner's textbook [26], left. Detail of a photo, right, with a joint appearance of Heinrich Obersteiner and Sigmund Freud as participants of the 66th General Meeting of the German Natural Scientists and Physicians on Psychiatry and Neurology held in Vienna on 24–30 September 1894. A keynote address at that meeting was given by the Swiss Professor Auguste Forel under the title "Brain and Mind" [65]. Front row, seated, left to right: Constantin von Monakow, Karl Ludwig Kahlbaum, Richard von Krafft-Ebing, Friedrich Jolly, Gabriel Anton, Heinrich Obersteiner, Salomon Stricker. Second row, standing: Sigmund Freud (third from right), with Olga von Leonowa and Auguste Forel to his left. Third row: Alois Alzheimer and Emanuel Mendel (second and third from left), Lothar von Frankl-Hochwart (third from right). Back row: Julius Wagner von Jauregg (third from right). Picture taken at the *Arkadenhof* of the University (credit: Sigmund Freud Museum, London; reproduced with permission)

neuroanatomical articles by prominent authors, including Bekhterev, Danilewsky, Mingazzini, Pal, Schaffer and Ziehen. Solms [24] generated an English translation of a previously unknown review by Freud, which focused on a monograph written by the versatile Obersteiner on hypnotism; this review represents one of Freud's earliest published references on the subject. Obersteiner was one of the neurologists who called attention to the experiences of Freud and Josef Breuer in hypnosis [9]. On the other hand, Freud [25] credits Obersteiner as the first to give an impetus to the scientific study of hypnosis.

Two other book reviews by Freud concerned anatomical works: the textbook on the central nervous system by Obersteiner [26] (Fig. 2), and the atlas of the human brain by the Polish neurologist Edward Flatau [27, 28] (Fig. 3). These two reviews were omitted by Freud from the bibliographical abstract of publications that he had compiled for his promotion dossier in May 1897, and were thus not included in the "*Standard Edition of the Complete Psychological Works*" [29] either. They are listed, respectively, as works "1887e" and "1894b" in the updated *Ausgewählte Bibliographie* by the Freud Museum in Vienna (http://www.freud-museum.at/cms/online/freud/themen/biblio.htm).

AUS DEM I. ANATOMISCHEN INSTITUT DER UNIVERSITÄT BERLIN.
(Director: Geh. Med.-Rat Prof. Dr. Waldeyer.)

SUPPLEMENT

zur ersten Auflage vom

ATLAS

des

Menschlichen Gehirns

und des

Faserverlaufes.

Von

Dr. EDWARD FLATAU

IN WARSCHAU

II. Mikroskopischer Theil.

BERLIN 1899
VERLAG VON S. KARGER
KARLSTRASSE 15.

Fig. 3: Obersteiner's personal copy of the 1899 "Microscopic Supplement" to Edward Flatau's atlas of the human brain [1] (author's archive)

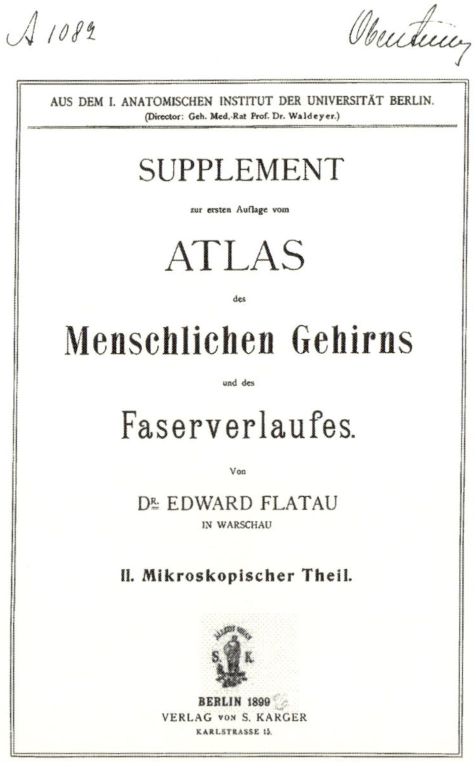

An English translation of Freud's critique [26] of Obersteiner's neuroanatomy follows (Fig. 2). The review of Flatau's atlas [28] has been already presented [30].

It is of interest to note that Freud's review is dated 1887 [26] whereas Obersteiner's book is dated 1888 [10], giving the impression that the critique might have preceded the book. The fact is that Freud's article [26] was published in issue 50 of volume 37 of the *Wiener Medizinische Wochenschrift*, i.e. in the second week of December 1887. Whereas Toeplitz & Deuticke, the book publisher, printed 1888 on the title page, Obersteiner's *Vorwort* is actually dated as October 1887. Even today, when a book is technically due to appear in print towards the end of a particular year, a publisher may sometimes indicate the new (upcoming) year as the year of publication.

The Review by Freud

The last three years have given us three accounts of the knowledge of brain structure, whereby a didactic intent immediately becomes evident. The first of them, Edinger's *Zehn Vorlesungen über den Bau der nervösen Centralorgane* ("Ten Lectures on the Structure of the Central Nervous Organs" [31]) is a short but successful attempt that highlights all those aspects of the anatomy of the brain that presently apply to its physiology and pathology, considerably relying upon results obtained through the use of Flechsig's method (study of fibre pathways in the forebrain). The second work, the *Traité élémentaire d'anatomie médicale du système nerveux* ("Elementary Textbook of Medical Anatomy of the Nervous System" [32]) by Féré, an adjunct at La Salpêtrière, is worthwhile insofar as it combines the clinical and pathological-anatomical findings of the school of Charcot, but it does not address the finer structure of the brain and the course of its fibres.

On the contrary, the new book by Obersteiner reviewed here can be described, as far as it goes, as the most reliable and complete of these new accounts of brain structure. Its comprehensiveness, clear layout and impartial approach allow one to express the expectation that this work will become, in due course, a reliable guide for anyone seeking to acquire a good anatomical understanding of the nervous system.

It would be appropriate to offer medical readers a better characterisation of this valuable book by means of some general remarks and a closer look at its contents. The first section deals with technical methods of studying brain anatomy, as well as various other sources that the knowledge on brain structure is derived from. In the discussion of the latter (a study of the incompletely formed and pathologically altered brain, a comparative-anatomical, experimental-physiological investigation), one will readily welcome the accompanying critical comments. In particular, the interpretation of results obtained by the Gudden method necessitates a critical approach, which researchers using this specific method do not always use. On the contrary, Obersteiner, as a general rule, limits himself to identifying certain points as being questionable instead of rebutting them, a trend that reveals his great discretion in reaching conclusions about the grand, contested questions. The second section, which deals with the morphology of the central nervous system, contains a large number of new, very good figures presented in woodcuts and several comments regarding the physiological meaning of the gyri of the cerebral hemispheres. One needs to emphasise the third section of the book, which constitutes a description of the histological elements of the central nervous system in health and in disease, accompanied by extremely accurate and especially successful figures. One realises in this, as well as in the remaining chapters of the book, that the author carefully avoids mentioning his own name, something that may not necessarily be praiseworthy. The fourth section on the finer structure of the spinal cord uses as an introduction a series of interesting approaches to the general anatomy of the central nervous system. Here one finds definitions of terms commonly used in describing the brain, such as nucleus, root, commissure,

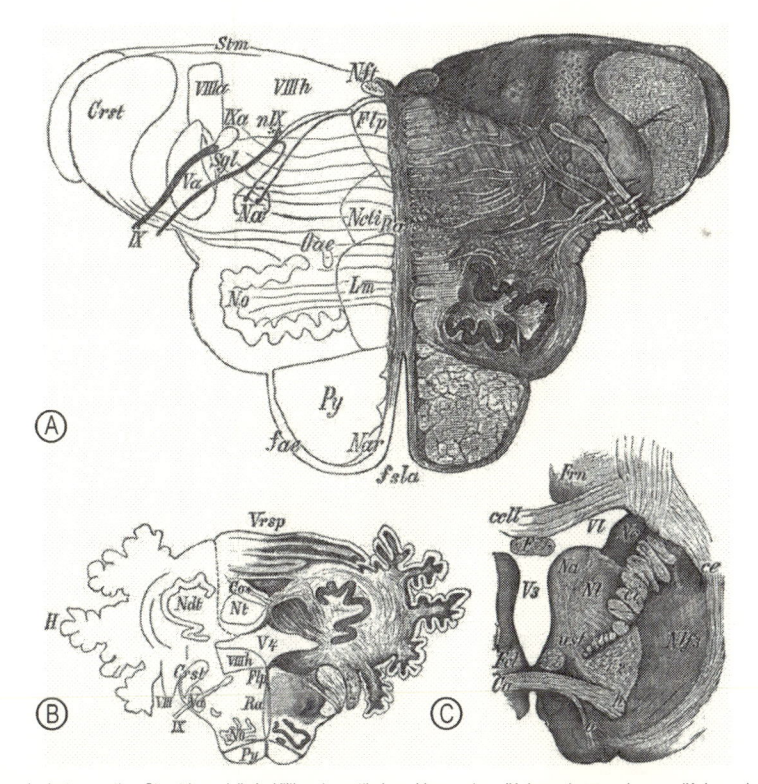

Fig. 4: (A) Transverse brainstem section. *Stm* stria medullaris; *VIIIh* main vestibulocochlear nucleus; *IX* glossopharyngeal nerve; *nIX* glossopharyngeal nucleus; *Flp* posterior longitudinal fasciculus; *Ncti* inferior central nucleus. Figure 116 in Obersteiner [10], also selected by the publisher for the promotion prospectus. Frontal sections through the monkey cerebellum and medulla oblongata **(B)** and rostral to the thalamus **(C)**. ×1.5. *H*, cerebellar hemisphere; *Vrsp*, superior vermis; *Ndt*, dentate nucleus; *Nt*, tectal nucleus; *Co+*, commissure; *V₄*, fourth ventricle; *Crst*, restiform body; *Py*, pyramid; *Flp*, posterior longitudinal fasciculus; *Ra* raphé; *No* olivary nucleus; *VIII*, vestibulocochlear nerve; *Va* ascending root of trigeminal. *Na*, anterior thalamic nucleus; *ust*, inferior thalamic peduncle; *h*, and *o*, hemispheric and olfactory portions of anterior commissure. Figures 123 and 131 in Obersteiner [10]

pathway and the like. What is lacking from the mention of the "fibre system" are those schematic terms that should be the most productive for a future presentation of "general brain anatomy". Nonetheless, a deeper look at the scientific ideas that should form the basis of brain anatomy in the future does not seem to be part of the plan of Obersteiner's book, which is defined as an "Introduction to the study of the central nervous system". Thus, attempts for an integrated view of brain structure, such as the system of Meynert and the schemes of Luys, Aeby and Flechsig, are dealt with in a few lines. The fifth section, "a topographic study of the brain", addresses the most difficult task of a textbook such as this, which is the depiction of orientation for the student, using a series of cross-sections throughout the brainstem. Figures 110-131 (figs. 118-139 in the English edition [12], Fig. 4), which accompany the text, are based on carmine preparations, and therefore show, first and foremost, the distribution of grey and white matter, and only secondarily depict the fibre system in cross-section. In this respect, these figures are less instructive than they could have been and less informative than e.g. the figures in the first volume of Meynert's *Psychiatry* [33]. The author was most likely aware of this, as one may deduce from the introduction. He opted, after all, to include in the figures precise reproductions of preparations that would be readily available to students. However, the Weigert preparations of adult human tissue, which depict fibre disposition in such an excellent way, do not allow for sufficient magnification to be useful for instructive purposes, and provide two series of images that would have raised the cost of the book to inappropriate heights for an educational text (The figures in Meynert's *Psychiatry* [33] are based on gold preparations, which are well suited for the demonstration of fibre disposition at low magnification). The sixth section contains, under the heading "Fibre tracts and pathways", a cohesive presentation of the previously known fibre pattern and is, accordingly, mostly based on results of secondary degeneration and

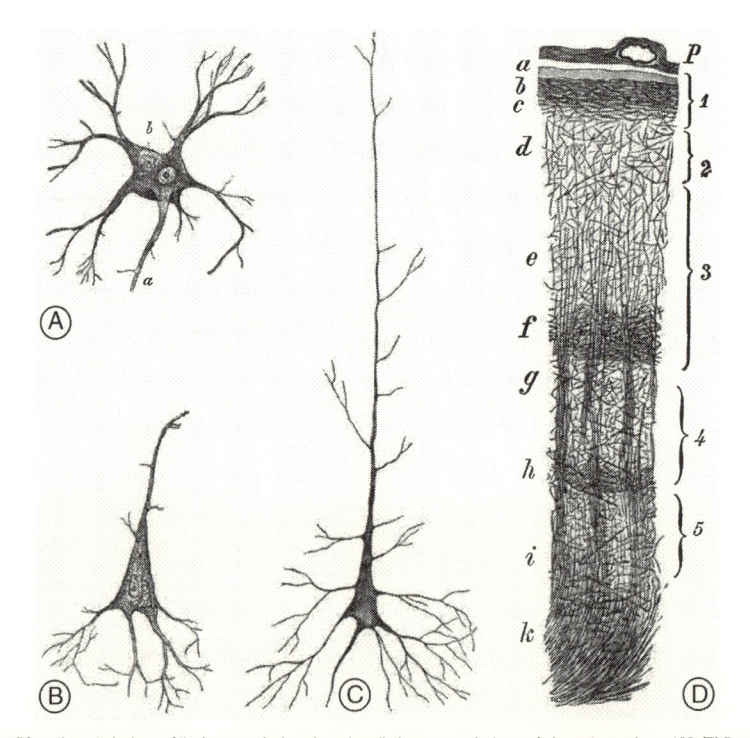

Fig. 5: (A) Nerve cell from the anterior horn of the human spinal cord; *a* axis-cylinder process; *b* clump of pigment granules. ×100. **(B)** Pyramidal cell from the human cerebral cortex. ×150. **(C)** Pyramidal cell from the cerebral cortex. Mercury preparation. ×150. Figures 45, 48 and 162 in Obersteiner [10]. **(D)** The "fig. 163" in Obersteiner [10] mentioned by Freud [26], showing the cerebral cortex of the frontal lobe with the Weigert method. *P*, pia mater; *1–5*, Meynert's five layers; *a*, layer of superficial connective tissue; *b*, layer of tangential myelinated fibres; *c*, deeper part of molecular layer; *d*, fibre network in small pyramidal layer; *e*, outer part of third layer; *f*, external stripe of Baillarger; *g*, fibre network of third and fourth layers; *h*, internal stripe of Baillarger; *i*, deepest part of fourth and fifth layers; *k*, white matter. ×50

incomplete myelination. At present, it is an exceedingly difficult task to deliver a presentation of this sort. The material available for this purpose is scanty, leaving big gaps, even in the chapters that appear to be the most complete, and a good part of the supposed facts still rely on the claims of individual researchers. The author, who was in a position to treat the contents of the other chapters of the book based on his own experience, has to appear as a compiler of information in the chapter on "Fibre tracts and pathways". However, it is this section of the book that displays the outstanding manner in which the author commands the material and literature contained therein. The chapter on fibre tracts and pathways contains a series of schematic drawings, several of which are new, e.g. the scheme of the central rhinencephalic apparatus and several new images of the cerebral cortex, e.g. fig. 163 (fig. 176 in the English edition [12], Fig. 5) (a Weigert preparation of the cortex of the frontal lobe), which turned out to be very beautiful and instructive. The fact that the section on the cerebellum is particularly rich (Fig. 6) can be explained by Obersteiner's long-standing involvement in studying this part of the brain, which had been essentially neglected since Stilling [34]. (Authors' note: The German anatomist and surgeon Benedikt Stilling (1810-1879) is also credited for introducing serial tissue sectioning in neurohistology [35].) A section on the meninges and brain vessels concludes this overall splendid and detailed new textbook, which has received a worthy layout from the publisher.

Dozent Dr. Sigmund Freud

[*Introduction to the Study of the Structure of the Central Nervous Organs in Health and Disease.* By Dr. H. Obersteiner. Toeplitz and Deuticke, Leipzig and Vienna 1888. (Literary Notices.)]

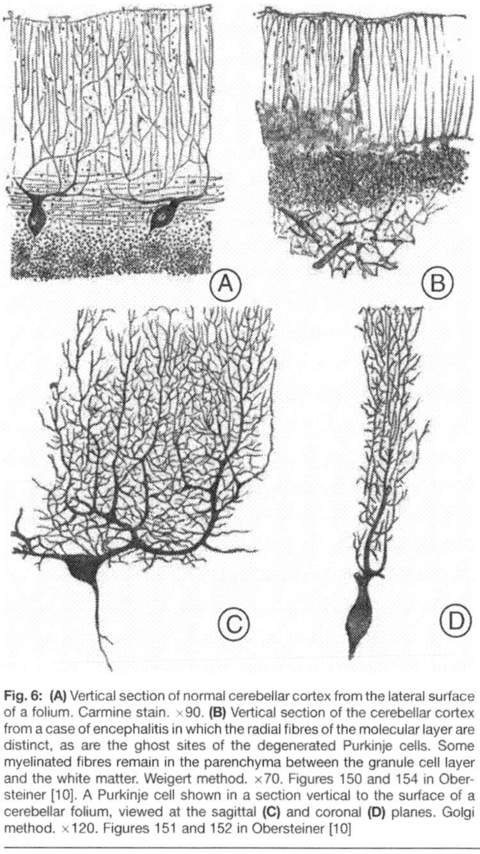

Comment

The value of Obersteiner's book largely rests on his personal observations and numerous original discoveries. In his worldwide famous textbook [16], he set the foundations for the era of brain research that followed. The book is thought to represent his most valuable work [9], having become "the Bible for generations of budding neurologists" [8]. In his preface, Obersteiner [12] notes:

> "Some decades ago, our knowledge of the intimate structure of the central nervous system was still very insufficient – so insufficient, indeed, that pathology was able to make little use of it. Hence, we can understand how, of the little that was known, the practitioners of the time, with very few exceptions, made use of the most striking facts only, and had to be content with an extreme poverty of data.

Since then, however, a succession of distinguished observers, supported by the improvements made in methods, have, with surprising rapidity, successively thrown more light into the chaos of manifold nerve paths and their nodal points; and therefore, it had to be acknowledged in practical medicine that the brain and spinal cord anatomy (until now so contemptuously set aside), despite their difficulty, are worthy of the most exhaustive consideration. Nay, more, regions which seem to stand far enough away from nerve-pathology – ophthalmology, osteology, and even dermatology – have come to feel the need of a fundamental orientation of the central nervous organs.

Fig. 6: **(A)** Vertical section of normal cerebellar cortex from the lateral surface of a folium. Carmine stain. ×90. **(B)** Vertical section of the cerebellar cortex from a case of encephalitis in which the radial fibres of the molecular layer are distinct, as are the ghost sites of the degenerated Purkinje cells. Some myelinated fibres remain in the parenchyma between the granule cell layer and the white matter. Weigert method. ×70. Figures 150 and 154 in Obersteiner [10]. A Purkinje cell shown in a section vertical to the surface of a cerebellar folium, viewed at the sagittal **(C)** and coronal **(D)** planes. Golgi method. ×120. Figures 151 and 152 in Obersteiner [10]

review

In the following pages, I have tried to provide the student with a trustworthy and reliable guide, with which, in the absence of any other teacher, he may undertake the troublesome journey through the several regions of the central nervous system ... The introduction of patho-anatomical observations, especially of the pathological changes in the cells, will prepare the road for the comprehension of the processes of disease in the central nervous system ... I suppose I need not point out that the presentation of the material rests throughout upon autoptical observations; when facts are stated on the ground of the observations of other authors, this is in every case noted ..."

Fully aware of the value of the recent introduction of the microtome and the importance of obtaining serial cross-sections for a mental reconstruction of anatomical structures towards a better understanding of the inner structure of the brain, Obersteiner [10] adopted another innovation in his textbook, i.e. the paired use of a histological picture on the right half of the figure of a brain section, and a schematic drawing in a mirror-image fashion on the left half [35] (Fig. 4).

Waldeyer [36] introduced the term "neuron" and popularised the neuron theory, largely based on the histological work of Ramón y Cajal, as well as on the substantial contributions of Forel, van Gehuchten, Gowers, His, Kölliker, von Lenhossék, Nansen, Nissl and Retzius, among others [37].

As a neurohistologist, Freud, with his studies on the lamprey [3, 38] and the river crayfish [39], became one of the early protagonists of the neuron theory. Carhart-Harris and Friston [40] have surmised that Freudian constructs, such as the primary and secondary processes (as functions of the id and the ego, respectively), have neurobiological substrates, owing in part to Freud's schooling in neuroanatomy and neurology, and the influence of teachers such as Theodor Meynert (1833–1892).

Meynert's thoughts are systematically exposed by Obersteiner [10, 12]:

"In formulating his scheme of brain and spinal cord structure, Meynert [41–43] commences with the cerebral cortex as being the organ devoted to conscious processes. All pathways that serve as media of communication between the cerebral cortex and the outer world are grouped together in a chief system. Through the fibres of this system, sensory images are projected on the perceptive cortex, and, further, not only are the movements of one's own body and the source of the sensations of movement represented in the brain in the same way as phenomena of the outer world, but the cortex also, by means of the motor tracts, reflects outwards again the states of stimulation, information with regard to which is transferred to it by means of sensory nerves. Therefore, Meynert terms the whole of these conducting paths as the *projection system.*"

The distinction of (ascending and descending) projection fibres (between the spinal cord and the cerebral cortex) and association fibres (intra- and interhemispheric connections) is regarded as being one of Meynert's main contributions to neuroanatomy [35], the other being the cytoarchitectonics of the cerebral cortex [44]. Meynert's quest at interpreting mental phenomena and psychiatric illness on a neuroanatomical basis justifies his fame during the period of the organic orientation of psychiatry in Vienna. Together with Wilhelm Griesinger (1817–1868) of Berlin, Meynert set the foundations of scientifically oriented psychiatry [21].

On the opposing views of Golgi and Forel, and what would eventually become the debate between the reticular and the neuron theories, Obersteiner [10, 12] wrote:

"Passing over earlier attempts in this direction, I shall mention Golgi's views alone. He distinguishes two kinds of nerve cells clearly characterised by their different behaviour under the corrosive sublimate method: (1) nerve cells whose axis-cylinder processes, although they give off many lateral branches, pass, without losing their independence, into myelinated fibres; (the doubt thrown upon the staining of nerve cells by this method should be borne in mind); (2) nerve cells, whose axis-cylinder processes resolve themselves eventually by frequent division into a network of fibres. Golgi finds cells of the first category in the regions in which motor fibres rise; the second category comprises the cells characteristic of the centres in which sensory fibres end. He, therefore, distinguishes the former as motor, and the latter as sensory cells. Hence, the curious result is reached that in the second class of cells, the axis-cylinder process is not distinguished by the only character that marks it as an axis-cylinder process, namely, its direct passage into a nerve fibre. This warns us to be careful in recognising axis-cylinder processes. Our concept of the relations of the finest ramifications of the cell process is in a very unstable condition. The most generally accepted view is that the cell processes break up into fibres that finally anastomose with the processes of neighbouring cells in a close felt-work from which, on the other side, the axis-cylinders of nerve fibres originate. Every, or almost every, nerve cell is, according to this view, in uninterrupted continuity with many others.

Forel's view of the arrangement of processes is quite different. He thinks that the processes of neighbouring cells grasp one another, like the branches of contiguous trees, without continuity of substance, but he does not indicate the way in which he thinks the ends of these branches terminate. From a physiological standpoint, it is not necessary to exact a direct continuity of cell processes. It is quite sufficient for the purposes of the physiological transference of impulses to imagine an interlocking of the filaments without continuity; something like the superposition of the spiral fibre upon the sympathetic cell as described by Ehrlich. Apart from genetic reasons, the appearances presented in successful sublimate preparations are rather in favour of the latter theory. Individual cells with their rich network are coloured, but no anastomosis between neighbouring cells is shown; (the metallic deposition does not surround the finest filaments of the felt-work)."

One notices the objectivity with which Obersteiner reviews the research findings of others. It becomes

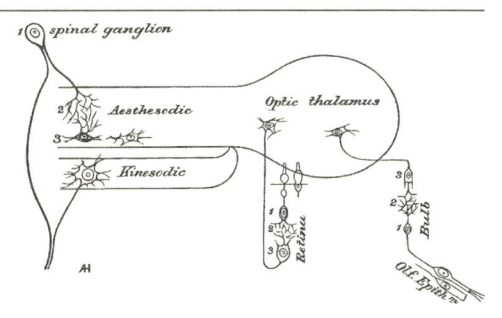

Fig. 7: Sketch showing the homology of "granules" of the olfactory bulb and retina and the cells of the spinal ganglia. *1* Bipolar cells; *2* plexus of "molecular" substance; *3* collecting or associating cells. Figure 57 in Obersteiner [12], initialled by Alex Hill

clear from the above that the contiguity of nerve cell processes (Figs. 5 and 7) suggested by Forel seems more logical than the continuity defended by Golgi. Thus, Obersteiner clearly verges on "neuronism" three years before Waldeyer's publication [36], supporting Cajal's doctrine of the neuron.

Cajal is not mentioned in the first edition of the book [10, 12]. There are nonetheless eleven citations to the anatomical studies of Freud, including the gold chloride impregnation modification [45], the histological experiments on the lamprey [3, 38] and the river crayfish [39], the study with Darkschewitsch on the human restiform body [46] and the origin of the eighth cranial nerve [47].

In the second edition, Obersteiner [11] cites Cajal's new discoveries on the embryonic spinal cord, which

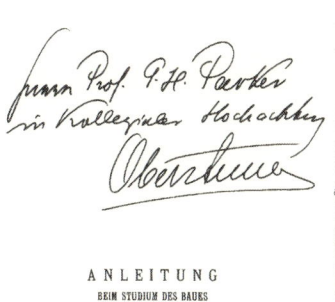

Fig. 8: The fifth German edition of Obersteiner's textbook [58], left, with hand-inscribed dedication to the zoology professor George Howard Parker (1864–1955) of Harvard University (author's archive). Ramón y Cajal's semidiagrammatic drawing of the cerebellar circuitry in a transverse section of a folium in the mammalian cerebellum, as adapted by Obersteiner, right. *A*, molecular layer; *B*, granular layer; *C*, white matter; *a*, Purkinje cells; *b*, basket cells with their baskets; *d*, *e*, small superficial (stellate) cells of the molecular layer; *f*, large nerve cells of the granular layer; *g*, granule cells with their ascending axons bifurcating; *h*, mossy fibres; *i*, cross-section of parallel fibres; *j*, glial cells of the molecular layer with a tuft; *m*, glial cells of the granular layer; *n*, climbing fibres; *o*, axis cylinder process of a Purkinje cell with collaterals. Figure 224 in Obersteiner [58]

would provide evidence for the autonomy of nerve cells [48].

One should note that the first German edition of Obersteiner's textbook [10] came out just before Cajal became aware of the Golgi method and began publishing his first studies with it [49-54]. The early editions of Obersteiner's book (English translator's *Preface* dated March 1890 [12], Obersteiner's *Vorwort* in the second German edition dated July 1891 [11]) were too early to reflect more than just Cajal's initial papers from January [50] and March of 1889 [55]. As already pointed out, Obersteiner's insightful comments on continuity *versus* contact were made three years before Waldeyer's 1891 review on the neuron [36]. In this sense Obersteiner's conceptual framework arose from the views of Forel against those of Golgi, as explained earlier, and it would have been hard for him to remodel it with the revolutionary new evidence.

Nonetheless, in the subsequent editions [56-58], Obersteiner expanded the section on the histology of the nerve cell and made repeated references to Cajal's findings. The overall book size was increased from 406 pages and 178 figures (first German edition of 1888 [10]) to 764 pages and 267 figures (fifth German edition of 1912 [58]). While the basic outline in seven chapters remained the same, the section on the histology of the nerve cell was doubled. In the third German edition [56], Obersteiner cited studies published by Cajal in German, French and Spanish [59-62], and in the fourth German edition [57] he referred to Cajal's "*Textura del Sistema Nervioso*" [63]. Obersteiner illustrated the morphological properties of neurons and their contiguity with the use of the Golgi silver method, with special emphasis on examples from the spinal cord, olfactory bulb and cerebellar and cerebral cortices. He even used Cajal's classic drawing of the cerebellar circuitry (Fig. 8). Thus, this historic textbook eventually fully built its histological section on the foundation of the neuron doctrine.

Later, the neuroanatomical tradition of the Viennese School, instigated by Theodor Meynert, saw its continuation in the "*Microscopic-Topographic Atlas of the Human Central Nervous System*" by Obersteiner's successor Otto Marburg [64] (who used microphotography for the histological documentation, thus departing from the older trend of woodcuts and lithographs), and even further in the masterful "*Atlas of Cytoarchitectonics of the Adult Human Cerebral Cortex*" by Constantin von Economo and Georg N. Koskinas [44], younger apprentices of Obersteiner and Marburg.

Conflict of interest

The authors declare that there is no conflict of interest regarding the work presented in the manuscript.

References

[1] Flatau E. Supplement zur ersten Auflage vom Atlas des menschlichen Gehirns und des Faserverlaufes. II. Mikroskopischer Theil. Berlin, Karger, 1899.
[2] Obersteiner H. Über Entwicklung und Wachstum der Sehne. Sitzungsber Kaiserl Akad Wiss – Math Naturwiss Kl (Wien), 56: 162-171, 1867.
[3] Freud S. Über den Ursprung der hinteren Nervenwurzeln im Rückenmark von Ammocoetes (*Petromyzon planeri*). Sitzungsber Kaiserl Akad Wiss - Math Naturwiss Kl (Wien), 75: 15-27, 1877.
[4] Marburg O. Heinrich Obersteiner zu seinem 70. Geburtstage, mit einer Porträtskizze von Olga Prager. Wien Med Wochenschr, 67: 2013-2016, 1917.
[5] Seitelberger F. Heinrich Obersteiner (1847-1922). In: Kolle K (ed) Grosse Nervenärzte, B and 3. G. Thieme, Stuttgart, pp 21-30, 1963.
[6] Marburg O. Heinrich Obersteiner. Gedenkrede anlässlich der am 5. Dezember 1922 stattgehabten Trauersitzung des Vereines für Psychiatrie und Neurologie in Wien. Arb Neurol Inst Univ Wien, 24: V-XXXII, 1963.
[7] Triarhou LC. Professor Otto Marburg, universal neurologist and the 'dean of teachers'. Wien Klin Wochenschr, 120: 622-630, 2008.
[8] Spiegel EA. Heinrich Obersteiner (1847–1922). In: Haymaker W, Baer KA (eds) The founders of neurology. Charles C Thomas, Springfield, pp 199-202, 1953.
[9] Schick A. The pluralism of psychiatry in Vienna. Psychoanal Rev, 65: 14-37, 1978.
[10] Obersteiner H. Anleitung beim Studium des Baues der nervösen Centralorgane im gesunden und kranken Zustande. Toeplitz & Deuticke, Leipzig-Wien, 1888.
[11] Obersteiner H. Anleitung beim Studium des Baues der nervösen Centralorgane im gesunden und kranken Zustande, 2. Aufl. Franz Deuticke, Leipzig-Wien, 1892.
[12] Obersteiner H. The anatomy of the central nervous organs in health and in disease (transl. by A Hill). Charles Griffin, London, 1890.
[13] Obersteiner H. Anatomie des centres nerveux: guide pour l'étude de leur structure á l'état normal et pathologique (trad. par JX Coroënne). Georges Carré, Paris, 1893.
[14] Seitelberger F. Heinrich Obersteiner and the Neurological Institute: foundation and history of Neuroscience in Vienna. Brain Pathol, 2: 163-168, 1992.
[15] Bernheimer H. Der Anfang – und wie es weiterging: 125 Jahre Klinisches Institut für Neurologie. Wien Klin Wochenschr, 120: 583-586, 2008.
[16] Stransky E. Erinnerungen an Heinrich Obersteiner zum 31. Juli 1957. Wien Klin Wochenschr, 69: 537-538, 1957.
[17] Marburg O. Zur Geschichte des Wiener neurologischen Institutes. In: Marburg O (ed) Festschrift zur Feier des 25jährigen Bestandes des Neurologischen Institutes (Institut für Anatomie und Physiologie des Zentralnervensystems) an der Wiener Universität. Vol 1. Leipzig-Wien, Franz Deuticke, pp VI-XIII, 1907.
[18] Richter J. The brain commission of the international association of academies: the first international society of neurosciences. Brain Res Bulletin, 52: 445-457, 2000.
[19] Waldeyer W. Document I of the report of the President of the Brain Commission (transl. by HH Donaldson). J Comp Neurol Psychol, 18: 87-90, 1908.
[20] Waldeyer W. Report on the present status of the Academic Institutes for Brain Study, together with a report of the meetings of the Executive Committee of the Brain Commission, held at Berlin, March 14, 1908 (transl. by HH Donaldson). Anat Rec, 2: 428-431, 1908.
[21] Jellinger KA. A short history of neurosciences in Austria. J Neural Transm, 113: 271-282, 2006.
[22] Triarhou LC, del Cerro M. Freud's contribution to neuroanatomy. Arch Neurol, 42: 282-287, 1985.
[23] Triarhou LC. Exploring the mind with a microscope: Freud's beginnings in neurobiology. Hellenic J Psychol, 6: 1-13, 2009.
[24] Solms M. A previously-untranslated review by Freud of a monograph on hypnotism. Int J Psychoanal, 70: 401-403, 1989.

[25] Freud S. Referate und literarische Anzeigen – Forel: Der Hypnotismus, seine Bedeutung und seine handhabung. Wien Med Wochenschr, 39: 1097–100, 1892–1896, 1889.
[26] Freud S. Literarische Anzeigen – Anleitung beim Studium des Baues der nervösen Centralorgane im gesunden und kranken Zustande. Von Dr. H. Obersteiner. Wien Med Wochenschr, 37: 1642–1644, 1887.
[27] Flatau E. Atlas des menschlichen Gehirns und des Faserverlaufes. Berlin, Karger, 1894.
[28] Freud S. Kritische Besprechungen und literarische Anzeigen – Atlas des menschlichen Gehirns und des Faserverlaufes. Von Ed. Flatau. Int Klin Rundschau, 8: 1131–1132, 1894.
[29] Freud S. The standard edition of the complete psychological works, vol I (1886–1899): pre-psycho-analytic publications and unpublished drafts (transl. by J Strachey and A Freud). Hogarth Press/Institute of Psycho-Analysis, London, 1966.
[30] Triarhou LC. A review of Edward Flatau's 1894 atlas of the human brain by the neurologist Sigmund Freud. Eur Neurol, 65: 10–15, 2011.
[31] Edinger L. Zehn Vorlesungen über den Bau der nervösen Centralorgane für Ärzte und Studirende. F. C. W. Vogel, Leipzig, 1885.
[32] Féré C. Traité élémentaire d'anatomie médicale du système nerveux. A. Delahaye et Lecrosnier, Paris, 1886.
[33] Meynert T. Psychiatrie. Klinik der Erkrankungen des Vorderhirns, begründet auf dessen Bau, Leistungen und Ernährung. Wilhelm Braumüller, Erste Hälfte. Wien, 1884.
[34] Stilling B. Untersuchungen über den Bau des kleinen Gehirns des Menschen. T. Kay, Cassel, 1864.
[35] Hakosalo H. The brain under the knife: serial sectioning and the development of late nineteenth-century neuroanatomy. Stud Hist Phil Biol Biomed Sci, 37: 172–202, 2006.
[36] Waldeyer HWG. Über einige neuere Forschungen im Gebiete der Anatomie des Centralnervensystems. Dtsch Med Wochenschr, 17: 1213–1218, 1244–1246, 1287–1289, 1331–1332, 1352–1356, 1891.
[37] Shepherd GM. Foundations of the neuron doctrine. Oxford University Press, New York, 1991.
[38] Freud S. Über Spinalganglien und Rückenmark des Petromyzon. Sitzungsber Kaiserl Akad Wiss – Math Naturwiss Kl (Wien), 78: 81–167, 1878.
[39] Freud S. Über den Bau der Nervenfasern und Nervenzellen beim Flusskrebs. Sitzungsber Kaiserl Akad Wiss – Math Naturwiss Kl (Wien), 85: 9–46, 1882.
[40] Carhart-Harris RL, Friston KJ. The default-mode, ego-functions and free-energy: a neurobiological account of Freudian ideas. Brain, 133: 1265–12683, 2010.
[41] Meynert T. Neue Untersuchungen uber den Bau der Grosshirnrinde und ihre örtlichen Verschiedenheiten. Allg Wien Med Ztg, 13: 419–428, 1868.
[42] Meynert T. Der Bau der Gross-Hirnrinde und seine örtlichen Verschiedenheiten, nebst einem pathologisch-anatomischen Corollarium. Neuwied-Leipzig, J. H. Heuser'sche Verlagsbuchhandlung, 1872.
[43] Meynert T. Die anthropologische Bedeutung der frontalen Gehirnentwicklung nebst Untersuchungen über den Windungstypus des Hinter hauptlappens der Säugethiere und pathologischen Wägungsresultaten der menschlichen Hirnlappen. Jahrb Psychiatr (Leipz), 7: 1–48, 1887.
[44] von Economo C, Koskinas GN. Atlas of cytoarchitectonics of the adult human cerebral cortex (transl., rev. and ed. by LC Triarhou). Karger, Basel, 2008.

[45] Freud S. A new histological method for the study of nerve-tracts in the brain and spinal cord. Brain, 7: 86–88, 1884.
[46] Darkschewitsch L, Freud S. Über die Beziehung des Strickkörpers zum Hinterstrang und Hinterstrangskern nebst Bemerkungen über zwei Felder der Oblongata. Neurol Cbl, 6: 121–129, 1886.
[47] Freud S. Über den Ursprung des N. acusticus. Monatsschr Ohrenheilk, 20: 245–251, 277–282, 1886.
[48] Ramón y Cajal S. Sur l'origine et les ramifications des fibres nerveuses de la moelle embryonaire. Anat Anz (Jena), 5: 85–95, 111–119, 1890.
[49] Ramón y Cajal S. Coloración por el método de Golgi de los centros nerviosos de los embriones de pollo. Bol Inst Méd Valenciano, 21: 53–58, 1889.
[50] Ramón y Cajal S. Coloración por el método de Golgi de los centros nerviosos de los embriones de pollo. Gaceta Méd Catalana, 12: 6–8, 1889.
[51] Ramón y Cajal S. Nuevas aplicaciones del método de coloración de Golgi. Bol Inst Méd Valenciano, 21: 302–305, 1889.
[52] Ramón y Cajal S. Nuevas aplicaciones del método de coloración de Golgi. Gaceta Méd Catalana, 12: 28–32, 1889.
[53] Ramón y Cajal S. Recollections of my life (translated by E. H. Craigie and J. Cano). The MIT Press, Cambridge, MA, 1989.
[54] Lopez Piñero JM, Terrada Ferrandis ML, Rodríguez Quiroga A. Bibliografía Cajaliana – Ediciones de los Escritos de Santiago Ramón y Cajal y Estudios sobre su Vida y Obra. Valencia, Albatros – Artes Gráficas Soler, 2000.
[55] Ramón y Cajal S. Contribución al estudio de la estructura de la médula espinal. Rev Trim Histol Normal Patol, 1: 79–106, 1889.
[56] Obersteiner H. Anleitung beim Studium des Baues der nervösen Centralorgane im gesunden und kranken Zustande, 3. Aufl. Franz Deuticke, Leipzig-Wien, 1896.
[57] Obersteiner H. Anleitung beim Studium des Baues der nervösen Centralorgane im gesunden und kranken Zustande, 4. Aufl. Franz Deuticke, Leipzig-Wien, 1901.
[58] Obersteiner H. Anleitung beim Studium des Baues der nervösen Zentralorgane im gesunden und kranken Zustande, 5. Aufl. Franz Deuticke, Leipzig-Wien, 1912.
[59] Ramón y Cajal S. Neue Darstellung vom histologische Bau des Centralnervensystems. Arch Anat Physiol Anat Abt, 17[Suppl.]: 319–428, 1903.
[60] Ramón y Cajal S. Les nouvelles idées sur la structure du système nerveux chez l'homme et chez les vertébrés. C. Reinwald & Cie, Paris, 1895.
[61] Ramón y Cajal S. Algunas conjeturas sobre el mecanismo anatómico de la ideación, asociación y atención. Rev Med Cirug Práct, 19: 497–508, 1895.
[62] Ramón y Cajal S. Apuntes para el estudio del bulbo raquídeo, cerebelo y origen de los nervios encefálicos. Anal Soc Españ Hist Nat (Madrid), 24: 1–118, 1895.
[63] Ramón y Cajal S. Textura del Sistema Nervioso del Hombre y de los Vertebrados, Tomo I. Nicolás Moya, Madrid, 1899.
[64] Marburg O. Mikroskopisch-topographischer Atlas des menschlichen Zentralnervensystems mit begleitendem Texte, 3. Aufl. Franz Deuticke, Leipzig-Wien, 1927.
[65] Forel A. Gehirn und Seele – Ein Vortrag. Emil Strauss, Bonn, 1894.

Christfried Jakob's 1921 Theory of the Gnoses and Praxes as Fundamental Factors in Cerebral Cortical Dynamics

Zoë D. Théodoridou · Lazaros C. Triarhou

Published online: 13 October 2010
© Springer Science+Business Media, LLC 2010

Abstract This study aims at reviving an important contribution by the pioneer neurobiologist and neurophilosopher Christfried Jakob (1866–1956) to the understanding of higher cortical functions. Jakob studied cortical dynamics at multiple levels by comparing gnoses and praxes and their corresponding pathological states, i.e. the agnosias and the apraxias. We herein provide a complete English translation of Jakob's original Spanish article dating to 1921, and further consider some key points under the scope of the neuropsychological knowledge available then, and the research evidence available 90 years later.

Keywords Christfried Jakob · Cerebral cortex · History of neuroscience · Gnosis · Praxis · Agnosia · Apraxia

Introduction

The progress in aphasiology effected since the second half of the 19th century has enhanced research on the cortical localization of mental functions. The description and the study of multiple forms of agnosia and apraxia have contributed to that end.

The term 'agnosia' was introduced by Sigmund Freud (1856–1939) in his monograph *On aphasia* (1891) to denote functional disturbances between the concept of an object and the concept of the word corresponding to it (Macmillan 2004; Goldberg 2005, p. 103). The first use of the term 'apraxia' is attributed to the

---

L. C. Triarhou (✉)
University of Macedonia, 156 Egnatia Ave., Rm. Z-312, 54006 Thessaloniki, Greece
e-mail: triarhou@uom.gr

Z. D. Théodoridou · L. C. Triarhou
Economo-Koskinas Wing for Integrative and Evolutionary Neuroscience, University of Macedonia, Thessaloniki, Greece

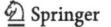

German psychiatrist Hugo Liepmann (1863–1925), who defined motor apraxia and distinguished it from agnosia and sensory apraxia in his 1900 classic *Das Krankheitsbild der Apraxie* (Devinsky and D'Esposito 2004, p. 236; Etcharry-Bouyx and Ceccaldi 2007, p. 36). The term had been used in 1871 in a similar sense by Heymann Steinthal (1823–1899) (Cockburn 2008, p. 210; Liepmann 1988, p. 3).

The pioneer neurobiologist-neurophilosopher Christfried Jakob (1866–1956) (Triarhou and del Cerro 2006a, b, 2007) studied agnosias and apraxias both clinically and anatomically in order to shed light on cortical dynamics from a structural, functional and evolutionary viewpoint (Jakob 1921). The present study aims at reviving a particular contribution of Jakob on the representation and production of higher gnosic-praxic functions.

Jakob was born in 1866 in Bavaria, Germany (Moyano 1957). He studied medicine at the University of Erlangen and graduated in 1890 (López Pasquali 1965; Orlando 1966; Triarhou and del Cerro 2006a). His doctoral dissertation dealt with aortitis syphilitica and was supervised by Albert von Zenker (1825–1898) (Triarhou and del Cerro 2007). In the early 1890s Jakob worked as assistant at the Erlangen Medical Clinic headed by Adolph von Strümpell (1853–1925), and also practised privately in Bamberg (Moyano 1957). Having attained worldwide renown through his early brain atlases, Jakob moved to Argentina in 1899 to head the Laboratory of the Psychiatric and Neurological Clinic of the Hospicio de Las Mercedes, affiliated with the University of Buenos Aires (López Pasquali 1965; Orlando 1966). His first name became 'castillianized' to Christofredo when he was naturalized as an Argentinian citizen (Orlando 1966). In 1922 Jakob occupied the chair of biology of the nervous system in the Department of Educational Sciences of the University of La Plata (Triarhou and del Cerro 2006b) and the following year he published his textbook of neurobiology (Jakob 1923). Overall, Jakob authored 30 books and 250 articles covering developmental, evolutionary, anatomical, pathological and philosophical topics in neurobiology (Triarhou and del Cerro 2006a).

Several of Jakob's papers have philosophical ramifications, with Kantian influences often conspicuous. The consideration of gnoses into the axes of space and time—the a priori conditions of our internal intuition (Kant 1999)—becomes apparent. Jakob wrote 14 philosophical works (López Pasquali 1965). Some of the issues he tackled include the relation between biogenesis and philosophy (Jakob 1914) and the philosophical meaning of the human brain (1945a). He authored a monograph entitled 'Biophilosophical Documents' (Jakob 1946), the fifth in the *Folia neurobiológica Argentina* series. In that sense, Jakob can be considered as one of the earliest neurophilosophers.

In a path of enquiry spanning over half a century, the frontal lobe occupied Jakob's thought constantly, forming a major motive that led to the formulation of a dynamic theory on cerebral cortical function (Pedace 1949). Within such a framework, gnoses play a key role as the preparatory acts, and praxes as the productive acts, of all psychogenetic processes (Jakob 1941). According to Jakob, psychogenesis (<Gk. *psyche*=soul and *genesis*=origin) refers to a structuralistic developmental process taking place in the human cortex and leading to the formation of abstract thought (Jakob 1941). The term became widely used in psychiatry (Freud 1955; Jung 1960) and it was adopted by Jean Piaget (1896–

1980) to denote the formation of knowledge (Piaget 1972, p. 19), an explanation not far from Jakob's. Figure 1 presents an outline of Jakob's evolutionary components of psychogenesis.

This work carries special weight because it underscores the emergence of Jakob's foremost theories regarding (a) the biological basis of memory and (b) the phylogeny of the kineses. Both of these theories were published in 1935 (Jakob 1935a, b) and are considered essential in understanding his psychobiological thought (Moyano 1957).

According to Jakob's postulate (Jakob 1935b), phylogeny occurs in two phases. The first, 'plasmodynamic' phase entails elementary biological phenomena such as tropism and pulsatility. The second ('neurodynamic') phase is divided into three stages: a phylogenetically older *archikinetic* stage, where reflex actions emerge; a *paleokinetic* stage characterized by instinctive reactions; and a *neokinetic* stage, which elaborates conscious motor responses. The *neokineses* include three kinds of complex neurocognitive processes: (a) *gnoses*, which secure the conscious orientation in one's environment, (b) *praxes*, which underlie active individual intervention and (c) *symbolisms*, which subserve the communication by means of abstract ideas. Each one of these three stages corresponds to different levels of organization in the vertebrate CNS. The archikinetic stage corresponds to the archineuronal, the paleokinetic to the paleoneuronal, and the neokinetic to the neoneuronal.

The original presented article, written in Spanish, was published in 1921 in the Peruvian journal *La Crónica Médica* (Fig. 2). It highlights the 'middle period' of Jakob's work on cortical dynamics. When it was published, the 55-year-old Jakob was at the prime of his neurobiological thought (Triarhou and del Cerro 2006b). An earlier version had been presented a couple of years earlier to the 'Argentinian Medical Circle and Medical Student Center' in Buenos Aires (Jakob 1919; López Pasquali 1965; Orlando 1966).

We provide an English translation of Jakob's full 1921 paper, followed by a discussion of some key points, considered under the scope of the neuropsychological knowledge available at the time, and the experimental evidence available today.

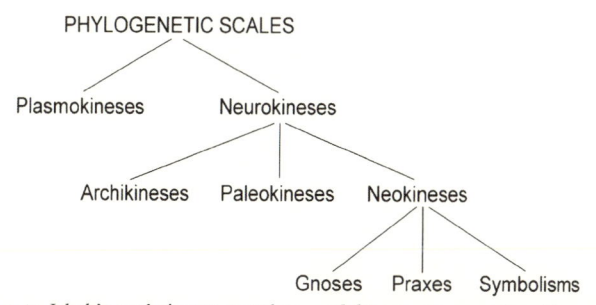

Fig. 1 According to Jakob's evolutionary postulate, *archikineses* represent hereditary reflex actions of psychism, *paleokineses* correspond to instinctive reactions, and *neokineses*—which represent the phylogenetically most recent type of the kineses—form the core of human consciousness (Jakob 1935b; c.f., Szirko 1995; Triarhou 2008; Triarhou and del Cerro 2006b)

Fig. 2 Frontispiece of Jakob's original 1921 article on gnoses and praxes (Jakob 1921)

LA CRONICA MEDICA

Año XXXVIII   LIMA - PERU - 1921   Sanmartí y Cía. Impresores.

La teoría actual de las gnosias y praxias como factores fundamentales en el dinamismo de la corteza cerebral

Por el Dr. CHRISTOFREDO JAKOB

Entre los múltiples problemas que ocupan la Fisiología moderna, no hay indudablemente ninguno más importante y complejo y que al mismo tiempo más interese al hombre como biotipo *sui géneris*, que el del dinamismo cerebro-cortical y su relación con las facultades mentales.

The Theory of the Gnoses and Praxes as Fundamental Factors in Cerebral Cortical Dynamics (1921)

by Christfried Jakob

Among the numerous problems that occupy modern physiology, there is undoubtedly no more important and complex a problem—and at the same time more interesting to man as a biotype sui generis—than that of cerebral cortical dynamics and its relation to the mental faculties.

A scientific concept on the psychophysiological conditions of cortical functions becomes equally necessary in psychology, in physiology, and in the neuropsychiatric clinic. With reasonable satisfaction, we may state that modern psychology owes its knowledge on the matter to medicine and its fosterers, both in the neurological clinic and laboratory, and in neurophysiological experimentation. On the other hand, psychology has only known to confuse and to entangle problems—which are sufficiently difficult on their own—with an imprecise terminology.

I present a short summary of the history of our relevant knowledge; it becomes clear how psychological concepts gradually disappear, and become replaced with clinical-physiological, and finally biological terms. Thus, concepts gradually turn from theoretical and fictitious into natural, capable of being subsequently subjected to critical scientific study.

Leaving aside the old theory of the 'animal spirits', a remnant of the theory of 'animism' sustained by the old philosophy and its localization (pneumatic ventricular theory), we find in principle scientific concepts only in the 17th and 18th centuries, with Bartholin and Willis and their schools localizing mental processes to the cerebral matter for the first time; they had only been precisely delineated by Gall and his disciples, in the cerebral gyri, i.e. in the internal organization. But what these authors localized were still extremely complex functions; sensitivity, will, memory, imagination or the various mental and moral qualities that distinguish humans. A localization of such abstract concepts, virtues and talents, was evidently psychological, but had nothing psychological about it.

Springer

It is to the clinic that we owe the rise of a new era: localization and language studies (Broca, Wernicke, Déjerine) [and] motor and sensory functional studies (Jackson, Hitzig, Munck, Goltz, etc.) rejected the psychological qualities and localized sensory-motor physiological functions of different modality and localization to projection areas for the first time. The shadow of old psychology continued to exert its influence, because in all those theories a zone (albeit smaller and smaller) was tacitly sustained for higher mental functions.

Such a view was presented concretely by Flechsig, based on embryological data, hastily interpreted as the frontal and temporoparietal 'association areas', like an 'ecclesiastic reserve'[1] for the elaboration of consciousness, ideation, abstraction, etc.

The normal and pathological anatomy rejected such theories and safely established that the so-called association areas receive important contingents of afferent pathways (of projection); projection areas have the same number of association pathways as well.

Thus, the functional dualism of both categories of areas could not be sustained anatomically. Besides, it has been impossible to find sufficient characteristic dispositions in regional cortical structure considered as projection and association, as I was able to show in my studies on cortical histoarchitecture.

One of the most difficult points in localization theories was the question of where does one localize the respective associative functions. A doubt persisted as to whether they are executed at the same time and place as perceptive processes. It is worth considering how such functions are distributed in sensory-motor projection areas, or even in areas considered as association; we can assume the existence of one or some memory areas or rather a mnemonic apparatus for each projection area. In the latter case, it would be necessary to interrupt the unity of association areas and to structure them into other such mnemonic areas, equalling in number the projection areas.

This last concept was mainly elaborated by Ramón y Cajal. In his cortical theory, Cajal established a mosaïc of projection areas surrounded by other mnemonic (association of first order), further surrounded by second and third order, committed to concrete and abstract ideative productions. Moreover, it is interesting to note the cortical functional unity established by Flourens's physiology, which has progressively resulted in much smaller dynamic centers, always correlated with each other. However, the resulting dualist criterion of the influence of psychology on different localization from the physiological phase on one hand, and from the mental on the other, was in essence still conserved. And it is with such inventory, more or less selectively fixed, that current psychology is handled. For the sake of curiosity, I mention here the recent creation—psychological rather than physiological—the occurrence of psycho-hormones,[2] a real resurrection of 'animal spirits' in the endocrine domain.

---

[1] According to the Peace of Augsburg (1555), a treaty between Charles V, Holy Roman Emperor, and the Lurtheran princes, German lay people could freely and unconditionally select their religion. In this respect Catholics recognized Lutheranism. Still, there was a clause consisting in the divestment of all the goods including the territory of an ecclesiastic in case one embraced Protestantism [translators' note].

[2] The author might conceivably be referring to von Monakow's contemporary concept of *horme*, i.e. 'a hypothetical, self-actualizing force that brought individual processes together into a moral and functional whole' (c.f., Finger 1994, p. 58) [translators' note].

While the above theories were being elaborated, the clinic began to bring new, fertile concepts to psychophysiolology, as it had done in the past. These are the pathological phenomena described as *agnosias and apraxias*; their clinical-anatomical analysis has shed new light on normal cortical dynamics. Thus, the so-called *astereognosis* or *stereoagnosia* that appears in certain cases of injuries to the parietal lobe has been known for a long time through the work of Wernicke, Déjerine, Horsley, Starr, and others. *Astereognosis* or *stereoagnosia* consists in an inability of the patient to recognize only by tact and grasp, objects that are given to him to hold, despite the fact that tactile sensitivity is not substantially altered. The patient feels that he takes something in his hand, but he cannot remember if this object is long, short, round, smooth, etc., with his eyes closed. Visual, auditory, olfactory, gustative agnosias, etc. have been described in an analogous form. In such cases, the respective sense, though injured, is not abolished. Thus, the patient cannot integrate sensory information—normally gotten by a certain number of isolated perceptions of distance, color, forms, intensity, etc.,—which characterizes an object one has seen, heard, tasted, etc. One then normally arrives at a state of 'apperceptive condensation and associative correlation' for the analogous impressions that allow one to finally construct 'the notion of the object', namely its *complete gnosis*.

It is evident that such agnosias result from injuries of complex cortical dynamics of momentary perceptions with previously fixed associations. Thus, *gnosis*, i.e. the positive process, consists in the synthetic condensation of a previous experience with an analogous current situation. In brief, it results from an intricate game of sequential cortical elaborations.

Tactile (haptognoses), thermal, tactile-muscular (stereognoses), visual, auditory, olfactory gnoses, etc. work then with isolated, experienced, correlated and repeated senses. They distribute and organize them in order as the securing of orientation in space and time demand it. Therefore, they stabilize one's experience of the external environment.

'Gnosic (or cognitive) processes' are not naturally the result of a special cortical power of gnosis. Indeed, that would bring us back to the old error, i.e. the theory of projection and association areas. In that theory, memory, consciousness, will and intellect were thought of as substantiated powers. On the contrary, it is only modalities here that accompany all cortical neurobiological processes to a greater or smaller intensity and extent.

The gnosic mechanism, like all nervous processes, is made up of a trilogy of elements: receptors, assimilators and combined effectors.

The receptive factors represent all sensory systems which, directed by the posterior half of the basal and dorsal thalamus, radiate towards the posterior half of the hemispheres. Thus, they include the entire cortex behind the central sulcus of Rolando: parietal, temporal and occipital (thalamo-parietal, temporal and occipital radiations).

The assimilator elements are formed by short and long inter- and intra-cortical pathways, and the association of these regions.

The effector elements represent the motor apparatus of attention, which, from auditory, visual, olfactory, tactile centers etc., stimulates the movements of attention of the ear and its accessory apparatus, of the eyes and their motor apparatus, of the nose and the related respiratory movements; for the tactile and muscular regions the effector apparatus represents the same pyramidal tract with its motor impulse on the limbs and body. The exact boundaries among different cortical gnosic centers cannot be drawn as yet; that is a question for future clinical study.

The gnosic dynamics in its turn rests fundamentally on the congruence of the analogous sensory-affective reactions. Similar percipient situations produce equal central reactions regarding the corresponding location, association and attention. Thus, they raise essentially equal affective states. Gnosis, then, is elaborated on the basis of the parallelism of outer and inner experiences through the matching of an identical perceptive situation with an analogous affective tone.

The intensity of the affection (I call it interest) during the elaboration of a gnosis of a new object gradually loses its initial tension and finally maintains a very reduced value in numerous gnosic acts that are then called automatic. Still, attention can always return to its initial value.

In my opinion, the fundamental fact is that all parieto-occipito-temporal cortical zones contribute in the elaboration of gnoses both in animals and in humans. Thus, we can crystallize the localization of the gnoses as represented in the posterior half of the cerebral hemispheres. Nevertheless, I insist that gnosis consists in the elaboration and condensation of sensory-motor acts, and not only sensory, as the old theory of the 'association and projection areas' claimed.

Specifically and in a detailed manner, there may plausibly be different gnoses with different localizations: labial, lingual, digital and tactile-gnoses localized in the posterior central gyrus; thermo-gnoses localized in the superior parietal gyrus; oral, manual and ocular stereo-gnoses localized in the supramarginal and angular gyri; visual-gnoses of form, color and perspective localized in the entire occipital lobe and the angular gyrus; auditory-gnoses of noises, sounds, rhythm and melodies localized in the posterior two-thirds of the temporal lobe; olfactory-gnoses localized in the hippocampus; and gustatory-gnoses possibly localized in the temporal pole. In sympathetic areas (cingulate gyrus) respective processes for visceral-gnoses etc. (condition of the bladder, of the stomach, endo-gnoses) will occur, as well (Fig. 3).

In this way, all these regions are unlashed into projection and association areas simultaneously. I absolutely reject the possibility of localizing perceptive and associative process, which combined characterize gnosis, into different zones for each function.

For example, when we have acquired the gnosis of a pencil, the momentary visual perception of a pencil evokes the acquired partial gnoses of form, color, surface, weight, hardness etc. The cortical constitutive elements reside in the nuclear complexes of visuoretinal, visuomotor, tactile-motor etc. areas, connected to each other in the certain combination that has been elaborated during childhood, the gnosic notion of the pencil.

Then, we do not need special mnemonic centers, because what distinguishes the mnemonic image and the immediate sensory perception is only the degree of affective tension, lower in the former case and greater in the latter. Nevertheless, they are the same elements combined in the same form that with their dynamics produce the image or the sensation.

This can be proven experimentally in animals and in humans, when partial resections of cortical segments only lead to transient gnosic alterations. This means that the neighboring zones, according to the old 'associative theory', gradually

Fig. 3 'Golden section' of the human cerebral hemisphere (frontal praxic sectors I, II, III; gnosic sectors I, II, III, IV, V) according to Jakob (1943, p. 37). Lateral **a** and midsagittal **b** views

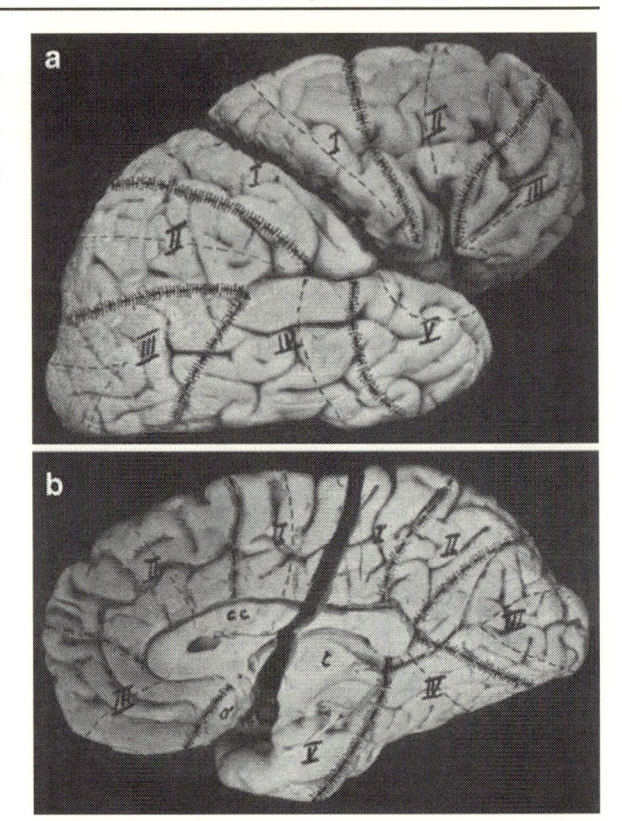

compensate for the defect. That would be impossible a priori; they would only have the ability to receive and store gnosic functions in equal form, exactly like the area previously destined to carry out such work.

In an analogous form, the study of the apraxias has contributed to our understanding of cortical function; their analysis offers a major importance to the concept of the gnoses, as a 'cortical faculty' sui generis.

Apraxia has been studied by Heilbronner, Liepmann, Pick, von Monakow, and others; I have also contributed to this field with several works. It consists in the oblivion of an act or a series of necessary acts, previously learned, to make any intentional movement without a real paralysis of the respective muscle. Thus, an apraxic does not know how to take the pencil, to wind the clock or to smoke etc., because he has forgotten the series of the necessary movements, coordinated to this end.

The complete analogy with the concept of gnosis can be immediately observed: the background of memory defects, objects or qualities, movements or their coordination.

Like in the gnoses, different forms of apraxias can be distinguished, e.g. manual, digital, oral, labial, limb, etc. There is always a certain sequence of associated movements that the patient has forgotten. Frontal ataxia belongs to this group, i.e. the inability to maintain balance in cases of lesions in the superior frontal gyrus (frontal astasia-abasia without paralysis). Furthermore, the motor aphasia of Broca type following injury of the inferior frontal gyrus, whereby the patient, without having paralysis of his articulator apparatus, does not find the necessary movements to produce the previously well-known word. The case of agraphia seems to belong to the apraxias as well.

If we now move on from the pathological process to its corresponding normal function, we must name as praxis the cortical process that associates in different combination the series of motor acts during the long learning process in infancy and childhood, to guarantee a determined movement of the limbs, the tongue, the lip, and the trunk or the entire body.

Thus, praxes are the walking, jumping and dancing regarding the lower limbs (localization in the superior frontal gyrus); the use of fork and knife, writing, and every technical-manual work for the hands (superior and mainly middle frontal gyrus); mastication, imitation, language, singing and whistling for mouth and tongue (middle frontal gyrus). The mechanism of praxis is formed by the apparatus of three systems, receptors, assimilators and effectors, just like in the gnoses. Its receiving systems formed by indirect pathways of cutaneous sense muscle (kinesthetic) crossing the cerebellum project via the red nucleus to the anterior thalamus; from there, the anterior, frontal and central radiations of the thalamus penetrate towards the cortical areas in front of the central sulcus of Rolando. It is virtually undoubted that the seat of the elaboration of praxes is the whole anterior half of the cerebral hemispheres, i.e. the anterior Rolandic and entire frontal lobe with its related associative systems (I shall not discuss the major dominion of the left hemisphere for both higher gnoses and praxes).

Their effector pathways are represented by the fronto-hypothalamic and pontine systems on the one hand, destined to strengthen the muscular coordination en bloc. Especially the pyramidal and the operculo-bulbar tract serve as effector systems as well. These turn out to be at the disposition of the two great cortical powers: gnoses and praxes become mainly discharged by means of the pyramidal tract. Hence results the great importance of such motor pathways among other secondary pathways.

Praxes become gradually automatic as well. The affective tone that initially accompanies and stimulates their acquisition finally occurs with a lesser effort. We see, then, that the gnosic and praxic cortical automatism cannot be explained, as it has been claimed by physiology and psychology [the famous polygon of Grasset (1912) shown in Fig. 4], through a mechanism of specific location, but through dynamics different from its constitutive elements.

Without entering into histophysiological details of such a process and the relative participation of cortical elements [cf. my previous study on cortical neurobiology (Jakob 1913)], I establish in summary that, with the theory of the gnoses and the praxes, clinical neurological studies have a new potential in analyzing pathological, nervous and mental phenomena. In physiology, the fact that we have once and for all closed the books on psychophysiological dualism is equally important, replacing the old concept of sensory areas with those of gnosic functions. Thus, we establish a real and reasonable physiological meaning for the puzzling frontal lobe.

The complete mental process results from the assimilating, energetic gnosic-praxic condensation, and the 'idea of the pencil' is equal to the correlation of the gnosic and praxic dynamics of that object elaborated in the cortex; this is a totally new fact in psychology, which has been unaware of the importance of praxic factors in ideative elaboration.

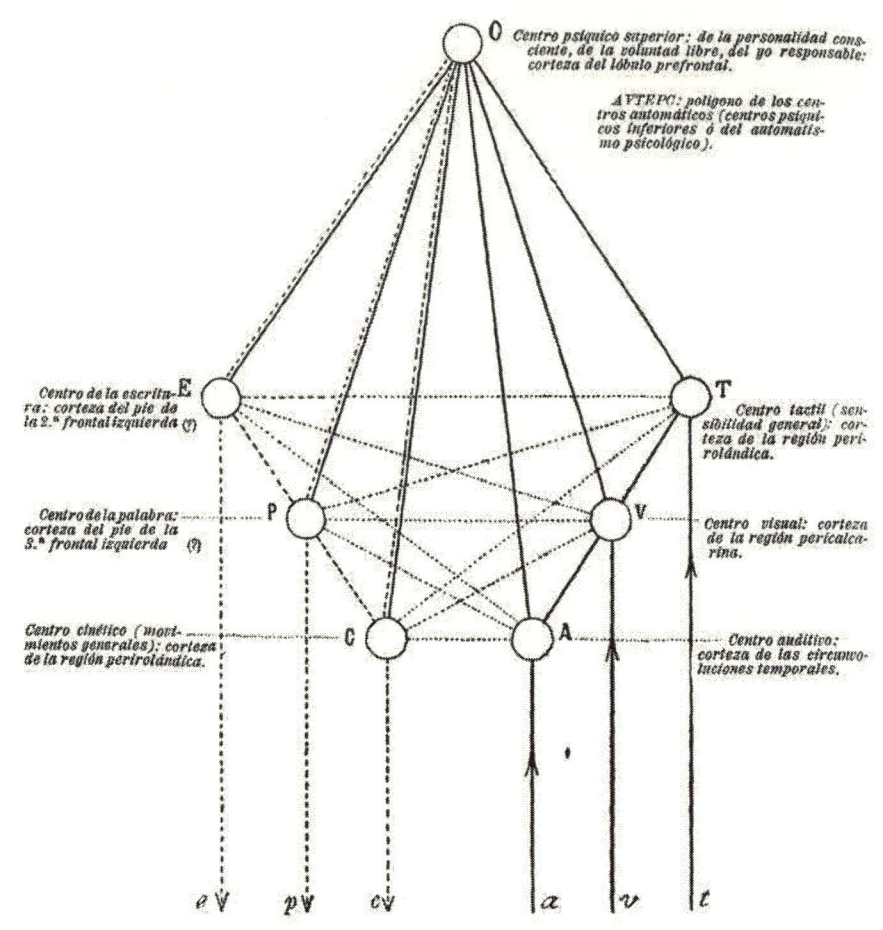

Fig. 4 General scheme of the higher anatomical centers (inferior and superior 'psychical' centers) according to Grasset (1912, p. 68). Abbreviations: *O*, superior psychical center of conscious personality, free will and responsible ego (prefrontal cortex); *AVTEPC*, polygon of automatic centers (inferior psychical centers) or of psychological automatism; *A*, auditory center (cortex of temporal gyri); *V*, visual center (cortex of pericalcarine region); *T*, tactile center or general sensitivity (cortex of perirolandic region); *C*, kinetic center or general movements (cortex of perirolandic region); *P*, language center (cortex of foot of left inferior frontal gyrus); *E*, writing center (cortex of foot of left middle frontal gyrus)

Gnoses and praxes are then neither sensory nor motor, but concomitantly sensory-motor processes and their a priori connection with the functions of the pyramidal tract give us the possibility of satisfactorily explaining the passage of gnosis and praxis to the definitive voluntary movement; a passage that the old physiology, and psychology to a lesser extent, had never been able to explain.

Mental functions cannot have for that reason localizations determined in 'associative areas' of first or third order. Rather, their characteristics reside in the transcortical dynamics that reunite isolated sensory-motor acts. Therefore, the only and true localizable elements of the process are physiological; existing primarily in the gnoses and praxes, they then create the mental phenomenon, the integrative fusion of both dynamics.

The intervention of language and its explanation by identical gnosic and praxic processes completes the objective and abstract mental elaboration. I reserve myself for such a study on another occasion, which will give me the opportunity to further deepen into what I have previously established on cortical dynamics, ideas also useful in the physiogenesis of that supreme function of humans.

Regarding the phylogeny of praxic gnosic centers, we are also led to a deeper biological concept by establishing that gnosic centers are much older, and presently exist in all animal species with cerebral cortical matter. On the contrary, praxic cortical dynamics developed much later and appear more extended in higher mammals and especially in primates. This in turn means that the intensity of mental elaboration rests essentially with the praxic components that complete the gnosic cortical product. Such a clue teaches us about human psychology in an incomparable way, with productive (praxic) mentality predominating over the merely representative (gnosic) mentality.

Discussion

The idea of studying pathology to shed light on normal brain function was not new when Jakob (1921) worked on agnosias and apraxias. His ingenuity rests on the combination of different approaches in formulating an integrated theory of cortical dynamics.

From an evolutionary perspective, Jakob conveyed the idea, still valid today, that productive mentality derives from the frontal lobes. In contemporary terms, 'Homo sapiens, knowing man, is issued from Homo habilis, handy man' (de Duve 2002, p. 192). Jakob pointed out that this brain region evolved and expanded in a unique way in primates: 'The great development of the frontal lobes is typical of the brain of primates and in no way an exclusively human characteristic' (Jakob 1943, p. 89). Jakob's extensive studies on human brains and over 100 species of the Patagonian fauna helped him propose a theory of cortical phylogeny (Jakob 1912a, b; Triarhou 2010). The fact that humans and the great apes share a large frontal cortex is backed by modern research. The possibility of a parallel functional reorganization of this region may account for the special cognitive abilities that distinguish primates from other species (Semendeferi et al. 2002). The evolutionarily older gnosic centers are thought to reside in the postcentral 'microdynamics' (Capizzano 2006).

Concerning the ontogeny of gnoses and praxes, Jakob placed their development in infancy and childhood. Thus, one herein encounters a striking similarity between Piagetian and 'Jakobian' concepts. The term 'assimilation' was introduced by Piaget (1952, p. 6) to describe 'structuring through incorporation of external reality into forms due to the subject's activity'. Nonetheless, an early use of the term appears in Jakob's 1921 article, being subsequently refined (Jakob 1935a, 1945a, b), to imply the process of changing of qualities, modalities and relations through which the individual incorporates the external and internal world of objects, processes and situations.

Jakob recorded in detail the various types of gnoses, including tactile, thermal, tactile-muscular (stereognoses), visual, auditory and olfactory, each one being further classified into subtypes. For example, labial, lingual and digital gnoses fall into the category of tactile gnoses. Accordingly, Jakob held the view that gnosic processes are accompanied by modalities, a concept close to the modern interpretation of agnosia, which is considered a modality-specific inability to access semantic knowledge of an object or any other stimulus which cannot be attributed to an impairment of basic perceptual processes (Greene 2005).

With regard to localization theory, Jakob defended the existence of Broca's area from an anatomical-clinical standpoint (Jakob 1906; Tsapkini et al. 2008). He argued that every gnosic and praxic mechanism comprises localizable elements, such as receptors, assimilators and effectors (Jakob 1921); however, he considered the strict localization of mental function or dysfunction as misleading. By attributing apraxias to the disturbance of transcortical dynamics, Jakob highlighted the role of cortical communication. He paralleled neurocognitive functions to electrical current: 'it is only possible to localize the source' (Jakob 1941). Carl Wernicke (1848–1905) opposed the localization of higher functions to specific regions as well, stressing the importance of association areas (Catani and ffytche 2005) and claimed that apraxia results from the separation of brain regions (Finger 1994). Wernicke's line of thought influenced Heinrich Lissauer (1861–1891), an assistant at the Breslau Psychiatric Clinic (Shallice and Jackson 1988). In his 1890 paper, Lissauer subdivided visual agnosia into two subtypes, 'apperceptive' and 'associative' (Lissauer 1890; Lissauer and Jackson 1988). Such a distinction is considered to be the most influential in the history of research in agnosia (Shallice and Jackson 1988). Apperceptive agnosia is accompanied by impaired object recognition due to deficits in perceptual processing, whereas in association agnosia the primary deficit lies in difficulties in accessing the relevant knowledge about objects from memory (Eysenck 2004, p. 251). Jakob seems to agree with Lissauer's work when he refers to a dual premise for the construction of a complete gnosis: 'apperceptive condensation and mnemonic correlation'. Associationist models produced disconnectionist accounts of disorders of higher functions. Liepmann's apraxia model and Déjerine's pure alexia description fall into this tradition, which was revived with Geschwind's neo-associationism. Geschwind (1965a, b) attributed higher function deficits to disconnections that result either from white matter lesions or lesions of association areas, whereas, more recently, Catani and ffytche (2005) updated that model into a hodotopic framework.

Jakob (1921) argued that 'gnoses and praxes are neither sensory nor motor, but concomitantly sensory-motor processes'. Similarly, the idea of 'occasionally fluid boundaries' between agnosia and apraxia has been developed by several authors (Lange 1988, p. 176). In his renowned work 'Matter and memory' (Bergson 1896), the French philosopher Henri Bergson (1859–1941) argued that it is impossible to define where perception ends and movement begins (Blumen and Blumen 2002). Contemporary researchers seem to agree with this view; limb apraxias are considered higher-order disorders of sensory-motor integration (Leiguarda and Marsden 2000). Since apraxia is viewed as a type of motor agnosia, Jakob (1921) aptly notes that 'it is impossible for the patient to integrate sensory information'.

An interesting point in Jakob's work concerns the localization of sensory and associative functions in relation to cortical plasticity. Jakob clearly rejected the separation of the cerebral cortex into independent projection and association areas (Jakob 1912a, b; Triarhou 2010). Specifically, he claimed that there are no special associative centers apart from sensory areas, where a stimulus is both perceived and revived, thus arguing against Cajal's hypothesis of 'mnemonic centers' (Azmitia 2007), namely, a three-order system of neural networks that subserve associative functions.

Jakob explained the compensatory functions of the cerebral cortex by arguing that a functional take-over is only possible whenever brain regions show a certain equipotentiality as far as the elaboration of modality-specific stimuli is concerned. The experimental data gathered from the advent of sophisticated imaging methods lend credence to Jakob's reasoning: for example, Grafman (2000) attributes primary and secondary functional assignments to cortical regions; secondary functional assignments are inhibited until the normally responsible area suffers a damage that renders necessary the activation of the backup region. Neuroimaging techniques further shed light to cases of cross-modal plasticity (Fujii et al. 2009; Sadato 2005). In view of those considerations, one may understand how Jakob's theorizing ability compensated for the technical limitations in his times.

Jakob rejected mechanistic concepts and adopted a dynamic approach in explaining cortical function; he argued for an active exchange between external environment and the adaptive brain. Such a dynamic approach first appeared in his 1918 paper 'From the mechanism to the dynamics of the mind: A critical historical study of organic psychology' (Jakob 1918). Although dynamic concepts prevailed in physics at that time, it took a while for such ideas to be applied to brain theory. York (2009) contends that an era's broader historical, political and cultural framework is reflected in scientific trends. Theoretical dynamic approaches became popular in many fields after the 1940s. To our knowledge, the first reference to neurodynamics is attributed to Trigant Burrow (1943). Influenced by computer science, modern theories use the metaphor of cognition as a dynamic system sustained on spatiotemporal topology (Ibañez and Cosmelli 2008). Wiener's (1948) critical work in cybernetics opened up new vistas (François 1999). The Chilean neurobiologist Francisco Varela (1946–2001), a herald of modern brain dynamics and cybernetics, argued against 'brain-bound neural events' that constitute the mind (Rudrauf et al. 2003); he supported the view that 'consciousness depends crucially on the manner in which brain dynamics are embedded in the somatic and environmental context of an animal's life' (Thompson and Varela 2001). Such trends are compatible with Jakob's views: López Pasquali (1965) underlines that Jakob's work seems to anticipate cybernetics in certain aspects.

Scientists today highlight the importance of the study of praxes in relation to (a) the localization of function, (b) hemispheric potential and (c) the ability of the brain to compensate for injury (Goldmann-Gross and Grossman 2008). Jakob addressed these problems and formulated an integrative theory on the function of gnosio-praxic systems. Some of his views may share commonalities with Wernicke and Lissauer. A point worth emphasizing is the multi-level approach that Jakob adopted, by combining anatomo-functional and phylo-ontogenetic data.

Acknowledgments The authors gratefully acknowledge the anonymous reviewers for their constructive criticism which led to an improved manuscript, and the courtesy of the staff at the National Library of Medicine of the United States, the Bibliotheek van de Universiteit van Amsterdam, and the Ibero-Amerikanisches Institut Preussischer Kulturbesitz zu Berlin.

References

Azmitia, E. C. (2007). Cajal and brain plasticity: insights relevant to emerging concepts of mind. *Brain Research Reviews, 55*, 395–405.

Bergson, H. (1896). *Matière et memoire: essai sur la relation du corps à l'esprit*. Paris: Félix Alcan.

Blumen, S. C., & Blumen, N. (2002). From the philosophy auditorium to the neurophysiology laboratory and back: from Bergson to Damasio. *The Israel Medical Association Journal, 4*, 163–165.

Burrow, T. (1943). The neurodynamics of behavior. A phylobiological foreword. *Philosophy of Science, 10*, 271–288.

Capizzano, A. (2006). Actualidad del pensamiento de Cristofredo Jakob. *Revista del Hospital Italiano de Buenos Aires, 26*, 71–73.

Catani, M., & ffytche, D. H. (2005). The rises and falls of disconnection syndromes. *Brain, 128*, 2224–2239.

Cockburn, J. (2008). Stroke. In B. Woods & L. Clare (Eds.), *Handbook of the clinical psychology of ageing* (pp. 201–218). West Sussex: John Wiley and Sons Ltd.

de Duve, C. (2002). *Life evolving: Molecules, mind, and meaning*. New York: Oxford University Press.

Devinsky, O., & D'Esposito, M. (2004). *Neurology of cognitive and behavioral disorders*. New York: Oxford University Press.

Etcharry-Bouyx, F., & Ceccaldi, M. (2007). Gestural apraxia. In O. Godefroy & J. Bogousslavsky (Eds.), *The behavioral and cognitive neurology of stroke* (pp. 36–52). Cambridge: Cambridge University Press.

Eysenck, M. W. (2004). *Psychology: An international perspective*. Hove: Psychology.

Finger, S. (1994). *Origins of neuroscience: A history of explorations into brain function*. New York: Oxford University Press.

François, C. (1999). Systemics and cybernetics in a historical perspective. *Systems Research and Behavioral Science, 16*, 203–219.

Freud, S. (1891). *Zur Auffassung der Aphasien—Eine kritische Studie*. Leipzig–Wien: Franz Deuticke.

Freud, S. (1955). The psychogenesis of a case of homosexuality in a woman (Translation by J. Strachey, A. Freud, A. Strachey and A. Tyson of *Über die Psychogenese eines Falles von weiblicher Homosexualität* [1920]). In: J. Strachey (Ed.), *The Standard Edition of the Complete Psychological Works of Sigmund Freud, Volume XVIII (1920–1922): Beyond the Pleasure Principle, Group Psychology and Other Works* (pp. 145–172). London: The Hogarth Press and the Institute of Psycho-Analysis.

Fujii, T., Tanabe, H. C., Kochiyama, T., & Sadato, N. (2009). An investigation of cross-modal plasticity of effective connectivity in the blind by dynamic causal modeling of functional MRI data. *Neuroscience Research, 65*, 175–186.

Geschwind, N. (1965a). Disconnexion syndromes in animals and man. Part I. *Brain, 88*, 237–294.

Geschwind, N. (1965b). Disconnexion syndromes in animals and man. Part II. *Brain, 88*, 585–644.

Goldberg, E. (2005). *The wisdom paradox*. New York: Gotham Books.

Goldmann-Gross, R. G., & Grossman, M. (2008). Update on apraxia. *Current Neurology and Neuroscience Reports, 8*, 490–496.

Grafman, J. (2000). Evidence for forms of neuroplasticity. *Journal of Communication Disorders, 33*, 345–356.

Grasset, J. (1912). *Tratado de fisiopatología clínica. III. Neurobiología, ontogenia y filogenia, herencia*. Barcelona: Salvat y Compañía.

Greene, J. D. W. (2005). Apraxia, agnosias, and higher visual function abnormalities. *Journal of Neurology, Neurosurgery and Psychiatry, 76*(Suppl 5), 25–34.

Ibañez, A., & Cosmelli, D. (2008). Moving beyond computational cognitivism: Understanding intentionality, intersubjectivity and ecology of mind. *Integrative Psychological & Behavioral Science, 42*, 129–136.

Jakob, C. (1906). Existe ó no un centro de Broca? *La Semana Médica (Buenos Aires), 13*, 677–678.

Jakob, C. (1912a). Über die Ubiquität der senso-motorischen Doppelfunktion der Hirnrinde als Grundlage einer neuen, biologischen Auffassung des corticalen Seelenorgans. *Journal für Psychologie und Neurologie (Leipzig), 19*, 379–382.

Jakob, C. (1912b). Über die Ubiquität der senso-motorischen Doppelfunktion der Hirnrinde als Grundlage einer neuen biologischen Auffassung des kortikalen Seelenorgans. *Münchener Medizinische Wochenschrift, 59*, 466–468.

Jakob, C. (1913). La psicología orgánica y su relación con la biología cortical. *Archivos de Psiquiatría. Criminología y Ciencias Afines (Buenos Aires), 12*, 680–698.

Jakob, C. (1914). Los problemas biogenéticos en sus relaciones con la filosofía moderna. *Revista del Círculo Médico Argentino y Centro Estudiantes de Medicina (Buenos Aires), 14*, 87–98.

Jakob, C. (1918). Del mecanismo al dinamismo del pensamiento: Estudio histórico-crítico de psicología orgánica. *Anales de la Facultad de Derecho y Ciencias Sociales de la Universidad de Buenos Aires, 18*, 195–238.

Jakob, C. (1919). La teoría actual de las gnosias y praxias como factores fundamentales en el dinamismo cortical. *Revista del Círculo Médico Argentino y Centro Estudiantes de Medicina (Buenos Aires), 19*, 1266–1275.

Jakob, C. (1921). La teoría actual de las "gnosias y praxias" como factores fundamentales en el dinamismo de la corteza cerebral. *La Crónica Médica, 38*, 17–24.

Jakob, C. (1923). *Elementos de neurobiología*. La Plata: Biblioteca Humanidades.

Jakob, C. (1935a). Sobre las bases orgánicas de la memoria. *Revista de Criminología, Psiquiatría y Medicina Legal (Buenos Aires), 127*, 84–114.

Jakob, C. (1935b). La filogenia de las kinesias: sobre su organización y dinamismo evolutivo. *Anales del Instituto de Psicología de la Facultad de Filosofía y Letras de la Universidad de Buenos Aires, 1*, 109–127.

Jakob, C. (1941). La función psicogenética de la corteza cerebral y su posible localización (Aspectos de la ontopsicogénesis humana). *Anales del Instituto de Psicología de la Facultad de Filosofía y Letras de la Universidad de Buenos Aires, 3*, 63–80.

Jakob, C. (1943). *Folia neurobiológica Argentina, tomo III. El lóbulo frontal: Estudio monográfico anatomoclínico sobre base neurobiológica*. Buenos Aires: Aniceto López–López y Etchegoyen.

Jakob, C. (1945a). El cerebro humano: su significación filosófica. *Revista Neurológica de Buenos Aires, 10*, 89–110.

Jakob, C. (1945b). Sobre el origen de la conciencia: investigaciones neurobiológicas sobre la dinámica cortical en relación con su sectorización conmemorativa. In E. Mouchet (Ed.), *Temas actuales de psicología normal y patológica, publicados bajo el patrocinio de la Sociedad de Psicología de Buenos Aires* (pp. 345–381). Buenos Aires: Editorial Médico-Quirúrgica/Talleres 'The Standard'.

Jakob, C. (1946). *Folia neurobiológica Argentina, tomo V. Documenta biofilosófica: Folleto I: Biología y filosofía A. Aspectos de sus divergencias y concomitancias; B. Ensayo de psicogenia orgánica*. Buenos Aires: López & Etchegoyen.

Jung, C. G. (1960). *The psychogenesis of mental disease* (Translation by R. F. C. Hull of *Zur Psychogenese der Geisteskrankheiten* [1906]). *Volume 3 of the Collected Works—Bollingen Series XX*. New York: Pantheon Books.

Kant, I. (1999). *Critique of pure reason* (Translation by P. Guyer & A. W. Wood of *Kritik der reinen Vernunft* [1781]) (1999th ed.). Cambridge: Cambridge University Press.

Lange, J. (1988). Agnosia and apraxia (Translation by G. Dean, E. Perecman & J. W. Brown of *Agnosie und Apraxie* [1936]). In J. W. Brown (Ed.), *Agnosia and apraxia: Selected papers of Liepmann, Lange, and Pötzl* (pp. 43–226). Hillsdale: Lawrence Associates.

Leiguarda, R. C., & Marsden, C. D. (2000). Limb apraxias: higher-order disorders of sensorimotor integration. *Brain, 123*, 860–879.

Liepmann, H. (1988). Apraxia (Translation by G. Dean & E. Franzen of *Apraxie* [1920]). In J. W. Brown (Ed.), *Agnosia and apraxia: Selected papers of Liepmann, Lange, and Pötzl* (pp. 3–39). Hillsdale: Lawrence Erlbaum Associates.

Lissauer, H. (1890). Ein Fall von Seelenblindheit nebst einem Beitrage zur Theorie derselben. *Archiv für Psychiatrie und Nervenkrankheiten, 21*, 222–270.

Lissauer, H., & Jackson, M. (1988). A case of visual agnosia with a contribution to theory. *Cognitive Neuropsychology, 5*, 157–192.

López Pasquali, L. (1965). *Christfried Jakob—Su obra neurológica, su pensamiento psicológico y filosófico*. Buenos Aires: López Libreros Editores S.R.L.

Macmillan, M. (2004). "I could see, and yet, mon, I could na' see": William MacEwen, the agnosias, and brain surgery. *Brain and Cognition, 56*, 63–76.

Moyano, B. A. (1957). Christfried Jakob, 25/12/1866–6/5/1956. *Acta Neuropsiquiátrica Argentina, 3*, 109–123.

Orlando, J. C. (1966). *Christofredo Jakob—Su vida y obra*. Buenos Aires: Editorial Mundi.

Pedace, E. A. (1949). Contribución de la escuela neurobiológica Argentina del Prof. Chr. Jakob en el estudio del lóbulo frontal. *Archivos de Neurocirugía, 6*, 464–466.

Piaget, J. (1952). *The origins of intelligence in children* (Translation by M. Cook of *La naissance de l'intelligence chez l'enfant, 2ème édition* [1948]). New York: International Universities Press.

Piaget, J. (1972). *The principles of genetic epistemology* (Translation by W. Mays of *Introduction à l'épistémologie génétique* [1950]). London: Routledge and Kegan Paul.

Rudrauf, D., Lutz, A., Cosmelli, D., Lachaux, J.-P., & Le Van Quyen, M. (2003). From autopoiesis to neurophenomenology: Francisco Varela's exploration of the biophysics of being. *Biological Research, 36,* 27–66.

Sadato, N. (2005). How the blind 'see' Braille: lessons from functional magnetic resonance imaging. *The Neuroscientist, 11,* 577–582.

Semendeferi, K., Lu, A., Schenker, N., & Damasio, H. (2002). Humans and great apes share a large frontal cortex. *Nature Neuroscience, 5,* 272–276.

Shallice, T., & Jackson, M. (1988). Lissauer on agnosia. *Cognitive Neuropsychology, 5,* 153–156.

Szirko, M. (1995). A la antropología ganglionar desde la kinesiología: un fallido ensayo de extrapolar lo orgánico. *Electroneurobiología, 2,* 101–191.

Thompson, E., & Varela, F. J. (2001). Radical embodiment: neural dynamics and consciousness. *Trends in Cognitive Sciences, 5,* 418–425.

Triarhou, L. C. (2008). Centenary of Christfried Jakob's discovery of the visceral brain: an unheeded precedence in affective neuroscience. *Neuroscience and Biobehavioral Reviews, 32,* 984–1000.

Triarhou, L. C. (2010). Revisiting Christfried Jakob's concept of the dual onto-phylogenetic origin and ubiquitous function of the cerebral cortex: a century of progress. *Brain Structure and Function, 214,* 319–338.

Triarhou, L. C., & del Cerro, M. (2006a). Semicentennial tribute to the ingenious neurobiologist Christfried Jakob (1866–1956). 1. Works from Germany and the first Argentina period, 1891–1913. *European Neurology, 56,* 176–188.

Triarhou, L. C., & del Cerro, M. (2006b). Semicentennial tribute to the ingenious neurobiologist Christfried Jakob (1866–1956). 2. Publications from the second Argentina period, 1913–1949. *European Neurology, 56,* 189–198.

Triarhou, L. C., & del Cerro, M. (2007). Pioneers in neurology: Christfried Jakob (1866–1956). *Journal of Neurology, 254,* 124–125.

Tsapkini, K., Vivas, A. B., & Triarhou, L. C. (2008). 'Does Broca's area exist?' Christofredo Jakob's 1906 response to Pierre Marie's holistic stance. *Brain and Language, 105,* 211–219.

Wiener, N. (1948). *Cybernetics or control and communication in the animal an the machine*. Paris: Hermann.

York, G. K., III. (2009). Localization of language function in the twentieth century. *Journal of the History of the Neurosciences, 18,* 283–290.

Zoë D. Théodoridou holds BA and MA degrees in Educational Policy from the University of Macedonia, Thessaloniki, Greece, where she is currently pursuing a doctorate in neuroeducation. She works as a special education teacher at the Second Elementary School in Chalastra, Greece.

Lazaros C. Triarhou is Professor of Neuroscience at the University of Macedonia, Thessaloniki, Greece. He obtained his MD from Aristotelian University (Greece), MSc from the University of Rochester, New York, and PhD from Indiana University. His research interests are centered on the evolution of ideas in neurobiology, mainly after the laboratory revolution.

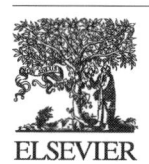

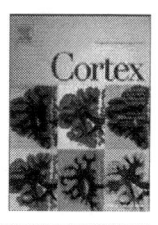

Special issue: Historical paper

Challenging the supremacy of the frontal lobe: Early views (1906—1909) of Christfried Jakob on the human cerebral cortex

Zoë D. Théodoridou and Lazaros C. Triarhou*

Economo-Koskinas Wing for Integrative and Evolutionary Neuroscience, University of Macedonia, Thessaloniki, Greece

ARTICLE INFO

Article history:
Received 14 July 2010
Revised 6 September 2010
Accepted 15 December 2010
Published online 21 January 2011

Keywords:
Christfried Jakob
cerebral cortex
history of neuroscience
frontal lobe
localization of cognitive functions

ABSTRACT

This article focuses on a series of six studies that address functional localization in the frontal lobe; they were published in Argentina between 1906 and 1909 by Christfried Jakob (1866—1956), one of the great thinkers in early 20th century neuropathology and neurophilosophy. At that time, the localization-holism controversy was at a peak, having been triggered by the historic Marie-Déjerine aphasiology debate. Jakob held the view that constitutive physiological elements of cognition are localized. Nonetheless, he cast doubt on phrenological approaches that considered the frontal lobe as 'superior' to the other cortical regions. Jakob studied the human frontal lobe from fetal life through senility, in normality and pathology, including tumors, injuries, softening, general paralysis and dementia. Based on those finds, he considered strict localization theories a dead-end. Taking a critical look at Flechsig's ideas on the parallel ontogenies of frontal association centers and intellect, Jakob argued that the frontal lobe does not carry any selective advantage over the remaining human cerebral lobes or even over the frontal lobe in non-human primates. Regarding lesion experiments in laboratory animals, he pointed to methodological caveats, such as insufficient recovery time, that may lead to disorientating conclusions, and rejected élite brain research, calling it superficial and inexact. Jakob was convinced that the verification of the anatomical connections of the frontal lobe would elucidate its functions. Thus, he viewed the frontal lobe as a central station receiving input via olfactory pathways and thalamic radiations, pertinent to muscular and cutaneous senses, and attributed a perceptive character to a brain region traditionally associated with productive functions. Modern neuroscience seems to support Jakob's rejection of distinguishable motor and sensory regions and to adopt a cautious stance concerning oversimplified localization views.

© 2011 Elsevier Srl. All rights reserved.

1. Introduction

After more than a century of cortical research, frontal lobe function still poses challenges. The complexity of the cerebral cortex has led authors to consider it anything from 'the apparatus of civilization' to an organ, the removal of which may not always lead to behavioral deficits (Teuber, 2009). The fact that the human frontal cortex occupies one-third of the

---

* Corresponding author. Neuroscience Wing, University of Macedonia, 156 Egnatia Ave., Bldg. Z-312, 54006 Thessaloniki, Greece.
E-mail addresses: ztheodoridou@hotmail.com (Z.D. Théodoridou), triarhou@uom.gr (L.C. Triarhou).
0010-9452/$ — see front matter © 2011 Elsevier Srl. All rights reserved.
doi:10.1016/j.cortex.2011.01.001

total cortical surface has instilled in researchers the expectation that the unveiling of frontal lobe function might explain the uniqueness of human behavior (Raichle, 2002).

A long debate has been taking place with regard to the functional localization of higher neurocognitive processes in the frontal lobe. Modern theoretical stances fall into a continuum that ranges from fractionated approaches to central concepts; at the same time, attempts are being made to reconcile contrasting views. The common denominator of fractionated approaches (cf. Koechlin et al., 2003; Shallice, 2002; Shallice and Burgess, 1996; Stuss et al., 2002) is the belief that there is no unitary frontal lobe process. The anterior part of the brain rather subserves multiple distinct control processes that underpin executive functions (Godefroy et al., 1999). Within such a framework, modularity and fractionation may even pertain to higher human abilities (Baddeley, 1996; Stuss et al., 2002). A more central concept has been put forth by Duncan and Miller (2002), who reject a fixed functional specialization and highlight the adaptability of select regions of the prefrontal cortex in order to complete a goal-directed activity. Finally, Stuss (2006) argues that the debate between fractionation and adaptability is a false debate and suggests that brain networks may be both locally segregated and functionally integrated (Yeterian et al., 2012, this issue; Catani et al., in press). Marshaled evidence showing the recruitment of the same frontal regions for different cognitive demands (Duncan and Owen, 2000) suggests that in spite of the fractionation, frontal processes are applicable to many domain-specific modules, and therefore are domain-general (Stuss, 2006).

However, the issue of functional localization has been at the core of neuropsychological research, as well as of philosophical delving, since the 19th century (Catani and Stuss, 2012, this issue). Although the idea of specific cerebral localizations of physiological functions was adopted before 1861 by several researchers including Gall and Bouillaud (cf. Finger, 2000), it was Broca's (1861) lecture to the Paris Anthropological Society that brought it forcefully to the scientific world (Lorch, 2008). The second of the two liveliest debates in the history of aphasiology took place when Marie questioned Broca's views, while Déjerine defended localization at a special joint meeting of the New York and the Philadelphia Neurological Societies and at the Neurological Society in Paris two years later, triggering a debate that spread internationally (cf. Tsapkini et al., 2008). At the same time, Jakob (1866–1956), a neurobiologist working in Buenos Aires, would adopt an integrative approach in his attempt to elucidate cortical function.

Born and educated in Germany, Jakob (Fig. 1) went to Argentina in July 1899. At that time, he had already made an international name for himself through his early brain Atlas (Figs. 2 and 3). Zülch (1975) credits Jakob (1899, 1901, Plate 15.5) for demonstrating that, at the direct corticospinal level, the pyramidal pathway is not yet myelinated in the newborn human; as Flechsig (1927) had described, only pathways that pass from motor cortex to the midbrain are myelinated at birth. In all, Jakob left 30 books and 250 articles that cover developmental, evolutionary, anatomical, pathological and philosophical issues in neurobiology (Barutta et al., 2011; Moyano, 1957; Triarhou and del Cerro, 2006a, 2006b; 2007).

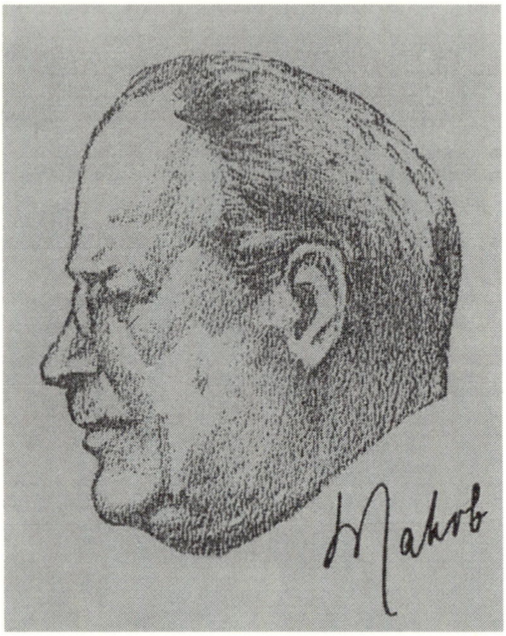

Fig. 1 — A sketch of Christfried Jakob by his student and biographer López Pasquali (1965). Signature from Orlando (1966).

The frontal lobe occupied Jakob's thought constantly in a path of enquiry spanning over five decades. Having studied the frontal lobe in its various developmental stages, and in neuropathological conditions, Jakob (1906a, 1907c) cast doubt on its 'supremacy' (Fig. 4). He pointed to potential historical reasons—linked to classical Greek philosophy—that might explain the importance attached to it. Jakob noted that physical characteristics, such as the upright posture, the extremities, and the extended forehead, distinguish humans from animals. In particular, Jakob (1943) considered the 'Olympian forehead', artistically expressed in the sculptures of Zeus, as the symbol of 'humanization'.

Jakob's contributions, written in German and Spanish, have been largely neglected in the English scientific literature. The present study aims at highlighting key concepts from his 'early' period. In that context, we provide selected translated passages from six papers, published between 1906 and 1909 (Jakob, 1906a, 1906b, 1906c, 1907a, 1907b, 1909), that address biological, anatomo-clinical and pathophysiological aspects of the frontal lobe. A psychobiological theory on the gnoses and praxes that culminated during Jakob's 'middle' period is presented elsewhere (Théodoridou and Triarhou, 2010).

2. Neuroanatomical studies

Jakob constantly viewed morphology in a functional context (Tsapkini et al., 2008). He believed that the elucidation of the

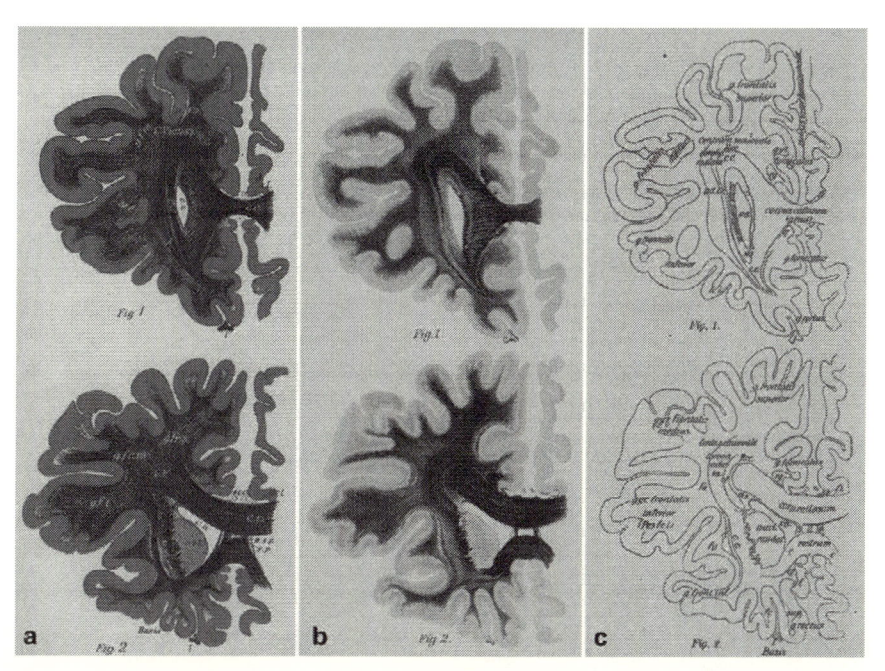

Fig. 2 — Drawings of coronal sections of the frontal lobe by Jakob for his early brain Atlases. (a) Plate 24 from the first edition (Jakob, 1895, 1896): frontal sections through the knee of the corpus callosum and the anterior segment of the frontal lobes (upper) and through the head of the caudate (lower). Abbreviations: g.f.s., superior frontal gyrus; g.f.m., middle frontal gyrus; g.f.i., inferior frontal gyrus; c.a., anterior horn of lateral ventricle; f.a., lateral association bundles; C.Vieuss., centrum semiovale; I, olfactory bulb; s.p., septum pellucidum; c.st., head of the caudate nucleus; c.i., anterior limb of the internal capsule. (b, c) Plate 28 from the second edition and explanatory diagram (Jakob, 1899, 1901). Abbreviations: Rcc., radiation of corpus callosum; pd.Cr., base of corona radiata; ft, tangential fibers; st.s, central gray matter of the ventricle; v, ventricle; of, occipitofrontal fasciculus; cg, cingulum; fa, arcuate fasciculus; fu, uncinate fasciculus; ce, external capsule; cl, claustrum; pes fr.i., foot of inferior frontal gyrus; sL, nerves of Lancisi; st.a., central gray matter.

anatomical connectivity of the frontal lobe would decipher its functions. Therefore, the anatomo-clinical approach was taken as the safest way in reaching conclusions on function. Jakob emphasized the importance of studying connections, an idea consistent with the current hodological trend (cf. Catani and ffytche, 2005; ffytche and Catani, 2005; Thiebaut de Schotten et al., 2012, this issue). Furthermore, his writings on connections seem attuned to more recent theories of frontal systems and neural networks, such as Alexander et al.'s (1986) influential concept of parallel but segregated frontal-subcortical circuits that has been put into a clinical framework. An in-depth discussion of the association between frontal-subcortical circuits and neurobehavioral disorders can be found in Chow and Cummings (1999) and other papers of the special issue (Krause et al., 2012, this issue; Cubillo in press, 2012; Langen et al., in press).

In studying the structure of the frontal lobe, Jakob did not see any substantial differences from the remaining lobes of the cerebral hemispheres: "The frontal lobe has three categories of fibers just like the other lobes: afferent and efferent projection fibers, association fibers and commissural fibers... Through the study of the afferent pathways we understand that in the major part of the frontal lobe, covering the whole of its convexity lies the great center of the muscular senses of a higher order" (Jakob, 1906b).

Concerning the connections between the frontal gyri and the Rolandic motor areas via 'U' fibers, Jakob (1906b) wrote: "These fibers join the superior frontal gyrus with motor foci that innervate the lower extremities, relate the middle frontal gyrus with the foci of the arms, and the inferior frontal gyrus with facial-lingual movements... Moreover, there exist short association fibers that connect the three gyri among them, and commissural fibers that, passing through the corpus callosum, enable the communication between the frontal gyri of the two sides... Thus, we come across the existence of an apparatus inserted between the muscles of the periphery and the cerebellum on one side and the Rolandic centers on the other" (Fig. 5).

Jakob (1906c) described the sensory-muscular pathways that arrive at the frontal lobe via the cerebellum, the red nucleus and the thalamus, concluding: "Although it is doubtful whether tactile senses arrive at the frontal lobe, it is true that numerous muscular sensory inputs enter the frontal lobe." In concordance with such an argument, Cappe et al. (2009) demonstrated the existence of thalamic projections to the cerebral cortex using neuroanatomical track-tracing

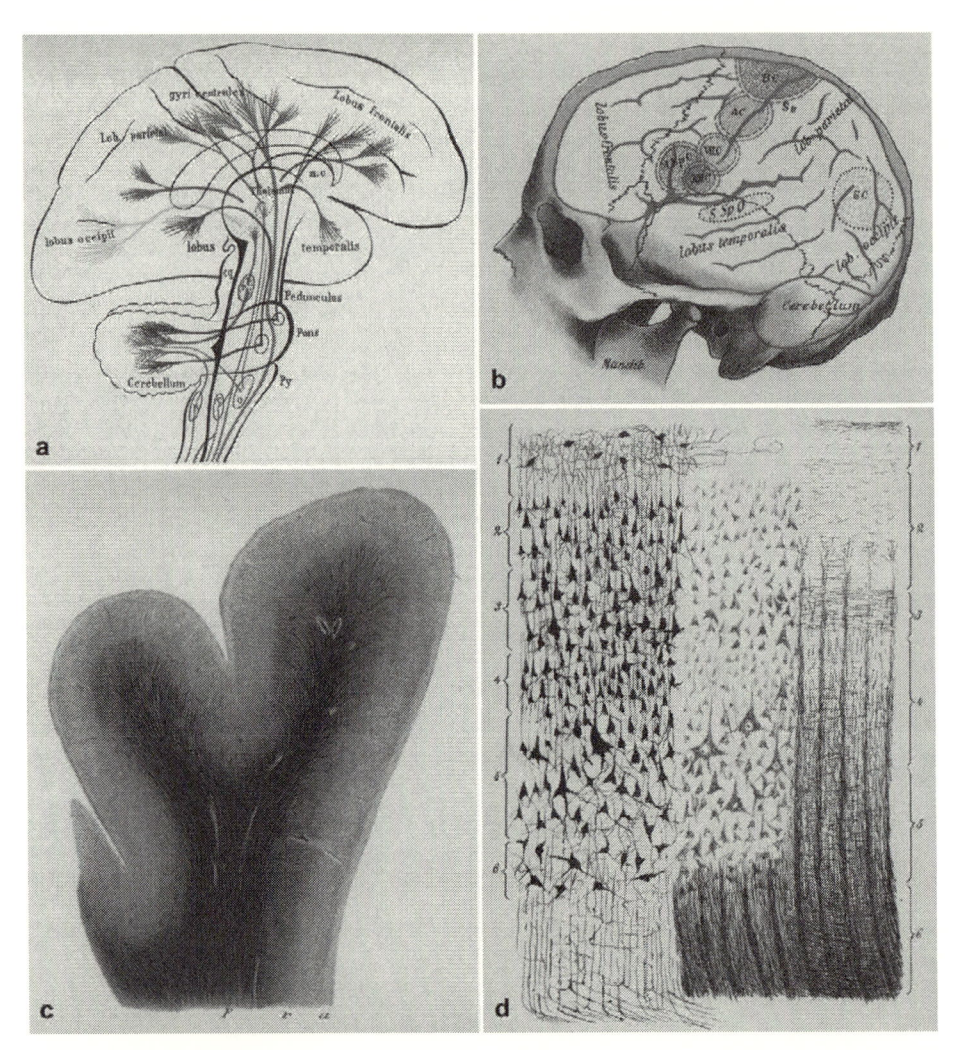

Fig. 3 — Additional drawings by Jakob from the second edition of his early brain Atlas (Jakob, 1899, 1901). (a) Plate 56.1 showing a general view of projection paths. Fibers forming the corona radiata enter the optic thalamus (brown). The frontal and temporal pontine pathway reaches the cerebellum through the contralateral middle cerebellar peduncle (blue). The pyramidal tract appears red, the sensory tract green, the cerebello-olivary tract violet, the optic radiation yellow, and the brachia brown. (b) Plate 21.3 depicting the position of psychomotor and psychosensory cortical centers in the cavity of the skull. Abbreviations: BC, motor center for lower extremities; AC, motor center for upper extremities; VIIC, XIIC, centers for muscles innervated by the facial and hypoglossal nerves; MSpC, SSpO, motor and sensory speech centers; SC, visual center. (c) Plate 20.1 showing a section from the center of the anterior central gyrus (carmin myelin sheath stain). White matter (F) appears blue-black; radial bundles (r) radiate in all directions and end in the cortex; a, outermost subpial layer. (d) Plate 19 showing the arrangement of cells (left and middle, stained with silver and methylene blue, respectively) and fibers (right) in the cerebral cortex. Cytoarchitectonic layer nomenclature: (1) Stratum zonale; (2) first layer of small pyramidal cells; (3) layer of medium-sized and large pyramidal cells; (4) second layer of small closely packed pyramidal cells; (5) second layer of medium-sized and large pyramidal cells with a few giant pyramidal cells; (6) layer of polymorphous cells.
Myeloarchitectonic layer nomenclature: (1) stratum zonale with superficial layer of tangential fibers; (2) superradial reticulum and Bekhterev-Kaes stripe; (3) coarser tangential fibers (stripes of Baillarger, Gennari, Vicq d'Azyr); (4) interradial reticulum of tangential fibers; (5) closely packed radial bundles; (6) medullary layer with radiating white fibers (projection, commissural, and long association tracts) and transverse short association bundles (arcuate fibers of Meynert). For the most part, nerve fibers pass from the cerebral white matter into the cortex; collected in bundles, they enter the second layer of cells, where their terminal fibrils end. These radial bundles (radii) therefore have a vertical arrangement. They are crossed at right angles by other fibers running parallel with the cortical surface and forming the plexus of tangential fibers — the superradial reticulum above the radii, and the interradial reticulum with the radii.

ANALYSES 595

1053) **La légende des Lobes Frontaux en tant que Centres supérieurs du Psychisme de l'Homme**, par Cristofredo Jakob (de Buenos-Aires). *Archivos de Psiquiatría y Criminología*, Buenos-Ayres, an V, p. 679-698, novembre-décembre 1906.

L'auteur donne plusieurs observations de lésions des lobes frontaux sans déficit psychique d'aucune sorte. La conclusion de son travail est que les lobes frontaux n'exercent aucune hégémonie sur le reste du cerveau; ce qui est perdu de la personnalité psychique à la suite des lésions étendues des lobes frontaux n'est qualitativement, ni quantitativement différent de ce qui est perdu à la suite de la destruction étendue de tout autre lobe cérébral.   F. Deleni.

Fig. 4 – Jakob's 1906 paper abstracted in French in the prestigious *Revue Neurologique* (Jakob, 1907c). The summary reiterates Jakob's conclusion, based on observations that lesions in the frontal lobes do not lead to any substantial mental deficit: "The frontal lobes do not exert any hegemony over the rest of the brain. Any mental deterioration after damage to the frontal lobe does not differ qualitatively or quantitatively from that seen after damage to any other cerebral lobe".

markers. Furthermore, Goldman-Rakic and Porrino (1985) showed that the prefrontal cortex is defined by multiple specific relationships with the thalamus. Performing retrograde tracing experiments, Mitchell and Cauller (2001) examined the corticocortical and thalamocortical afferents to layer I of the rat frontal cortex and affirmed the existence of afferent projections from thalamic nuclei to the frontal lobe.

Based on his anatomical observations, Jakob (1906c) viewed the major part of the frontal lobe as a central station with multiplier and combinatorial characteristics, constantly receiving stimuli from all the motility organs via multiple pathways (Fig. 6). According to Jakob (1911), the various centripetal pathways course into all sectors; thus, the cortex has a perceptive activity over its entire extent (Triarhou, 2010). Jakob's position is compatible with modern views on the function of the anterior parts of the human brain: the prefrontal cortex is considered a locus of synthesis of the outputs of various brain systems which provides the basis for the orchestration of complex behavior (Duncan & Miller, 2002). Furthermore, the role of the frontal lobe in integrating

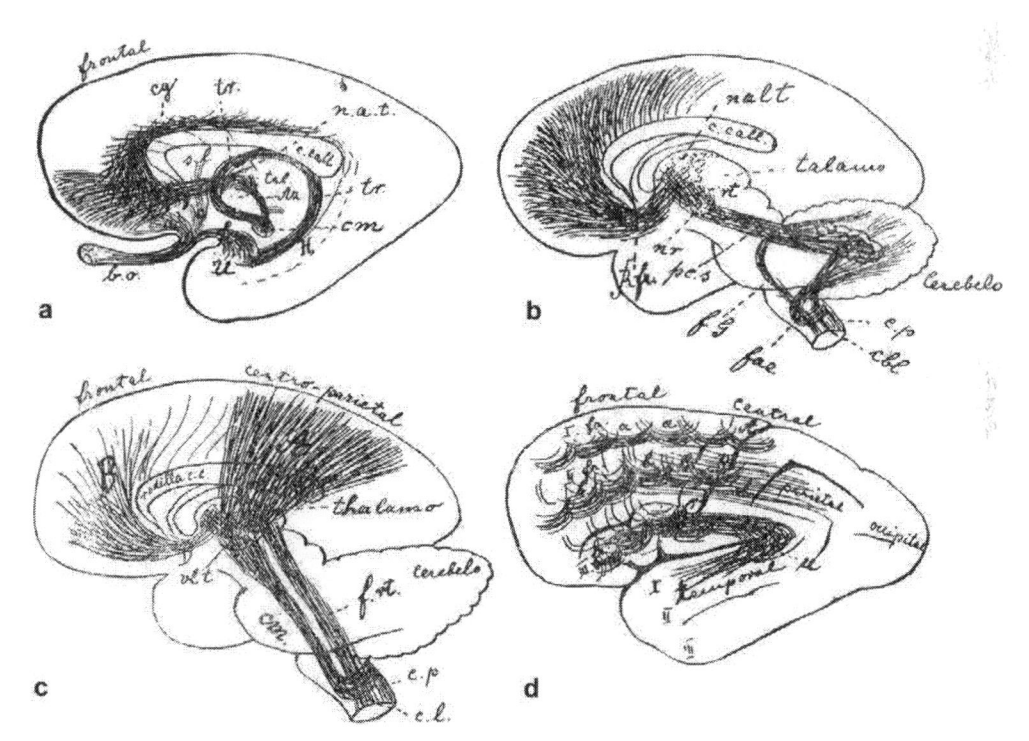

Fig. 5 – Schematic drawings by Jakob (1906b) showing: (a) Olfactory pathways in the frontal lobe. Abbreviations: b.o., olfactory bulb; a, internal root; b, lateral root; sl, septum pellucidum; u, uncus; h, hippocampus; tr, trigonum; cm, mamillary body; Az, bundle of Vicq d'Azyr; nat, anterior nucleus of thalamus; Rf, thalamo-frontal radiation; cg, cingulum. (b) Cerebello-frontal pathways. Abbreviations: cp, posterior spinal fasciculus; cbl, lateral cerebellar bundle; fG, bundle of Gowers; pcs, superior cerebellar peduncle; nr, red nucleus; rt, rubro-thalamic pathway; nalt, anterior lateral thalamic nucleus; Rfr frontal radiation. (c) Direct medullo-thalamo-frontal pathways. Abbreviations: cp, posterior spinal bundle; cl, lateral bundle; frt, reticular formation; cm, median band of Reil; vlt, ventral nuclei of thalamus; A, thalamo-Rolandic pathway; B, thalamo-frontal pathway. (d) Association pathways in the frontal lobe. Abbreviations: A, Rolandic center of crus; a, U-fibers of superior frontal gyrus (I); B, brachial center; b, U-fibers of middle frontal gyrus (II); C, facio-lingual center; c, U-fibers of inferior frontal gyrus (III); u, uncinate fasciculus; d, superior longitudinal fasciculus.

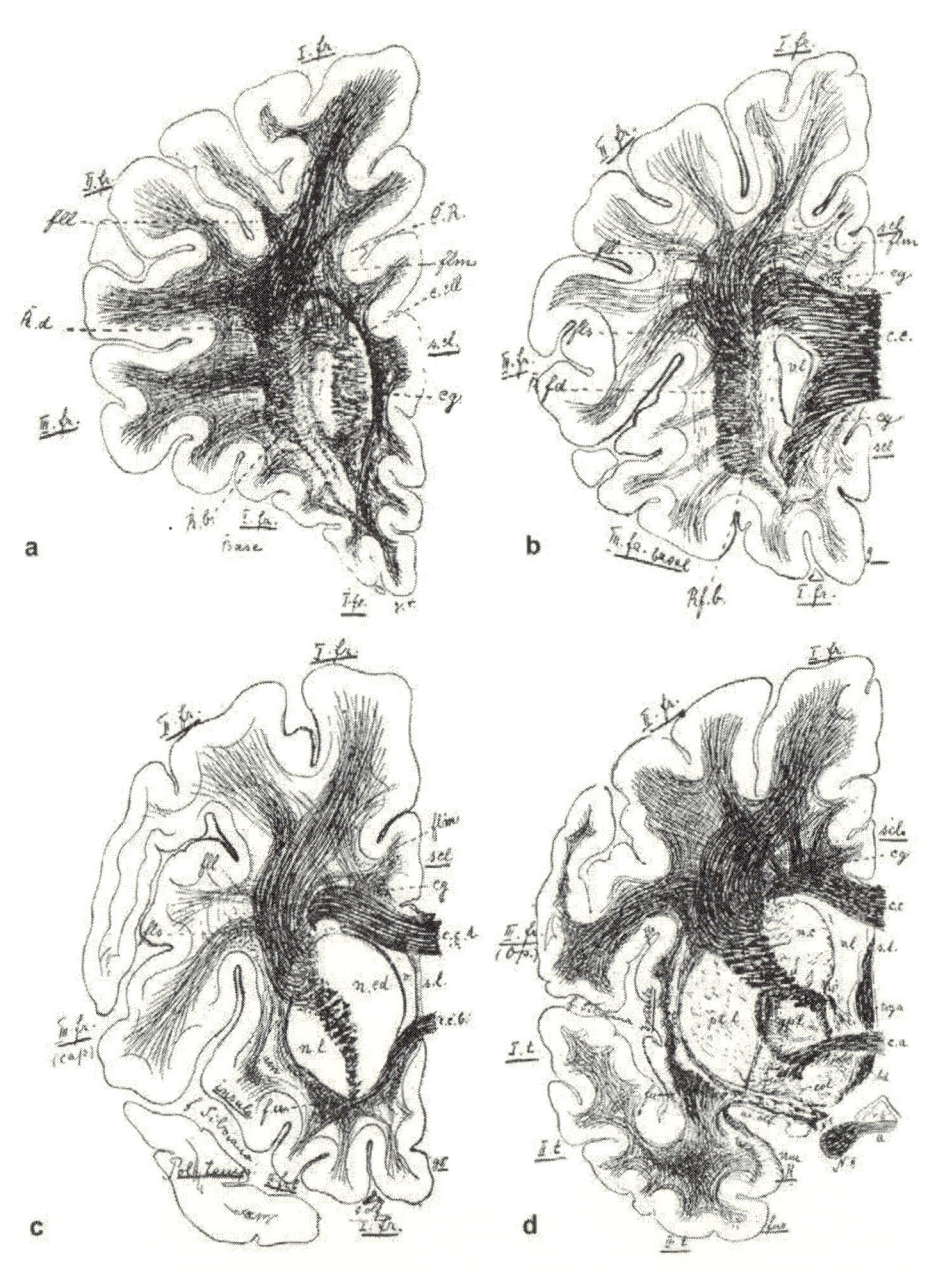

Fig. 6 — Schematic drawings by Jakob (1906c) based on a complete series of serial sections through the frontal lobe; Weigert method to depict fiber pathways. (a) Frontal section (no. 1154) in front of the corpus callosum. (b) Long projection, commissural and association pathways; section (no. 1076) through the knee of the corpus callosum. (c) Projection and commissural pathways and the formation of the internal capsule (frontal radiation); section (no. 948) through the corpus striatum. (d) Section (no. 882) through the posterior region of the frontal lobe with all its long frontal pathways. Abbreviations: *fr*, frontal; *t*, temporal; *v*, ventricle; *l*, lateral; *nc*, caudate nucleus; *ptl*, putamen-lenticular nucleus; *gpl*, globus pallidus; CR, corona radiata; RD, dorsal radiation of internal capsule; Rb, basal radiation of internal capsule; *gr*, rectal gyrus; *cg*, cingulum; *flm*, *fll*, *fls*, medial, lateral and superior longitudinal fasciculus; *fu*, uncinate fasciculus; *cc*, corpus callosum; *sl*, septum pellucidum; *am*, claustrum; *scl*, supracallosal gyrus; *nl*, lenticular nucleus; *ca*, anterior commissure; v_{III}, third ventricle; NI, olfactory nerve; NII, optic nerve; *ar.olf*, olfactory area; *trga*, anterior pillars of trigonum; *col*, coliculi of corpus striatum.

information from multiple brain areas supports its crucial involvement in learning, comprehension and reasoning (Baddeley, 2002). Frontal and prefrontal regions have been linked to visual, auditory and somatosensory inputs (Fogassi et al., 1996; Graziano et al., 1994, 1999; Wallace et al., 1992). Sensory, mnemonic and response signals that a single neuron displays provide strong evidence that prefrontal neurons behave as sensorimotor integrators (Goldman-Rakic, 2000). Prefrontal cortical neurons are considered to be a part of integrative neural systems that subserve cross-modal interactions across time (Fuster et al., 2000). According to Fuster's (2006) theorizing, actions related to human behavior, reasoning, and language are organized by means of interactions between prefrontal and posterior networks at the top of the 'perception–action cycle.' In non-human primates, multisensory integration takes place in frontal, parietal and temporal areas (Avillac et al., 2005). Thus, mounting evidence shows that much if not all of the neocortex is involved in multisensory integration (Ghazanfar and Schroeder, 2006).

3. Histological studies

3.1. Cytoarchitectonics

Based on the argument that structural differences signal functional specialization, Jakob studied human brain cytoarchitecture (Fig. 3d). Jakob (1906c) summed up his research as follows: "The frontal cortex is organized in the same cell layers, in the same associations of pyramidal cells that are differentiated only by their size, as we notice in the parietal and temporal lobe as well. The only thing that distinguishes the frontal cortex is the restricted variation of the size of the pyramidal cells due to the lack of large and giant pyramidal cells. My studies allow me to admit that toward the feet of the frontal gyri appear the large pyramidal cells covering the background of the precentral sulcus. Moreover, I managed to prove that the frontal cortex contains more cells per square millimeter compared with the Rolandic and the temporal regions. I could not deduce from this fact that the absolute number of cells would be greater in the frontal region compared to the Rolandic or the temporal regions, because the latter have a very high density".

At about the same time, Campbell (1905), a pioneer of cortical cytoarchitectonic parcellation, compiled clinical, anatomical and physiological evidence as a guide to function (ffytche and Catani, 2005). However, it was Brodmann's (1909) opus magnum that changed the view of histological localization in the human cerebral cortex once and for all (cf. Garey, 2006). Brodmann (1913) also produced a subsequent study concentrating on the frontal cortex (Elston and Garey, 2004).

3.2. Myeloarchitectonics

Having studied preparations with the Weigert method (Fig. 6), Jakob (1906c) argued: "As far as frontal myeloarchitectonics is concerned I notice the same disposition of radiating fibers as in other regions... The so-called association layers are identical to the ones of the other lobes and the tangential layer is well developed. On the contrary, the supraradial layer stands out in showing remarkably fewer myelinated fibers... I am inclined to see a structural inferiority, an idea that is reinforced by the following facts: a diminished total density and density of the various layers, a smaller average cell volume and a less developed supraradial layer." Regarding Flechsig's proposal of a parallel development of myelination pathways and intellect, Jakob wrote: "While the central tracts of the frontal lobe are not completed until several months after birth, Flechsig demonstrated that other regions of the brain develop in a similar fashion, for instance parts of the parietal and temporal lobes, the insula, and the so-called associative centers... Any chronological difference is not of much importance since a child has his frontal center perfectly myelinated before reaching six months of age. However, a newborn infant and one of six months are not easily differentiated with respect to their cognitive development" (Jakob, 1906a).

Myelination in humans continues well into the second decade of life (Yakovlev and Lecours, 1967). Structural magnetic imaging studies have shown gray matter changes in the frontal lobe from adolescence to adulthood (Sowell et al., 1999). In support of Flechsig's claim, the myelination of the frontal lobe has been repeatedly correlated with the development of higher cognitive functions, such as working memory (Nagy et al., 2004) and language (Pujol et al., 2006), while incomplete myelination has been blamed as the underpinning of weak decision-making skills in adults (Giedd, 2004).

Campbell's cytoarchitectonic data led to conclusions close to those of Jakob: "The structural development of the prefrontal cortex is exceedingly low. It presents an extreme of fibre poverty; all its fibre elements are of delicate calibre, and its association system is particularly deficient. Its cell representation is on a similar scale. The cortex is also shallow" (Campbell, 1905).

4. Pathophysiological studies

For the most part of the 19th century, the literature emphasized the role of the frontal lobe based on cases of damage that resulted in profound personality changes. Having studied human brains with frontal lobe tumors, injuries and degeneration, Jakob (1909) pointed to the rareness of 'pure cases'; he highlighted the characteristics that may render pathological specimens inappropriate for drawing secure conclusions. He emphasized that (a) the appearance of symptoms does not necessarily coincide with the onset of the disease; thus, progression may be difficult to determine; (b) tumors compress the brain parenchyma; (c) lesions of vascular origin lead to widespread degeneration; and (d) brain damage may cause inflammation or concussion which may affect the whole brain (Jakob, 1906c, 1909).

von Monakow (1904, 1910) underlined certain factors that had been overlooked by other investigators who studied lesions, i.e., the effects of inflammation, the lack of aseptic conditions during surgery, and the distant effects of local damage over time (Finger, 1994). Further caution has been expressed by Teuber (2009) about the contradictions found in the clinical literature: case studies may involve either massive lesions extending beyond the frontal lobe or small, unilateral, or asymmetric lesions with correspondingly small and easily compensated effects.

5. Comparative studies

Jakob's phylogenetic studies, from the human brain to over 100 species of the Patagonian fauna (Jakob, 1912a, 1912b; Jakob and Onelli, 1913, Triarhou, 2010), provided him with the bases for formulating the following ideas:

> "The development of the frontal lobes increases from lower to higher mammals in a continuous and constant relation, whereas in other vertebrates there are no hemispheres with a cortex comparable to those of mammals. It is obvious that the region located in front of the cruciate sulcus (a structure homologous to the central sulcus) increases in size and in the number of gyri it possesses from the marsupial to the rodent, from the rabbit to the dog, from the dog to the monkey, and approaches the size and complexity of humans only in anthropomorphous apes…[1] Although the external morphology progresses from lower to higher scale in a constant manner, the same process does not occur in the internal structure… We see, then, that what is true about the process of comparative development in the frontal lobe is true in all the other lobes as well. Perhaps there are greater variations in one structure than another; but such variations are slight and it would be a highly difficult, if not impossible, venture to find a fundamental exception for the frontal lobe" (Jakob, 1906a).

Elsewhere, he wrote: "When the frontal lobes of the different mammals, of ape and man are compared, the concord of the fine cortical structure strikes our attention; it is hard to encounter well defined differences… I myself noticed that the radiating fibers of the frontal lobe in apes are of a smaller calibre in comparison to other regions, a fact that has already been mentioned for humans. As far as the pyramidal cells are concerned ape shows all the different human types… What distinguishes the human frontal lobe is only the number of large and giant pyramidal cells… If the frontal lobe were such a superior center that it would differentiate by its functions humans from animals, then we should have met more evident differences in histological structure. According to my studies, I am inclined to believe that the similarities between the frontal cortical regions of some higher animals (for example apes) and humans are greater than the differences. This fact comes to demonstrate that the problem of the superior human functions does not lie in their localization in this or that lobe, but in factors of another nature" (Jakob, 1906c).

From the beginning of the 20th century, the extraordinary human cognitive development has been attributed to the large size of the frontal lobes. Cytoarchitectonic studies show a very similar organization between human and macaque monkey prefrontal cortex (Petrides, 2005; Petrides et al., 2012, this issue). Magnetic resonance imaging studies (Semendeferi et al., 2002) show that the frontal cortex of humans and great apes occupies a similar proportion of the cortex of the cerebral hemispheres. Accordingly, the enlargement of the human brain has generally preserved the relationship between its major lobes (Risberg, 2006). A relative increase of association cortex due to encephalization cannot lead to a regional expansion of the frontal association areas since all four cerebral lobes have both primary and association cortices; therefore, such an expansion should be common to all (Allen, 2009). For further discussion see also Petrides et al., (2012, this issue), Yeterian et al., (2012, this issue) and Thiebaut de Schotten et al., (2012, this issue).

6. Experimental animal studies

Laboratories where experiments on animals were conducted have been one of the most vivid battlefields in the localizationist–antilocalizationist controversy. The experimental confirmation of motor cortex in dog brain by Fritsch and Hitzig (1870) was a landmark in the history of functional localization (Catani and Stuss, 2012, this issue). This tradition continued with new mosaïcists and holists. Jakob (1906b) points out: "Goltz, Ferrier, Hitzig and Bianchi observed that animals that had both frontal lobes removed present remarkable alterations in intellect and character, such that they become irritable and have an increased tendency to bite… These experimenters did not sufficiently prolong their observations, and neither were they able to exclude as an explanation the consecutive inflammation or infections caused by the operation. New experimental verification, performed with meticulous care by Munk, Grossglik, Horsley and Schafer (1888), did not absolutely verify any of the previous observations. They found that once the animals had passed the first moments of postoperative excitation, they all returned to their status quo".

The vulnerability of the first series of experiments was also highlighted by Jacobsen et al. (1936), who attributed it to (a) the lack of objective measures of the degree and nature of behavioral deficits and (b) the lack of the demonstration that lesions of equal extent in other cortical regions do not cause dementia of the same severity.

7. Frontal lobe and higher cortical functions

According to Jakob's model, intelligence, memory and the like are needed for handling abstract concepts (Jakob, 1906c). Similarly, the view that psychical terms do not have localizable physiological correlates was expressed by Jackson and embraced by Freud, Goldstein, Pick, and Head (Meyer, 1974).

In 1906 Jakob wrote: "Consciousness is formed gradually as a result of the chaining of different cortical operations. It is impossible to view it as a localizable, special power separate from such processes. Consciousness is the manifestation of the synchronization of its components, since it is afflicted whenever any one of such components is afflicted. Intelligence is a quality par excellence that represents the rapid and safe function of the sensory, motor and associative apparatus. It cannot be localized, because it is a phenomenon inseparable from the overall cerebral process. Character is a mode of motor reactions congenitally imprinted on cortical elements. It intervenes in the transformation of the sensory and the motor functions and it is manifested in every action. Character is a quality, not a substantial power; therefore it could

---

[1] This was not a new observation: it is found, for instance, in the anatomy of Owen (1866–1868).

not be localizable. With the word 'memory' we designate an essential function that touches upon all the biological processes in the wider sense and especially upon the cortical processes. Will is the result of the inhibitory or productive influence that is exerted by gradually acquired associations on the inferior reflex actions via the motor centers. It has its origin in the association centers that cover the entire cortex. Only a determined voluntary act may be limited in a specific portion of the grand apparatus; nevertheless, for the production of such an act all the hemispheric regions intervene with greater or lesser intensity" (Jakob, 1906c).

Jakob's neurophilosophical writings became gradually refined and expanded in the course of his career. Well before neurophilosophy emerged as a formal scientific discipline, Jakob had written at least 14 philosophical works (López Pasquali, 1965), touching upon issues such as the relation between biogenesis and philosophy (Jakob, 1914) and the philosophical meaning of the human brain (Jakob, 1945; Théodoridou and Triarhou, 2010). Today, theories seek to elucidate the neural correlates of consciousness (cf. Crick & Koch, 1990). The so-called 'hard problem' lies in the consideration of consciousness as an 'emergent' property 'arising' from functional elements of the neurocognitive structure without attributing a dualistic character to it (Kouider, 2009). For example, according to Edelman and Tononi's model of a constantly shifting dynamic core (cf. Edelman, 1992; Tononi and Edelman, 1998), consciousness arises from the fast integration within a dynamic core of interacting elements. Other neurobiological theories, such as the global neuronal workspace (Dehaene et al., 1998; Dehaene and Naccache, 2001) highlight the interconnection between multiple cerebral modules that enables the broadcasting of information (Kouider, 2009). Whereas "proving the case for synchronization in the human brain" is still considered technically demanding (Zeman, 2001), Jakob conceived, in an impressive manner, the idea of synchronization of neuronal activity as the underlying mechanism of consciousness, more than a hundred years ago. Jakob's interpretation is consistent with the view that consciousness is to be correlated with a non-continuous event determined by synchronous activity in the thalamocortical system (Ribary et al., 1994). The transient synchronization of brain operations is considered to have the potential to construct unified and relatively stable neural states that underlie conscious states (Fingelkurts et al., 2005). The perception of volition seems to be generated in specific networks with the parallel activation of the global neuronal workspace (Hallett, 2007). The role of inheritance in behavior has been shown by selection and strain studies for animal behavior and by twin and adoption studies for human behavior (Plomin, 1990). Further evidence for the endogenous nature of traits derives from studies of behavior genetics, parent-child relations, personality structure, animal personality, and the longitudinal stability of individual differences (McCrae et al., 2000).

To conclude, Jakob tackled the 'terra incognita' of cognition with a multi-level approach in order to avoid bias. He was critical of oversimplifying localization explanations. Further, Jakob understood that it is essential to realize the limitations and misdirections involved in any attempt to decipher the brain–mind relationship. Being aware of such limitations, he searched for diverse clues, and largely relied on the anatomo-clinical approach. His concrete knowledge of neuroanatomy, coupled with his ingenuity, enabled him to produce knowledge that can be corroborated today via sophisticated tracing techniques. In a broad framework, studying Jakob's papers helps to correct and reconstruct an important episode in neurological history. Moreover, new English translations of such works will make them accessible by a wider audience. Given that the riddle of the human frontal lobe remains a central issue in modern neurobiology, Jakob's early views, a century later, may still provide meaningful clues.

Acknowledgments

Part of this work was presented at the 15th Annual Meeting of the International Society for the History of Neurosciences, Paris, France, June 15–19, 2010. The authors gratefully acknowledge the courtesy of the staff at the Ibero-Amerikanisches Institut and Staatsbibliothek Preussischer Kulturbesitz zu Berlin, the Library of Congress and the National Library of Medicine of the United States, as well as the anonymous reviewers for their constructive criticism.

REFERENCES

Alexander GE, DeLong MR, and Strick PL. Parallel organization of functionally segregated circuits linking basal ganglia and cortex. *Annual Review of Neuroscience*, 9: 357–381, 1986.

Allen JS. *The Lives of the Brain: Human Evolution and the Organ of Mind*. Cambridge, MA: Belknap Press of Harvard University Press, 2009.

Avillac M, Denève S, Olivier E, Pouget A, and Duhamel JR. Reference frames for representing visual and tactile locations in parietal cortex. *Nature Neuroscience*, 8(7): 941–949, 2005.

Baddeley AD. Exploring the central executive. *Quarterly Journal of Experimental Psychology*, 49A(1): 5–28, 1996.

Baddeley AD. Fractionating the central executive. In Stuss DT and Knight RT (Eds), *Principles of Frontal Lobe Function*. Oxford: Oxford University Press, 2002: 246–260.

Barutta J, Hodges J, Ibanez A, Gleichgerrcht E, and Manes F. Argentina's early contributions to the understanding of frontotemporal lobar degeneration. *Cortex*, 47(5): 621–627, 2011.

Broca P. Perte de la parole, ramollissement chronique et destruction partielle du lobe antérieur gauche du cerveau. *Bulletin de la Société d'Anthropologie (Paris)*, 2: 235–238, 1861.

Brodmann K. *Vergleichende Lokalisationslehre der Grosshirnrinde in ihren Prinzipien dargestellt auf Grund des Zellenbaues*. Leipzig: Barth, 1909.

Brodmann K. Neue Forschungsergebnisse der Grosshirnrindenanatomie mit besonderer Berücksichtigung anthropologischer Fragen. *Verhandlungen der Gesellschaft Deutscher Naturforscher und Ärzte*, 85: 200–240, 1913.

Campbell AW. *Histological Studies on the Localisation of Cerebral Function*. Cambridge: University Press, 1905.

Cappe C, Rouiller EM, and Barone P. Multisensory anatomical pathways. *Hearing Research*, 258(1/2): 28–36, 2009.

Catani M and Stuss DT. At the forefront of clinical neuroscience. *Cortex*, 48(1): 1–6, 2012.

Catani M, Dell'Acqua F, Vergani F, Malik F, Hodge H, Roy P, et al. Short frontal lobe connections of the human brain. *Cortex*, doi: 10.1016/j.cortex.2011.12.001.

Catani M and ffytche DH. The rises and falls of disconnection syndromes. *Brain*, 128(10): 2224–2239, 2005.

Chow TW and Cummings JL. Frontal subcortical circuits. In Miller BL and Cummings JL (Eds), *The Human Frontal Lobes: Functions and Disorders*. New York: Guilford Press, 1999: 25–43.

Crick F and Koch C. Towards a neurobiological theory of consciousness. *Seminars in Neuroscience*, 2: 263–275, 1990.

Cubillo A, Halari R, Smith A, Taylor E, and Rubia K. A review of fronto-striatal and fronto-cortical brain abnormalities in children and adults with Attention Deficit Hyperactivity Disorder (ADHD) and new evidence for dysfunction in adults with ADHD during motivation and attention. *Cortex*, doi:10.1016/j.cortex.2011.04.007.

Dehaene S, Kerszberg M, and Changeux JP. A neuronal model of a global workspace in effortful cognitive tasks. *Proceedings of the National Academy of Sciences of USA*, 95(24): 14529–14534, 1998.

Dehaene S and Naccache L. Towards a cognitive neuroscience of consciousness: Basic evidence and a workspace framework. *Cognition*, 79(1–2): 1–37, 2001.

Duncan J and Miller EK. Cognitive focus through adaptive neural coding in the primate prefrontal cortex. In Stuss DT and Knight RT (Eds), *Principles of Frontal Lobe Function*. Oxford: Oxford University Press, 2002: 278–291.

Duncan J and Owen AM. Common regions of the human frontal lobe recruited by diverse cognitive demands. *Trends in Neurosciences*, 23(10): 475–483, 2000.

Edelman GM. *Bright Air, Brilliant Fire: On the Matter of the Mind*. New York: Basic Books, 1992.

Elston GN and Garey L. *New Research Findings on the Anatomy of the Cerebral Cortex of Special Relevance to Anthropological Questions*. Australia: University of Queensland Press, 2004.

ffytche DH and Catani M. Beyond localization: From hodology to function. *Philosophical Transactions of the Royal Society of London (Biology)*, 360(1456): 767–779, 2005.

Fingelkurts AA, Fingelkurts AA, and Kahkonen S. Functional connectivity in the brain – Is it an elusive concept? *Neuroscience and Biobehavioral Reviews*, 28(8): 827–836, 2005.

Finger S. *Origins of Neuroscience: A History of Explorations Into Brain Function*. New York: Oxford University Press, 1994.

Finger S. *Minds Behind the Brain: A History of the Pioneers and Their Discoveries*. Oxford: Oxford University Press, 2000.

Flechsig P. *Meine myelogenetische Hirnlehre mit biographischer Einleitung*. Berlin: Julius Springer, 1927.

Fogassi L, Gallese V, Fadiga L, Luppino G, Matelli M, and Rizzolatti G. Coding of peripersonal space in inferior premotor cortex (area F4). *Journal of Neurophysiology*, 76(1): 141–157, 1996.

Fritsch GT and Hitzig E. On the electrical excitability of the cerebrum. In Von Bonin G (Ed), *Some Papers on the Cerebral Cortex*. Springfield, IL: Charles C. Thomas, 1870. p. 1960.

Fuster JM, Bodner M, and Kroger JK. Cross-modal and cross-temporal association in neurons of frontal cortex. *Nature*, 405(6784): 347–351, 2000.

Fuster J. The cognit: A network model of cortical representation. *International Journal of Psychophysiology*, 60(2): 125–132, 2006.

Garey LJ. *Brodmann's Localisation in the Cerebral Cortex*. New York: Springer, 2006.

Ghazanfar AA and Schroeder CE. Is neocortex essentially multisensory? *Trends in Cognitive Sciences*, 10(6): 278–285, 2006.

Giedd JN. Structural magnetic resonance imaging of the adolescent brain. *Annals of the New York Academy of Sciences*, 1021: 77–85, 2004.

Godefroy O, Cabaret M, Petit-Chenal V, Pruvo JP, and Rousseaux M. Control functions of the frontal lobes. Modularity of the central-supervisory system? *Cortex*, 35(1): 1–20, 1999.

Goldman-Rakic PS and Porrino LJ. The primate mediodorsal (md) nucleus and its projection to the frontal lobe. *Journal of Comparative Neurology*, 242(4): 535–560, 1985.

Goldman-Rakic P. Localization of function all over again. *NeuroImage*, 11(5): 451–457, 2000.

Graziano MSA, Reiss LA, and Gross CG. A neuronal representation of the location of nearby sounds. *Nature*, 397(6718): 428–430, 1999.

Graziano MSA, Yap GS, and Gross CG. Coding of visual space by premotor neurons. *Science*, 266(5187): 1054–1057, 1994.

Hallett M. Volitional control of movement: The physiology of free will. *Clinical Neurophysiology*, 118(6): 1179–1192, 2007.

Horsley V and Schafer EA. A record of experiments upon the functions of the cerebral cortex. *Philosophical Transactions of the Royal Society of London (Biology)*, 179: 1–45, 1888.

Jacobsen CF, Elder JH, and Haslerud GM. Studies of cerebral function in primates. *Comparative Psychology Monographs*, 13: 1–60, 1936.

Jakob C. *Atlas des gesunden und kranken Nervensystems nebst Grundriss der Anatomie, Pathologie und Therapie desselben*. München: J. F. Lehmann, 1895.

Jakob C. *An Atlas of the Normal and Pathological Nervous Systems. Together With a Sketch of the Anatomy, Pathology, and Therapy of the Same* (transl. by J. Collins). New York: William Wood & Co., 1896.

Jakob C. *Atlas des gesunden und kranken Nervensystems nebst Grundriss der Anatomie, Pathologie und Therapie desselben*. 2. Aufl. München: J. F. Lehmann, 1899.

Jakob C. *Atlas of the Nervous System Including an Epitome of the Anatomy, Pathology, and Treatment* (transl. by E. D. Fisher). 2nd edn. Philadelphia–London: W. B. Saunders & Co, 1901.

Jakob C. La leyenda de los lóbulos frontales cerebrales como centros supremos psíquicos del hombre. *Arquivos de Psiquiatría, Criminología y Ciencias Afines*, 5: 679–699, 1906a.

Jakob C. Nueva contribución á la fisio-patología de los lóbulos frontales. *La Semana Médica*, 13(50): 1325–1329, 1906b.

Jakob C. Estudios biológicos sobre los lóbulos frontales cerebrales. *La Semana Médica*, 13(52): 1375–1381, 1906c.

Jakob C. Sobre la sintomatología de las afecciones del lóbulo frontal. *La Semana Médica*, 14(43): 1285, 1907a.

Jakob C. Sobre apraxia. *La Semana Médica*, 14(44): 1344, 1907b.

Jakob C. La légende des lobes frontaux en tant que centres supérieurs du psychisme de l'homme (abstracted by F. Deleni). *Revue Neurologique*, 15: 595, 1907c.

Jakob C. Estudios anátomoclínicos sobre los lóbulos frontales del cerebro humano (Comunicación presentada al IV Congreso Médico Latinoamericano, Rio de Janeiro, 1–8 de agosto de 1909). *Argentina Médica*, 7(36): 463–472, 1909.

Jakob C. *Das Menschenhirn: Eine Studie über den Aufbau und die Bedeutung seiner grauen Kerne und Rinde*. München: J. F. Lehmann, 1911.

Jakob C. Über die Ubiquität der senso-motorischen Doppelfunktion der Hirnrinde als Grundlage einer neuen, biologischen Auffassung des corticalen Seelenorgans. *Journal für Psychologie und Neurologie (Leipzig)*, 19(1): 379–382, 1912a.

Jakob C. Ueber die Ubiquität der senso-motorischen Doppelfunktion der Hirnrinde als Grundlage einer neuen biologischen Auffassung des kortikalen Seelenorgans. *Münchener Medizinische Wochenschrift*, 59(9): 466–468, 1912b.

Jakob C. Los problemas biogenéticos en sus relaciones con la filosofía moderna. *Revista del Círculo Médico Argentino y Centro Estudiantes de Medicina (Buenos Aires)*, 14(150): 87–98, 1914.

Jakob C. *Folia neurobiológica Argentina, tomo III. El lóbulo frontal: Estudio monográfico anatomoclínico sobre base neurobiológica*. Buenos Aires: Aniceto López - López y Etchegoyen, 1943.

Jakob C. El cerebro humano: Su significación filosófica. Ensayo de un programa psico-bio-metafísico, después de 50 años de dedicación neurobiológica. *Revista Neurológica de Buenos Aires*, 10(2): 89–110, 1945.

Jakob C and Onelli C. *Atlas del cerebro de los mamíferos de la República Argentina: Estudios anatómicos, histológicos y biológicos comparados sobre la evolución de los hemisferios y de la corteza cerebral*. Buenos Aires: Guillermo Kraft, 1913.

Koechlin E, Ody C, and Kouneiher F. The architecture of cognitive control in the human prefrontal cortex. *Science*, 302(5648): 1181–1185, 2003.

Kouider S. Neurobiological theories of consciousness. In Banks W (Ed)Encyclopedia of Consciousness. Amsterdam: Elsevier, 2009: 87–100.

Krause M, Mahant N, Kotschet K, Fung VS, Vagg D, Wong CH, et al. Dysexecutive behaviour following deep brain lesions – A different type of disconnection syndrome. Cortex, 48(1): 96–117, 2012.

Langen M, Leemans A, Johnston P, Ecker C, Daly E, Murphy CM, et al. Fronto-striatal circuitry and inhibitory control in autism: Findings from diffusion tensor imaging tractography. Cortex, doi:10.1016/j.cortex.2011.05.018.

López Pasquali L. Christfried Jakob. Su obra neurológica, su pensamiento psicológico y filosófico. Buenos Aires: López Libreros Editores S.R.L, 1965.

Lorch MP. The merest Logomachy: The 1868 Norwich discussion of aphasia by Hughlings Jackson and Broca. Brain, 131(6): 1658–1670, 2008.

McCrae RR, Costa PT, Ostendorf F, Angleitner A, Hrebićkovać M, Avia MD, Sanz J, Saćnchez-Bernardos ML, Kusdil ME, Woodfield R, Saunders PR, and Smith PB. Nature over nurture: Temperament, personality, and life span development. Journal of Personality and Social Psychology, 78(1): 173–186, 2000.

Meyer A. The frontal lobe syndrome, the aphasias and related conditions: A contribution to the history of cortical localization. Brain, 97(3): 565–600, 1974.

Mitchell BD and Cauller LJ. Corticocortical and thalamocortical projections to layer I of the frontal neocortex in rats. Brain Research, 921(1): 68–77, 2001.

von Monakow C. Über den gegenwärtigen Stand der Frage nach der Lokalisation im Grosshirn. Ergebnisse der Physiologie, 3(2): 100–122, 1904.

von Monakow C. Neue Gesichtspunkte in der Frage nach der Lokalisation im Grosshirn. Zeitschrift für Physiologie der Sinnesorgane, 34: 161–182, 1910.

Moyano BA. Christfried Jakob, 25/12/1866–6/5/1956. Acta Neuropsiquiátrica Argentina, 3: 109–123, 1957.

Nagy Z, Westerberg H, and Torkel K. Maturation of white matter is associated with the development of cognitive functions during childhood. Journal of Cognitive Neuroscience, 16(7): 1227–1233, 2004.

Orlando JC. Christofredo Jakob: su vida y obra. Buenos Aires: Editorial Mundi, 1966.

Owen R. On the Anatomy of Vertebrates. London: Longmans, Green, and Co, 1866–1868.

Petrides M, Tomaiuolo F, Yeterian EH, and Pandya DN. The prefrontal cortex: Comparative architectonic organization in the human and the macaque monkey brains. Cortex, 48(1): 45–56, 2012.

Petrides M. Lateral prefrontal cortex: Architectonic and functional organization. Philosophical Transactions of the Royal Society of London (Biology), 360(1456): 781–795, 2005.

Plomin R. The role of inheritance in behaviour. Science, 248(4952): 183–188, 1990.

Pujol J, Soriano-Mas C, Ortiz H, Sebastian-Galles N, Losilla JM, and Deus J. Myelination of language-related areas in the developing brain. Neurology, 66(3): 339–343, 2006.

Raichle ME. Foreword. In Stuss DT and Knight RT (Eds), Principles of Frontal Lobe Function. Oxford: Oxford University Press, 2002. vii-ix.

Ribary U, Llinaćs R, and Joliot M. Human oscillatory brain activity near 40Hz coexists with cognitive temporal binding. Proceedings of the National Academy of Sciences of USA, 91(24): 11748–11751, 1994.

Risberg J. Evolutionary aspects on the frontal lobes. In Risberg J and Grafman J (Eds), The Frontal Lobes: Development, Function, and Pathology. Cambridge: Cambridge University Press, 2006: 1–20.

Semendeferi K, Lu A, Schenker N, and Damasio H. Humans and great apes share a large frontal cortex. Nature Neuroscience, 5(3): 272–276, 2002.

Shallice T. Fractionation of the supervisory system. In Stuss DT and Knight RT (Eds), Principles of Frontal Lobe Function. Oxford: Oxford University Press, 2002: 261–277.

Shallice T and Burgess P. The domain of supervisory processes and temporal organization of behaviour [and discussion]. Philosophical Transactions of the Royal Society of London (Biology), 351(1346): 1405–1412, 1996.

Sowell ER, Thompson PM, Holmes CJ, Jernigan TL, and Toga AW. In vivo evidence for postadolescent brain maturation in frontal and striatal regions. Nature Neuroscience, 2(10): 859–860, 1999.

Stuss DT. Frontal lobes and attention: Processes and networks, fractionation and integration. Journal of the International Neuropsychological Society, 12(2): 261–271, 2006.

Stuss DT, Alexander MP, Floden D, Binns MA, Levine M, McIntosh AR, Rajah N, and Hevenor SJ. Fractionation and localization of distinct frontal lobe processes: Evidence from focal lesions in humans. In Stuss DT and Knight RT (Eds), Principles of Frontal Lobe Function. Oxford: Oxford University Press, 2002: 392–407.

Teuber HL. The riddle of frontal lobe function in man. Neuropsychology Review, 19(1): 25–46, 2009.

Théodoridou ZD and Triarhou LC. Christfried Jakob's 1921 theory of the gnoses and praxes as fundamental factors in cerebral cortical dynamics. Integrative Psychological and Behavioral Science, doi:10.1007/s12124-010-9145-4 (online first) 2010.

Thiebaut de Schotten M, Dell'Acqua F, Valabregue R, and Catani M. Monkey to human comparative anatomy of the frontal lobe association tracts. Cortex, 48(1): 81–95, 2012.

Tononi G and Edelman GM. Consciousness and complexity. Science, 282(5395): 1846–1851, 1998.

Triarhou LC. Revisiting Christfried Jakob's concept of the dual onto-phylogenetic origin and ubiquitous function of the cerebral cortex: A century of progress. Brain Structure and Function, 214(4): 319–338, 2010.

Triarhou LC and del Cerro M. Semicentennial tribute to the ingenious neurobiologist Christfried Jakob (1866–1956). 1. Works from Germany and the first Argentina period, 1891–1913. European Neurology, 56(3): 176–188, 2006a.

Triarhou LC and del Cerro M. Semicentennial tribute to the ingenious neurobiologist Christfried Jakob (1866–1956). 2. Publications from the second Argentina period, 1913–1949. European Neurology, 56(3): 189–198, 2006b.

Triarhou LC and del Cerro M. Pioneers in Neurology: Christfried Jakob (1866–1956). Journal of Neurology, 254(1): 124–125, 2007.

Tsapkini K, Vivas AB, and Triarhou LC. 'Does Broca's area exist?' Christofredo Jakob's 1906 response to Pierre Marie's holistic stance. Brain and Language, 105(3): 211–219, 2008.

Wallace MT, Meredith MA, and Stein BE. Integration of multiple sensory modalities in cat cortex. Experimental Brain Research, 91(3): 484–488, 1992.

Yakovlev PI and Lecours AR. The myelogenetic cycles of regional maturation of the brain. In Minkowski A (Ed), Regional Development of the Brain in Early Life. London: Blackwell, 1967: 3–70.

Yeterian EH, Pandya DN, Tomaiuolo F, and Petrides M. The cortical connectivity of the prefrontal cortex in the monkey brain. Cortex, 48(1): 57–80, 2012.

Zeman A. Consciousness. Brain, 124(7): 1263–1289, 2001.

Zülch KJ. Pyramidal and parapyramidal motor systems in man. In Zülch KJ, Creutzfeldt O, and Galbraith GC (Eds), Cerebral localization: An Otfrid Foerster symposium. Berlin-Heidelberg: Springer, 1975: 32–47.

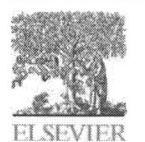

Brain and Cognition 78 (2012) 179–188

Brain and Cognition

journal homepage: www.elsevier.com/locate/b&c

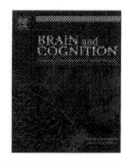

Theoretical Integration

Christfried Jakob's late views (1930–1949) on the psychogenetic function of the cerebral cortex and its localization: Culmination of the neurophilosophical thought of a keen brain observer

Zoë D. Théodoridou, Lazaros C. Triarhou *

Economo-Koskinas Wing for Integrative and Evolutionary Neuroscience, Department of Educational and Social Policy, University of Macedonia, 54006 Thessaloniki, Greece

ARTICLE INFO

Article history:
Accepted 14 November 2011
Available online 30 January 2012

Keywords:
Neurophilosophy
Christfried Jakob
Consciousness
History of neuroscience

ABSTRACT

This article follows the culmination of the scientific thought of the neurobiologist Christfried Jakob (1866–1956) during the later part of his career, based on publications from 1930 to 1949, when he was between 64 and 83 years of age. Jakob emphasized the necessity of bridging philosophy to the biological sciences, neurobiology in particular. Thus, we consider him as one of the early protagonists in the emergence of neurophilosophy in the 20th century. The topics that occupied his mind were the foundations for a future philosophy of the brain, and the 'neurobiogenetic', 'neurodynamic', and 'neuropsychogenetic' problems in relation to how consciousness emerges. Jakob's views have many elements in common with great thinkers of philosophy and psychology, including Immanuel Kant, William James, Edmund Husserl, Henri Bergson, Jean Piaget and Willard Quine. A common denominator can also be discerned between Jakob's dynamic approach and certain aspects of cybernetics and neurophenomenology. Jakob propounded the interdisciplinarity of sciences as an indispensable tool for ultimately solving the enigma of consciousness.

© 2011 Elsevier Inc. All rights reserved.

1. Introduction

With the progress effected in the brain sciences over the past 20 years, traditional philosophical questions have been steered into new directions (Churchland, 2008). Thus, the field of consciousness studies has been opened up to a growing body of biologists, neuroscientists, psychologists and philosophers (Blackmore, 2005). The investigation of philosophical theories in relation to neuroscientific hypotheses falls within the 'modern' domain of neurophilosophy (Northoff, 2004). Formalized by Churchland (1986), the term 'neurophilosophy' denotes the interdisciplinary attempt at unifying cognitive neurobiology. In the years following its foundation, neurophilosophy has grown exponentially. Its main theses have centered around: (a) psychological and neuroscientific theories, as well as intertheoretical relationships; (b) the opposition to the autonomy of either psychology or functionalism alone; and (c) a trend of rendering the cognitive neurosciences accessible to and comprehensible by a broader audience (Bickle, 2009, p. 3).

On the other hand, philosophy of neuroscience has gradually become a distinguishable field reflecting "an inquiry into foundational (especially epistemic and metaphysical) questions that apply to neuroscience" (Bechtel, 2001, p. 7). Such questions can be approached either descriptively, i.e. by depicting how neuroscience proceeds, or normatively, i.e. by implying how neuroscience should proceed (Bickle, Mandik, & Landreth, 2010).

The fluidity of the boundaries between neurophilosophy and the philosophy of neuroscience has led Brook and Mandik (2007) and Bickle (2009) to use the term 'Philosophy and Neuroscience', which entails ongoing transdisciplinary interactions, accommodating both endeavors. That is the definition we adopt in the present article.

Not until recently have philosophers started paying close attention to the data provided by the neurosciences. A few exceptions prior to the 1980s include the work of Nagel (1971), von Eckardt-Klein (1975), and Dennett (1978) as pointed out by Brook and Mandik (2007). The establishment and dissemination of reductionistic approaches in the 20th century, prompted to a great extent by Jacques Loeb (1859–1924) and Ivan P. Pavlov (1849–1936), relegated consciousness studies to philosophy, mysticism or 'soft' science, thus diminishing the influence of more integrated contemporary approaches, such as those of Sherrington and Lashey (Greenspan & Baars, 2005). As behaviorists were reacting to the earlier introspection—as exemplified e.g. in the thought of Wundt, James and Freud—with a desire for objectivity, they devised animal experiments, resolutely leaving the human mind out of the picture;

---

* Corresponding author. Address: University of Macedonia, Egnatia 156, Bldg. Z-312, 54006 Thessaloniki, Greece. Fax: +30 2310891388.
E-mail addresses: zoitheo@uom.gr (Z.D. Théodoridou), triarhou@uom.gr (L.C. Triarhou).

0278-2626/$ - see front matter © 2011 Elsevier Inc. All rights reserved.
doi:10.1016/j.bandc.2011.11.005

only around the middle of the 20th century did psychological theorizing swing back to studying the mind in the realm of cognitive psychology (Ochs, 2004, p. 356).

About a century ago, Christfried Jakob (1866–1956), a neurobiologist with an extraordinary scope of interests, put consciousness under scientific scrutiny, arguing that philosophy should be linked to the biological sciences (Triarhou & del Cerro, 2006b).

The son of Godofredo and Babette (née Körber) Jakob, Christfried Jakob was born on December 25, 1866 in Bavaria. His father, a cultivated teacher, recognized and encouraged Christfried's inclination in the natural sciences (Orlando, 1966). Jakob graduated in medicine in 1890 from the University of Erlangen with a prize of 1000 DEM, offered to the most distinguished student (Moyano, 1957). He next carried out his doctorate under the supervision of Friedrich Albert von Zenker (1825–1898), studying aortitis syphilitica (Triarhou & del Cerro, 2007). In the early 1890s he worked as an assistant to Adolf von Strümpell at the Erlangen Medical Clinic and privately practised medicine in Bamberg (Orlando, 1966). Jakob made a name for himself through his first brain atlas (Jakob, 1895; Jakob, 1899), which was translated into several languages (for details, see Triarhou & del Cerro, 2006a).

In 1899, Jakob accepted an offer from Domingo Cabred (1859–1929), the Argentinian Professor of Psychiatry, to direct the Laboratory of the Psychiatric and Neurological Clinic of the Hospital of Mercedes at the National University of Buenos Aires (Orlando, 1966). He went to Argentina having signed a three-year contract. One determining factor in his decision to leave Europe was the prospect of having 300 brains available for pathological study annually (López Pasquali, 1965). At that time, the Argentine population as well as the country's economy grew fervently as a result of immigration and a decreasing mortality (Véganzonès & Winograd, 1997), as Argentina was emerging as one of the ten richest countries in the world. By 1910, Jakob had produced critical works in anatomy, neurology, psychopathology and anthropology (Triarhou & del Cerro, 2007).

When his Argentinian contract expired in 1910, Jakob returned to Germany, where he promoted his original idea on the ubiquity of the dual sensory-motor function of the cerebral cortex (Jakob, 1911, 1912a, 1912b; Triarhou, 2010b). The works of his 'early' period (1890–1912) mostly centered around neuroanatomy, reflecting Jakob's training in the 'German school' (López Pasquali, 1965). His anatomical thinking during that early period has been presented elsewhere (Théodoridou & Triarhou, 2012).

The 'middle' period of Jakob's work (1913–1935) began with his permanent move to Argentina, where he assumed clinical, research and teaching duties. He was appointed Chief of the Neuropathological Institute at the National Psychiatric Hospital for Women in the Federal Capital, and Professor and Director of the Institute of Biology at the Faculty of Philosophy and Letters of the National University of La Plata. In 1922, Jakob was appointed Professor of Neurobiology at the Faculty of Humanities and Educational Sciences of the National University of La Plata. From 1921 to 1933, he held a joint appointment as Professor of Pathological Anatomy at the School of Medical Sciences of La Plata (Triarhou & del Cerro, 2006b).

The development of Jakob's 'dynamic approach' emerged in a 1918 article entitled 'From the mechanism to the dynamics of the mind: A critical historical study of organic psychology'. In his 1919–1921 work on gnoses and praxes as fundamental factors in cerebral cortical dynamics (Jakob, 1919, 1921) he further built on his original psychobiological ideas. Two subsequent studies (Jakob, 1935a, 1935b) have been considered by his colleague and biographer Moyano (1957) as vital constituents of Jakob's psychobiological theorizing; they were titled, 'On the biological bases of memory' (Jakob, 1935b) and 'The phylogeny of the organization and the evolutionary dynamics of the kineses' (Jakob, 1935a). An account of the 'middle' period of Jakob's thought has been published as well (Théodoridou & Triarhou, 2011).

In the 'late' phase of his life, Jakob's thought became more synthetic. He blended his philosophical background with the clinical and research experience, maintaining that the utmost problem of science and philosophy converges in cerebral function (Théodoridou & Triarhou, in press). He suggested a scientific psychology and a corpus of philosophy (López Pasquali, 1965).

Jakob retired in 1945 (Orlando, 1966). However, he kept his formal appointment in Buenos Aires as Chairman of Pathological Anatomy and continued to work in his laboratory at the National Psychiatric Hospital for Women until 1954; he died in Buenos Aires in 1956 at the age of 90 (Triarhou & del Cerro, 2006a, 2006b, 2007).

In all, Jakob authored 30 monographs and 200 papers that cover developmental, evolutionary, anatomical, pathological and philosophical themes in neurobiology (Triarhou & del Cerro, 2006a). He is viewed as the father of Argentinian neuroscience (Pedace, 1949) and one of the great thinkers of the 20th century. His scientific caliber was such that von Economo and Koskinas (1925) express the view that future research on the cortex would have to be based on the fundamental works of three investigators: Theodor Kaes (1852–1913), Santiago Ramón y Cajal (1852–1934) and Christfried Jakob, further considering Jakob's ideas on cortical phylo-ontogeny as 'ingenious' (Triarhou & del Cerro, 2006a).

The present study examines the culmination of his neurophilosophical thought during the 'late' period of his life and career. Jakob's involvement with philosophy was neither superficial nor based on improvisations (López Pasquali, 1965). Quite the contrary. We consider Jakob as an 'early neurophilosopher' for the following reasons.

Firstly, he was most likely one of the first academics to formally teach neurobiology in a School of Education, at the National University of La Plata, Argentina. Thus, he introduced fundamentals of neuroeducation decades before that discipline was formalized in the current era. Fischer et al. (2007) have defined the fervently growing field of mind, brain and education as "the quest for the integration of disciplines that investigate human learning and development bringing together education, biology, and cognitive science".

Secondly, Jakob's philosophical background is evident throughout his work. It peaked during his late years. Jakob published 20 articles in philosophy and neuroscience, besides philosophical papers on Kant and Descartes (Jakob, 1926, 1937, 1938).

Thirdly, Jakob (1943a) proposed the term 'psychophilosophy' in an imaginative conference of philosophical discussions among a small number of interlocutors ('*Conferencia magistral de introducción a la psicofilosofía*') that recalls the Socratic dialogs. Jakob (1943a), being the professor alongside six alumni, deals with issues such as the existence and the perception of God by the human mind, the nature of philosophy and science, the scientific basis of psychology, the nature of ideas, and the existence of a priori conditions of our internal intuition.

In the following sections we highlight some of Jakob's most important ideas on philosophy and neuroscience.

2. The diffusion of neurobiological knowledge into philosophy

In the first part of his 'Biophilosophical Documents' ('*Documenta Biofilosófica*') (Fig. 1), Jakob (1946) presented the following arguments for the necessity of diffusing common and divergent aspects of neurobiology into philosophy:

(A) Issues concerning life, from general aspects of evolution to heredity and the diversity of the human species, form a justified base for an objective, rational and scientific development of the philosophical orientations.

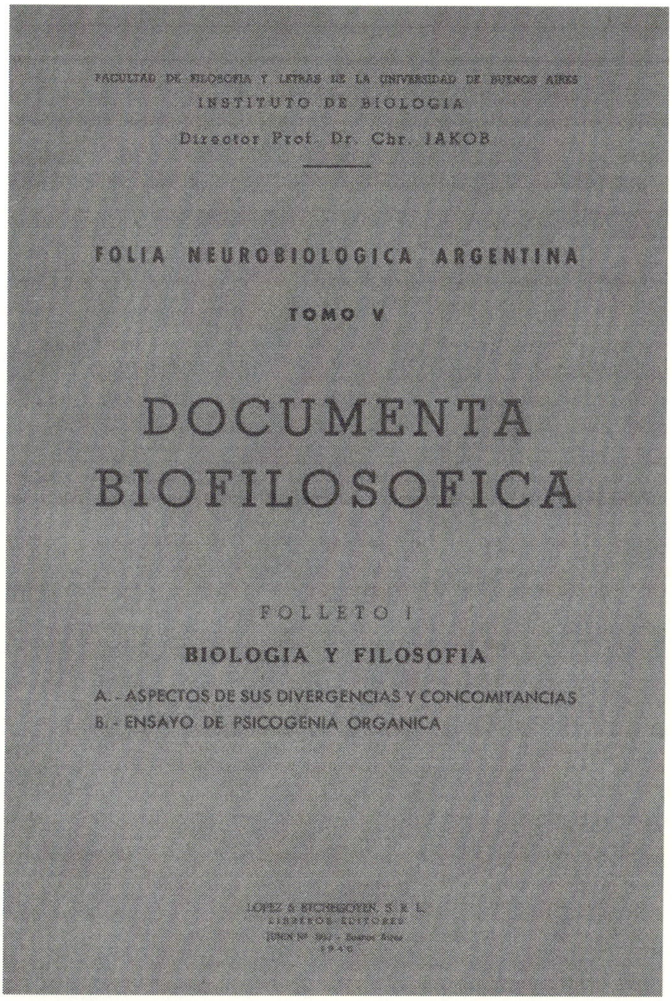
FACULTAD DE FILOSOFIA Y LETRAS DE LA UNIVERSIDAD DE BUENOS AIRES
INSTITUTO DE BIOLOGIA
Director Prof. Dr. Chr. JAKOB

FOLIA NEUROBIOLOGICA ARGENTINA

TOMO V

DOCUMENTA BIOFILOSOFICA

FOLLETO I

BIOLOGIA Y FILOSOFIA

A. - ASPECTOS DE SUS DIVERGENCIAS Y CONCOMITANCIAS
B. - ENSAYO DE PSICOGENIA ORGANICA

Fig. 1. Frontispiece of Jakob's monograph *Biophilosophical Documents*, being volume 5 of the *Folia Neurobiológica Argentina* series (Jakob, 1946).

(B) The scientific field of neurobiology that studies nervous structure and function (see e.g. Jakob, 1906b) under normal or pathological conditions, both evolutionarily and developmentally, is indispensable for psychology and its related sciences (cf. also Jakob, 1913).
(C) The knowledge of the morphophysiological evolution of the human brain in correlation with psychogenetic maturation, as well as brain alterations and their sequelae on memory, behavior, language and other abstract processes form the natural foundation of a conscious learning science.
(D) The creation and the preservation of higher cognitive functions (intellect, volition and emotions), instincts and reflexes depend on our cerebral organization.

Jakob (1946) argued that philosophical reasoning consists in elaborations stemming from a germ cell. Therefore, neurobiology should provide the organic basis of epistemology, logic, phenomenology, axiology, ethics, esthetics and metaphysics.

In that respect, Jakob (1945a) maintained that sciences dealing with the empirically accessible reality and philosophy which examines the possibilities that arise beyond experience need a philosopher who would above all master the former in order to treat the latter with composure.

3. Foundations for a future philosophy of the brain

Jakob (1945b) considered himself "a groundworker of a biocentric epistemology" (*'Como preliminares de una gnoseología biocéntri-*

ca...'). He described the theoretical background and main points that a future philosophy of the brain would have to treat. Along this line, he suggested that such a future discipline should consist of a synthesis of proven as universally valid neuro-psycho-dynamic theories concerning: (a) a universal, central organization; (b) heredity; and (c) the evocation and transformation of physical processes into psychological phenomena by means of neurohistological and physiological processes (Jakob, 1945b).

In this endeavor, Jakob (1945b) considered the following issues of primary importance:
(A) The laws that govern cerebral phylogeny and ontogeny and their stages.
(B) The microoganization of neuroblasts and the dynamics of their functional derivatives in normal and pathological conditions.
(C) The polyenergetic transformation at cosmological, biological, neurological and psychological levels in the integrative creation of the external (objective) and the internal (subjective) environment (see also Jakob, 1920).

Moreover, Jakob (1945b) argued that a philosophy of brain should shed light on the 'neurobiogenetic', 'neurodynamic', and 'neuropsychogenetic' problems. The first of these problems implies the various stages of the biological development of the nervous system, which is beyond the scope of the present article. The other two problems are detailed next.

4. The neurodynamic problem

In his neurodynamic postulate, (Jakob, 1921, 1935a; Théodoridou & Triarhou, 2011) explores psychogenesis from an evolutionary perspective (Fig. 2), with phylogeny occurring in two phases. The first or 'plasmodynamic' phase entails elementary biological phenomena such as tropism and pulsatility. The second or 'neurodynamic' phase is divided into three stages that correspond to different levels of organization in the vertebrate CNS: the 'archikinetic' stage corresponds to the archineuronal level; the 'paleokinetic' stage corresponds to the paleoneuronal level; and the 'neokinetic' stage corresponds to the neoneuronal level.

The phylogenetically older, archikinetic stage entails reflex actions that lead to the emergence of 'archipsychism'. The paleokinetic stage is characterized by the appearance of instinctive reactions that constitute 'paleopsychism'. The neokinetic stage is responsible for the elaboration of conscious responses, in other words it underpins 'neopsychism'. Neopsychism comprises three kinds of neurocognitive processes: (a) *gnoses*, which secure the conscious orientation in one's environment; (b) *praxes*, which underlie active individual intervention; and (c) *symbolisms*, which subserve the communication of abstract ideas by means of human language.

Jakob held that the notion of space results from the direction of a movement, the notion of time from its duration and, finally, the notion of causality from its intensity. From the angle of psychogenesis, space and time are deeply rooted psychogenetically in the gnosic sphere, whereas causality rests in the praxic sphere (Jakob, 1945b).

Topographically, gnoses are mostly positioned in retrorolandic regions, precisely in parieto–occipito–temporal regions. However, for the construction of the notion of a concrete object the dynamic collaboration of all cortical sectors (Fig. 3) is indispensable. Besides, gnoses maintain their sensory-motor character. Jakob (1921) wrote:

"Gnoses and praxes are then neither sensory nor motor, but concomitantly sensory-motor processes and their a priori connection with the functions of the pyramidal tract give us the possibility of satisfactorily explaining the passage of gnosis and praxis to the definitive voluntary movement...Mental functions cannot have for that reason localizations determined in such-and-such associative areas of the first or third order. Rather, their characteristics reside in transcortical dynamics that reunite isolated sensory-motor acts. Therefore, the only and true localizable elements of the process are physiological, existing primarily in gnoses and praxes; they then create the psychic phenomenon, the integrative fusion of both dynamics".

Gnoses express the reconstructive thinking and they are necessarily orientated in space and time. The praxic zone is apparent in the brains of lower mammals. Still, it crescents in primates with the appearance of functions of active intervention individually

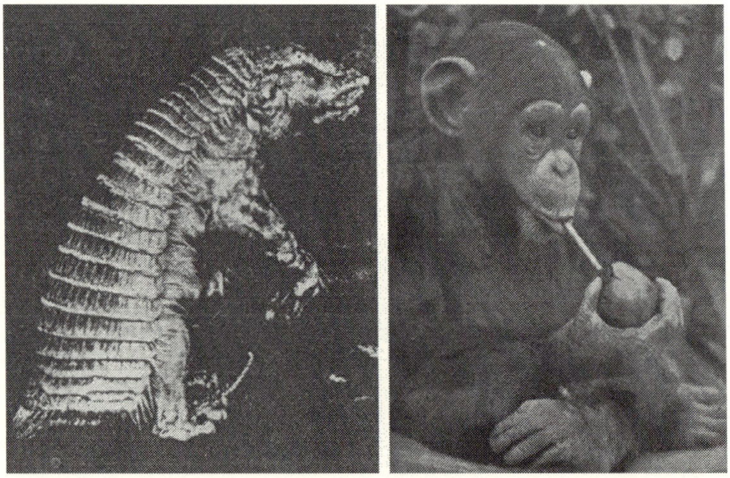

Fig. 2. *Left:* The edentate 'pichiciego pampeano' *(Chlamyphorus truncatus)*, the pink fairy of the armadillo species also known as *ratoncito cascarudo*, shown at a ½ scale (Jakob, 1943, p. 12). *Right:* Manual praxis in a chimpanzee (Jakob, 1943b, p. 22; photo by Clemente Onelli).

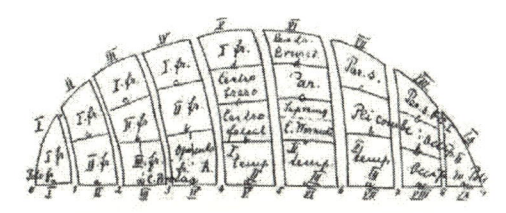

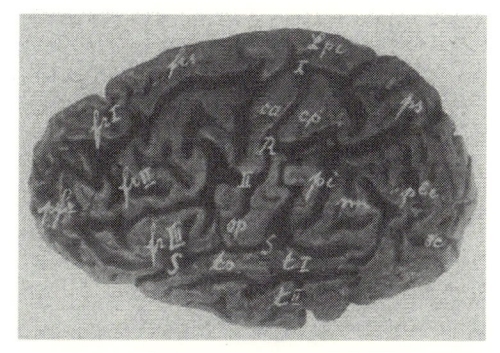

Fig. 3. *Upper:* Jakob's (1906b, p. 363) neuroanatomical procedure for studying hemispheric 'sectors' in the human cerebrum, consisted in defining a line, which he took as a basis, with the brain situated in its normal position, and dividing it through a system of coordinates dictated by the plan of cerebral morphology itself. *Lower:* A human brain with two atypical interruptions of the Rolandic area (x, x), fully encompassing the trigyral type of the hemispheric convexity in the Rolandic region (Jakob, 1941, p. 77). See also Fig. 3 in Théodoridou and Triarhou (2011) for lateral and midsagittal views of the human cerebral hemispheres and the 'golden section' concept with its praxic and gnosic sectors (Jakob, 1943, p. 37).

acquired by means of motor responses (for example, walking and language).

Jakob maintained that a higher mental activity that enables the emergence of the neopsychic sphere is reached only in primates, and especially humans, due to symbolic language, whereby the sphere of inner (visceral) feelings becomes integrated with environmental gnosio-praxic experiences (Triarhou, 2010a). He associated the emergence of conscious processes with the appearance of "the organ of consciousness, the cerebral cortex that allows the individual elaboration of the essential condition of memory" (Jakob, 1945b). Jakob (1945b) argued that the first commemorative sector and therefore creator of something conscious is the Ammonic cortex, termed 'paleocortex'. He attributed the commemorative ability of the Ammonic cortex to the fact that it houses two layers of cortical elements, one receiving stimuli (dentate area) and one effector (Ammonic area), that form reciprocal sets of fixation, residual of elaborated experiences (Jakob, 1945b).

By arguing that only in the human brain the commemorative cortical superiority enables the elevation of comparative thought to abstract reasoning, Jakob highlighted memory as a basic component or prerequisite for conscious processes. In fact, he claimed that the sense of continuity that is given by memory underpins the emergence of the conscious self. Jakob (1941, 1946) tackled the development of such processes in his neuropsychogenetic postulate.

5. The neuropsychogenetic problem

Jakob delved into the neuropsychogenetic problem in his 1941 article entitled: 'The psychogenetic function of the cerebral cortex and its possible localization: aspects of human ontopsychogenesis'. He used much of the text in the second part of his 'Biophilosophical Documents' (Jakob, 1946) under the title 'An essay on organic psychogenesis'.

Jakob (1941, 1946) theorized that two great worlds, 'like battlefields', create our cortical organ during its ontogeny forming an a priori unit: the external ('*ambiental*') and the internal ('*introyental*') milieu. The external, environmental factors act as stimulating material and the internal as hereditary germ capital, the maturation of which gives birth to the adequate central organic assimilation system. The external and internal domains were considered to enable the elaboration of personal and conscious experiences through a process of "internal-environmental frontalization", whereas the "commemorative accumulation" of such experiences was thought to allow an individual to plan and execute future actions (Barutta, Hodges, Ibáñez, Gleichgerrcht, & Manes, 2010). The endogenous sector is represented on the medial facies of the mammalian cerebral hemispheres, including the cingulate gyrus, and is charged with vegetative-autonomic functions, whereas the exogenous is represented on the convexity of the cerebral hemispheres and serves somatic functions (Triarhou, 2008). Nonetheless, Jakob (1906a, 1906–1908) rejected strict localization, arguing that it is impossible to view consciousness as a localizable, special power separate from processes chaining cortical operations.

The external and the internal milieux differentiate and complement each other via two essential psychogenetic acts, 'somatization', i.e. a course of action that leads to the formation of the position toward the external milieu, and 'sympathization', i.e. the course of action that leads to the formation of the position toward the internal milieu. A somatic act consists in a process of acceptance or rejection accompanied by the corresponding affective intonation. For example, when the infant encounters an obstacle (stimulus), unity becomes divorced: this 'object' will be 'environmental', and the organ that hits against the obstacle with all its neuromuscular organization will be 'internal'. On the other hand, a sympathetic act corresponds to a process of emotional intonation of pleasure or pain. For example, the infant satisfies its hunger by sucking. Milk, along with mother and chest, will be environmental; the tranquilization of the visceral needs, along with all of the glandulo-musculo-neural apparatus, belongs to the internal milieu.

Jakob (1941, 1946) suggested that psychogenesis is effected in three developmental stages—an 'infantile', a 'juvenile', and a 'mature' stage—and eventually leads to the construction of the external milieu and the creation of the somatic ego ("*La psicogenia realiza, en general, en su fase evolutiva, las siguientes tres etapas: una infantil, otra juvenil y uno última de maduración*").

In the first or *infantile* stage, there is a primitive perception of constellations of objects and processes. This stage elaborates the elementary knowledge of experience via cortical macro–microdynamic successions and associations. ("*La primera etapa representa la fijación de situaciones enteras que en sucesión macro–microdinámica cortical y colaboración asociativa primitiva gnoseo-práxica, elaboran las nociones elementales de la experiencia y en donde objeto y proceso están completamente fusionados formando un solo complejo conjunto..., una «situación completa»—constelación.*")

Therefore, the elemental reflex formation is created through a process of cortical 'synergy'. Memory provides accumulated material transferred via cortical elements organized in macro- and micro-dynamic systems (Fig. 4) for the emergence of orientation and intervention processes, i.e. gnoses and praxes. For this to happen, constellations must be transformed into differentiated objects and processes, forming concrete phenomena of the experienced world through a process of comparison and identification in the second or *juvenile* stage. ("*Enlazando y comparando tales «complejos» se separan poco a poco los elementos estacionarios de la situación de los movidos, transformándolos en objeto y proceso y creándose así,* a human ability that Jakob termed 'symbolism'. ("*En la tercera fase psicogenética de maduración mental, se procede a la seriación de objetos y procesos, creándose por la subsumpción simbolizante del lenguaje de los fenómenos concretos, la ideación abstracta. Situaciones complejas aisladas, nociones concretas totalizadas y, finalmente, seriadas en ideas abstractas simbolizadas son, entonces, sucesivamente los productos psicogeneticos de la labor gnoseo-práxica-cortical.*")

Jakob (1945b) described a cortical apparatus organized in such a way that accumulates and guards its traces in the form of cortical microdynamisms, linking them in a continuous and therefore conscious current.

Jakob (1906a) defined consciousness as the manifestation of the synchronization of its components. He argued that consciousness does not just emerge, but it is gradually formed as a result of cortical elaborations, attributing an adaptive character to the brain. ("*La conciencia se forma en el niño poco á poco como resultante del encadanamiento de las diferentes operaciones corticales...Ella es la manifestación den sincronismo de sus componentes...*")

He thought that there is a circular, reactive process between the object and the subject. The dynamics of consciousness—stemming from his views on cerebral cortical dynamics (Fig. 4)—consist in the simultaneous evocation of somatic reactions orientated to the external environment and sympathetic reactions orientated to the internal environment. Their synthesis links the external with the internal world in a constant adaptation.

6. Discussion

Jakob's understanding of evolutionary anatomy and biological mechanisms led him into viewing the cerebral cortex as a historical product of the external environment and at the same time as the human organ of active adaptation (López Pasquali, 1965). In a similar way, Ochs (2004) argues that the accumulated historical experiences have allowed the evolution of human social groups and subsequently the emergence of civilization.

Jakob supported the idea of a constant dynamic exchange between the internal and the external milieu, sensation and motion, perception and action (Théodoridou & Triarhou, in press). He developed such views especially throughout his 'middle' and 'late' periods. In his 1921 article he described explicitly his dynamic approach that highlights a circular flow, wherein the brain gets informed, updated and finally orientated in its environment in order to actively intervene in it. Such an approach anticipated, in certain aspects, the field of cybernetics (cf., Wiener, 1948), which, in turn, is considered as one of the critical antecedents of contemporary cognitive science (Gardner, 1985).

In defining 'systemics and cybernetics' we follow François (1999): "a metalanguage of concepts and models for transdisciplinarian use still evolving within a slow process of accretion through inclusion and interconnection of many notions, which came and are still coming from very different disciplines". Some common points between Jakob's ideas and the theories of cybernetics are discussed next.

Jakob and Copello (1948) wrote: "Life in general and the human organism in particular receive stimuli for their reactive neuronal phylogeny and ontogeny from two sources: an endogenous, generic, inner source that gives rise to the vegetative-sympathetic sphere, and an exogenous, individually orientated one that gives rise to the environmental-somatic sphere. They both create the neurodynamic nature and the personal consciousness of their carrier in a continuous reciprocal amalgamation. Neurobiology demonstrates that the same structurally bipartite and functionally integrated neural plan is applied as much on amoebae as on men. Even in protozoa there is a mutual contact of the organism with the external milieu and an internal regulatory mechanism

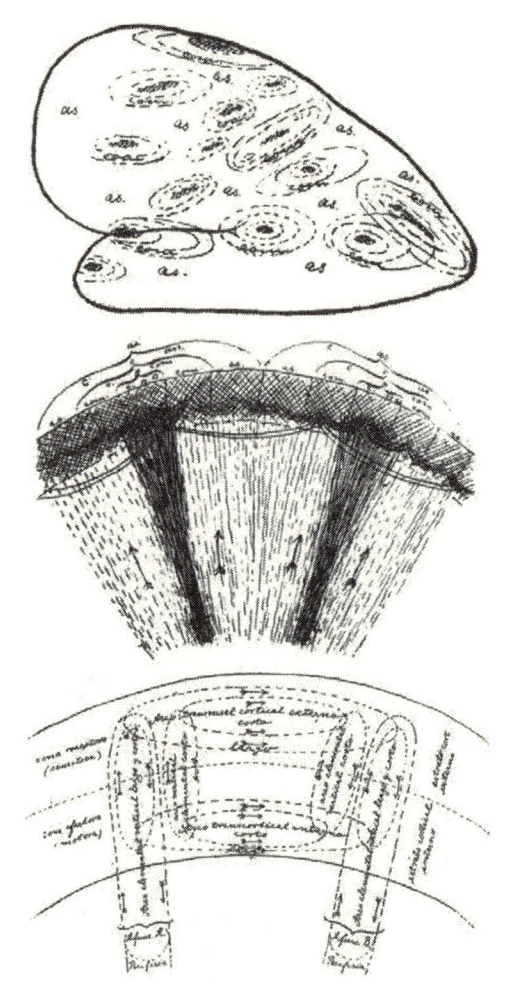

Fig. 4. *Upper:* A schematic drawing of perception areas by Jakob (1906–1908, p. 301), outlining the annular commemorative and the association centers. *Middle:* Schematic drawing by Jakob (1906–1908, p. 304) of two adjacent centers of perception, *v.o.* and *v.a.*, representing the central afferent pathways; within their confines, the other centripetal and centrifugal fibers of the commemorative (*c. com.*) and the association center (*c. acc.*); *c.p.o.* and *c.p.a.*, perception (centrofocal) center. *Lower:* Outline of the major cortical streams (elementary long and short vertical arc, external or internal cross-arc, long and short) according to Jakob (1913, p. 694). See also Figs. 5 and 6 in Triarhou and del Cerro (2006b) for Jakob's depiction of neocortical histotopography with its microdynamic organization and macrodynamic events (Jakob, 1945a, pp. 99–100).

por encima de situaciones análogas o diferentes, las ideas concretas del mundo objetivo experimentado.")

The third or *mature* stage reflects human consciousness, or according to Jakob's terminology 'neopsychism'. Within this phase objects and processes are organized in the dimensions of space, time and causality by means of complex neurocognitive processes, i.e. gnoses and praxes. The human mind then becomes capable of generating abstract ideas through the symbolic code of language, that secures the preservation of the organism". Furthermore, within the tripartite model that he presented in his neurodynamic postulate, Jakob conceived 'psychism' as "the neurobiophylactic [neural life-protecting] complex of neuroenergetic reception, assimilation and reaction, which regulates the organism's vital necessities against variable factors in the external and internal milieu" (Jakob, 1939, p. 8). In addition, López Pasquali (1965) underlines the fact that Jakob's studies on assemblies of circuits might have anticipated the concept of autoregulation in cybernetics.

Bernard (1878, 1974) had formulated his ideas on the internal environment to unify the explanations concerning the fundamental physiologies of the body under the general principle of the preservation of stability (Gross, 1998). Bernard's momentous pronouncements, including his final account of the conception of an internal environment ("*le milieu intérieur*"), were gathered and published posthumously in the first volume of the 'Lectures on the Phenomena of Life Common to Animals and Plants' (Olmsted & Olmsted, 1952). At the time, the general concepts of 'living system' and 'regulation' were latent (François, 1999).

Jakob's hypothesis on the integrated function of perception and action may have parallels in diverse fields. The concept that higher processes enter at the most elementary stage of sensation was introduced by Kant; perception is then far from a simple construct following on passively received sensory reception (Ochs, 2004). von Uexküll (1934) described a functional cycle of perceptual and motor field, considered as an early account of Biocybernetics. Within his theory, perceptual and effector fields together form a closed unit, a systematic whole, the *Umwelt* (von Uexküll, 1934). von Weizsäcker (1950) attempted to represent the unit of perception and movement in the theoretical basis of Gestalt psychology introducing the concept of *Gestaltkreis* (Théodoridou & Triarhou, in press).

The idea of a 'perception–action cycle' flourished within the confines of ecological psychology. Gibson (1986) saw perception in dynamic terms and emphasized the importance of sensory feedback from movement (Hurley, 2001). Arbib (1981) put the concept into the framework of computational neuroscience, whereas Fuster (2006) is credited with the designation of the perception–action cycle in the cerebral cortex. According to the latter's theorizing (Fuster, 2006), the upper stages of the biocybernetic cycle compose the perception–action cycle, where sensory information is analyzed in the context of existing perceptual 'cognits', i.e. basic units of memory or knowledge comprised of distributed, interactive, and overlapping networks of neurons, and processed in the context of existing executive 'cognits'.

In a biocybernetic framework, Maturana and Varela (1980, 1987) developed the concepts of 'autopoiesis' and 'operational closure'. Autopoiesis, a multi-connected concept significant for problems of cognition but also for the self-reproduction of living systems is associated with the concepts of self-closure, self-reference and self-production (François, 1999).

Varela introduced neurophenomenology arguing against 'brain-bound neural events' that constitute the mind (Rudrauf, Lutz, Cosmelli, Lachaux, & Le Van Quyen, 2003); he supported the view that "consciousness depends crucially on the manner in which brain dynamics are embedded in the somatic and environmental context of an animal's life" (Thompson & Varela, 2001). Varela's conception of mind and ultimately of experience is concerned with the constraints exerted by the specific phenomenology of our concrete coping upon our internal dynamics as autonomous systems, and reciprocally, the effects of the latter upon the former, in a circular framework (Rudrauf et al., 2003). In this sense, one could argue that Jakob's views herald neurophenomenology (cf., Varela, 1996).

As far as the neuropsychogenetic problem is concerned, Jakob (1941) perceived psychogenesis (<Gk. *psyche* = soul and *genesis* = origin) as a dynamic process leading to the formation of abstract thought. Piaget shared a common view relating 'psychogenesis' to cognitive development, maintaining the literal meaning of the word contrary to its wide and popular psychiatric use (Freud, 1920; Jung, 1960).

Further similarities are found between the mechanisms and laws that rule Jakob's stages of organic psychogenesis and concepts encountered in Piaget's formulations. In particular, in his attempt to explain how the forms of intellectual activity are constructed at the sensory-motor level and subsequently how the world is constructed in the child's mind, Piaget (1952, 1954) conceived and described the functions of assimilation and accommodation that proceed from a state of chaotic undifferentiation to a state of differentiation with correlative coordination: "At first the universe consists in mobile and plastic perceptual images centered about personal activity...The external world, therefore, begins by being confused with the sensations of a self unaware of itself, before the two factors become detached from one another and are organized correlatively" (Piaget, 1954).

In Jakob's theoretical framework, the conscious self arises while one elaborates interacting internal (sympathetic) and external (somatic) experiences; external experiences issue from the external milieu, the notion of which is created when the child realizes that his/her body is separate from the objects found in his/her environment (López Pasquali, 1965). Jakob (1941, 1946) argued that the first notion of something external, the divorce between the self and the world, comes with the satisfaction of hunger, an internal need. In the first stage of the construction of the external milieu "object and process are completely fused to form a single, joint complex consisting of blurred, moving or variable elements" (Jakob, 1941, 1946). Elsewhere (Jakob & Copello, 1948), he argued that neither in an evolutionarily primitive nor in a developmentally infantile stage do humans discriminate the 'inner' from the 'outer' being subjected to a 'genuine monism'. Such a monism turns into the dualism of the two milieux, internal and external, only by means of experience.

To Piaget (1954) "assimilation ceases merely to incorporate things in personal activity and establishes, through the progress of that activity, an increasingly tight web of coordinations among the schemata that define it and consequently among the objects that such schemata are applied to. From this time on, the universe is built up into an aggregate of permanent objects connected by causal relations that are independent of the subject and are placed in objective space and time."

Jakob (1941, 1946) described the second psychogenetic stage of the somatic ego as a process that enables the separation and differentiation of the stable and unaltered elements of a situation from the blurred, moving, or variable elements through the connection and comparison of the 'complexes' of the first stage. The complexes are thus transformed into objects and processes, and they create concrete ideas of the experienced objective world through a process of identification or differentiation within the juvenile phase. This process seems to share a common element with Quine's (1960) 'similarity standard', i.e. the ability to relate things to the world as similar to or different from one another, according to their properties and the state of our perceptual scheme at the time.

The third psychogenetic phase of mental maturation elaborates the "sequencing of objects and processes". Eventually, "isolated complex situations, integrated concrete notions, and series of symbolized abstract ideas successively comprise the psychogenetic products of the gnosio-praxico-cortical work" (Jakob, 1941, 1946). According to Jakob (1941, 1946), our psycho-dynamic creation moves forward to three correlated dimensions: the spatial, the temporal, and the causal.

Maintaining that inherited dynamics are organized in the dimensions of space, time and causality, Jakob (1921, 1943a,

1943b, 1945b)—like Piaget—adopted Kant's (1781) a priori conditions. However, this aprioristic conservative principle is counterbalanced by the aposterioristic flexible principle that rises due to the openness of the brain to the stimuli of the external world (Capizzano, 2006).

Living an ocean apart, Jakob and Piaget left their marks of interdisciplinarity in biopsychology and philosophy, and formulated convergent propositions. For instance (Szirko, 1999), they adopted a similar approach to the study of the procedure through which extramental organic regulations prolong themselves into certain cognitive processes (Jakob, 1906–1908, 1922, 1948; Piaget, 1967, 1976). The two scientists were born and died almost a quarter-century apart. We do not know whether they ever communicated or exchanged ideas directly. An extra degree of difficulty stems from Jakob's rather informal style of citing references—like many authors in his era, and a common trend in scientific writing at the time. Thus, he refers e.g. to ideas conceived by Kant or Aristotle, without quoting specific sources. Piaget published his first relevant work in the 1920s (Fondation Jean Piaget, 2011), and Jakob was fluent in French (see for example Jakob, 1905, 1907). Some of the statements made by Jakob early on could clearly be independent of Piaget's writing. On the other hand, might some later statements and terminology, in the 1940s and 1950s, have been conceivably influenced by reading Piaget? That interpretation, and the question whether Jakob borrowed ideas from Piaget or vice versa, remain open to future historical research.

Jakob argued that the conscious self is born through the binding of the external and internal spheres and it becomes manifest by the synchronization of its components. Whereas "proving the case for synchronization in the human brain" is still considered technically demanding (Zeman, 2001), Jakob conceived the idea of synchronization of neuronal activity as the underlying mechanism of consciousness more than a hundred years ago (Théodoridou & Triarhou, 2012).

Jakob seems to have conceived ideas that were much ahead of his time; he anticipated the emergence of critical aspects in the incessant attempt to elucidate the neural correlates of consciousness. For example, the idea that consciousness crucially depends on memory was expressed by Crick and Koch (1990) in their theory of consciousness, where attentional mechanisms render possible the firing of neurons in a coherent semi-oscillatory way, so that a global unity would be imposed on the brain with the subsequent activation of working memory. The role of memory in consciousness was also stressed by Bergson (1934), who claimed that the continuous growth of memory equals consciousness.

Two landmark works particularly stand out with regard to the psychological and philosophical study of the experience of time (Andersen & Grush, 2009). These are William James' 'Principles of Psychology' (James, 1952), first published in 1890, and Edmund Husserl's (1928) papers on the 'Phenomenology of Inner Time Consciousness', compiled by Heidegger. They both convey the idea that the contents grasped by consciousness are built upon duration and therefore they are temporally solid (Andersen & Grush, 2009). In line with James' 'stream of consciousness' the 'Cartesian theater model' assumes that there is a locus of synthesis in the brain where experience enters consciousness (Dennett, 1991).

On the other hand, the 'multiple drafts' model (Dennett, 1991), which appeared as an alternative to the dualistic 'Cartesian theater model', holds that neural events that discriminate various perceptual contents are distributed in both space and time in the brain. However, none of these temporal properties is thought to determine subjective order, since there is no single, constitutive 'stream of consciousness' but rather a parallel stream of conflicting and continuously revised contents (cf. Dennett & Kinsbourne, 1992).

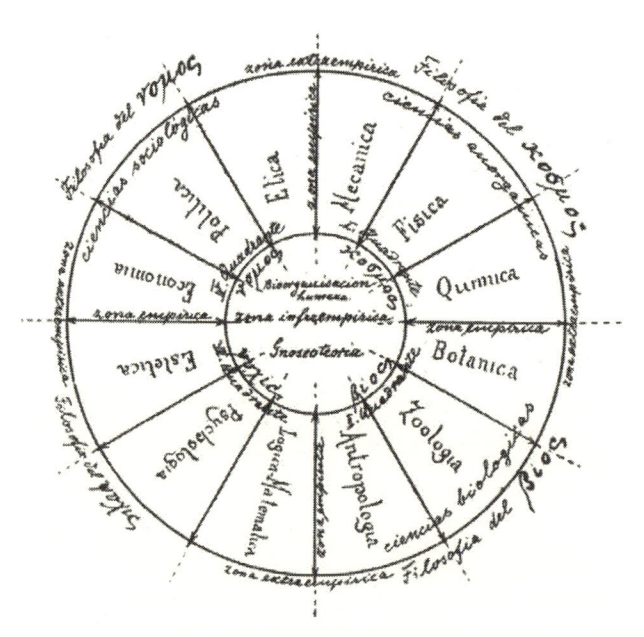

Fig. 5. Schematic synopsis of the zone of experience with the four quadrants of the exact sciences and their infra- and extra-empirical philosophical projections according to Jakob (1920, p. 30). See also Fig. 4 in Triarhou and del Cerro (2006b), based on Jakob (1945a, p. 90).

It has been further suggested that the function of time in human consciousness primarily resides in systems that maintain synchrony and allow the 'binding' between the internal environment as it is shaped by the brain's chemicals and the influence of the external environment (Dawson, 2004). Thus, time is considered as an organizing parameter to the binding problem (Dawson, 2004). The binding problem, i.e. the generation of the unity of conscious experience, may have made its first appearance in Kant's 'Critique of Pure Reason' where the "principle of transcendental unity of apperception" describes the synthesis of the "knowledge of the manifold" (Mashour, 2004).

The richness and variety of mechanisms by which animals and humans, including infants, can represent the dimensions of space, time and number to integrate diverse sensory elements for the creation of conscious experience is complex and suggests the existence of evolutionary processes and neural mechanisms by which Kantian intuitions might universally arise (Dehaene & Brannon, 2010). The evolution of the concept of time carries special weight due to its role in promoting the biological ability of the species to survive and adapt to environmental demands. From a developmental viewpoint, its importance is further reflected in the consequences of temporal disorganization on consciousness as they are observed in psychopathological conditions (Broome, 2005), aging and drug use (Dawson, 2004).

In spite of remarkable advances in neuroscience and the diffusion of biological evidence into philosophy in the modern field of neurophilosophy, the so-called 'hard problem of consciousness', i.e. the problem of explaining why and how cerebral elaborations give rise to conscious phenomenal experience (cf. Chalmers, 1995) remains a puzzle for scientists, philosophers and lay people to date.

Jakob's (1945b) stance towards such a puzzle is summarized in the following paragraph: "The origin of errors and misconceptions in the attempt to explain consciousness lies in the excessive though inevitable specialization of the diverse scientific fields that are getting involved in this attempt. Given that the external and the internal spheres, the environment and the brain or macrocosmos and microcosmos, create a cycle, the answers can be found only in a synthetic approach. Therefore, physics, histology, physiology, psychology and philosophy should form a new arena of scientific exploration" (Fig. 5).

The aim of this article has been to shed light on some early key works that fall within the domain of 'Philosophy and Neuroscience', largely overlooked. The introduction of philosophical ideas into neuroscience can be considered as some of the most critical and pioneering among Christfried Jakob's contributions. We further attempted to draw parallels and to provide evidence of convergence between the ideas of Jakob and other great thinkers of the 20th century; a definite documentation of precedence remains open to future research. In any case, Jakob's synthesis may be meaningful in the formulation of new theories of cortical function.

Disclosure statement

The authors declare that there is no conflict of interest regarding the work presented in the manuscript.

Acknowledgments

These results were included in the dissertation submitted by Z.D.T. to the University of Macedonia in partial fulfillment of the requirements for the Doctorate in Educational and Social Policy. The authors gratefully acknowledge the anonymous reviewers for their constructive criticism, and the courtesy of the staff at the Ibero-Amerikanisches Institut Preussischer Kulturbesitz zu Berlin, the British Library, the Library of Congress and the National Library of Medicine of the United States.

References

Andersen, H. K., & Grush, R. (2009). A brief history of time-consciousness: Historical precursors to James and Husserl. *Journal of the History of Philosophy, 47*, 277–307.
Arbib, M. A. (1981). Perceptual structures and distributed motor control. In V. B. Brooks (Ed.). *Handbook of physiology; Nervous system* (Vol. II, pp. 1448–1480). Bethesda, MD: American Physiological Society.
Barutta, J., Hodges, J., Ibáñez, A., Gleichgerrcht, E., & Manes, F. (2010). Argentina's early contributions to the understanding of frontotemporal lobar degeneration. *Cortex, 47*, 621–627.
Bechtel, W. (2001). *Philosophy and the neurosciences: A reader*. Malden, MA: Blackwell.
Bergson, H. (1934). *La pensée et le mouvant: Essais et conférences*. Paris: Félix Alcan.
Bernard, C. (1878). *Leçons sur les phénomènes de la vie communs aux animaux et aux végétaux, tome premier* (pp. 113–114). Paris: J.-B. Baillière et fils.
Bernard, C. (1974). *Lectures on the phenomena common to animals and plants* [1878] (translated by H.E. Hoff, R. Guillemin, L. Guillemin). Springfield, IL: Charles C. Thomas.
Bickle, J. (2009). *The Oxford handbook of philosophy and neuroscience*. Oxford: Oxford University Press.
Bickle, J., Mandik, P., & Landreth, A. (2010). The philosophy of neuroscience. In E. N. Zalta (Ed.), *The Stanford encyclopedia of philosophy*. <http://plato.stanford.edu/archives/sum2010/entries/neuroscience> Accessed 24.06.11.
Blackmore, S. J. (2005). *Consciousness: A very short introduction*. Oxford: Oxford University Press.
Brook, A., & Mandik, P. (2007). The philosophy and neuroscience movement. *Analyse und Kritik, 26*, 382–397.
Broome, M. R. (2005). Suffering and eternal recurrence of the same: The neuroscience, psychopathology, and philosophy of time. *Philosophy, Psychiatry, & Psychology, 12*, 187–194.
Capizzano, A. (2006). Actualidad del pensamiento de Cristofredo Jakob. *Revista del Hospital Italiano de Buenos Aires, 26*, 71–73.
Chalmers, D. J. (1995). The puzzle of conscious experience. *Scientific American, 273*, 80–86.
Churchland, P. S. (1986). *Neurophilosophy: Toward a unified science of the mind-brain*. Cambridge, MA: MIT Press.
Churchland, P. S. (2008). The impact of neuroscience on philosophy. *Neuron, 60*, 409–411.
Crick, F., & Koch, C. (1990). Towards a neurobiological theory of consciousness. *Seminars in the Neurosciences, 2*, 263–275.
Dawson, K. A. (2004). Temporal organization of the brain: Neurocognitive mechanisms and clinical implications. *Brain and Cognition, 54*, 75–94.
Dehaene, S., & Brannon, E. M. (2010). Space, time, and number: A Kantian research program. *Trends in Cognitive Sciences, 14*, 517–519.
Dennett, D. C. (1978). Why you can't make a computer that feels pain. *Synthese, 38*, 415–449.
Dennett, D. C. (1991). *Consciousness explained*. Boston: Little, Brown and Co.
Dennett, D. C., & Kinsbourne, M. (1992). Time and the observer: The where and when of consciousness in the brain. *Behavioural and Brain Sciences, 15*, 183–247.
Fischer, K. W., Daniel, D. B., Immordino-Yang, M. H., Stern, E., Battro, A., & Koizumi, H. (2007). Why mind, brain, and education? Why now? *Mind, Brain and Education, 1*, 1–2.
Fondation Jean Piaget (2011). Bibliographie. <http://www.fondationjeanpiaget.ch/fjp/site/bibliographie> Accessed 10.11.11.
François, C. (1999). Systemics and cybernetics in a historical perspective. *Systems Research and Behavioral Science, 16*, 203–219.
Freud, S. (1920). The psychogenesis of a case of homosexuality in a woman. *Standard Edition, 18*, 145–172.
Fuster, J. (2006). The cognit: A network model of cortical representation. *International Journal of Psychophysiology, 60*, 125–132.
Gardner, H. (1985). *The mind's new science: A history of the cognitive revolution*. New York: Basic Books.
Gibson, J. J. (1986). *The ecological approach to visual perception*. Hillsdale, NJ: Lawrence Erlbaum.
Greenspan, R. J., & Baars, B. J. (2005). Consciousness eclipsed: Jacques Loeb, Ivan P. Pavlov, and the rise of reductionistic biology after 1900. *Consciousness and Cognition, 14*, 219–230.
Gross, C. G. (1998). Claude Bernard and the constancy of the internal environment. *Neuroscientist, 4*, 380–385.
Hurley, S. (2001). Perception and action: alternative views. *Synthese, 129*, 3–40.
Husserl, E. (1928). *Vorlesungen zur Phänomenologie des inneren Zeitbewusstseins* [1893–1917] (herausgegeben von Martin Heidegger). Halle: Max Niemeyer.
Jakob, C. (1895). *Atlas des gesunden und kranken Nervensystems nebst Grundriss der Anatomie, Pathologie und Therapie desselben*. München: J.F. Lehmann.
Jakob, C. (1899). *Atlas des gesunden und kranken Nervensystems nebst Grundriss der Anatomie, Pathologie und Therapie desselben* (2nd ed.). München: J.F. Lehmann.
Jakob, C. (1905). Contribution à l'étude de la morphologie des cerveaux des Indiens. *Revista del Museo de La Plata, 12*, 59–72.
Jakob, C. (1906a). Estudios biológicos sobre los lóbulos frontales cerebrales. *La Semana Médica (Buenos Aires), 13*, 1375–1381.

Jakob, C. (1906b). Estudio anátomo-topográfico acerca de las relaciones entre los hemisferios cerebrales y el cráneo. *Revista de la Sociedad Médica Argentina (Buenos Aires), 14*, 353–378.

Jakob, C. (1906–1908). Localización del alma y de la inteligencia, pt. I–IX. *El Libro–Órgano de la Asociación Nacional del Profesorado (Buenos Aires), 1*, 151–159, 281–291, 433–445, 553–567; *2*, 3–16, 171–186, 293–308, 537–552, 695–710.

Jakob, C. (1907). Problèmes actuels de l'embryologie humaine. *Revue de la Clinique Obstétricale et Gynécologique (Buenos Aires), 2*, 19–32, 105–120.

Jakob, C. (1911). *Das Menschenhirn: Eine Studie über den Aufbau und die Bedeutung seiner grauen Kerne und Rinde*. München: J.F. Lehmann.

Jakob, C. (1912a). Über die Ubiquität der senso-motorischen Doppelfunktion der Hirnrinde als Grundlage einer neuen, biologischen Auffassung des corticalen Seelenorgans. *Journal für Psychologie und Neurologie (Leipzig), 19*, 379–382.

Jakob, C. (1912b). Ueber die Ubiquität der senso-motorischen Doppelfunktion der Hirnrinde als Grundlage einer neuen biologischen Auffassung des kortikalen Seelenorgans. *Münchener Medizinische Wochenschrift, 59*, 466–468.

Jakob, C. (1913). La psicología orgánica y su relación con la biología cortical. *Archivos de Psiquiatría, Criminología y Ciencias Afines (Buenos Aires), 1*, 680–698.

Jakob, C. (1919). La teoría actual de las gnosias y praxias como factores fundamentales en el dinamismo cortical. *Revista del Círculo Médico Argentino y Centro de Estudiantes de Medicina (Buenos Aires), 19*, 1266–1275.

Jakob, C. (1920). Filosofía de la naturaleza: Un curso de conferencias dictadas en la Facultad de Filosofía y Letras en 1920, Cátedra de Biología. *Revista del Jardín Zoológico de Buenos Aires [Época II], 16*, 28–55.

Jakob, C. (1921). La teoría actual de las gnosias y praxias como factores fundamentales en el dinamismo de la corteza cerebral. *Crónica Médica (Lima), 38*, 17–24.

Jakob, C. (1922). Del tropismo a la teoría general de la relatividad. *Revista Humanidades (La Plata), 3*, 45–58.

Jakob, C. (1926). El espíritu de la música en la filosofía pre y postkantiana. *Revista Humanidades (La Plata), 13*, 119–132.

Jakob, C. (1935a). La filogenia de las kinesias: Sobre su organización y dinamismo evolutivo. *Anales del Instituto de Psicología de la Facultad de Filosofía y Letras de la Universidad de Buenos Aires, 1*, 109–127.

Jakob, C. (1935b). Sobre las bases orgánicas de la memoria. *Revista de Criminología, Psiquiatría y Medicina Legal, 127*, 84–114.

Jakob, C. (1937). Descartes en la biología. In L. J. Gerrero (Ed.), *Descartes—Homenaje en el tercer centenario del "Discurso del método", tomo I* (pp. 57–66). Buenos Aires: Instituto de Filosofía de la Facultad de Filosofía y Letras.

Jakob, C. (1938). La psicología de Descartes a través de tres siglos. *Anales del Instituto de Psicología de la Facultad de Filosofía y Letras de la Universidad de Buenos Aires, 2*, 297–327.

Jakob, C. (1939). *El neoencéfalo: Su organización y dinamismo*. La Plata – Buenos Aires: Universidad Nacional de La Plata, Facultad de Humanidades y Ciencias de la Educación – Imprenta López.

Jakob, C. (1941). La función psicogenética de la corteza cerebral y su posible localización: Aspectos de la ontopsicogénesis humana. *Anales del Instituto de Psicología de la Facultad de Filosofía y Letras de la Universidad de Buenos Aires, 3*, 63–80.

Jakob, C. (1943a). *Folia Neurobiológica Argentina, Tomo II. El pichiciego (Chlamydophorus truncatus): Estudios neurobiológicos de un mamífero misterioso de la Argentina*. Buenos Aires: Aniceto López.

Jakob, C. (1943b). *Folia Neurobiológica Argentina, Tomo III. El lóbulo frontal: Un estudio monográfico anatomoclínico sobre base neurobiológica*. Buenos Aires: Aniceto López.

Jakob, C. (1945a). El cerebro humano: Su significación filosófica. *Revista Neurológica de Buenos Aires, 10*, 89–110.

Jakob, C. (1945b). Sobre el origen de la conciencia: Investigaciones neurobiológicas sobre la dinámica cortical en relación con su sectorización conmemorativa. In: Mouchet, E. (Ed.), *Temas actuales de psicología normal y patológica, publicados bajo el patrocinio de la Sociedad de Psicología de Buenos Aires* (pp. 345–381). Buenos Aires: Editorial Médico-Quirúrgica/Talleres 'The Standard'.

Jakob, C. (1946). *Folia Neurobiológica Argentina, Tomo V. Documenta Biofilosófica, Folleto I. Biología y filosofía. (A) Aspectos de sus divergencias y concomitancias. (B) Ensayo de psicogenia orgánica*. Buenos Aires: López y Etchegoyen.

Jakob, C. (1948). La psicointegración introyento-ambiental orgánica y sus problemas para la neuropsiquiatría y psicología, primera parte: su filogenia constructiva. *Revista Neurológica de Buenos Aires, 13*, 115–141.

Jakob, C., & Copello, A. R. (1948). La psicointegración introyento-ambiental orgánica y sus problemas para la neuropsiquiatría y psicología. *Revista Neurológica de Buenos Aires, 13*, 63–79.

James, W. (1952). *The principles of psychology* [1890]. Chicago: University of Chicago Press – Encyclopaedia Britannica.

Jung, C. G. (1960). *The psychogenesis of mental disease*. New York: Pantheon Books.

Kant, I. (1781). *Critik der reiner Vernunft*. Riga: Johann Friedrich Hartknoch.

López Pasquali, L. (1965). *Christfried Jakob: Su obra neurológica, su pensamiento psicológico y filosófico*. Buenos Aires: López.

Mashour, G. A. (2004). The cognitive binding problem: From Kant to quantum neurodynamics. *NeuroQuantology, 2*, 29–38.

Maturana, H. R., & Varela, F. J. (1980). *Autopoiesis and cognition. The realization of the living*. Dordrecht: Reidel.

Maturana, H. R., & Varela, F. J. (1987). *The tree of knowledge: The biological roots of human understanding*. Boston, MA: New Science Library – Shambhala Publications.

Moyano, B. A. (1957). Christfried Jakob, 25/12/1866–6/5/1956. *Acta Neuropsiquiátrica Argentina, 3*, 109–123.

Nagel, T. (1971). Brain bisection and the unity of consciousness. *Synthese, 22*, 396–413.

Northoff, G. (2004). What is neurophilosophy? A methodological account. *Zeitschrift für Allgemeine Wissenschaftstheorie, 35*, 91–127.

Ochs, S. (2004). *A history of nerve functions: From animal spirits to molecular mechanisms*. Cambridge – New York: Cambridge University Press.

Olmsted, J. M. D., & Olmsted, E. H. (1952). *Claude Bernard and the experimental method in medicine*. New York: Henry Schuman.

Orlando, J. C. (1966). *Christofredo Jakob: Su vida y obra*. Buenos Aires: Editorial Mundi.

Pedace, E. A. (1949). Contribución de la escuela neurobiológica Argentina del Prof. Chr. Jakob en el estudio del lóbulo frontal. *Archivos de Neurocirugía, 6*, 464–466.

Piaget, J. (1952). *The origins of intelligence in children*. New York: International Universities Press.

Piaget, J. (1954). *The construction of reality in the child*. New York: Basic Books.

Piaget, J. (1967). *Biologie et connaissance. Essai sur les relations entre les régulations organiques et les processus cognitifs*. Paris: Gallimard.

Piaget, J. (1976). *Le comportement, moteur de l'évolution*. Paris: Gallimard.

Quine, W. (1960). *Word and object*. Cambridge, MA: MIT Press.

Rudrauf, D., Lutz, A., Cosmelli, D., Lachaux, J.-P., & Le Van Quyen, M. (2003). From autopoiesis to neurophenomenology: Francisco Varela's exploration of the biophysics of being. *Biological Research, 36*, 27–66.

Szirko, M. (1999). Constructivism is not pantopoiesis. *Karl Jaspers Forum*. <http://www.kjf.ca/15-C32SZ.htm> Retrieved 08.11.11.

Théodoridou, Z. D., & Triarhou, L. C. (in press). Evolution of Christfried Jakob's views on the frontal lobe, 1899–1949. In: Cavanna, A.E. (Ed.), *Frontal lobe: Anatomy, function and injury*. Hauppauge, NY: Nova Science Publishers.

Théodoridou, Z. D., & Triarhou, L. C. (2011). Christfried Jakob's 1921 theory of the gnoses and praxes as fundamental factors in cerebral cortical dynamics. *Integrative Psychological and Behavioral Science, 45*, 247–262.

Théodoridou, Z. D., & Triarhou, L. C. (2012). Challenging the supremacy of the frontal lobe: Early views (1906-1909) of Christfried Jakob on the human cerebral cortex. *Cortex, 48*, 15–25.

Thompson, E., & Varela, F. J. (2001). Radical embodiment: Neural dynamics and consciousness. *Trends in Cognitive Sciences, 5*, 418–425.

Triarhou, L. C. (2008). Centenary of Christfried Jakob's discovery of the visceral brain: An unheeded precedence in affective neuroscience. *Neuroscience and Biobehavioral Reviews, 32*, 984–1000.

Triarhou, L. C. (2010a). Final publications of Christfried Jakob: On the frontal lobe and the limbic region. In C. E. Flynn & B. R. Callaghan (Eds.), *Neuroanatomy research advances* (pp. 165–169). Hauppauge, NY: Nova Science Publishers.

Triarhou, L. C. (2010b). Revisiting Christfried Jakob's concept of the dual onto-phylogenetic origin and ubiquitous function of the cerebral cortex: A century of progress. *Brain Structure and Function, 214*, 319–338.

Triarhou, L. C., & del Cerro, M. (2006a). Semicentennial tribute to the ingenious neurobiologist Christfried Jakob (1866–1956). 1. Works from Germany and the first Argentina period, 1891–1913. *European Neurology, 56*, 176–188.

Triarhou, L. C., & del Cerro, M. (2006b). Semicentennial tribute to the ingenious neurobiologist Christfried Jakob (1866–1956). 2. Publications from the second Argentina period, 1913–1949. *European Neurology, 56*, 189–198.

Triarhou, L. C., & del Cerro, M. (2007). Pioneers in neurology: Christfried Jakob (1866–1956). *Journal of Neurology, 254*, 124–125.

Varela, F. (1996). Neurophenomenology: A methodological remedy to the hard problem. *Journal of Consciousness Studies, 3*, 330–350.

Véganzonès, M.-A., & Winograd, C. (1997). *Argentina in the 20th century: An account of long-awaited growth*. Paris: Development Centre of the Organisation for Economic Co-operation and Development.

von Eckardt-Klein, B. (1975). Some consequences of knowing everything (essential) there is to know about one's mental states. *Review of Metaphysics, 29*, 3–18.

von Economo, C., & Koskinas, G. N. (1925). *Die Cytoarchitektonik der Hirnrinde des erwachsenen Menschen*. Wien: Springer.

von Uexküll, J. (1934). A stroll through the worlds of animals and men. In C. Schiller (Ed.), *Instinctive behavior* (pp. 5–80). New York: International Universities Press.

von Weizsäcker, V. (1950). *Der Gestaltkreis*. Stuttgart: Thieme.

Wiener, N. (1948). *Cybernetics or control and communication in the animal and the machine*. Paris: Hermann.

Zeman, A. (2001). Consciousness. *Brain, 124*, 1263–1289.

Ramón y Cajal Erroneously Identified as Camillo Golgi on a Souvenir Postage Stamp

LAZAROS C. TRIARHOU[1] AND MANUEL DEL CERRO[2]

[1]University of Macedonia, Thessaloniki, Greece
[2]University of Rochester, Rochester, NY, USA

Focusing on a philatelic oddity that erringly identifies a picture of Santiago Ramón y Cajal as that of Camillo Golgi, this brief article examines official and unofficial stamp issues honoring the two great neuroanatomists, one from Spain and the other from Italy, who were early Nobel Prize winners in Physiology or Medicine.

Keywords Neuroscience in philately, neurological stamp, Nobel Prize, Golgi method, neuron theory, philatelic error

The celebrated 1906 Nobel Prize in Physiology or Medicine, jointly awarded to Camillo Golgi (1843–1926) of the University of Pavia, Italy, and Santiago Ramón y Cajal (1852–1934) of the University of Madrid, Spain, recognized "their work on the structure of the nervous system" (Bentivoglio, 1998). Golgi gave his Nobel Lecture entitled *La doctrine du neurone—théorie et faits* on Tuesday, December 11, 1906; Cajal delivered his on Wednesday, December 12, 1906, under the title *Structure et connexions des neurones* (Hasselberg et al., 1908).

Twenty-five years before the 1898 discovery of the Golgi apparatus ("internal reticular apparatus"), Golgi had published, in 1873, the silver impregnation method ("black reaction"), which he, Cajal, and numerous other histologists put to ample use in deciphering the secrets of nervous tissue structure (Bentivoglio, 1998, 1999; Berciano & Lafarga, 2001; Pannese, 1999; van Gijn, 2001). The two opposing concepts, born out of that work, came to be known as the "reticular theory" (propounded by Golgi) and the "neuron theory" (upheld by Cajal) (Jones, 2006; Mazzarello, 2006; Swanson et al., 2007). Definite proof of the contiguity of neurons, as originally suggested by Cajal, was established in the 1950s with the advent of electron microscopy and the demonstration of the ultrastructural features of synapses (De Robertis & Bennett, 1955).

These two illustrious scientists have been repeatedly honored by stamp issues from several countries (Loevy & Kowitz, 1990; Mazzarello, 1998; Richelmi et al., 2006; Shah, 2010) (Figures 1 and 2). Only on two occasions have the "twins" (as Cajal referred to himself and Golgi in some moment of irony) been shown together on the same stamp,

---

We thank the editors of the *Journal* and the anonymous reviewers for their expert guidance and constructive feedback. Special thanks to Professors Paolo Mazzarello and Plinio Richelmi of the University of Pavia, Italy, for generously providing material related to Camillo Golgi.

Address correspondence to Lazaros C. Triarhou, University of Macedonia, Egnatia 156, Bldg. Z-312, Thessaloniki, GR 54006, Greece. E-mail: triarhou@uom.gr

Cajal, Golgi, and a Souvenir Postage Stamp 133

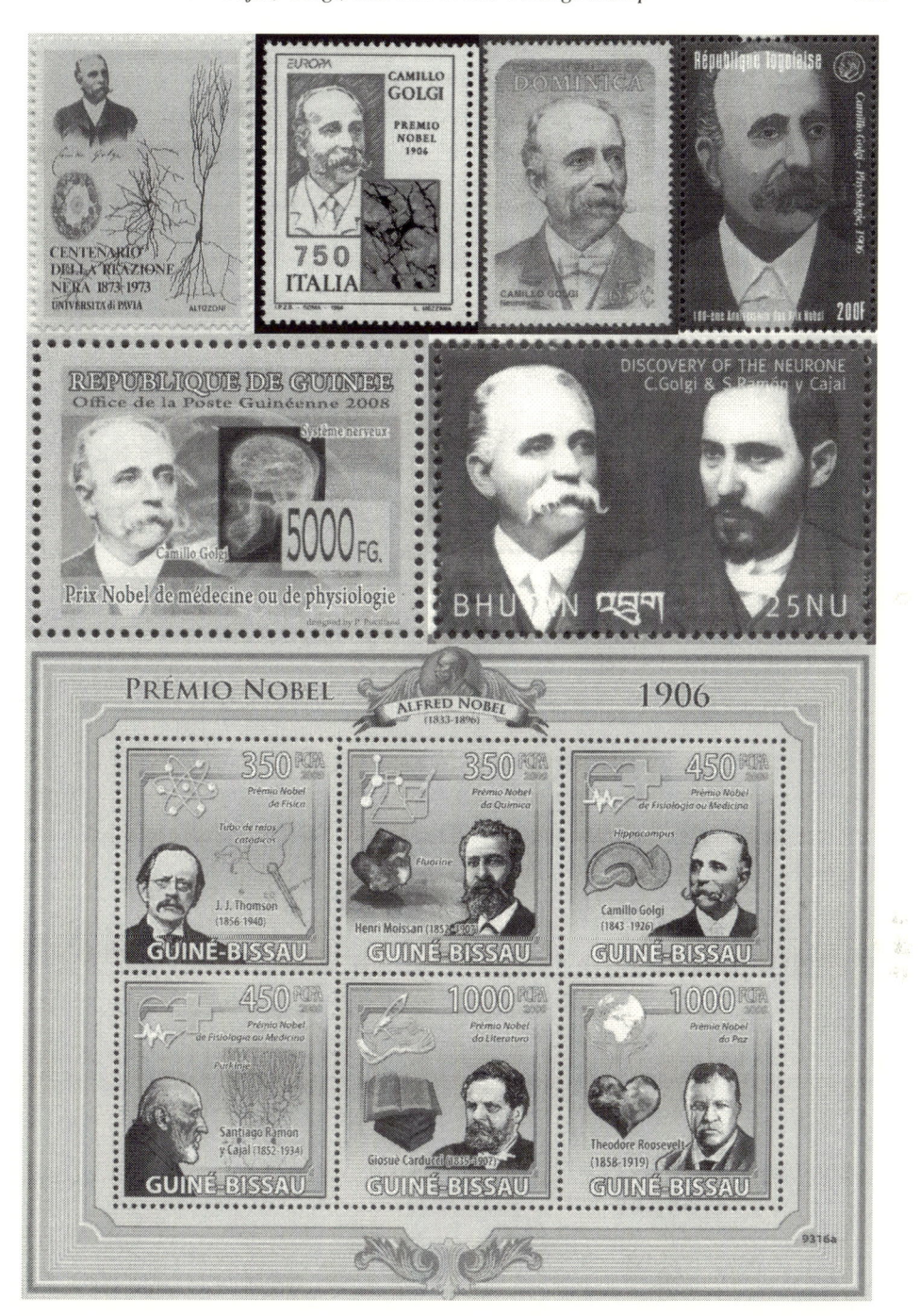

Figure 1. Postage stamps in honor of Camillo Golgi. Top row, left to right: a private 1973 printing by the University of Pavia (no postal value) to mark the centennial of the invention of the Golgi method, and an Italian 1994 stamp (Scott 1976) issued for the 33rd International Philatelic Exposition—the companion stamp honored the Italian chemist Giulio Natta (1903–1979), co-winner with Karl Ziegler (1898–1973) of the 1963 Nobel Prize in Chemistry for their discoveries in the field of the

that is, on the 2000 issue from Bhutan (Figure 1) and on the 1966 issue from Sweden (Figure 2). A 2009 Guinea-Bissau issue (Figure 1) has included separate stamps of Golgi and Cajal on the same souvenir sheet in the context of all the 1906 Nobel laureates. All the remaining issues have portrayed either Golgi or Cajal solo, without mention of the other scientist (five instances for Golgi, cf. Figure 1, and eight instances for Cajal, cf. Figure 2).

However, when one is identified by the name of his adversary, then the occurrence is worth noting. Such is the case with a private 2001 issue of Angola at a denomination of KRZ 10.5 *(kwanza reajustado)*, showing a classic portrait of Ramón y Cajal with a "Camillo Golgi" caption (Figure 3). It was bought by us, over the Internet, from three different vendors independently operating in Estonia, the Netherlands, and the United Kingdom, a fact that logically makes us lean towards the impression of an error—likely committed by the artist or the printer—rather than a forgery or a prank. Were this article the subject of a philatelic journal, one would have to discuss pertinent points about authenticity in depth. Nevertheless, the question in our mind is: Who would go into the trouble of faking an item of such limited exposure as this?

The Cajal/"Golgi" misnomer stamp forms part of a nine-stamp sheet titled "Millennium 2001" and subtitled "Nobel Prize Winners"—obviously commemorating the centennial of the first Nobel Prizes in 1901. The sheet also depicts Walter Rudolf Hess, Baruch S. Blumberg, Johannes V. Jensen, Jane Addams, The Curies, Frits Zernike, Teddy Roosevelt, and Winston Churchill (Figure 3). A complementary souvenir sheet shows portraits of Elie Wiesel, Albert Einstein, Bertrand Russell, Hideki Yukawa, Mother Teresa, Otto Hahn, Martin Luther King, Albert Schweitzer, and the Dalai Lama.

It remains unknown to what extent the Angolan government was involved in the production. One may ponder whether the printer was told to come up with something on a specific theme and then to sign off on it, or whether a zealous printer might perhaps have gone to the Angolan government with a possible product, asking if the country would like to put its name on it. These thoughts are nothing more than conjectures.

Figure 1. (Continued) chemistry and technology of high polymers (courtesy of Professor Paolo Mazzarello, University of Pavia); a 1997 issue from the Commonwealth of Dominica (Scott 2003) and a 2001 issue from the Togolese Republic (Scott A361) to commemorate the centennial of the first Nobel Prizes in 1901 (courtesy of Professor Plinio Richelmi, University of Pavia); for additional details cf. Richelmi et al. (2006). The 1997 Dominica series also included stamps depicting Pasteur, Barnard, Fleming, Salk, Khorana, and MacFarlane Burnet. Second row, left: Golgi in a 2008 issue by the Republic of Guinea (from a souvenir sheet 7B-890 "Prix Nobel de médecine ou physiologie" also honoring Thomas Hunt Morgan, Peyton Rous, Edmond Fischer, Arvid Carlsson, and Andrew Fire); right, Golgi and Cajal on a 2000 Bhutan millennium souvenir sheet (Scott A171) titled "Breakthroughs in Modern Medicine—100 Years" (the other scientists on the sheet are Albert Calmette, Alexander Fleming, Jonas Salk, Christiaan Barnard, and Luc Montagnier). Lower half: a sheetlet of six stamps, issued by Guinea-Bissau in 2009, depicting all Nobel Prize laureates of 1906, that is, British physicist Joseph J. Thomson, French chemist Henri Moissan, Golgi (upper right), Cajal (lower left), Italian poet Giosuè Carducci (literature), and the 26th U.S. President Theodore Roosevelt (peace).

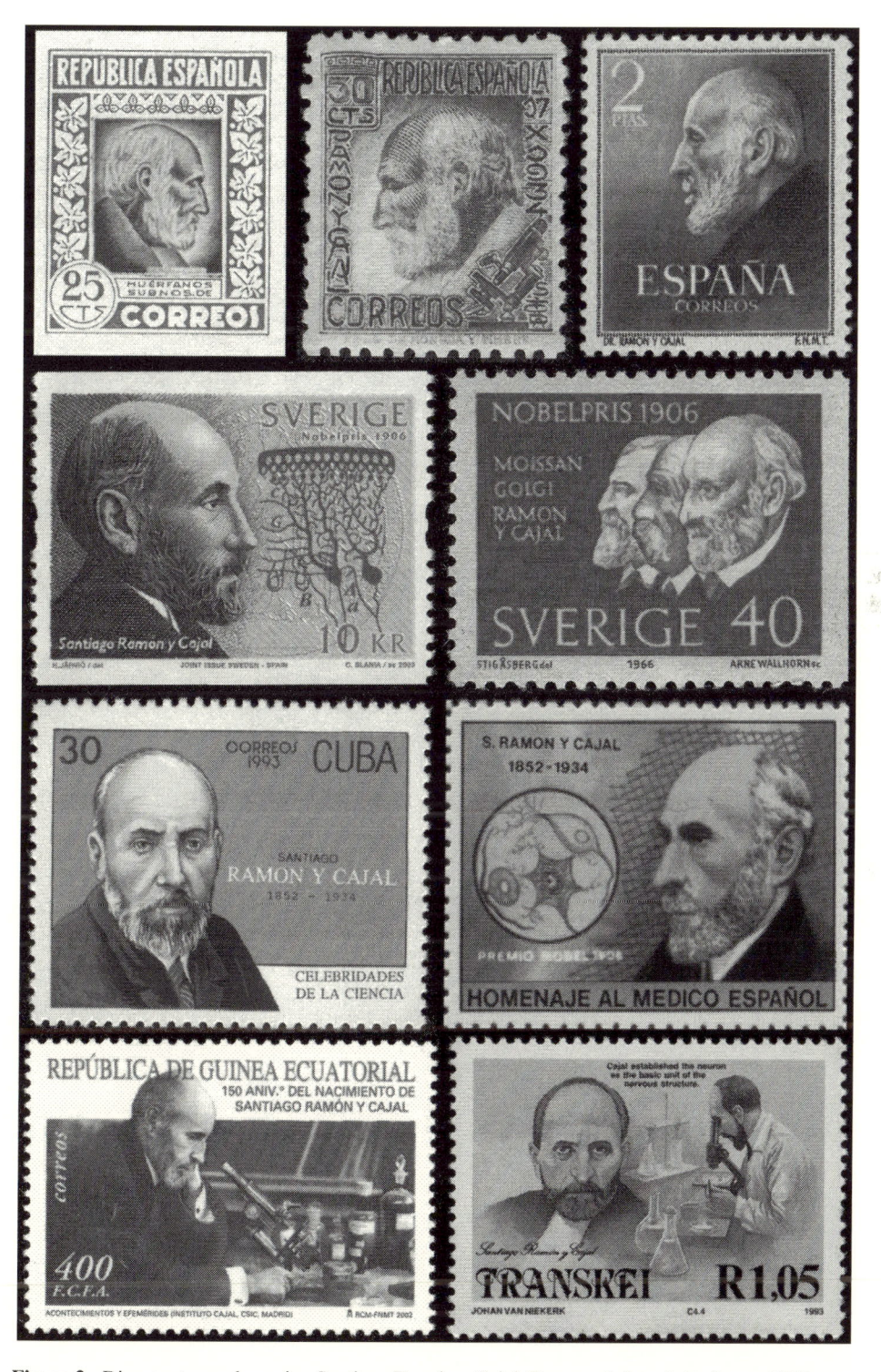

Figure 2. Diverse stamps honoring Santiago Ramón y Cajal. Top row, left to right: from a 1937 commemorative leaf (unserrated and uncatalogued) by *España Telégrafos*; official stamps by the Spanish Government from 1934 (year of Cajal's death; Edifil 680) and 1952 (Cajal Centennial; Edifil 1119).

The particular stamps (Figure 3) are not listed in common philatelic catalogues, such as Scott's. They appear to be what many collectors call "wallpaper,"[1] privately printed by a company that makes stamps for several countries without a full-fledged postal operation.

The first stamp of independent Angola was a 1.50-escudo value issued in 1975, as soon as the country ceased to be a colony under Portuguese rule. Initially the stamp program was conservative, with 20–30 stamps per year, but starting in the mid-1990s, large numbers of designs began to come out each year, eventually joined by adhesive labels inscribed "Angola," but not authorized by postal authorities and not valid for postage.

Among the countries represented in our figures, Angola, Bhutan, Dominica, and Guinea are client nations of the *Inter-Governmental Philatelic Corporation* or IGPC (www.igpc.net). In reviewing other products, one realizes that similar types of souvenir sheets are made for several client countries, that is, a "mish-mash" of Nobel laureates of different nationalities, years, and fields of award, not always with tighter integrating themes.

The Cajal/"Golgi" stamp lapse is confounding for a very good reason: Who was really the intended investigator of honor? One may only guess. Was it Cajal presented instead of Golgi—or perhaps Golgi's name misplaced when it should have been Cajal? The fact that only one person of the two (Golgi and Cajal) is on that souvenir sheet would not make sense to people familiar with their achievements, especially in the neurosciences. We could not find another Angola stamp with the other gentleman on it (of course, absence of evidence is not evidence of absence, as Carl Sagan used to teach). One would think that both scientists should have been included on the sheet, instead of picking only one of the two. Regardless, don Santiago would not have been amused by the error. On the other hand, *el sabio de*

Figure 2. (Continued) Second row, left: a joint 2003 issue by Sweden and Spain (Edifil 3964)—the companion stamp (Edifil 3965) honored the Spanish biochemist Severo Ochoa (1905–1993), who was jointly awarded the 1959 Nobel Prize in Medicine with Arthur Kornberg (1918–2007) for their discovery of the mechanisms in the biological synthesis of RNA and DNA; right, a 1966 Swedish issue (Scott 711) marking the sixtieth anniversary of the 1906 Nobel Prizes, portraying Moissan, Golgi, and Cajal (the companion stamp depicted Thomson and Carducci). Third row, left: an official 1993 Cuban stamp marked "Celebrities of Science" (Scott 3488); right: from the series "Homage to Spanish Physicians" (undated) issued by Beecham Research Laboratories—the series also included Cajal's students and biographers Pío del Río Hortega (1882–1945) and Gregorio Marañón (1887–1960). Fourth row: a 2002 issue by Equatorial Guinea for Cajal's sesquicentennial—the series also included Émile Zola (centennial of his death) and Victor Hugo (bicentennial of his birth); right, a 1993 stamp by Transkei in South Africa (Scott 294)—the series also honored James Lind, Alexis Carrel, Alexander Fleming, and Howard Florey.

---

[1] "Wallpaper" refers to unnecessary postal issues, where the "unnecessary" implies that the stamps issued go well beyond the reasonable needs of a country's actual postal issues and are instead aimed at collectors. Such issues typically depict subjects unrelated to any aspect of life in the particular country, for example, classic automobiles from a small Pacific island country or animals not found in the region. They are issued to generate revenue from collectors of theme stamps (on themes such as scientists, artists, flora, fauna, U.S. Presidents, etc.) and are not printed for posting letters. The stamps are typically produced "CTO" (cancelled-to-order); that is, cancellation marks may be printed on the stamp as part of the printing process, unlike conventional postal issues. Stamps in this category often have little monetary worth and typically draw little interest from more sophisticated professional collectors, even those interested in the specific theme.

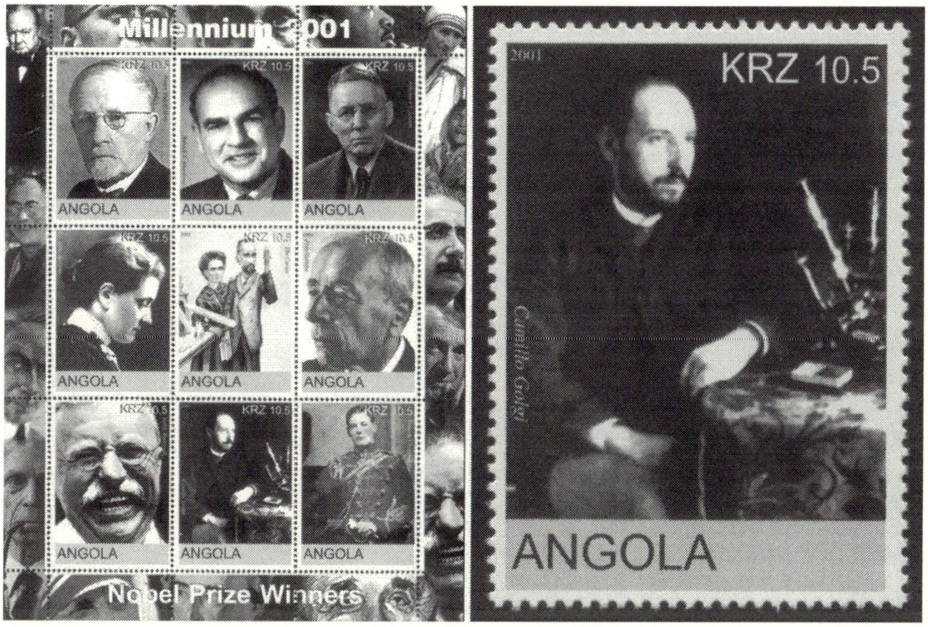

Figure 3. Ramón y Cajal by his microscopes, "denominated" Camillo Golgi in this millennium souvenir stamp (entire sheet on the left; detail on the right). Self-portrait from the Valencia years, circa 1887; the original photograph is in the Cajal Museum (Albarracín, 1982; De Felipe & Jones, 1988).

Pavia ("the learned man of Pavia")[2]—as Cajal used to call his feisty opponent—might have erupted in rage like the Vesuvius. The stamp, whether legitimate postage or "wallpaper," stands as a neuroscience collector's relic.

To summarize, there exists a stamp (Figure 3), which carries the name of a nation and the name of a Nobel laureate, except that the image of the person on the stamp represents the arch-rival of the person named. These facts are undeniable. The reality that the individuals in question are two epic figures in brain research should be of more than passing interest for readers in the history of the neurosciences.

References

Albarracín A (1982): *Santiago Ramón y Cajal o la Pasión de España.* Barcelona, Editorial Labor.
Bentivoglio M (1998): Life and discoveries of Camillo Golgi. *Nobelprize.org*. [Online]. Retrieved from http://nobelprize.org/nobel_prizes/medicine/articles/golgi/index.html [4 December 2010].
Bentivoglio M (1999): The discovery of the Golgi apparatus. *Journal of the History of the Neurosciences* 8: 202–208.

[2]The word has a dual connotation. Used in an expression such as *hombres sabios*, it can be translated exactly as "wise men", that is, persons characterized by consistent good and thoughtful judgment. Instead, used as *el sabio*—such as in King Alfonso X *el Sabio* (1221–1284), the poet king—it means "learned" as in "a learned man." This is most likely the meaning don Santiago tried to convey every time he referred to Golgi, and there were many such occasions. We know that don Santiago was fond of using the word to refer to some other investigators as well.

Berciano J, Lafarga M (2001): Santiago Ramón y Cajal (1852–1934). *Journal of Neurology 248*: 152–153.

De Felipe J, Jones EG (1988): *Cajal on the Cerebral Cortex: An Annotated Translation of the Complete Writings*. New York & Oxford, Oxford University Press.

De Robertis ED, Bennett HS (1955): Some features of the submicroscopic morphology of synapses in frog and earthworm. *Journal of Biophysical and Biochemical Cytology 1*: 47–58.

Hasselberg KB, Pettersson SO, Mörner KAH, Wirsén CD, Santesson MCG (1908): *Les Prix Nobel en 1906*. Stockholm, Imprimerie Royale P. A. Norstedt & Söner.

Jones EG (2006): The impossible interview with the man of the neuron doctrine. *Journal of the History of the Neurosciences 15*: 326–340.

Loevy HT, Kowitz A (1990): Dentistry on stamps: Santiago Ramón y Cajal. *Journal of the American Dental Association 120*: 582.

Mazzarello P (1998): Neurological stamp: Camillo Golgi (1843–1926). *Journal of Neurology, Neurosurgery and Psychiatry 64*: 212.

Mazzarello P (2006): The impossible interview with the man of the hidden biological structures. *Journal of the History of the Neurosciences 15*: 318–325.

Pannese E (1999): The Golgi Stain: Invention, diffusion and impact on neurosciences. *Journal of the History of the Neurosciences 8*: 132–140.

Richelmi P, Angelini P, Pizzala R, Mazzarello P (2006): Camillo Golgi and his Nobel Prize in philately. *Journal of the History of the Neurosciences 15*: 417–418.

Shah SN (2010): Medical Philately: Camillo Golgi and Ramón y Cajal who peeped into the mysterious world of the nervous system. *Journal of the Association of Physicians of India 58*: 200.

Swanson LW, Grant G, Hökfelt T, Jones EG, Morrison JH (2007): Introduction to "A century of neuroscience discovery": Reflecting on the Nobel Prize awarded to Golgi and Cajal in 1906. *Brain Research Reviews 55*: 191–192.

van Gijn J (2001): Camillo Golgi (1843–1926). *Journal of Neurology 248*: 541–542.

1

Cytoarchitectonics of the Human Cerebral Cortex: The 1926 Presentation by Georg N. Koskinas (1885–1975) to the Athens Medical Society

Lazaros C. Triarhou
University of Macedonia, Thessaloniki
Greece

1. Introduction

The Greek neurologist-psychiatrist Georg N. Koskinas (1885–1975) is better known for his collaboration with Constantin von Economo (1876–1931) on the cytoarchitectonic study of the human cerebral cortex (von Economo & Koskinas, 1925, 2008). Koskinas seems to have been one of those classically unrecognised and unrewarded figures of science (Jones, 2008, 2010). Such an injustice has been remedied in part in recent years (Triarhou, 2005, 2006). The

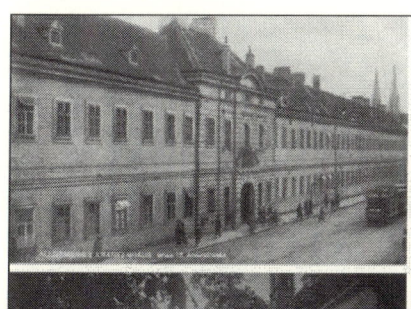

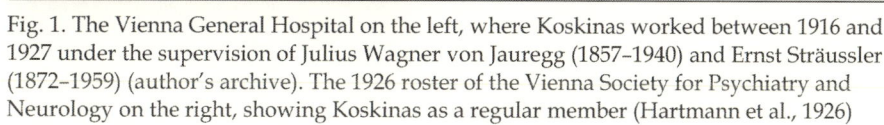

Fig. 1. The Vienna General Hospital on the left, where Koskinas worked between 1916 and 1927 under the supervision of Julius Wagner von Jauregg (1857–1940) and Ernst Sträussler (1872–1959) (author's archive). The 1926 roster of the Vienna Society for Psychiatry and Neurology on the right, showing Koskinas as a regular member (Hartmann et al., 1926)

year 2010 has marked the 125th birthday anniversary of Koskinas (1 December 1885) and the centennial of his graduation from the University of Athens (M.D., 1910).

As soon as the Atlas and Textbook of Cytoarchitectonics were published in 1925, Koskinas briefly returned to Greece and donated a set to the Athens Medical Society. On that occasion, he delivered a keynote address, which summarises the main points of his research with von Economo. That address (Koskinas, 1926) forms the main focus of this paper. There are only two other presentations known to have been made by Koskinas: one with von Economo at the Society for Psychiatry and Neurology in Vienna in February 1923 (von Economo & Koskinas, 1923), presenting an initial summary of cytoarchitectonic findings on the granularity of sensory cortical areas especially in layers II and IV; and the other with Sträussler at the 88th Meeting of the German Natural Scientists and Physicians in Innsbruck in September 1924 (Sträussler & Koskinas, 1925), reporting histopathological findings on the experimental malaria treatment of patients with general paralysis from neurosyphilis.

2. The 1926 presentation by Koskinas

The following is an exact English translation of the *Proceedings* of the Athens Medical Society, Session of Saturday, 23 January 1926, rendered from the original Greek text (Koskinas, 1926) by the author of the present chapter.

2.1 Introductory comment by Constantin Mermingas, presiding

"I am in the gratifying position of announcing an exceptional donation, made to the Society by the colleague Dr. G. Koskinas, sojourning in Athens; having temporarily come from Vienna, he brought with him a copy, as voluminous as you see, but also as valuable, of the truly monumental compilation, produced by the two Hellenic scientists in Vienna, C. Economo and G. Koskinas, who is among us today. It involves the book—text volume and atlas—*Cytoarchitektonik der Hirnrinde des erwachsenen Menschen*, about the value of which we had learnt from reviews published in foreign journals, but also convinced directly. Dr. Koskinas deserves our warm thanks, as well as our gratitude, for being willing to deliver a synopsis of that original scientific research and achievement."

2.2 Main lecture by Georg N. Koskinas, keynote speaker

"Thanks to the ardour of the honourable President of the Society, Professor Dr. Mermingas, who is meritoriously making every attempt to highlight the Society as a centre of noble emulation in scientific research and the promotion of science and at the encouragement of whom I have the honour of being a guest at the Society today. Enchanted by that, I owe acknowledgments because you are offering me the opportunity to briefly occupy you in person about the work published by Professor von Economo and myself in German, and deposited to the chair of the Society, "The Cytoarchitectonics of the Human Cerebral Cortex" *(Die Cytoarchitektonik der Hirnrinde des erwachsenen Menschen)*. An attempt on my behalf to analyse that work requires much time and many auxiliary media which, simply hither passing through, I lack. That is why I wish to confine myself, such that I very briefly cover the following simply and to the extent possible.

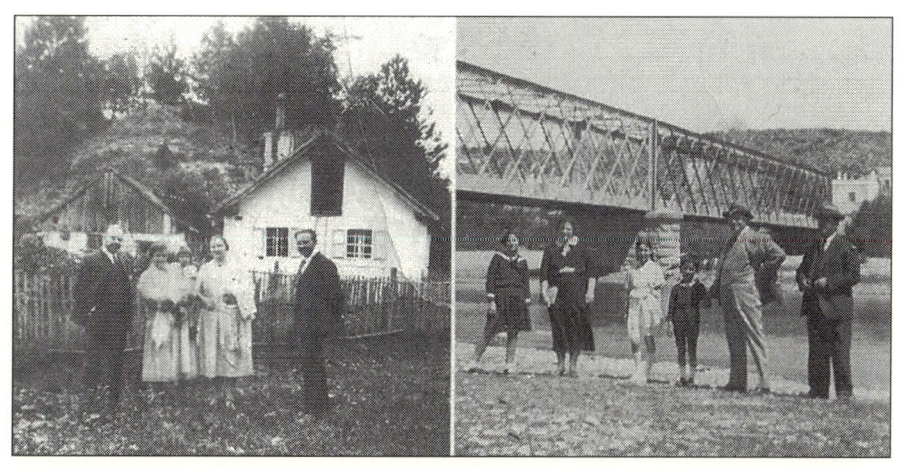

Fig. 2. Previously unpublished photographs of Koskinas and family members. The left photograph, taken in Vienna around 1926, shows Koskinas (first from the right) with his wife Stefanie, their daughter, his sister Paraskevi and her husband. The right photograph shows Koskinas (second from the right) in the Peloponnese in the 1940s — the bridge of the Eurotas River appears in the background — with his wife and daughter (left), and the children of his sister Irene and their father (photos courtesy of Rena Kostopoulou)

2.2.1 Incentives and aim

The incomplete and largely imperfect knowledge of the histological structure of the brain constituted the main reason that led us to its detailed architectonic research, and its ultimate goal was the localisation, to the extent possible, of the various cerebral functions and the pathological changes in mental disorders, as well as the interpretation of numerous problems, such as individual mental attributes, i.e. the talent in mathematics, music, rhetoric, etc.

2.2.2 Methods

At the outset of our studies we came across various obstacles and difficulties deriving on one hand from the very structure of the brain and on the other from the deficiency of the hitherto available research means. That is why we were obliged to modify numerous of the known means, to incise absolutely new paths, taking advantage of any possible means towards a precise, reliable and indelible rendition of nature. We modelled an entire system of new methods of brain research from the autopsy to the definitive photographic documentation of the preparations. Thus, we were able to not only solve many of the problems, but also, and above all, to provide to anyone interested various topics for investigation, as well as the manner for exploring them.

Allow me to mention some of the employed research means.

Sectioning method. Instead of the hitherto used method of sectioning the whole brain serially perpendicular to its fronto-occipital axis (Fig. 5), whereby gyri are rarely sectioned perpendicularly, we effected the sections always perpendicular to the surface of each gyrus and in directions corresponding to their convoluted pattern (Fig. 6). We arrived at that act by the idea that, in order to compare various parts of the brain cytoarchitectonically, sections must be oriented perpendicularly to the surface of the gyri, insofar as only then is provided precisely the breadth of both the overall cerebral cortex and of each cortical layer.

Ἱστολογία καὶ φυσιολογία τοῦ ἐγκεφάλου. Κατὰ τὴν συνεδρίαν τῆς 23ης Ἰανουαρίου 1926 ὁ Γ. Κοσκινᾶς ἐδώρησε τῇ Ἑταιρείᾳ ἓν ἀντίτυπον τοῦ συγγράμματος «Ἡ κυτταροαρχιτεκτονικὴ τοῦ φλοιοῦ τοῦ ἐγκεφάλου τοῦ ἀνθρώπου», ἐν συνεργασίᾳ μετὰ τοῦ Οἰκονόμου, ἐν Βιέννῃ δημοσιευθέντος, καὶ ἀνέπτυξεν ἀκολούθως τὴν ἀφετηρίαν καὶ τὸν σκοπὸν τοῦ ἔργου, τὸν τρόπον τῆς ἐρεύνης, τὰ ἐπιτευχθέντα καὶ προσδοκώμενα ἀποτελέσματα. Κατὰ τὴν συνεδρίαν τῆς 12ης Ἀπριλίου 1930 ὁ M. Minkowski, Καθηγητὴς τῆς Νευρολογίας ἐν τῷ Πανεπιστημίῳ τῆς Ζυρίχης διαλέγεται τὸ θέμα «ὀφθαλμὸς καὶ ἐγκέφαλος» προσκομίσας τῇ Ἑταιρείᾳ τὰ πορίσματα τῶν ἐρευνῶν του ἀπὸ φυλοοντογονικῆς, ἀνατομικῆς, φυσιολογικῆς ἅμα δὲ καὶ κλινικῆς ἀπόψεως.

ΣΥΝΕΔΡΙΑ 23ΗΣ ΙΑΝΟΥΑΡΙΟΥ 1926

ΠΡΟΕΔΡΕΙΑ Κ. ΜΕΡΜΗΓΚΑ

Γίνονται (παμψηφεὶ) δεκτοὶ ὡς τακτικοὶ ἑταῖροι οἱ Κοι Α. Θρουβάλας, Α. Κατσαρός, Κ. Μαχαίρας, Α. Φραγκοῦλης καὶ ἡ Δὶς Σ. Λεμπέση.

1) ***Πρόεδρος:*** *Εὑρίσκομαι εἰς τὴν εὐάρεστον θέσιν ὅπως ἀναγγείλω ἐξαιρετικὴν δωρεάν, γενομένην πρὸς τὴν Ἑταιρείαν ἐκ μέρους τοῦ παρεπιδημοῦντος ἐν Ἀθήναις συναδέλφου Κου Γ. Κοσκινᾶ, ὅστις, ἐλθὼν προσκαίρως ἐκ Βιέννης, ἐκόμισε μεθ' ἑαυτοῦ ἵνα δωρήσῃ πρὸς τὴν Ἑταιρείαν ἡμῶν ἓν ἀντίτυπον, τοσοῦτον ὀγκῶδες ὡς βλέπετε, ἀλλὰ καὶ τοσοῦτον πολύτιμον, τῆς ὄντως μνημειώδους συγγραφῆς, ἣν παρήγαγον δύο Ἕλληνες ἐπιστήμονες ἐν Βιέννῃ, ὁ Κ. Οἰκονόμος καὶ ὁ μεταξὺ ἡμῶν σήμερον εὑρισκόμενος Γ. Κοσκινᾶς. Πρόκειται περὶ τοῦ συγγράμματος, βιβλίου καὶ ἄτλαντος,* «Cytoarchitektonik der Hirn-

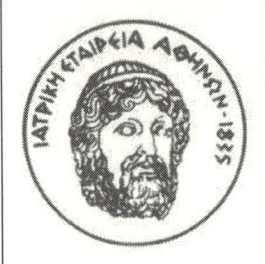

Fig. 3. The *Proceedings* of the Athens Medical Society for the Session of 23 January 1926

Staining method. The staining of the preparations was perfected by us such that a uniform tone was achieved not only of a single section, but of all the countless series of sections into which each brain was cut for study. And that was absolutely mandatory, on one hand in order to define the gradual differences of the histological elements of the neighbouring areas of the cerebral cortex, and on the other hand to achieve a consistent photographic representation.

Specimen depiction method. The hitherto occasional histological investigations of the brain depicted things schematically and therefore subjectively. Instead of such a schematic depiction, aiming at a precise representation of the preparations with all the relationships of the countless and polymorphous cells, we used photography. Photographic documentation constitutes the most truthful testimony of the exact depiction of nature, providing truly objective images of things as they bear in natural form, size and arrangement (Fig. 7). But to succeed in the photographic method it became necessary to turn to the study of branches foreign to medicine, such as advanced optics and photochemistry. We took advantage of both of these as much as we could. Lenses, light beams, filters, photographic plates and finally the photographic paper itself were all adopted towards the accomplishment of the intended goal of the most perfect, i.e. the photographic, depiction.

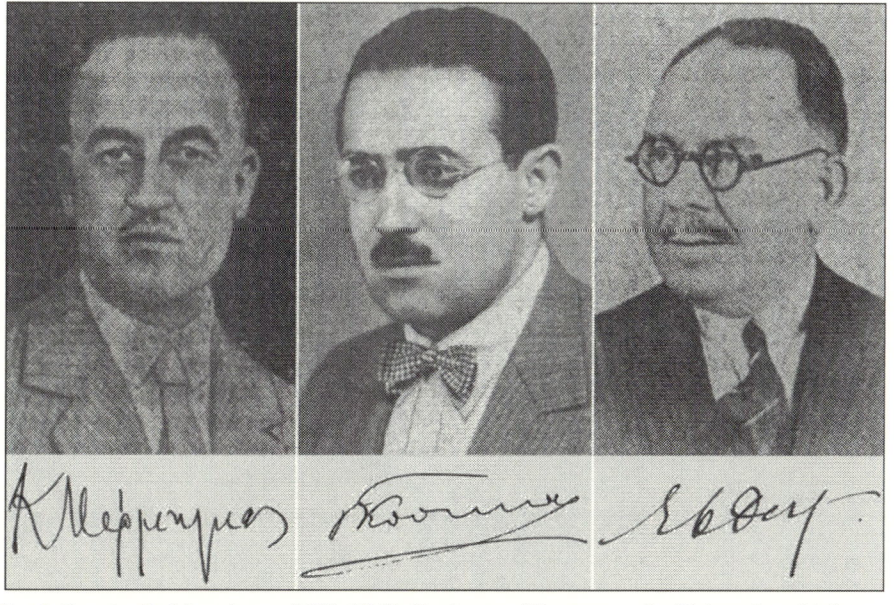

Fig. 4. Constantin Mermingas (1874–1942), Professor of Surgery at the University of Athens and President of the Athens Medical Society (left), Georg N. Koskinas (1885–1975) in the centre, and Spyridon Dontas (1878–1958), Professor of Physiology and Pharmacology at the University of Athens and President of the Academy of Athens (right). © 1957 *Helios Encyclopaedical Lexicon* (signatures from the author's archive)

2.2.3 Accomplished and anticipated results

Through our work an extremely precise and detailed description was achieved of the normal histological structure of the cerebral cortex as it is depicted in the photographic plates and explained in the text. Our photographic plates in the atlas, as such, constitute an ageless, imprescriptible opus, the basis and the control of any future research on the cerebral cortex. Whatever in such research is in agreement with the plates, must be considered as normal, and whatever diverges constitutes a pathological condition. From that precise knowledge of the architectonic structure of the cerebral cortex, which we achieved, it is allowable to anticipate the solution of numerous and different questions and issues of utmost importance; from their endless number I suffice in mentioning e.g. the following.

a. *The problem of problems, i.e. the problem of the psyche.* When, as anatomists and physiologists, we speak of the psyche, we do not refer to it as a metaphysical being that finds itself a priori outside any anatomical and physiological weight, but as a moral, mental, active and historical personality which interacts with others and influences ourselves.

b. *The problem of individual mental attributes, i.e. intellectual talents,* such as rhetoric, music, mathematics, delinquency and the variations in the mental development of human phyla on the earth. By comparing e.g. the centres of music in individuals who genetically present a total lack of music perception to individuals who possess an evolved musical talent we may exactly pinpoint differences in such music centres.

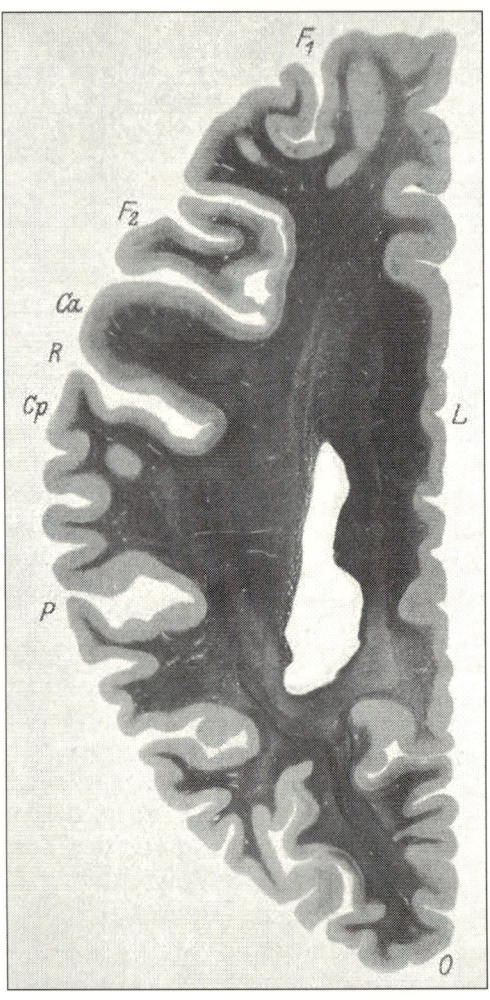

Fig. 5. Horizontal section through the left human cerebral hemisphere, depicting the sizeable regional differences in cortical thickness and the random orientation of the gyri (Koskinas, 2009). Weigert method. F_1 and F_2, superior and middle frontal gyrus; Ca, precentral gyrus; R, central sulcus; Cp, postcentral gyrus, P, parietal lobe; O, occipital lobe; L, limbic gyrus

c. *The problem of pathological lesions in numerous mental disorders* both primarily and secondarily encountered in the brain.
d. *The problem of the localisation of various centres.* The various localisations of sensation, movement, stereognosis, speech, etc., which thus far were mostly defined without an exact histological control, from now on, admittedly, can be readily and precisely defined on the basis of the cerebral cortical areas that we have designated, which from a total number of 52 known thus far we brought to 107 (Fig. 8–10). The solution of this

problem also possesses utmost sense, insofar as in that way diagnosis can be readily effected, foci can be defined with precision and brain surgery can be enhanced.

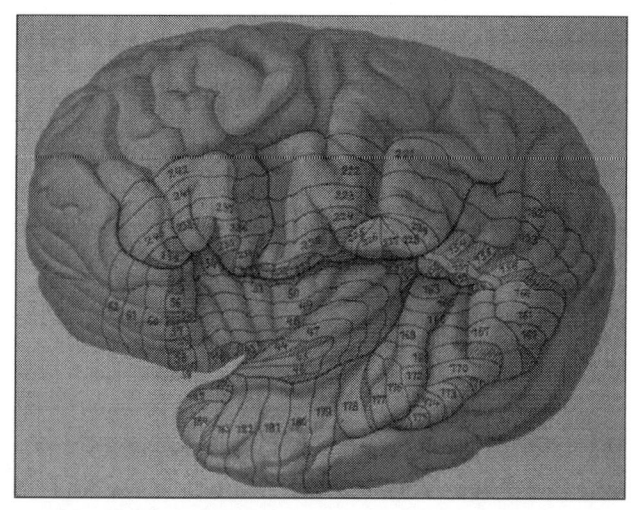

Fig. 6. Indication on the convex cerebral facies around the lateral (Sylvian) fissure of the von Economo & Koskinas (1925, 2008) method for dissecting each hemisphere into an average of 280 4mm-thick blocks perpendicular to the course of each gyrus for cytoarchitectonic study; hatched areas indicate the "cancelled" tissue

Sirs, in the phylogenetic line of living beings, nature, at times acting slowly and at times saltatorily, but always continually, produces new complex and viable animal forms. The same resourceful force that has given over the eons wings to the eagle to fly, has indirectly bestowed humans, by understanding their mind, with the capacity to construct wings themselves in order to defeat the law of gravity and to conquer the air. Nonetheless, the mind has its organic locus, its seat, its altar in the cerebral cortex. That is why one would be justified in saying that the anatomical and the physiological exploration of that noblest of organs deserves the utmost attention of science. The mind which explores and tends to subjugate everything, which tames everything and cannot be tamed, has to fall."

2.3 Response by Spyridon Dontas, annotator

"The work of Drs. Economo and Koskinas is monumental and constitutes a milestone of science, opening up new pathways towards the understanding of the brain from an anatomical, physiological and pathological viewpoint. It further forms the first comprehensive reference on the architecture of the adult human brain. And because the most precise of known methods was used, the optical, and through it a reproduction of the structure of the brain was achieved, in the natural, I reckon that this work will persevere as an everlasting possession of science. I further wish that Drs. Economo and Koskinas continue and complement their work, studying the remaining parts of the nervous system as well, to the great benefit of science."

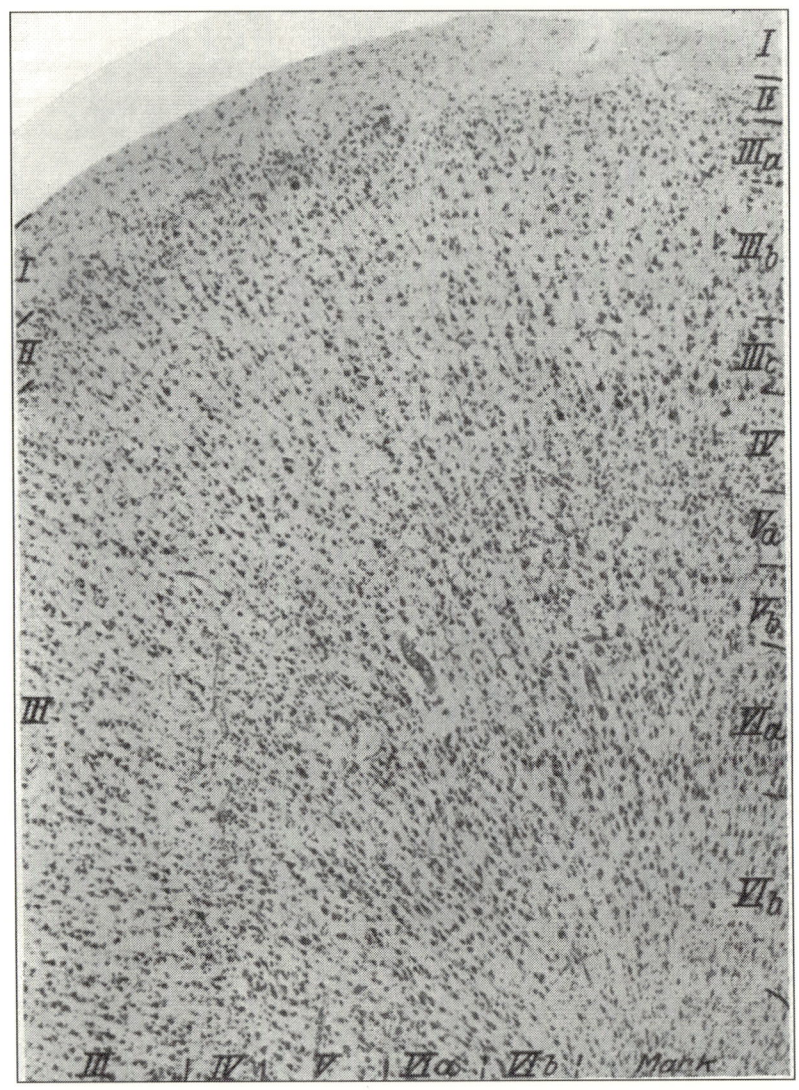

Fig. 7. Section of the dome of a gyrus from the frontal lobe of a human cerebral hemisphere, showing the normal six-layered (hexalaminar) cortex. The white matter (*Mark* in German), which is devoid of nerve cells, is seen on the lower-right hand corner. The six superimposed cortical cell layers are denoted in Latin numbers (I–VI). Photographed with a Carl Zeiss 2.0 cm Planar, a special objective lens with a considerably larger field than could be obtained with common microscopy objectives, especially valuable for large area objects under comparatively large magnifications and an evenly illuminated image free from marginal distortion. Planar micro-lenses are used without an eyepiece. ×50 (von Economo, 2009)

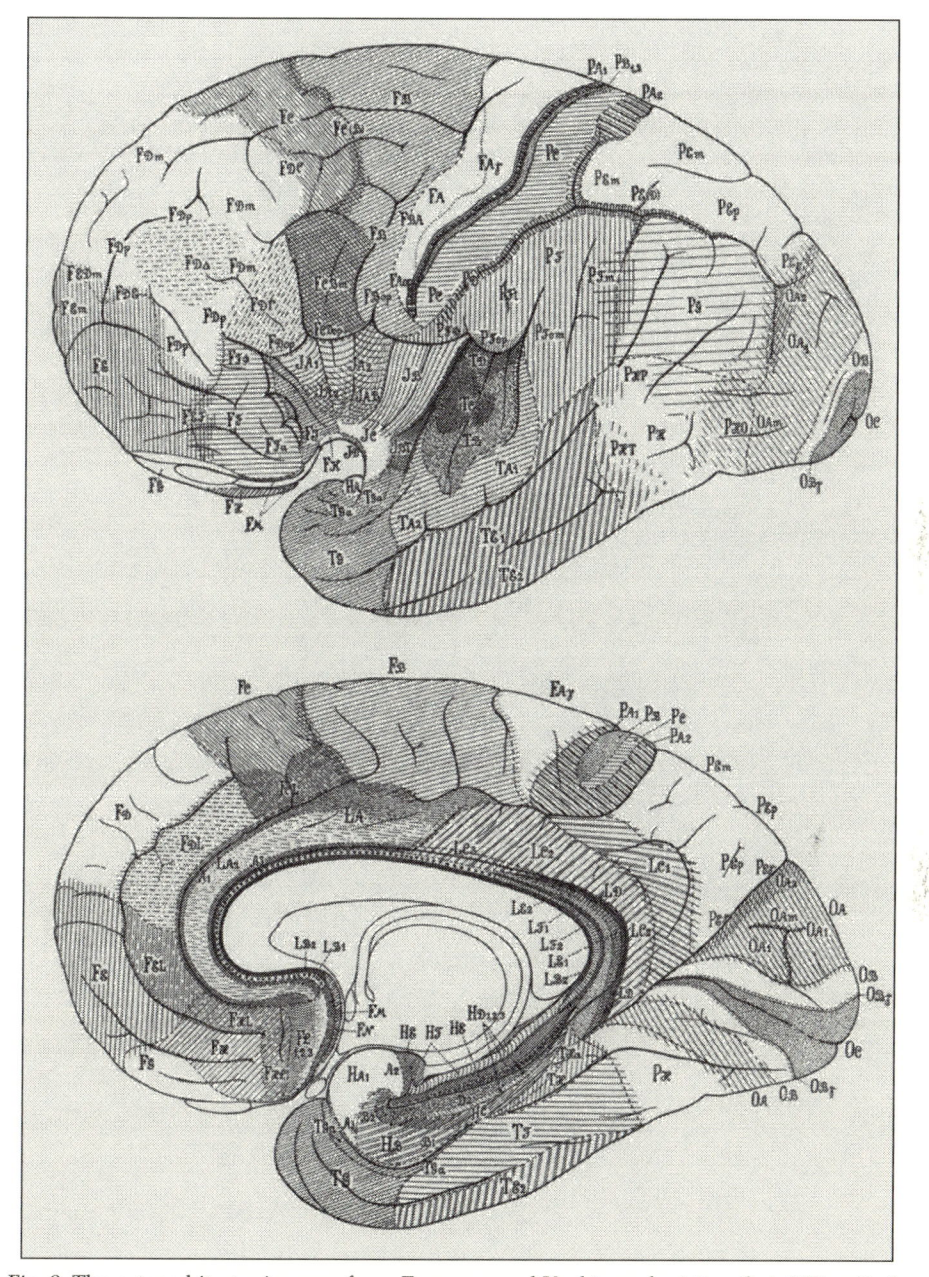

Fig. 8. The cytoarchitectonic map of von Economo and Koskinas, depicting their 107 cortical modification areas on the convex and median hemispheric facies of the human cerebrum

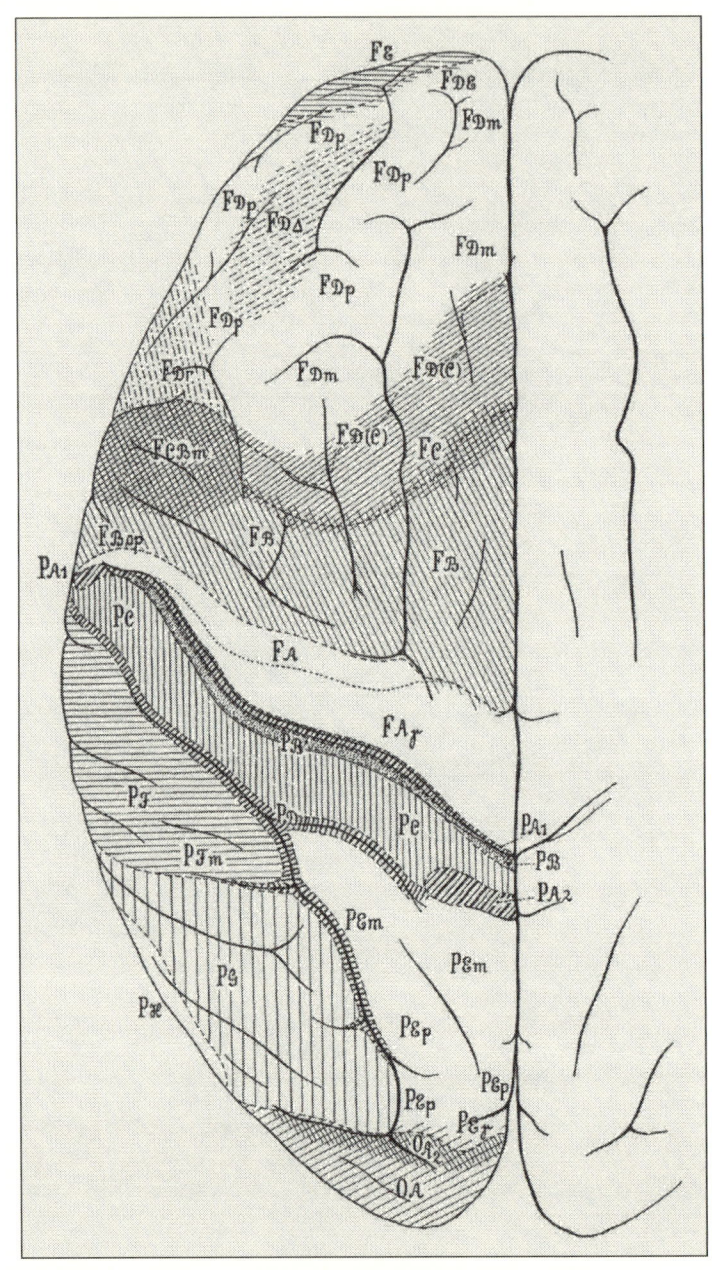

Fig. 9. The cytoarchitectonic map of von Economo and Koskinas, depicting their 107 cortical modification areas on the dorsal hemispheric surface of the human cerebrum

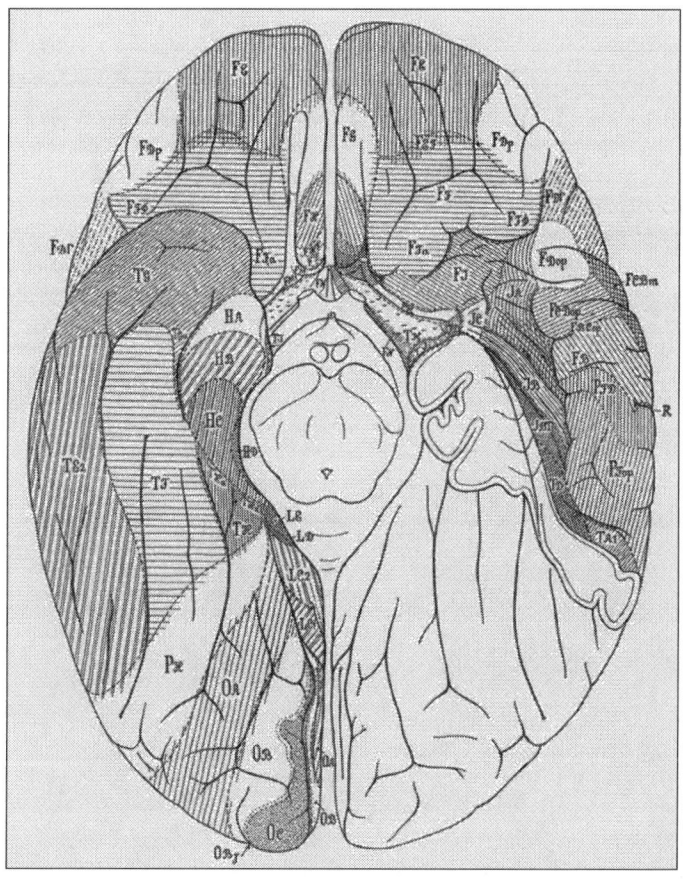

Fig. 10. The cytoarchitectonic map of von Economo and Koskinas, depicting their 107 cortical modification areas on the ventral hemispheric surface of the human cerebrum

3. Conclusion

Besides a histological mapping criterion, variations in cellular structure (cytoarchitecture) of the mammalian cerebral cortex reflect regional functional specificities linked to individual cell properties and intercellular connections. With the current interest in functional brain imaging, maps of the human cerebral cortex based on the classical cytoarchitectonic studies of Korbinian Brodmann (1868-1918) in Berlin are still in wide use (Brodmann, 1909; Garey, 2006; Olry, 2010; Olry & Haines, 2010; Zilles & Amunts, 2010). The Brodmann number system comprises 44 human cortical areas subdivided into 4 postcentral, 2 precentral, 8 frontal, 4 parietal, 3 occipital, 10 temporal, 6 cingulate, 3 retrosplenial, and 4 hippocampal.

Following in the footsteps of the Viennese psychiatrist and neuroanatomist Theodor Meynert (1833-1892), who is considered to be the founder of the cytoarchitectonics of the cerebral cortex (Meynert, 1872), von Economo and Koskinas, also working at the University of Vienna (Triarhou, 2005, 2006), took cytoarchitectonics to a new zenith almost two decades after Brodmann's groundwork by defining 5 "supercategories" of fundamental structural types of cortex (agranular, frontal, parietal, polar, and granulous or *koniocortex*), subdivided into 54 *ground*, 76 *variant* and 107 cytoarchitectonic *modification* areas (von Economo & Koskinas, 1925, 2008), plus more than 60 additional intermediate *transition* areas (von Economo, 2009; von Economo & Horn, 1930).

Topographically, the 107 Economo-Koskinas modification areas are subdivided into 35 frontal, 13 superior limbic, 6 insular, 18 parietal, 7 occipital, 14 temporal, and 14 inferior limbic or hippocampal. Moreover, the frontal lobe is subdivided into prerolandic, anterior (prefrontal), and orbital (orbitomedial) regions; the superior limbic lobe into anterior, posterior and retrosplenial regions; the parietal lobe into postcentral (anterior parietal), superior, inferior and basal regions; and the temporal lobe into supratemporal, proper, fusiform and temporopolar regions (von Economo, 2009; von Economo & Koskinas, 2008).

The detailed cytoarchitectonic criteria of von Economo & Koskinas (1925, 2008) confer a clear advantage over Brodmann's scheme; their work represents a gigantic intellectual and technical effort (van Bogaert & Théodoridès, 1979), an attempt to bring the existing knowledge into a more orderly pattern (Zülch, 1975), and the only subdivision to be later acknowledged by von Bonin (1950) and by Bailey & von Bonin (1951). It is meaningful that basic and clinical neuroscientists adopt the Economo-Koskinas system of cytoarchitectonic areas over the commonly used Brodmann areas (see also discussion by Smith, 2010a, 2010b).

Brodmann (1909; Garey, 2006) described the comparative anatomy and cytoarchitecture of the cerebral cortex in numerous mammalian orders, from the hedgehog—with its unusually large archipallium—up to non-human primate and human brains; he introduced terms such as *homogenetic* and *heterogenetic formations* to denote two different basic cortical patterns, which, respectively, are either derived from the basic six-layer type or do not demostrate the six-layer stage. Brodmann was intrigued by the phylogenetic increase in the number of cytoarchitectonic cortical areas in primates, and was astute in pointing out the phenomenon of phylogenetic regression as well (Striedter, 2005). Vogt & Vogt (1919) laid the foundations of fiber pathway architecture; they defined the structural features of allocortex, proisocortex, and isocortex, and extensively discussed the differences between paleo-, archi-, and neocortical regions (Vogt & Vogt, 1919; Vogt, 1927; Zilles, 2006).

Combining cyto- and myeloarchitectonics, Sanides (1962, 1964) placed emphasis on the transition regions *(Gradationen)* that accompany the "streams" of neocortical regions coming from paleo- and archicortical sources (Pandya & Sanides, 1973). [Vogt & Vogt (1919) had already spoken of "areal gradations".] The idea of a "koniocortex core" and "prokoniocortex belt areas" in the temporal operculum (Pandya & Sanides, 1973) was modified by Kaas & Hackett (1998, 2000), who speak of histologically and functionally distinct "core", "belt" and "parabelt" subdivisions in the monkey auditory cortex, with specified connections.

There are three major advantages in using the system of cytoarchitectonic areas defined by von Economo and Koskinas as opposed to the maps defined by Brodmann (von Economo, 2009; Triarhou, 2007a, 2007b):

3.1 Timing of publication

Brodmann published his monograph in 1909. Von Economo began work on cytoarchitectonics in 1912, with Koskinas joining in 1919; their *Textband* and *Atlas* were published in 1925, almost two decades after Brodmann, and comprised 150 new discoveries

(Koskinas, 1931, 2009), including the description of the large, spindle-shaped bipolar cells in the inferior ganglionic layer (Vb) of the dome of the transverse insular gyrus, currently referred to as "von Economo neurons" (Watson et al., 2006) — although a more accurate term would be "von Economo-Koskinas neurons". Ngowyang (1932) appears to be the first author to refer to fusiform neurons as "von Economo cells".

3.2 Defined cytoarchitectonic fields

Brodmann defined 44 cortical areas in the human brain. Von Economo and Koskinas defined 107 areas (von Economo, 2009; von Economo & Koskinas, 2008), plus another more than 60 *transition* areas (von Economo, 2009), thus providing a greater "resolution" over the Brodmann areas for the human cerebral hemispheres by a factor of four. Brodmann correlations can be found in the *Atlas* (von Economo & Koskinas, 2008) and in a related review (Triarhou, 2007b).

3.3 Extrapolated versus real surface designations

Brodmann maps are commonly used to either designate cytoarchitectonic areas as such, or as a "shorthand system" to designate some region on the cerebral *surface* (DeMyer, 1988). Macroscopic extrapolation of Brodmann projection maps are effected on the atlas of Talairach & Tournoux (1988), rather than being based on real microscopic cytoarchitectonics. Such a specification of Brodmann areas is inappropriate and may lead to erroneous results in delineating specific cortical regions, which may in turn lead to erroneous hypotheses concerning the involvement of particular brain systems in normal and pathological situations (Uylings et al., 2005). On the other hand, the unique sectioning method of von Economo and Koskinas, whereby each gyrus is dissected into blocks *always perpendicular to the gyral surface*, be it dome, wall or sulcus floor, essentially offers a "mechanical" solution to the generalized mapmaker's problem of flattening nonconvex polyhedral surfaces (Schwartz et al., 1989), one of the commonest problems at the epicentre of cortical research.

Furthermore, microscopically defined borders usually differ from gross anatomical landmarks, cytoarchitectonics reflecting the inner organisation of cortical areas and their morphofunctional correlates (Zilles, 2006). Despite the integration of multifactorial descriptors such as chemoarchitecture, angioarchitecture, neurotransmitter, receptor and gene expression patterns, as well as white matter tracts, it is clear that the knowledge of the classical anatomy remains fundamental (Toga & Thompson, 2007). The structure of cortical layers incorporates, and reflects, the form of their constitutive cells and their functional connections; the underpinnings of neuronal connectivity at the microscopic level are paramount to interpreting any clues afforded by neuroimaging pertinent to cognition.

4. Acknowledgment

I thank the Aristotelian University Central Library for providing a copy of the *Proceedings*, as well as Ms. Rena Kostopoulou and Dr. Vassilis Kostopoulos for providing archival material of the Koskinas family.

5. References

Bailey, P. & von Bonin, G. (1951). *The Isocortex of Man*, University of Illinois Press, Urbana, IL, U.S.A.

Brodmann, K. (1909). *Vergleichende Lokalisationslehre der Großhirnrinde,* J.A. Barth, Leipzig, Germany

DeMyer, W. (1988). *Neuroanatomy,* Harwal Publishing Company, ISBN 0-683-06236-0, Malvern, PA, U.S.A.

Garey, L.J. (2006). *Brodmann's Localisation in the Cerebral Cortex,* Springer Science, ISBN 978-0-387-26917-7, New York, U.S.A.

Hartmann, F.; Mayer, C.; Pötzl, O.; Wagner-Jauregg, J.; Pollak, E. & Raimann, E. (1926). Mitgliederverzeichnis des Vereines für Psychiatrie und Neurologie in Wien (Stand: Juli 1926). *Jahrbücher für Psychiatrie und Neurologie,* Vol. 45, pp. 80–84

Jones, E.G. (2008). Cortical maps and modern phrenology. *Brain,* Vol. 131, No. 8, (August 2008), pp. 2227–2233, ISSN 0006-8950

Jones, E.G. (2010). Cellular structure of the human cerebral cortex. Brain, vol. 133, No. 3, (March 2010), pp. 945–946, ISSN 0006-8950

Kaas, J.H. & Hackett, T.A. (1998). Subdivisions of auditory cortex and levels of processing in primates. *Audiology and Neuro-Otology,* Vol. 3, No. 2–3, (March-June 1998), pp. 73–85, ISSN 1420-3030

Kaas, J.H. & Hackett, T.A. (2000). Subdivisions of auditory cortex and processing streams in primates. *Proceedings of the National Academy of Sciences of USA,* Vol. 97, No. 22, (24 October 2000), pp. 11793–11799, ISSN 0027-8424

Koskinas, G.N. (1926). Cytoarchitectonics of the human cerebral cortex [in Greek]. *Proceedings of the Athens Medical Society,* Vol. 92, pp. 44–48

Koskinas, G.N. (1931). *Scientific Works Published in German – Their Analyses and Principal Assessments by Eminent Scientists* [in Greek], Pyrsus, Athens, Greece

Koskinas, G.N. (2009). An outline of cytoarchitectonics of the adult human cerebral cortex, In: *Cellular Structure of the Human Cerebral Cortex,* C. von Economo (translated and edited by L. C. Triarhou), pp. 194–226, S. Karger, ISBN 978-3-8055-9061-7, Basel, Switzerland

Meynert, T. (1872). *Der Bau der Gross-Hirnrinde und Seine Örtlichen Verschiedenheiten, Nebst Einem Pathologisch-Anatomischen Corollarium,* J.H. Heuser, Neuwied, Germany

Ngowyang, G. (1932) Beschreibung einer Art von Spezialzellen in der Inselrinde zugleich Bemerkungen über die v. Economoschen Spezialzellen. *Journal für Psychologie und Neurologie,* Vol. 44, pp. 671–674

Olry, R. (2010). Korbinian Brodmann (1868–1918). *Journal of Neurology,* Vol. 257, No. 12, (December 2010), pp. 2112–2113, ISSN 0340-5354

Olry, R. & Haines, D.E. (2010) Korbinian Brodmann: The Victor Hugo of cytoarchitectonic brain maps. *Journal of the History of the Neurosciences,* Vol. 19, No. 2, (May 2005), pp. 195–198, ISSN 0964-704X

Pandya, D.N. & Sanides, F. (1973). Architectonic parcellation of the temporal operculum in rhesus monkey and its projection pattern. *Zeitschrift für Anatomie und Entwicklungs-Geschischte,* Vol. 139, No. 2, (20 March 1973), pp. 127–161, ISSN 0044-2232

Sanides, F. (1962) *Die Architektonik des Menschlichen Stirnhirns,* Springer-Verlag, Berlin-Göttingen-Heidelberg, Germany

Sanides, F. (1964) The cyto-myeloarchitecture of the human frontal lobe and its relation to phylogenetic differentiation of the cerebral cortex. *Journal für Hirnforschung,* Vol. 47, pp. 269–282, ISSN 0944-8160

Schwartz, E.L., Shaw, A. & Wolfson, E. (1989) A numerical solution to the generalized mapmaker's problem: Flattening nonconvex polyhedral surfaces. *IEEE Transactions on Pattern Analysis and Machine Intelligence*, Vol. 11, No. 9, (September 1989), pp. 1005-1008, ISSN 0162-8828

Smith, C.U.M. (2010a). Does history repeat itself? Cortical columns: 1. Introduction. *Cortex*, Vol. 46, No. 3, (March 2010), pp. 279-280, ISSN 0010-9452

Smith, C.U.M. (2010b). Does history repeat itself? Cortical columns: 4. Déjà vu? *Cortex*, Vol. 46, No. 8, (September 2010), pp. 947-948, ISSN 0010-9452

Sträussler, E. & Koskinas, G.N. (1925). Untersuchungen zwecks Feststellung des Einflusses der Malariabehandlung auf den histologischen Prozeß der progressiven Paralyse. *Zentralblatt für die Gesamte Neurologie und Psychiatrie*, Vol. 39, pp. 471-480

Striedter, G.F. (2005) *Principles of Brain Evolution*, Sinauer Associates, ISBN 0-87893-820-6, Sunderland, MA, U.S.A.

Talairach, J. & Tournoux, P. (1988). *Co-planar Stereotaxic Atlas of the Human Brain. 3-Dimensional Proportional System: An Approach to Cerebral Imaging* (translated by M. Rayport), G. Thieme Verlag, ISBN 3-13-711701-1, Stuttgart, Germany

Toga, A.W. & Thompson, P.M. (2007). What is where and why it is important. *NeuroImage*, Vol. 37, No. 4, (1 October 2007), pp. 1045-1049, ISSN 1053-8119

Triarhou, L.C. (2005). Georg N. Koskinas (1885-1975) and his scientific contributions to the normal and pathological anatomy of the human brain. *Brain Reseach Bulletin*, Vol. 68, No. 3, (30 December 2005), pp. 121-139, ISSN 0361-9230

Triarhou, L.C. (2006). Georg N. Koskinas (1885-1975). *Journal of Neurology*, Vol. 253, No. 10, (October 2006), pp. 1377-1378, ISSN 0340-5354

Triarhou, L.C. (2007a). The Economo-Koskinas Atlas revisited: Cytoarchitectonics and functional context. *Stereotactic and Functional Neurosurgery*, Vol. 85, No. 5, (August 2007), pp. 195-203, ISSN 1011-6125

Triarhou, L.C. (2007b). A proposed number system for the 107 cortical areas of Economo and Koskinas, and Brodmann area correlations. *Stereotactic and Functional Neurosurgery*, vol. 85, No. 5, (August 2007), pp. 204-215, ISSN 1011-6125

Uylings, H.B.M.; Rajkowska, G.; Sanz-Arigita, E.; Amunts, K. & Zilles, K. (2005). Consequences of large interindividual variability for human brain atlases: Converging macroscopical imaging and microscopical neuroanatomy. *Anatomy and Embryology*, Vol. 210, No. 5-6, (December 2005), pp. 423-431, ISSN 0340-2061

van Bogaert, L. & Théodoridès, J. (1979). *Constantin von Economo: The Man and the Scientist*, Verlag der Österreichischen Akademie der Wissenschaften, ISBN 3-7001-0284-4, Vienna, Austria

Vogt, C. & Vogt, O. (1919). Allgemeinere Ergebnisse unserer Hirnforschung. *Journal für Psychologie und Neurologie*, Vol. 25, pp. 279-461

Vogt, O. (1927). Architektonik der menschlichen Hirnrinde. *Zentralblatt für die Gesamte Neurologie und Psychiatrie*, Vol. 45, pp. 510-512

von Bonin, G. (1950). *Essay on the Cerebral Cortex*, Charles C Thomas, Springfield, IL, U.S.A.

von Economo, C. (2009). *Cellular Structure of the Human Cerebral Cortex* (translated and edited by L. C. Triarhou), S. Karger, ISBN 978-3-8055-9061-7, Basel, Switzerland

von Economo, C. & Horn, L. (1930). Über Windungsrelief, Maße und Rindenarchitektonik der Supratemporalfläche, ihre individuellen und ihre Seitenunterschiede. *Zeitschrift für die Gesamte Neurologie und Psychiatrie*, Vol. 130, pp. 678-757

von Economo, C. & Koskinas, G.N. (1923). Die sensiblen Zonen des Großhirns. *Klinische Wochenschrift,* Vol. 2, No. 19, (7 May 1923), p. 905
von Economo, C. & Koskinas, G.N. (1925). *Die Cytoarchitektonik der Hirnrinde des Erwachsenen Menschen – Textband und Atlas mit 112 Mikrophotographischen Tafeln,* J. Springer, Vienna, Austria
von Economo, C. & Koskinas, G.N. (2008). *Atlas of Cytoarchitectonics of the Adult Human Cerebral Cortex* (translated, revised and edited by L. C. Triarhou), S. Karger, ISBN 978-3-8055-8289-6, Basel, Switzerland
Watson, K.K.; Jones, T.K. & Allman, J.M. (2006). Dendritic architecture of the von Economo neurons. *Neuroscience,* Vol. 141, No. 3, (1 September 2006), pp. 1107–1112, ISSN 0306-4522
Zilles, K. (2006). Architektonik und funktionelle Neuroanatomie der Hirnrinde des Menschen, In: *Neurobiologie Psychischer Störungen,* H. Förstl, M. Hautzinger & G. Roth (eds.), pp. 75–140, Springer Medizin, ISBN 978-3-540-25694-6, Heidelberg-Berlin, Germany
Zilles, K. & Amunts, K. (2010). Centenary of Brodmann's map – Conception and fate. *Nature Reviews Neuroscience,* Vol. 11, No. 2, (February 2010), pp. 139–145, ISSN 1471–003X
Zülch, K.J. (1975). Critical remarks on "Lokalisationslehre", In: *Cerebral Localization,* K.J. Zülch, O. Creutzfeldt & G.C. Galbraith (eds.), pp. 3–16, Springer-Verlag, ISBN 0-387-07379-5, Berlin-Heidelberg, Germany

PIONEERS IN NEUROLOGY

Alfred Fuchs (1870–1927)

Lazaros C. Triarhou

Received: 18 December 2011 / Revised: 17 January 2012 / Accepted: 18 January 2012 / Published online: 2 February 2012
© Springer-Verlag 2012

Alfred Fuchs (Fig. 1) was born on August 2, 1870, in Karolinenthal, outside of Prague (today Karlín, Czech Republic), into a Jewish family. He was the only son of Albert Fuchs (1825–1899), a district doctor in Prague, and Rosa, née Kornfeld (1843–1906). He had three sisters, Frieda, Elsa, and Mitzi [7].

Fuchs studied medicine at the Universities of Prague and Vienna, graduating from the latter in 1894. After 2 years of hospital service in internal medicine under Rudolf von Jaksch (1855–1947) in Prague and Hermann Nothnagel (1841–1905) in Vienna, he took a position as Secondary Physician at the Nervensanatorium Purkersdorf in Vienna's Umgebung District [6]. A few years later he published his first book, *Therapie der anomalen Vita sexualis bei Männern mit specieller Berücksichtigung der Suggestivbehandlung* (Enke, Stuttgart, 1899), with a preface by Richard von Krafft-Ebing (1840–1902).

In 1900, Fuchs left his post at the Nervensanatorium to pursue research at the University of Vienna. He joined the Second Psychiatric and Neurological Clinic as a Clinical Assistant, under Krafft-Ebing until 1902, and under Julius Wagner-Jauregg (1857–1940) thereafter. Fuchs published one of his early papers, 'On the meaning of remissions in the course of certain forms of acute psychosis' [1] in the *Festschrift* celebrating Krafft-Ebing's 30-year professorial anniversary.

Fuchs became habilitated in psychiatry and neurology in 1905, upon completing his 'Dozentenarbeit' (*Die Messung der Pupillengrösse und Zeitbestimmung der Lichtreaktion*

L. C. Triarhou (✉)
Economo-Koskinas Wing for Integrative and Evolutionary Neuroscience, University of Macedonia, Thessaloniki, Greece
e-mail: triarhou@uom.gr

der Pupillen bei einzelnen Psychosen und Nervenkrankheiten: Eine klinische Studie, Deuticke, Leipzig—Vienna, 1904). In 1909 he reported on 'Electrical studies with the aid of myographic curves' [2], concluding that paralysis agitans was to some extent analogous to diseases of the pyramidal pathway, such as hemiplegia, in that myographs did not indicate any anatomical or physiological perturbation of muscle tissue per se.

In 1912, Fuchs was appointed Titular Professor, and in 1919 Professor Extraordinarius. Apart from Wagner-Jauregg's Psychiatric Clinic, he worked at the Institute for Experimental Pathology, headed by Richard Paltauf (1858–1924). He published an experiment on guanidine-induced chorea in cats and a monkey [4] in the *Festschrift* for Wagner-Jauregg's silver professorship jubilee.

During World War I, Fuchs was asked by Wagner-Jauregg to direct the men's Division for the Wounded in the Neurology Department, which he did with the utmost devotion, despite the scarcity of staff. The division grew into the Station for Head Injuries, accommodating nearly 1,000 patients. After the war, the station was relocated to the Obersteiner Hospital in Döbling, where Fuchs worked until the end of his life [6, 10].

Fuchs was viewed by his peers as a knowledgeable, reliable, and conscientious scholar [10]. He contributed numerous and valuable papers to the medical literature.

In 1916, Constantin von Economo (1876–1931) had been summoned back to the Vienna hospitals from the Lavis Squadron in the South Tyrol front, "where he was serving as a reconnaissance mission pilot", to attend to patients with head injuries; that is when he commenced his observations on encephalitis lethargica. With Fuchs and Otto Pötzl (1877–1962) they published 'The sustained care following head injuries' [9] in the *Festgabe* for the 70th birthday of Auguste Forel (1848–1931). The following

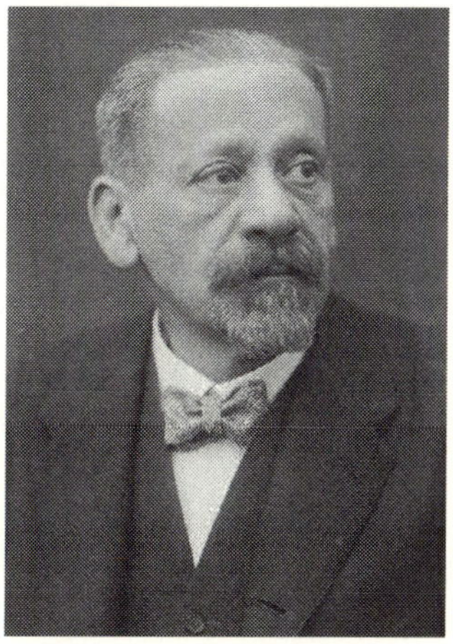

Fig. 1 Alfred Fuchs (1870–1927), Professor Extraordinarius of Psychiatry and Neurology at the University of Vienna. Courtesy Bildarchiv und Grafiksammlung der Österreichischen Nationalbibliothek. Used by permission and protected by copyright law. Copying, redistribution or retransmission without the author's express written permission is prohibited

year, von Economo and Fuchs published a series of studies on the long-term care of patients with head trauma [8]. In 1917, Fuchs and Pötzl contributed to the *Festschrift* for Heinrich Obersteiner (1847–1922) with a paper on the clinical and anatomical findings in patients with gunshot wounds affecting the visual fields.

Best known among Fuchs' works were his studies on the CSF, the exact measurement of pupil size, and the diagnosis of pituitary tumors. He was the co-inventor of the Fuchs–Rosenthal hemocytometer, still used today for manually obtaining cell counts in CSF samples. Other important contributions dealt with the relationship of tetany to ergotism [3], experimentally induced encephalitis [5], congenital defects of the lower spinal cord, reflex epilepsy, tabes, and the effects of an artificial anastomosis between the portal vein and the vena cava inferior (Eck fistula) on the nervous system [6, 10].

His books comprise an introductory text on nervous diseases (*Einführung in das Studium der Nervenkrankheiten für Studierende und Ärzte*, Deuticke, Leipzig—Vienna, 1911; second edition, 1925) and a monograph on the management of sexual disturbances (*Die konträre Sexualempfindung und andere Anomalien des Sexuallebens: Behandlung und Ergebnisse derselben*, Enke, Stuttgart, 1926). Moreover, he edited posthumous versions of Krafft-Ebing's *Psychopathia sexualis* (1907, 1912, and 1918).

Fuchs and his wife Bertha, née Ritter (1870–1929) had three sons, Felix, Albert, and Georg [7]. In the 1926 roster of the Vienna Society for Psychiatry and Neurology Fuchs is listed as a regular member, living at Garnisongasse 10 in Vienna's Ninth District.

Fuchs bore a prolonged illness with remarkable tranquility [10]. He succumbed on October 5, 1927 in Vienna, at about the time that the Nobel Committee in Stockholm deliberated about awarding the 1927 physiology or medicine prize to his chairman Wagner-Jauregg, for the "discovery of the therapeutic value of malaria inoculation in the treatment of dementia paralytica."

Conflicts of interest None.

References

1. Fuchs A (1902) Zur Frage nach der Bedeutung der Remissionen im Verlaufe einzelner Formen von acuten Psychosen. Jahrb Psychiatrie Neurol 22:390–410
2. Fuchs A (1909) Elektrische Untersuchungen mit Zuhilfenahme der myographischen Kurven. Jahrb Psychiatrie Neurol 30:201–208
3. Fuchs A (1911) Analogien im Krankheitsbilde des Ergotismus und der Tetanie. Wiener Med Wochenschr 61:1853–1858, 1920–1924, 1974–1980
4. Fuchs A (1914) Über einen experimentell-toxischen, choreiformen Symptomenkomplex beim Tiere. Jahrb Psychiatrie Neurol 36:165–176
5. Fuchs A (1921) Experimentelle Enzephalitis. Wiener Med Wochenschr 71:709–716
6. Jantsch M (1961) Fuchs Alfred, Neurologe. Neue Dtsch Biogr (Berl) 5:676–677
7. Rohel P, Kornfeld RR, Lowe P (2004–2011) Kornfeld family genealogy. http://freepages.genealogy.rootsweb.ancestry.com/~prohel/names/fried/kornfeld.html. Retrieved 11 Dec 2011
8. von Economo C, Fuchs A (1919) Nachbehandlung der Kopfverwundeten. Wiener Med Wochenschr 69:1885–1890, 1942–1948, 1995–2001
9. von Economo C, Fuchs A, Pötzl O (1918) Die Nachbehandlung der Kopfverletzungen. Z Gesamte Neurol Psychiatr 43:276–341
10. Wagner-Jauregg J (1927) Professor Dr. Alfred Fuchs. Wiener Klin Wochenschr 40:1367

PIONEERS IN NEUROLOGY

Erwin Stransky (1877–1962)

Lazaros C. Triarhou

Received: 31 January 2012 / Revised: 6 February 2012 / Accepted: 16 February 2012 / Published online: 8 March 2012
© Springer-Verlag 2012

This year marks the 50th anniversary of the death of Erwin Stransky (Fig. 1), one of the last "universal savants" of the Viennese School of Neurology and Psychiatry.

Stransky was born in Vienna on July 3, 1877, the son of Moritz Stransky, a Jewish manufacturer, and Mathilde (née Schönauer). He graduated from Leopoldstadt Community High School (currently *Sigmund-Freud-Gymnasium*) in 1894 and finished his medical studies at the University of Vienna in 1900. Realizing an interest in brain research during his student years, he trained under Heinrich Obersteiner, Lothar von Frankl-Hochwart, and Hermann Nothnagel. Following a 2-year internship at Vienna General Hospital, he joined the *Psychiatrische und Nervenklinik* of Julius Wagner-Jauregg in 1902 as an assistant. Stransky was habilitated in psychiatry and neuropathology in 1908; his thesis dealt with schizophrenia, then called dementia praecox [5]. Stransky was appointed *außerordentlicher Professor* of psychiatry and neurology in 1915. During World War I he served as an army physician, reaching the rank of major and decorated with the Knight's Cross of the Order of Franz Joseph [1].

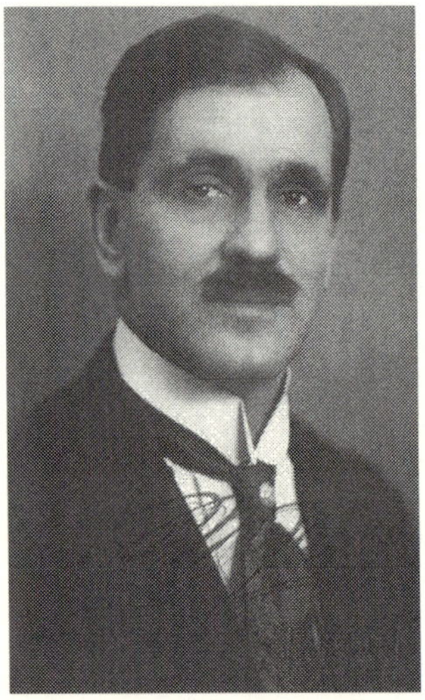

Stransky's *venia legendi* (right to teach) was revoked in 1938, following the *Anschluss*. He avoided deportation and survived the Third Reich unharmed owing to his "Aryan" wife [1, 10]. He was reinstated as full Professor in 1946, and retired as Professor Emeritus a year later. Subsequently, Stransky headed the Rosenhügel Neuropsychiatric Hospital; he was succeeded by Reisner [5] in 1951, but continued to be involved in the clinic and in research.

Between 1899 and 1962, Stransky produced 300 publications in neuropathology, neurology, psychiatry, clinical and medical psychology, psychotherapy, and mental health.

In his early years, he developed histological staining methods and investigated peripheral neuropathies [7], aphasia, asymbolia, thalamic tumors, and therapeutic blood transfusion in multiple sclerosis [9]. The "Stransky sign", a variant of the Babinski sign, denotes pyramidal tract damage: vigorous abduction of the little toe and its sudden release may elicit an extensor response of the great toe [8].

In 1903, Stransky formulated a "dissociation process" [6] and in 1904 "intrapsychic ataxia" (the incongruity

Fig. 1 Unpublished photograph of Erwin Stransky taken before World War I by Max Schneider, Vienna (author's archive). Copying, redistribution, or retransmission without the author's express written permission is prohibited

L. C. Triarhou (✉)
Economo-Koskinas Wing for Integrative and Evolutionary Neuroscience, University of Macedonia, Thessaloniki, Greece
e-mail: triarhou@uom.gr

between *thymopsyche* and *noopsyche*—or between affect and cognition in modern terms) as a pathogenetic hallmark of schizophrenia. His ideas were credited by Emil Kraepelin, Carl Jung, and Eugen Bleuler [3].

In 1932, Stransky reported the case of an electrocution accident that killed a catatonic patient; a temporary remission of clinical signs before the patient's death helped Stransky to foresee the potential value of shock therapy [5].

In a lecture to the Swiss Society for Neurology and Psychiatry ("From dementia praecox to schizophrenia") Stransky reviewed five decades of schizophrenia research. According to Hoff [2], the transcript of that talk (published in the *Swiss Archives of Neurology and Psychiatry* in 1953) belongs to the rare classical milestones that no serious researcher in the field may ignore.

He contributed the chapter on manic–depressive disorder to Aschaffenburg's *Handbuch der Psychiatrie* (1911). An opponent of psychoanalysis, Stransky published in the 1920s papers on hysteria, neuroses, psychiatric fashion trends, and subordination-authority-psychotherapy [10].

An outstanding clinician for organic diseases as well, Stransky studied progressive paralysis, Korsakoff's syndrome, and epilepsy.

Stransky suggested revisions of the Austrian Criminal Law and wrote on unjustified confinement, preventive measures against juvenile delinquency, and the psychiatrist as a criminologist [4]. He was often called as a medical expert to high-publicity trials [1]. His interest in mental health extended from medical consultation to studies on leadership, the idea of peace, and the psychopathology of statesmanship; he lectured at Vienna's high schools on mental health during maturation [2]. A final topic he delved into was the psychology and psychopathology of the aged, also observing his own aging process.

His books include a two-volume *Textbook of General and Special Psychiatry* (1914/1919), *War and Mental Illness* (1918), *Psychopathology of States of Emergency and Psychopathology of Everyday Life* (1921), and *Mental Health* (1955). As a medical historian, Stransky authored biographical notes on Heinrich Obersteiner, Emil Redlich, Sigmund Freud, Emil Kraepelin, Julius Wagner-Jauregg, Constantin von Economo, Anton Gabriel, and Alexander Pilcz.

He joined numerous societies, including the Société Médico-Psychologique in Paris, and became the first Austrian, in 1933, to be granted honorary membership by the American Psychiatric Association [10].

An eloquent public speaker, Stransky lectured undaunted until the end, despite a protracted physical hardship [2]. He died in Vienna on January 26, 1962 of an inoperable carcinoma of the stomach [5] and was interred at Vienna's *Zentralfriedhof*.

Students and colleagues, including Hans Hoff, Erich Menninger von Lerchenthal, Herbert Reisner, Franz Seitelberger, Walter Spiel, Helmut Tschabitscher and Milo Tyndel, extolled his vivacious eloquence, kindness, and medical ethos.

Stransky was married to the soprano Josefine Stransky (née Holas, 1899–1978). In the 1930s, she participated in the Salzburg Festival with performances of Bruckner's *Third Mass* and Mozart's *Requiem*.

Conflicts of interest None.

References

1. Angetter D (2012) Erwin Stransky, Mitbegründer der modernen Schizophrenielehre. Institute of the Austrian Biographical Lexikon and Documentation, Vienna. http://www.oeaw.ac.at/oebl/Bio_d_M/bio_2012_01.htm. Retrieved January 11, 2012
2. Hoff H (1962) In Memoriam Univ.-Professor Dr. Erwin Stransky. Wien Med Wochenschr 112:181–182
3. Kretzschmar C, Petit M (1994) Erwin Stransky et l'ataxie intrapsychique. Encéphale 20:377–383
4. Menninger-Lerchenthal E (1962) Die Bedeutung Stranskys als psychiatrischer Sachsverständiger. Wien Z Nervenheilkd Grenzgeb 20:13–16
5. Reisner H (1962) Dem Andenken Univ.-Prof Dr. Erwin Stranskys. Wien Klin Wochenschr 74:213–214
6. Scharfetter C (2001) Eugen Bleuler's schizophrenias—synthesis of various concepts. Schweizer Arch Neurol Psychiatrie 152:34–37
7. Seitelberger F (1962) Stransky als Neuropathologe. Wien Z Nervenheilkd Grenzgeb 20:11–13
8. Stransky E (1933) Eine Abart des Babinskischen Reflexes. Nervenartzt 6:595
9. Tschabitscher H (1962) Stransky als Neurologe. Wien Z Nervenheilkd Grenzgeb 20:8–11
10. Tyndel M (1962) Erwin Stransky, M.D. Am J Psychiatry 119:287–288

Historical Note

Eur Neurol 2012;67:338–351
DOI: 10.1159/000337953

Received: February 10, 2012
Accepted: March 4, 2012
Published online: May 9, 2012

Professor Bernhard Pollack (1865–1928) of Friedrich Wilhelm University, Berlin: Neurohistologist, Ophthalmologist, Pianist

Lazaros C. Triarhou

University of Macedonia, Thessaloniki, Greece

Key Words
Berlin Doctors' Orchestra · Histological staining methods · Moritz Moszkowski · Artist-physicians · Paul Silex · University of Berlin · Carl Weigert

Abstract
This article highlights the life and work of Bernhard Pollack (1865–1928), a pioneer neurohistologist, ophthalmologist, and world-class pianist. In 1897, Pollack published the first standard manual on staining methods for the nervous system. Born into a Prussian-Jewish family, he received his piano education from the composer Moritz Moszkowski and his pathology education from Carl Weigert. Pollack worked in the Institutes of Wilhelm Waldeyer (anatomy), Emanuel Mendel (neuropsychiatry), the later Nobel laureate Robert Koch (infectious diseases), and the Eye Policlinic of Paul Silex (ophthalmology), becoming a Professor of Ophthalmology at Berlin's *Friedrich-Wilhelms-Universität* in 1919. The study also chronicles the founding by Pollack of the Berlin Doctors' Orchestra in 1911.

Copyright © 2012 S. Karger AG, Basel

In his account of the foundations of neuroscience in Vienna, the neuropathologist Franz Seitelberger (1916–2007) wrote: 'Modern writers seem to be most interested in the economic, social and political circumstances of scientific progress. Not the least important condition, however, appears to be the role individual personalities have played in the history of sciences. The qualities and performances of these outstanding individuals have promoted scientific knowledge and life' [1].

Despite a substantial modern corpus on the history of European neurology, gaps and inconsistencies remain, stemming in part from the disappearance of the permanent records of 'non-Aryan' professors in German universities during the Third Reich. Pieces of the puzzle therefore have to be pieced together indirectly from bibliographic and other sources.

Such seems to be the case with Bernhard Pollack (fig. 1), one of the most esteemed *Künstlerärzte* (artist-physicians) in pre-war Berlin, remembered by peers and socialites as a distinguished ophthalmologist, splendid pianist, and kindhearted genius [2]. He authored one of the earliest manuals on histological staining methods for studying the brain, published by Karger in the 1890s [3].

The present article details Pollack's medical and artistic endeavors, as well as his founding of the *Berliner Ärzte-Orchester* (Berlin Doctors' Orchestra) in 1911.

Family and Academic Life

Biographical resources for Bernhard Pollack are scanty [2, 4, 5] and at times incongruous [6, 7]. Kreuter [6] mentions 'Bernhard Pollack (1888–1929)' as a neurologist and attributes to him a 1888 paper on 'A case of hysteroepi-

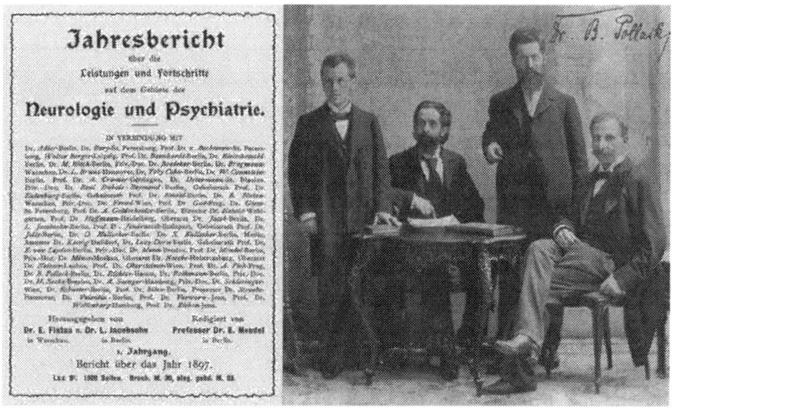

Fig. 1. Editorial board of the inaugural issue of 'Annual Report on Accomplishments and Progress in the Fields of Neurology and Psychiatry' (left). The names of Vladimir M. Bekhterev (1857–1927), Max Bielschowsky (1869–1940), Sigmund Freud (1856–1939), Ludwig Jacobsohn (1863–1941), Emanuel Mendel (1839–1907), Lazar S. Minor (1855–1942), Heinrich Obersteiner (1847–1922), Arnold Pick (1851–1924), Paul Silex (1858–1929) and Theodor Ziehen (1862–1950) appear alongside with those of the four gentlemen shown in the right photo (taken in 1901 in Berlin). Left to right: neuropathologist Siegfried Kalischer (1862–1954) ('Sturge-Kalischer-Weber syndrome'), neurologist Edward Flatau (1868–1932) ('Redlich-Flatau disease' and 'Flatau-Sterling syndrome'), neuroanatomist Ludwig Jacobsohn (1863–1941) ('Bekhterev-Jacobsohn reflex'), and Bernhard Pollack, seated. Credit: Wikimedia Commons; photo traced by Eisenberg [65] in the Berta Lask Archive of the Berlin Academy of Arts. Pollack's signature digitally etched from personal copy of Flatau's *Atlas* (author's archive).

lepsy in a man' [8], which was actually authored by Julius Pollak – an associate of psychiatrist Károly Laufenauer and neuropathologist Friedrich von Korányi of Budapest. The publication year of that paper [8] and of Pollack's last paper [9] could well explain the erroneous dates (they imply that Pollack received his doctorate at the age of 5, and published his book on staining methods at the age of 9). Elsewhere, Pollack was described as a 'Viennese neuroanatomist' [7] rather than a Berlin ophthalmologist [5]. There was also a Bernhard Pollack von Parnau (1847–1911) in Vienna, an industrialist-financier and art collector, known for his philanthropism [10].

Bernhard Pollack was born on August 14, 1865, into a Jewish family [4, 5]. He had two elder brothers, Joseph and Paul, and two sisters, Clara Lichtheim (née Pollack) [11], who was the mother of the political activist and author Richard Lichtheim (1885–1963), and Betty Friedmann (née Pollack), who was later murdered at Auschwitz, along with her daughter and son-in-law, when she was over 80 years old [4].

Clara Pollack-Lichtheim's father-in-law, Health Councilor *(Sanitätsrat)* Heinrich Lichtheim, was a cousin of Professor Ludwig Lichtheim (1845–1904) of the Universities of Bern and Königsberg; his Internal Medicine Department at Königsberg was an 'oracle' for Russian Jews, who traveled great distances to be treated [4]. Lichtheim, and the Prussian neuropathologist Carl Wernicke (1848–1905), formulated prevailing views on aphasia, later discussed by Freud in his *Critical Study* [12].

Pollack enjoyed a privileged education. He grew up in Berlin and studied medicine in Heidelberg [13], where he was particularly fond of the lectures of Professor Julius Arnold (1835–1915) ('Arnold-Chiari malformation').

After becoming a certified physician, Pollack pursued graduate studies in pathology at the University of Leipzig. He defended his doctoral dissertation 'On Metastatic Lung Tumors' (fig. 2) on April 17, 1893, during the period when Felix Victor Birch-Hirschfeld (1842–1899) was chairing the Pathology Department. Pollack's thesis [13] was supervised by Carl Weigert. Weigert and Pollack studied vascular lesions in lung metastases from diverse primary carcinomas in autopsy material from 16 patients aged 30–79 years [13, 14].

Following his graduation, Pollack settled in Berlin and prepared ophthalmological specimens for the State Collection of Medical Instruction Aids [15]. He worked at the Institutes of Wilhelm Waldeyer [16], Emanuel Mendel [17], and the later Nobel laureate Robert Koch [18], and the Eye Policlinic of Professor Paul Silex (1858–1929) [19–21], who, in 1914, had founded with the blind singer Betty Hirsch (1873–1957) the first school for the blind in Berlin. Silex attracted students from abroad, even from countries hostile to Germany as a result of World War I [22]. Pollack practiced as an *Oberarzt* (chief physician), kept a research laboratory [23], and attained a reputation as one of Silex's most distinguished colleagues [22]. Together they saw an estimated 300,000 eye patients over 30 years [9]. Pollack also collaborated with Max Bielschowsky [17, 24] and Edward Flatau [25], who described him as 'the man with the great work on the nervous system' (fig. 3).

Pollack was 'a man of life'; a gentleman of the old school, he hardly ever drank a glass of wine and always enjoyed good table conversation [4]. He was briefly married to the Viennese soubrette Fritzi Massary, the Operetta's *Primadonna assoluta* of the Weimar Republic [26]. Massary left Pollack [4] and in 1917 married the actor Max Pallenberg. Being Jewish, Massary fled Germany in 1933 and eventually moved to California [27]. Bruno Walter treasured Massary's voice, casting her as 'Adele' in the Salzburg production of *Die Fledermaus* and in the title role in Bizet's *Carmen* [26]. A street is named after her in Berlin (Fritzi-Massary-Strasse, zip code 12057, for the interested reader).

Pollack lived in one of the most fashionable residential avenues, still remembered by old Berliners, not far away from Potsdamer Platz and the old Philharmonie [28]. In 1906, he moved from Linkstrasse 41 to Blumeshof 15 in Lützow. In 1912, Pollack remarried, to the Viennese Baronin Marie Elisabeth (Miky) Popper von Podhrágy, daughter of Berthold Popper von Podhrágy and Katharina (née Löwenstein).

Pollack's father-in-law Berthold was born in Kotessó (Kotešová), Slovakia, the seventh of eight children. He had inherited a respectable sum from his father and worked in the timber trade with his younger brother Armin Freiherr Popper von Podhrágy, who held a Doctorate in Philosophy from the University of Freiburg [29, 30].

In 1910, Berlin's *Friedrich-Wilhelms-Universität* marked its centennial, Rector Emil Fischer welcoming the Emperor and his wife to the festivities. In 1919, Pollack became Professor of Ophthalmology while Julius Hirschberg (1843–1925), the noted medical historian, was chair of the Ophthalmology Department [31].

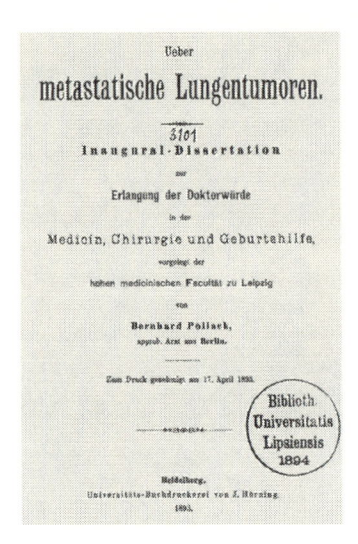

Fig. 2. Pollack's 47-page doctoral dissertation [13] (courtesy of Bibliotheca Albertina, Universität Leipzig). The acknowledgements read (my translation): 'In closing, I take the liberty to express my heartfelt gratitude to Professor Weigert for the gracious kind loan of the material and for his kind support in the preparation of this work. Likewise, let me offer my sincere thanks to Councilor Arnold, whose special instruction and guidance I had the opportunity to enjoy during my student years in Heidelberg'. Copying, redistribution or retransmission without the author's express written permission is prohibited.

Staining Methods for the Nervous System

Within the first few years of founding his Publishing House in Berlin, Samuel Karger solicited young but acknowledged scholars to write state-of-the-art compendia, surveying important fields of medicine for the practicing physician [32–34].

The compendium produced by Pollack [3] was part of that series. Considered to be the first of its kind [35], it was intended as a convenient reference for the neurologist and assumed some theoretical and practical knowledge of microscopic technique. Pollack dedicated it to Waldeyer and Weigert. A second, enlarged edition was written within 9 months [36], and a third 6 years later [37] (fig. 4). Specific instructions covered most neurohistological methods known at the time, with special emphasis on stains [35], accompanied by a comprehensive bibliography of 40 references, expanded to 100 in the second, and

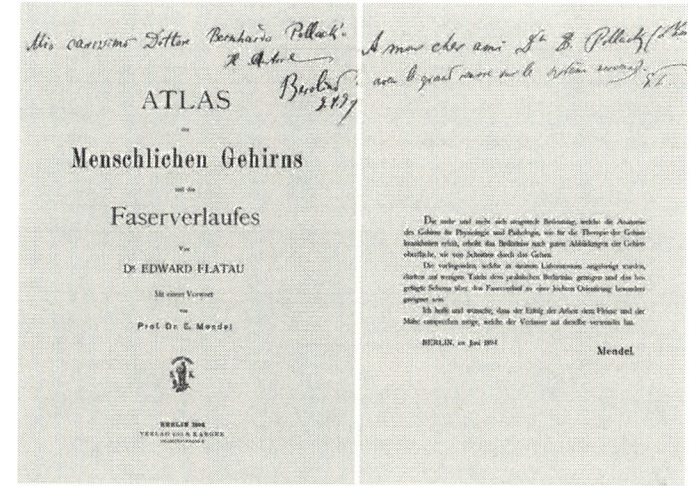

Fig. 3. Flatau's handwritten dedications of his 1894/1899 'Atlas of the Human Brain' [41] to Pollack in Italian and in French. The inscriptions read: 'To my dearest doctor Bernhard Pollack. The Author, Berlin' (left) and 'To my dear friend Dr. B. Pollack (the man with the great work on the nervous system). E.F.' (right). Author's library. Copying, redistribution or retransmission without the author's express written permission is prohibited.

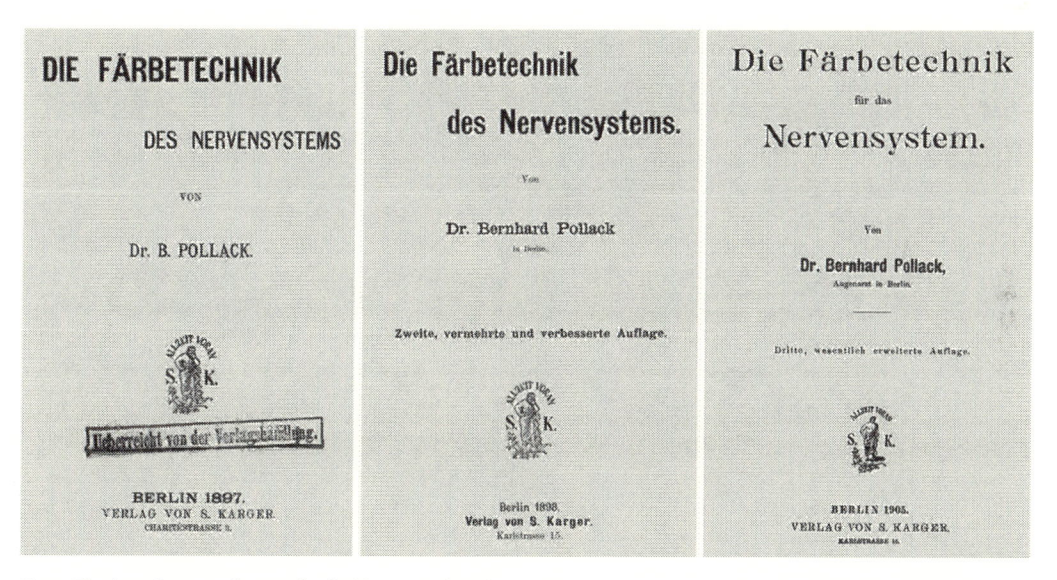

Fig. 4. The three German editions of Pollack's compendium [3, 36, 37]. Credits: Staatsbibliothek zu Berlin Preussischer Kulturbesitz (left); author's library (middle and right). Copying, redistribution or retransmission without the author's express written permission is prohibited.

300 in the third edition. The second edition was translated into English, French and Russian, and the third into Italian [37–39].

The book was structured in five parts: (1) removal of the brain, dissection of the central and peripheral nervous system, macroscopic examination, and conservation for museum purposes; (2) fixation, embedding, sectioning, and microscopic technique; (3) changes in brain weight depending on fixative, micrographic and photographic documentation; (4) methods of staining the main elements of the nervous tissue, i.e. neurons, myelin, axons and glia; and (5) general remarks and practical suggestions on choice of technique for normal or pathological neurohistology.

A few years earlier, Waldeyer [40] had coined the term 'neuron' and supported the theory of Ramón y Cajal on the autonomy of nerve cells as structural and functional units of the nervous system. Working in Waldeyer's Institute, Pollack commanded the chemical basis of each staining method and went over the postulates of fixation for improving microscopic specimens. He described the methods of Ehrlich, Nissl, Weigert, Golgi, Cajal, Marchi, Flechsig, Freud, Nansen, von Lenhossék, Frey, Roncoroni, and Azoulay, among others, and covered the macrophotographic methods developed by Flatau, who had published his 'Atlas of the Human Brain' [41, 42] 3 years earlier (fig. 3).

The separate chapter on the structure of nerve cells in the retina of vertebrates [36, 38] and a subsequent study on the innervation of the mammalian eye [17] were early comprehensive and groundbreaking works on staining methods applied to ocular microscopy.

Pollack received a positive review from Theodor Ziehen, who commented that the book 'meets an urgent necessity in an excellent manner with its detailed coverage' [43].

The book's merits were praised by the *British Medical Journal* [44]. The review of the first German edition stated: 'The author has wisely adopted the method so successfully used in Kahlden's *Histologische Technik*, of giving a summary in most cases of how the method is precisely carried out ... This book will no doubt prove of much service to those interested in the subject, and can be thoroughly recommended'. The review of the second German edition commented:

'The call for a second edition of this little book within 12 months of its first appearance is sufficient evidence of its value. The author has increased this value in the new edition by some judicious omissions and additions. The method of preserving the brain for museum purposes by a 2% solution of formalin in glycerine, as suggested by Laskowski, is a wise addition to the older methods ... The value of the book is greatly increased by the list of references appended, and the author has brought this thoroughly up to date. The book is excellent, and we venture to think it will have a wide circulation.'

Of the third German edition, the reviewer wrote: 'This book is up to date and trustworthy. An important feature is that the writer distinguishes between the methods he considers of first importance and those of second-rate value. We have no hesitation in again recommending Dr. Pollack's handbook in its latest edition'.

Alfred W. Campbell, the cortical cytoarchitectonics pioneer, found the third edition [45] a useful companion to the general histology *vade mecum* of Arthur Bolles Lee [46, 47], which had been published in March 1885 and seen six editions by June 1905 (chapters 31–35, or 65 pages, were devoted to the nervous system). Campbell [45] remarked that Pollack's running commentaries on each staining procedure were full of sound suggestions and proved the author to be a 'thoughtful, accomplished, and well-practised microscopist'.

Of the English edition, the *British Medical Journal* [44] wrote:

'The author has increased the value of his book by some omissions and several useful additions, notably a chapter on the retina, set forth with admirable clearness. To those who are working at the histology of the nervous system some of the newer methods added in this edition will probably be of value, and no doubt to English readers the English edition will be a boon.'

The review of the French version observed [44]:

'The needs of a handbook of neurohistological technique giving useful and practical methods have been met by the publication of Dr. Pollack's work. Methods are clearly detailed. The general remarks on methods and processes are suggestive and full of information, and an up-to-date bibliography is appended. The present edition will be welcome, it shows clearness of topography and of meaning, and the little work has merits of a decided and practical character.'

The French translation [39] was prompted by the international success of the manual, according to Professor Pierre-Émile Launois of Paris, who emphasized the revolution witnessed over the preceding 25 years in the knowledge on the structure of nerve and glial cells and their histophysiological relationships in health and disease, largely owing to the perfection of microscopes, and fixation and staining techniques. Golgi published his breakthrough discovery of the potassium dichromate-silver nitrate method in 1873, Cajal putting it to full use from 1888 onwards; in 1886, Ehrlich discovered that nervous elements could be colored after intravenous injections of methylene blue; Nissl, Marchi and Weigert registered equally important advances, and Flechsig was deciphering brain ontogeny by studying myelination. All that knowledge was used by Waldeyer [40] to systematize the 'neuron theory', which further explained secondary degenerative phenomena reported by Charcot, von Monakow, von Gudden and others. Launois argued that Pollack's comprehensive and practical book, with its orderliness, precision and clarity, would lead to scientific progress through the betterment of research methods.

As Pollack was finalizing the third edition, word arrived of the death of Weigert. Pollack wrote in the foreword [37]:

'Carl Weigert, the man who was a mentor to all of us, has eternal merits especially in our field of neurological research, as in so many other sectors. There is a profound need to extend to this man, beyond the grave, my deepest thanks from the heart for all he has always accorded me from a scientific, as well as a purely human perspective.'

Scientific Papers

Pollack carried out experimental and clinical studies in brain and eye research in addition to practicing ophthalmology. His first published article, based on research carried out in Waldeyer's Anatomical Institute, was 'Some remarks on neuroglia and neuroglia staining' [16]. Pollack reviewed the modifications of the Weigert and the Golgi-Cajal impregnation methods and their relative merits for studying the human and animal nervous system under normal and pathological conditions. He discussed the debate between Golgi, Cajal and most anatomists, who attributed nervous-like functions to neuroglia, against the views of Weigert and Ranvier, who absolutely rejected such a role.

Soon after the *Bacillus botulinus* was discovered, Kempner and Pollack [18], working at Koch's Institute for Infectious Diseases, were among the first, along with Marinesco [48], to study neuron lesions in cranial and spinal motor nuclei after experimental botulinum intoxication [49]. The clinical picture did not parallel the severity of the histopathological findings. Kempner and Pollack [18] found an early stage of cytoplasmic degeneration that they described as a 'clumpy swelling' of cell granules, but no evidence of glia proliferation; they further noted that in cases in which a lethal dose was administered that was sufficient to kill an animal in 48 h, its life could be saved if it received antitoxin within 24 h. In any event, neuronal lesions persisted 2 weeks later and disappeared very slowly. Evidently, cells were damaged for a long time after the disappearance of the clinical signs, and there was a discrepancy between lesion severity and clinical picture [50, 51]. Dickson [50] credits the work of Kempner and Pollack [18] as the only record of *B. botulinus* being isolated from nature, having recovered a strain from the intestinal contents of a normal hog.

In tuberculous panophthalmitis, Pollack [20] found that the inner layers of the sclera are stained blue instead of red by hematoxylin (metachromasia) and considered such a reaction typical, owing to degeneration, with mucin playing a possible role.

Working at Silex's clinic, Kurzezunge and Pollack [19] presented a case to the Berlin Ophthalmological Society on July 16, 1903, considered unique in the literature at the time, of a primary tumor of the optic disc in a 21-year-old man (fig. 5). The ophthalmoscopic examination revealed a shiny reddish-yellow growth on the right side, sharply protruding by about 1 mm from the fundus into the vitreous humor; it was rich in capillaries, had a cauliflower-like shape with a blue-gray margin pigment, and a diameter double that of the disc. Right vision was 5/50 with a central 10–20° scotoma. Since the growth did not change 6 months after intensive mercury and potassium iodide treatment, it was interpreted as a neurofibroma or myxosarcoma of childhood origin.

Waterman and Pollack [21] published the case of a railroad worker with an injury to the upper left orbital region that led to visual impairment, striking personality changes, and a belated atrophy of the optic nerves, which the authors attributed to a contre-coup fracture of the base of the skull (fig. 5). Additional signs resulted from damage to the cranial nerves, including left anosmia, anacusia, trigeminal paresis; motor and sensory disturbances were noted on the left side of the body.

Working in Mendel's laboratory, Bielschowsky and Pollack [24] presented histological results (Berlin Society for Psychiatry and Nervous Diseases, session of June 9, 1896) applying the Weigert glia method to study the spinal cord, medulla and optic chiasm; in the same session, Pollack described glial preparations of the optic nerve and spinal cord [52]. Six years later, Bielschowsky and Pollack [17] published a paper on the innervation of the retina, optic nerve, iris and cornea in the rabbit, dog, horse and human, using a silver-impregnation modification of Bielschowsky's fiber method with success; in line with Cajal [53], they refuted the interpretation of Embden [54] which favored the reticular theory regarding the horizontal cells of the retina, viewing them as discrete neuron entities instead [55].

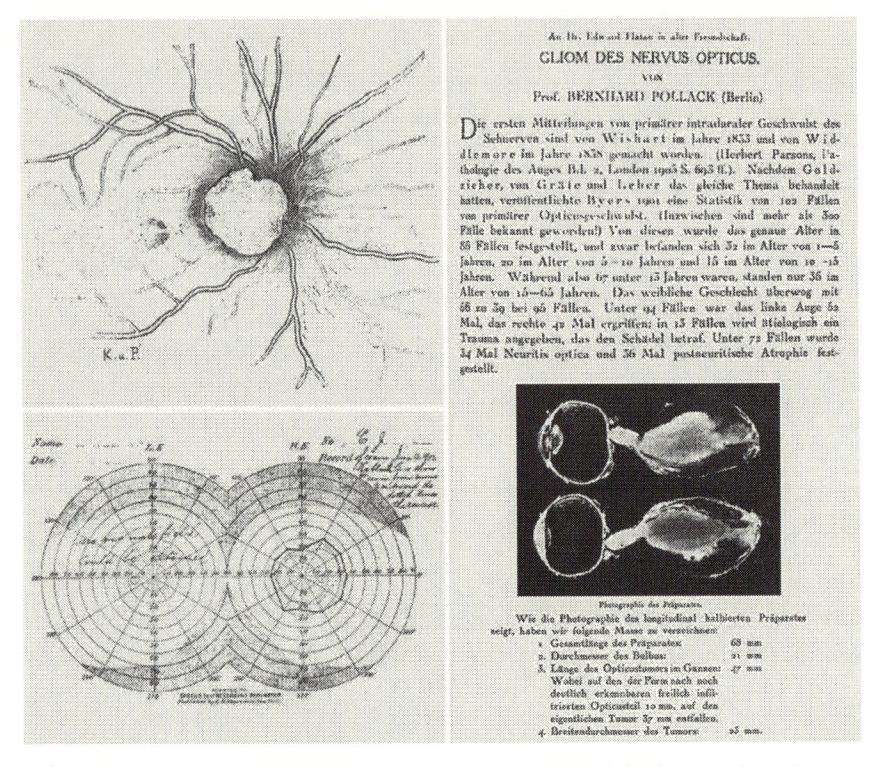

Fig. 5. Case reports of a primary tumor of the optic disc [19] (upper left) and of a head injury with visual impairment [21] (lower left). Pollack's final paper [9] (right), the posthumously published chapter in the *Festschrift* for Flatau (courtesy of Ruth Lilly Medical Library, Indiana University).

In an essay titled 'Costless eye examination' [56], Pollack warned about the perils of relying on opticians for free eye examinations instead of visiting the ophthalmologist. He stressed the value of ophthalmoscopy, as well as the timely diagnosis of glaucoma, retinal detachment, diabetic complications, kidney disease, cerebrospinal degeneration, internal hemorrhage and tumors. From the several hundred opticians operating in Berlin, to his knowledge, only three or four consulted an ophthalmologist. Pollack proposed a mandatory prescription for glasses by a physician and described the abuse of eye glasses (especially brand names) by crooks to treat anything from insomnia and obesity to diabetes and hemorrhoids; they charged anything up to 200 marks. He mentions the case of a young girl suffering from a gonorrheal eye infection, who lost her sight, following a hocus-pocus treatment by a local charlatan, who turned out to be mentally ill. Pollack came down hard on Christian 'science' imported from America, which he said shamed scientific knowledge.

Pollack's last paper [9] is a chapter on an optic nerve gliosarcoma in a woman, with macroscopic and histological finds, which appeared posthumously in the *Festschrift* for Flatau (fig. 5).

Conferences and Editorial Activities

Pollack presented cases to the Berlin Ophthalmological Society on ocular filariasis [57, 58], optic nerve glioma in a 20-year-old woman [59], spindle cell sarcoma of the frontal sinus [60], metastatic choroidal carcinoma [61], and Mikulicz disease (Sjögren syndrome) [62].

In August 1897, Pollack attended the Twelfth International Congress for Internal Medicine in Moscow [63–65] and participated in the discussion on cellular pathology [63]. Attendants included prominent figures in international neurology and psychiatry, such as Richard von Krafft-Ebing, Heinrich Obersteiner, Hippolyte Bernheim, Lazar S. Minor, Alfred Goldscheider, Hermann Oppenheim, Arthur van Gehuchten, and Georges Marinesco [63, 64].

In September 1904, Pollack attended the Tenth International Congress of Ophthalmologists in Lucerne and summarized its proceedings [66].

Pollack served on the editorial board of the *Centralblatt für Praktische Augenheilkunde*, edited by Julius Hirschberg [31], and the *Jahresbericht über die Leistungen und Fortschritte auf dem Gebiete der Neurologie und Psychiatrie*, edited by E. Mendel and L. Jacobsohn [67], by contributing literature reviews on the staining and anatomical methods of neurological research [25, 68].

Between 1897 and 1909, Pollack wrote literature reviews on microscopic methods for the study of the nervous system for the *Monatsschrift für Psychiatrie und Neurologie* [69, 70] and compiled the proceedings of the Berlin Ophthalmological, Physiological, Medical and Psychiatric-Neurological Societies for the *Zeitschrift für Augenheilkunde*, currently *Ophthalmologica* [71, 72].

Musical Life

Besides being an established neuroanatomist and eye surgeon, Pollack was a pianist of the highest rank. He took piano lessons in the 1870s from the composer Moritz Moszkowski [73, 74], the enlightened music pedagogue who taught at the *Neue Akademie der Tonkunst* in Berlin between 1871 and 1896 [75]. In 1890, Pollack published a four-hand piano transcription of his teacher's *Second Suite for Orchestra*, op. 47 (fig. 6).

Pollack's elder brother Joseph, who died young in a railway accident [4], was also musically gifted. A brilliant pianist with an impressive memory, he had been accepted for piano audition by Franz Liszt. Moszkowski dedicated his *Gondoliera*, op. 41, to Joseph Pollack, and piano arrangements of the *Scherzo-Valse* and *Maurischer Marsch* from *Boabdil* – his opera on the capture of Granada – to Bernhard Pollack (fig. 7).

Bernhard Pollack could have been as good a pianist as a physician [4]. Following the death of his father Jakob, and having inherited a fortune of several hundred thousand marks, he hardly practiced medicine at all and instead lived to indulge his musical inclinations. Only in later years, after using up much of the fortune, did he resume clinical practice.

Pollack had many artist friends, whom he frequently hosted. As a student, Lichtheim [4] spent time with his uncle Bernhard. In Pollack's bachelor dwelling – a rendez-vous of prominent figures from the music world – Lichtheim met Emil von Sauer, Moriz Rosenthal, Teresa Carreño, Josef Hofmann (to whom Moszkowski had dedicated his *Piano Concerto* in E major, op. 59, and Rachmaninoff his *Piano Concerto* in D minor, op. 30), and Fritz Kreisler (who had briefly studied medicine after being rejected by the Vienna Philharmonic, to return to the violin in 1899 with an acclaimed concert by the Berlin Philharmonic under conductor Arthur Nikisch).

The Hungarian violinist Joseph Szigeti recalls Pollack as his 'kindhearted pilot' and one of the finest chamber music pianists; they played together at salon style musicales in Berlin [2]. The young Dr. Pollack had anonymously accompanied Kreisler on one of the latter's early tours of the United States [2, 4]. Kreisler dedicated his violin and piano arrangement of Giuseppe Tartini's *Devil's Trille Sonata* in G minor to Pollack: '*Meinem lieben Freunde Dr. B. Pollack herzlichst zugeeignet*' [76].

Leibbrand [77] mentions Pollack's masterly performance of a Beethoven piano concerto in Berlin. Lichtheim [4] recalls a concert by the Berlin Philharmonic, when his uncle Bernhard moved from the parquet to the podium after the performance by a famous cellist to accompany him at the piano encores that the public forced upon the soloist impromptu, even when the orchestra had left.

On March 8, 1897, Pollack [78] gave a lecture to the Berlin Society for Psychiatry and Nervous Diseases on 'Musical memory'. After briefly describing memory function in painters, mathematical geniuses and chess players, he moved on to the musical memory of musicians. The musician, he claimed, upon hearing a piece of music for the first time, recognizes its key (e.g. C minor or E-flat major) and visualizes the composition. Such a complex function, often impossible for the dilettante, enhances perception and explains the precision, ease and consistency of musicians' ability to reproduce a piece. Some people further experience *audition colorée*, a topic little investigated. Besides the ear, the musician quasi uses the eye to mentally visualize notes without actually seeing them. A third substantial element involves rhythm, the characteristic of primeval music (music and dance of the wild), which adds substance to any melody, from a simple waltz to an endless Wagnerian phrase.

Fig. 6. Moritz Moszkowski (1854–1925) (left). Photo by Foetisch Frères S.A., éditeurs, Lausanne (courtesy Lebrecht Music & Arts, London, reproduced with permission; signature from an autographed copy of *Études de Virtuosité*, op. 72, dated January 26, 1918, author's archive). Title page of Pollack's piano arrangement for four hands of the *Second Suite for Orchestra*, op. 47 (right), with dedication to Hans von Bülow (1830–1894), Professor of Piano at the Stern Conservatory and Principal Conductor of the Berlin Philharmonic from 1887 to 1893 [28]. Credit: Sibley Music Library, Eastman School of Music of the University of Rochester, New York. Copying, redistribution or retransmission without the author's express written permission is prohibited.

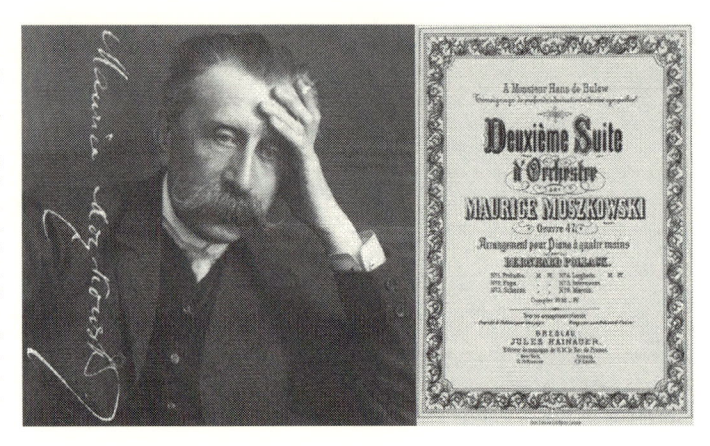

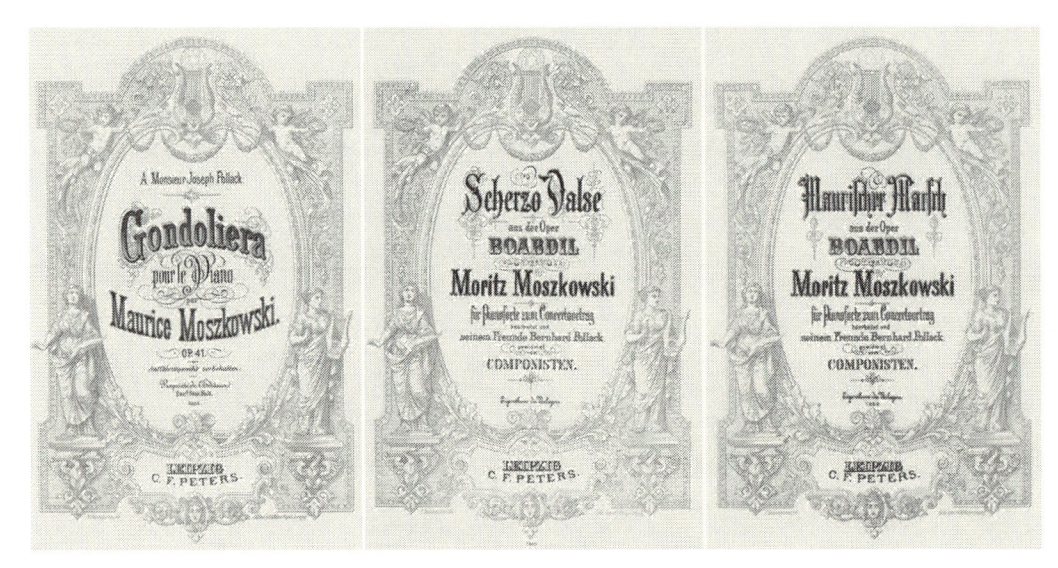

Fig. 7. Moszkowski's *Gondoliera for piano*, op. 41, dedicated by the composer to Pollack's brother Joseph (left); author's library. *Scherzo-Valse* and *Maurischer Marsch* ('Moorish March') from the opera *Boabdil*, op. 40, arranged for pianoforte concert performance and dedicated by the composer 'to his friend Bernhard Pollack' (center and right). Courtesy of Chicago Public Library *(Scherzo-Valse)* and of Biblioteca del Conservatorio di Musica 'G. Verdi' di Milano *(Maurischer Marsch)*. Copying, redistribution or retransmission without the author's express written permission is prohibited.

Pollack argued that experiments might help to better understand musical memory, citing Hermann Ebbinghaus and Emil Kraepelin. He revisited the problem of localization and the work of Hermann Oppenheim and Martin Bernhardt. With insight, Pollack suggested that the observed occurrence of amusia without aphasia excludes an identical localization of the corresponding cortical areas. In conclusion, Pollack mentioned the work published in Russian by Alexander N. Bernstein, who, on the basis of anatomical data on the sensory pathways of vision and olfaction, assumed the existence of a similar center for audition. Finally, he made reference to Friedrich Jolly, who contended that, in spite of neither having musical training nor knowing what C minor or E-flat major meant, he could nonetheless recite a simple melody [78].

In reviewing Rietsch's monograph on 'The Tone-Art in the Second Half of the 19th Century' – based on lectures at the University of Vienna – Pollack [79] expressed concern that the book was too technical and, although professionals would certainly appreciate its ascetic form, 'music, the most popular of all arts, should be accessible by a wider audience'.

The Berlin Doctors' Orchestra

The famous Berlin Philharmonic was founded by 54 musicians in 1882 [28]. In 1911, Pollack had the idea of forming an orchestra of 60 physicians with the talent and the courage to perform symphonic works [5, 80–83]. The *Berliner Ärzte-Orchester-Verein* was placed under the auspices of the Berlin Internal Medicine Association as a charitable ensemble.

The constitutive assembly convened on June 10, 1911, at the *Langenbeckhaus* in Berlin-Mitte. A temporary board was appointed, which extended an invitation for another assembly on October 11, 1911, at the *Kaiserin-Friedrich-Haus*. Heinrich Joachim, physician, medical historian and public officer in Berlin and Brandenburg, and a distinguished Egyptologist who had provided in 1890 the first commentary and translation of the Ebers papyrus, made the *Berliner Ärzte-Correspondenz* available as the official journal of the Orchestra Society [80].

In a board meeting on October 1, 1911, it was agreed to hold rehearsals from 9:15 to 11:00 p.m. on Tuesdays. The October 11, 1911, assembly elected a nine-member advisory committee. The conductors were to be Bernhard Pollack and Carl Weibgen and the concert-master Alfred Lewandowski. The first two rehearsals, with Pollack conducting, took place on October 24 and 31, 1911, at the *Kaiserin-Friedrich-Haus*; the program comprised Haydn's *London Symphony* and Grieg's *Elegiac Melodies* [80].

Regular performances took place at the *Beethovensaal* of the old Berlin Philharmonic Hall (Köthener Strasse 32, Berlin-Kreuzberg), which had been built by the architect Ludwig Heim in 1898 with a seating capacity of 1,066. The proceeds benefited widows and orphans of deceased colleagues.

Thus, Berlin joined Vienna and Paris [81, 82] in having a Doctors' Orchestra. Heinrich Obersteiner, the founder of Vienna's Neurological Institute in 1882 [1] and a gifted musician, conducted the *Wiener Ärzte-Orchester* [84]. On a cheerful note, the Vienna Doctors' Orchestra once asked a famous singer to perform two arias with them. The tenor, skeptical about the physicians' talent, replied: 'Before I sing the arias with the Doctors Orchestra, I shall let my colleagues at the Vienna Philharmonic remove my appendix!' [85].

The apogee of the Berlin Doctors' Orchestra came in the 1920s, before the advent of radio and the record. In the setting of the old Philharmonie, a wide repertory of works was performed with famous soloists. The example has been repeated internationally, such that a European Doctors' Orchestra was founded in 2004 and a World Doctors' Orchestra in 2007, apart from national Doctors' Orchestras in Switzerland, Spain, Romania, Finland, Australia, Japan, Taiwan and the United States.

The Composer Moszkowski

Pollack became a key figure in Berlin's artistic circles, closely associated with Hermann Wolff, the influential concert manager of the Berlin Philharmonic [86]. Until 1905, Pollack lived at Linkstrasse 41, next to the old Bechstein Hall, which was inaugurated in 1892 at Linkstrasse 42.

Moritz Moszkowski, Pollack's piano teacher (fig. 6), was a composer of refined music. A key figure in music history of the late nineteenth century, he has often been 'crowded' into a small paragraph, rather condescendingly, as a composer of 'salon' or 'genre' music [87]. He knew his orchestra as well as his piano, in fact. In his playing 'there was not attempt to astonish' and his elegant compositions are distinguished by graceful melodic veins and piquant rhythms [88]. Between the turn of the century and the outbreak of World War I, there was hardly a salon orchestra that did not perform the 'hit' *Spanish Dances*, and the *Virtuose Studies* became mandatory reading in Russian Conservatories.

In the 1880s, a neurological problem with Moszkowski's arm curtailed his career as a pianist, and he became increasingly devoted to composition [75, 89]. In 1884, he married Henriette Chaminade, the youngest sister of Cécile Chaminade; they had two children, Marcel and Sylvia. In 1890, Henriette left Moszkowski for the poet Ludwig Fulda, and a divorce was issued 2 years later. In 1897, Moszkowski moved to Paris. Henriette died in 1900. Moszkowski's own health deteriorated, and in 1906, he lost his 17-year-old daughter.

Yet Moszkowski never abandoned his wit. Noted for his *bon mots*, he once looked at the title page of a work by Raoul Gunsbourg that ran, *Ivan the Terrible, Opera by R. Gunsbourg*, and commented: 'It is a matter of a misplaced comma. It should read, *Ivan, the Terrible Opera by R. Gunsbourg*' [88]. Responding to a request by the German-American composer Ernst Perabo for an autobiography, he replied: '... I should be happy to send you my piano concerto but for two reasons: first, it is worthless; second, it is most convenient (the score being 400 pages long) for making my piano stool higher when I am engaged in studying better works ...' [90].

After World War I, Moszkowski was financially ruined, having invested all his capital in the crashing Austrian and German economies, and became seriously ill. Two former pupils came to the help of their ailing teacher: Josef Hofmann and Bernhard Pollack. Through Pollack's mediation in 1921, the Peters Publishing House in Leipzig offered a gift of 10,000 marks to Moszkowski, besides personal donations of 10,000 marks from Hofmann and 5,000 marks from Pollack. Pollack further sent piano arrangements of *Boabdil* to Peters, who supported the composer with an extra 10,000 francs, camouflaged as royalties [74].

A benefit concert for Moszkowski was given on December 21, 1921, in Carnegie Hall by 15 distinguished pianists, playing in ensemble under Walter Damrosch [91]. Among the artists were W. Backhaus, I. Friedmann, O. Gabrilowitsch, P. Grainger, J. Lhevinne and E. Ney. The concert netted 13,275 USD; one sum was transferred to the manager of the Paris branch of the National City Bank of New York with the instruction to use it for the needs of Moszkowski, and an annuity was purchased at Metropolitan Life Insurance Company, whereby the composer would receive 1,250 USD (or 15,000 francs) annually for the rest of his life, with the first monthly payment on March 1, 1925. On March 4, 1925, Moszkowski died in Paris of stomach cancer, in poverty and in comparative obscurity.

Ten days after his teacher's death, Pollack published the 'Recollections of Moritz Moszkowski' in a Berlin newspaper [73]. That article is a substantial testimony, because, even today, few biographical essays exist on Moszkowski. In addition to an overview of Moszkowski's output, Pollack, as an insider, recounts several anecdotes that convey the composer's spirit. For example: '... Larger works soon followed, such as the *First Suite for Orchestra* in F major, a charming work from happier days. The *Suite* had become a sensational success in the mid-1880s and the joyous composer was repeatedly invited to conduct it in big cities in England and Germany. In those days, Moszkowski told with amusement how he would check into hotels as *Moszkowski with the Suite*' [73].

Conclusion

Pollack died on March 3, 1928, in the *Franziskus Krankenhaus* (St. Francis Hospital or *Vereinslazarett Franziskus-Sanatorium*, Burggrafenstrasse 1, Berlin), 3 years to the day after Moszkowski. His renown transcended continental Europe [92]. In the years that followed, Mrs. Pollack suffered hardship. When the National Socialists came to power, she fled to Paris in 1933. Apparently, Bernhard and Marie Elisabeth Pollack had a son, Hanns, who stayed in Berlin with friends [29, 30]. Richard Lichtheim, the two children of Pollack's brother Paul, and the grandchildren of Pollack's sister Betty were able to escape abroad [4].

Pollack left this world with Berlin in one piece. The events of 1938–1945 halted Europe's progress and led academic institutions to disaster. There is one regret that will always remain, apart from the bestial slaughter: the deprivation of humanity of an intellectual, cultural and scientific heritage that might have been.

Postscript

On Sunday, May 2, 2010, the *Berliner Ärzte-Orchester* gave their spring concert at the *Kammermusiksaal* of the Philharmonie in Berlin, performing Beethoven's *Fourth Piano Concerto* and Brahms's *Fourth Symphony*.

On the following morning, a rainy Monday, surmising that Pollack's burial site could be the *Jüdischer Friedhof* in Berlin-Weissensee, my brother and I took off for Herbert-Baum-Strasse 45. As soon as the gentleman at the office typed 'Bernhard Pollack' in the system, a microfilm record appeared: *Feld H Abteilung II. Beerdigt am 6.3.1928* ('Field H Row 2. Interred on March 6, 1928').

In the serenity of the *Friedhof*, amidst the musky flora and the avian song, we reached Field H. A partially

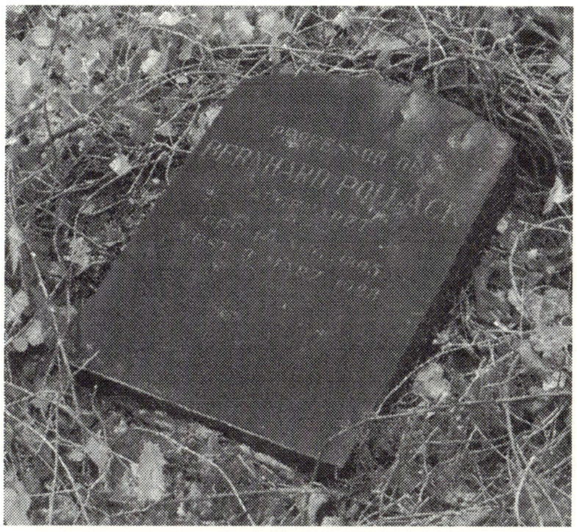

Fig. 8. Bernhard Pollack's tombstone at the *Jüdischer Friedhof* in Berlin-Weissensee, documenting the correct dates of his birth and death. Discovered and photographed by the author and his brother on May 3, 2010. Copying, redistribution or retransmission without the author's express written permission is prohibited.

exposed tombstone engraved 'George Lichtheim (1849–1908)' was the only obvious clue to the Pollack family site. To the right, less conspicuous, was 'Clara Lichtheim (1857–1896)' – Pollack's sister. To the left, an inconspicuous black marble, apparently unnoticed for decades, shyly revealing 'EN' through the overgrown vine: the middle characters of AUGENARZT. We cleaned the plaque with water from the nearby faucet. A little orange-bellied bird landed on the lower-right corner of the shiny marble and drank a couple of droplets. Memorable. We stayed silent, lost in time, warmed at heart, pondering over the *antiqui huomini*, and a life full of notes and accord (fig. 8).

I made another supposition, that the *Berliner Ärzte-Correspondenz* must have mentioned Pollack's death. I traced the 1928 volume at the Berlin State Library and at the Humboldt University Library. There was a memoir, in the March 17 issue, authored by Dr. Else Wolfsohn-Jaffé [93] – an assistant to Professor Adolf Gutmann. An English translation of that note concludes the present article:

'On March 3, 1928 the Berlin ophthalmologist Professor Dr. Bernhard Pollack, well-known and highly regarded by his colleagues, died. An agonizing malady, which cast its shadow over a long period of time, put an early end to a rich life.

From inner conviction, Pollack chose the medical profession, for which he was exceptionally suited. He began as a devoted student of Weigert in anatomic pathology. He published a groundbreaking comprehensive work on the staining methods applied to ocular microscopy. Moreover, he was outstanding as a practicing ophthalmologist; the circle of his activity expanded soon, and he became increasingly influential after settling in Berlin. He combined great ability with the finest psychology and artistic intuition and was thus able to treat and help anyone, from the common folk to the highly trained artist.

The dual nature of the physician and the artist added a special note to his personality. He was a pianist of the highest rank and mastered virtually the entire piano repertory as a virtuoso performer. Moszkowski called him the greatest memory in existence. He would readily register any request by heart. Once he saw the manuscript of a newly composed piece on a composer's grand piano; he read the score unnoticed and later played it from memory to the astonishment of the composer. The composer immediately remarked, 'You would really impress me, if you could play the compositions I have not composed yet'. Pollack was a close friend of the greatest in the music world. As a young man he journeyed with Kreisler to America. There he enjoyed his first triumph as an accompanist and soloist and became a very welcome guest at the homes of the dollar kings. He was most entertaining and sociable, and with his effusive spirit and wit injected life into any circle.

Those great intellectual qualities were only exceeded by a deep goodness and inner amiability toward others, what one of his friends called a 'charming heart'. Such goodness was his hallmark. Whenever he could, he supported colleagues in need. He would sacrifice himself for his friends anytime they needed it. He lived their destiny as his own, and only those who were close to him can appreciate that his passing leaves a void that can never be filled.'

Acknowledgements

The following individuals and organizations provided valuable input and are gratefully acknowledged: Dipl.-Archivarin Sabine Hank, Centrum Judaicum, Stiftung Neue Synagoge Berlin; Jüdischer Friedhof, Berlin-Weissensee; Cimetière Parisien de Bagneux, Mairie de Paris; Staatsbibliothek zu Berlin Preussischer Kulturbesitz; Jacob und Wilhelm Grimm Zentrum, Humboldt Universitätsbibliothek zu Berlin; Bibliotheca Albertina der Universität Leipzig; Universität der Künste Berlin (former Kullak and Stern Academies); Literaturarchiv der Akademie der Künste Berlin; Biblioteca del Conservatorio di Musica 'G. Verdi' di Milano; Chicago Public Library; Mrs. Dorothee Köhncke, Berliner Ärzte-Orchester. This work was carried out in part during a sabbatical leave of absence from the University of Macedonia to Berlin in spring semester 2010. It is a joy to thank my brother Michalis for insightful ideas and invaluable help in rendering complex German passages into sensible English.

Disclosure Statement

The author reports no proprietary or commercial interest in any product mentioned or concept discussed in this article.

References

1 Seitelberger F: Heinrich Obersteiner and the Neurological Institute: foundation and history of neuroscience in Vienna. Brain Pathol 1992;2:163–168.
2 Szigeti J: With Strings Attached – Reminiscences and Reflections. New York, A.A. Knopf, 1947.
3 Pollack B: Die Färbetechnik des Nervensystems. Berlin, S. Karger, 1897.
4 Lichtheim R: Rückkehr – Lebenserinnerungen aus der Frühzeit des deutschen Zionismus. Stuttgart, Deutsche Verlags-Anstalt GmbH, 1970.
5 Triarhou LC: Bernhard Pollack (1865–1928). J Neurol 2010;257:1585–1586.
6 Kreuter A: Deutschsprachige Neurologen und Psychiater – Ein Biographisch-Bibliographisches Lexikon von den Vorläufern bis zur Mitte des 20. Jahrhunderts, Bd. 3. München, K.G. Saur, 1996, p 1122.
7 Stahnisch F: Mind the gap: Synapsen oder keine Synapsen? – Bildkontrolle, Wortwechsel und Glaubenssätze im Diskurs der morphologischen Hirnforschung; in Stahnisch F, Bauer H (eds): Bild und Gestalt – Wie formen Medienpraktiken das Wissen in Medizin und Humanwissenschaften? Münster, LIT Verlag, 2007, pp 101–124.
8 Pollak J: Ein Fall von Hysteroepilepsie bei einem Manne. Cbl Nervenheilk Psychiatr Gerichtl Psychopathol 1888;11:2–5.
9 Pollack B: Gliom des Nervus opticus; in Bornsztajn M (ed): Księga Jubileuszowa Edwarda Flataua. Warszawa, Gebethner i Wolff, 1929, pp 595–600.
10 Mentschl J: Pollack von Parnau, Bernhard. Österr Biogr Lexikon 1983;8:174.
11 Levenson A: The conversionary impulse in fin de siècle Germany. Leo Baeck Inst Yearbk 1995;40:107–122.
12 Freud S: Zur Auffassung der Aphasien; eine kritische Studie. Leipzig – Vienna, F. Deuticke, 1891.
13 Pollack B: Über metastatische Lungentumoren (Inaugural-Dissertation, Medizinische Fakultät zu Leipzig). Heidelberg, J. Hörning, 1893.
14 Kaufmann E: Lehrbuch der Speciellen Pathologischen Anatomie für Studirende und Ärzte, 2nd ed. Berlin, G. Reimer, 1901.
15 Kutner R: Die staatliche Sammlung ärztlichen Lehrmittel. Chronik Königl Friedrich Wilhelms Univ Berlin 1905;18:139–141; 1906;19:153–156.
16 Pollack B: Einige Bemerkungen über die Neuroglia und Neurogliafärbung. Arch Mikrosk Anat 1896;48:274–280.
17 Bielschowsky M, Pollack B: Zur Kenntniss der Innervation des Säugethierauges. Neurol Cbl 1904;23:387–394.
18 Kempner W, Pollack B: Die Wirkung des Botulismustoxins (Fleischgiftes) und seines specifischen Antitoxins auf die Nervenzellen. Dtsch Med Wschr 1897;23:505–507.
19 Kurzezunge D, Pollack B: Ein Fall von primärer Neubildung auf der Papille des Opticus. Z Augenheilk 1903;10:302–308.
20 Pollack B: Ueber das Verhalten der Sclera bei Panophthalmie. Z Augenheilk 1903;9:218–223.
21 Waterman O, Pollack B: Fracture of the basis cranii followed by atrophy of both optic nerves and peculiar psychic phenomena. J Nerv Ment Dis 1904;31:250–257.
22 Pollack B: Geheimrat Professor Dr. Silex. Berl Tagebl 1918(Mar 18);47:3.
23 Pines L: Untersuchungen über den Bau der Retina mit Weigerts Neurogliamethode. Z Augenheilk 1899;2:252–256.
24 Bielschowsky M, Pollack B: Demonstration von Präparaten welche nach der Weigert'schen Neurogliamethode angefertigt sind. Arch Psychiatr Nervenkrankh 1898;30:984–985.
25 Pollack B, Flatau E: Anatomische Untersuchungsmethoden des Nervensystems. Jber Leist Fortschr Geb Neurol Psychiatr 1900;3:1–11; 1902;5:1–10.
26 Bollert W: Massary, Fritzi. Neue Dtsch Biogr 1990;16:357.
27 Schneidereit O: Fritzi Massary – Versuch eines Porträts. Berlin (East), VEB Lied der Zeit, 1970.
28 Stresemann W: The Berlin Philharmonic from Bülow to Karajan – Home and History of a World-Famous Orchestra (translated by J. Stresemann). Berlin, W. Stapp, 1979.
29 von Blaschek WR: Die Freiherren Popper von Podhrágy – Schicksale und Lebensbilder einer Familie. Vienna, Private Manuscript, 1936.
30 Popper WA: Wolf A. Popper Family Collection (AR 25312). New York, Leo Baeck Institute Archives – Center for Jewish History, 1974. http://digital.cjh.org (accessed May 28, 2010).
31 Hirschberg J: Vermischtes – 4) Ernennungen. Cbl Prakt Augenheilk (Leipz) 1919;43:19–20.
32 Karger S: Verlags-Katalog 1890–1930: Vierzig Jahre Verlagstätigkeit der Firma S. Karger in Berlin auf dem Gebiete der Medizin und Naturwissenschaften. Berlin, S. Karger, 1930.
33 Karger T: A short history of the Karger publishing firm. Bull Med Libr Assoc 1981;69:254–257.
34 Schmeck HM: Karger – Turning Medical Progress into Print: A Mirror of a Century of Medical and Scientific Publishing. Basel, S. Karger, 1990, pp 13–14.
35 Bracegirdle B: A History of Microtechnique – The Evolution of the Microtome and the Development of Tissue Preparation. Ithaca, NY, Cornell University Press, 1978.
36 Pollack B: Die Färbetechnik des Nervensystems, 2nd ed. Berlin, S. Karger, 1898.
37 Pollack B: Die Färbetechnik für das Nervensystem, 3rd ed. Berlin, S. Karger, 1905.
38 Pollack B: Methods of Staining the Nervous System (translated by W.R. Jack). Glasgow, F. Bauermeister, 1899.
39 Pollack B: Les méthodes de préparation et de coloration du système nerveux (traduit par J. Nicolaïdi; préface de P.-É. Launois). Paris, G. Carré et C. Naud, 1900.
40 Waldeyer HWG: Über einige neuere Forschungen im Gebiete der Anatomie des Centralnervensystems. Dtsch Med Wschr 1891; 17:1213–1218, 1244–1246, 1287–1289, 1331–1332, 1352–1356.
41 Flatau E: Atlas des menschlichen Gehirns und des Faserverlaufes. Berlin, S. Karger, 1894/1899.
42 Triarhou LC: A review of Edward Flatau's 1894 Atlas of the Human Brain by the neurologist Sigmund Freud. Eur Neurol 2011;65:10–15.
43 Ziehen T: Buch-Anzeigen – Die Färbetechnik des Nervensystems, von B. Pollack. Mschr Psychiatr Neurol 1897;1:509–510.
44 Editorial: Reviews and notes on books. Br Med J 1897;2:139–140; 1898;1:1269–1271; 1899;1:92; 1901;2:19–20; 1905;2:1528–1529.
45 Campbell AW: Die Färbetechnik für das Nervensystem, by Bernhard Pollack (book review). Brain 1905;28:88–89.
46 Bolles Lee A: The Microtomist's Vade-Mecum – A Handbook of the Methods of Microscopic Anatomy. London, J. & A. Churchill, 1885.
47 Bolles Lee A, Henneguy L-F: Traité des méthodes techniques de l'anatomie microscopique – Histologie, embryologie et zoologie. Paris, O. Doin, 1887.
48 Marinesco G: Pathologie générale de la cellule nerveuse, lésions secondaires et primitives. Presse Méd 1897;5:41–47.
49 Swab CM, Gerald HF: The ophthalmic lesions of botulism: additional notes and research. Br J Ophthalmol 1933;17:129–144.
50 Dickson EC: Botulism – a clinical and experimental study. Monogr Rockefeller Inst Med Res 1918;8:1–117.
51 Cowdry EV, Nicholson FM: An histological study of the central nervous system in experimental botulinus poisoning. J Exp Med 1924;39:827–836.
52 Pollack B: Einige erläuternde Bemerkungen zu den Neurogliapräparaten des Nervus opticus und der Medulla spinalis. Arch Psychiatr Nervenkrankh 1898;30:985.
53 Ramón y Cajal S: Das Neurofibrillennetz der Retina. Int Mschr Anat Physiol 1904;21:369–399.
54 Embden G: Primitivfibrillenverlauf in der Netzhaut. Arch Mikrosk Anat 1901;57:570–583.
55 Wässle H, Peichl L, Boycott BB: Topography of horizontal cells in the retina of the domestic cat. Proc R Soc Lond (Biol) 1978;203:269–291.

56 Pollack B: Kostenlose Augenuntersuchung. Prakt Arzt Repert Prakt Med (Leipz) 1916; 56:215–221, 248–250.
57 Pollack B: Filaria loa. Z Augenheilk 1906;16: 84–85.
58 Pollack B: Demonstration einer Filaria Loa. Klin Wschr 1923;2:1621.
59 Pollack B: Gliom des Optikus. Berl Klin Wschr 1921;58:210–211.
60 Pollack B: Ein Spindelzellensarcom des Sinus frontalis. Cbl Prakt Augenheilk (Leipz) 1905;29:51.
61 Pollack B: Ein 60jähriger Mann mit Metastatischem Chorioideal-Carcinom. Z Augenheilk 1905;13:66–67.
62 Pollack B: Mikulicz'sche Krankheit. Cbl Prakt Augenheilk (Leipz) 1905;29:298.
63 Flatau E, Jacobsohn L: XII. Internationaler medicinischer Congress zu Moskau; Section für Geistes- und Nervenkrankheiten. Arch Psychiatr Nervenkrankh 1897;30:295–322.
64 Flatau E, Jacobsohn L: XII. Internationaler medicinischer Congress in Moskau; Sitzungsbericht über die Sektion für Nerven- und Geisteskrankheiten. Mschr Psychiatr Neurol 1897;2:307–314, 392–404, 451–474.
65 Eisenberg U: Vom 'Nervenplexus' zur 'Seelenkraft'. Werk und Schicksal des Berliner Neurologen Louis Jacobsohn-Lask (1863–1940). Frankfurt a.M., P. Lang, 2005.
66 Pollack B: Bericht über den X. Internationalen Ophthalmologen-Kongress in Luzern. Z Augenheilk 1904;12:686–719.
67 Eisenberg U: Home away from home: the Berlin neuroanatomist Louis Jacobsohn-Lask in Russia; in Solomon SG (ed): Doing Medicine Together; Germany and Russia between the Wars. Toronto, University of Toronto Press, 2006, pp 407–460.
68 Pollack B: Färbetechnik und anatomische Untersuchungsmethoden des Nervensystems. Jber Leist Fortschr Geb Neurol Psychiatr 1903;6:1–10; 1904;7:1–10; 1905;8:1–13; 1906;9:1–7; 1907;10:1–6; 1908;11:1–5.
69 Pollack B: Fortschritte der microscopischen Technik für die Untersuchung des Nervensystems. Mschr Psychiatr Neurol 1897;2: 299–306.
70 Pollack B: Neuere Arbeiten aus dem Gebiete der mikroskopischen Anatomie des Nervensystems, mit Einschluss der Faserverlaufs. Mschr Psychiatr Neurol 1898;3:196–201.
71 Pollack B: Referate und Berichte aus den Berliner Gesellschaften. Z Augenheilk 1899;2: 90–92, 218–219.
72 Pollack B: Berliner Ophthalmologische Gesellschaft – Sitzung vom 17. November 1904. Z Augenheilk 1905;13:66–69.
73 Pollack B: Erinnerungen an Moritz Moszkowski. Berl Tagebl Handels-Ztg 1925(Mar 14);54:2–3.
74 Assenov B: Moritz Moszkowski – eine Werkmonographie. Berlin, Geisteswissenschaftliche Fakultät der Technischen Universität, 2009.
75 Kolb F: Moszkowski, Moritz/Maurice; in Finscher L (ed): Die Musik in Geschichte und Gegenwart, Personenteil 12, 2nd ed. Kassel – Basel, Bärenreiter-Verlag/Stuttgart – Weimar, J.B. Metzler, 2004, pp 541–543.
76 Widgery CJ: Fritz Kreisler Collection. Washington, DC, Library of Congress – Music Division, 1992, box 9/folder 9.
77 Leibbrand W: Musik und Medizin; in Schwarz V (ed): Der Musik-Almanach. München, K. Desch, 1948, pp 212–227.
78 Pollack B: Musikalisches Gedächtniss. Neurol Cbl (Leipz) 1897;16:335–336.
79 Pollack B: Besprechungen – Heinrich Rietsch. Die Tonkunst in der zweiten Hälfte des neunzehnten Jahrhunderts. Z Ästhetik Allg Kunstwiss (Stuttg) 1908;3:609–610.
80 Pollack B: Aerzte-Orchester-Verein. Berl Aerzte Corresp 1911;16:112, 116, 120, 197, 212, 216, 248.
81 Williams D: Literary notes. Br Med J 1911;2: 305.
82 Weinfield E: Medical men who have attained fame in other fields of endeavor. I. Medical men as musicians. Ann Int Med 1930;3: 1046–1054.
83 Nickling HG: Berliner Gesellschaft für Innere Medizin e.V. – Versuch einer unvermeidlich lückenhaften chronologischen Zusammenstellung. Berlin, C. Boldt, 1999.
84 Schick A: The pluralism of psychiatry in Vienna. Psychoanal Rev 1978;65:14–37.
85 Bürgermeister JF: Wissenswertes-Unterhaltsames. Wesenitztaler Landbote 2009;19:27. http://www.duerrroehrsdorf-dittersbach.de/Haupt-seite/Service/Mitteilungsblatt_Mai09.pdf (accessed June 24, 2010).
86 Godowsky L: Letter to Freda Godowsky dated Apr 21, 1901; in Benko G (ed): International Piano Archives. College Park, MD, University of Maryland Libraries, 2005.
87 Seeber L: Music Notes – Moritz Moszkowski (1854–1925): Piano Concerto in E Major, op. 59. Englewood Cliffs, NJ, Moss Music Group, 1992.
88 Downes O: The passing of Moritz Moszkowski – Traits of a brilliant personality. The New York Times 1925(Mar 22); Section: Drama Music Screen Art, p 132.
89 Sohn J: Moszkowski, Moritz; in Singer I (ed): The Jewish Encyclopedia, vol. IX. New York – London, Funk & Wagnalls, 1905, p 97.
90 Moszkowski M: Moritz Moszkowski on himself. Etude Music Magazine. Philadelphia, Theodore Presser Co., 1910 (Jan). http://scriabin.com/etude/1910/01/moritz-moszkowski-on-himself.html (accessed June 20, 2010).
91 Aldrich R: 15 Noted pianists play in ensemble. The New York Times, 1921(Dec 22); Section: Amusements, p 21.
92 Horner NG: Memoranda. Br Med J 1928;1: 1003–1005.
93 Wolfsohn-Jaffé E: Professor Doktor Bernhard Pollack. Berl Aerzte Corresp 1928;33: 97–98.

Ramón y Cajal as an Analytical Chemist of Bottled Water? Use (and Misuse) of the Great Savant's Repute by the Industry

Lazaros C. Triarhou[1] and Manuel del Cerro[2]

Abstract
The name of the eminent neurohistologist Santiago Ramón y Cajal (1852-1934) was occasionally mentioned in commercial labels by the Spanish industry advertising mineral waters from natural spring sources and their medical benefits. Concomitantly with his landmark neuroanatomical research, Cajal had served as director of the Alfonso XIII National Institute of Hygiene. In that capacity, his name had to be included in certificates as a mere bureaucratic formality. Cajal had an early interest in bacteriology, and introduced a pioneering chemical vaccine against cholera during the 1885 epidemic in Spain. However, in a letter to the Madrid press, he vehemently denied any involvement with actual chemical analyses or commercial promotion of products such as bottled water, medicinal wines, disinfectants, and even toothpaste. In this episode, we realize that Cajal's view was absolutely contrary to the impression one might have gathered on the basis of the commercial documents alone.

Keywords
cholera epidemic, history of neuroscience, Santiago Ramón y Cajal (1852-1934)

Introduction

The life of the ingenious neurohistologist Santiago Ramón y Cajal (1852-1934), Spain's restive spirit fittingly hailed as "El gran sabio Español" or great Spanish savant (Caullery, 1934; Ferrari Billoch, 1957; Hasselberg, Pettersson, Mörner, Wirsén, & Santesson, 1908), remains an inexhaustible repository of history bits. As a child, he painted and experimented with explosives (Ramón y Cajal, 1988; Triarhou & del Cerro, 2008a). As an academic physician, besides studying nervous tissue, he pioneered the invention of a cholera vaccine (Ramón y Cajal, 1885a, 1885b), practiced hypnosis for labor analgesia (Stefanidou, Solà, Kouvelas, del Cerro, & Triarhou, 2007), analyzed cross-sections of photographic film under the microscope (Triarhou & del Cerro, 2008b), and conjectured on the psychology of poets (Triarhou & Vivas, 2009).

The present article examines certain claims made by the bottled water industry in commercial documents, implying Cajal's involvement in the capacity of an analytical chemist. Among other things, Cajal is mentioned as director by the *Cabreiroá* mineral water company of Verín, Galicia, and as having performed chemical analyses for the *Carabaña* mineral water company of Madrid.

Cajal had entered the Spanish medical corps after obtaining the doctor's degree in 1873. Having a strong national character and being in excellent physical shape, he served as a lieutenant physician in the Third Carlist War, and subsequently as a captain in the Cuban War. His stay in Cuba was marked by hardship and disease. The decline of Spain's colonial policy, a war fought in a hostile climate, and corruption among military officers led Cajal to be stationed in a theater of operations with a rigid logistical system of "trails," which would end up in military failure and a loss of the colony. Disappointed and seriously ill from malaria, Cajal returned to Spain on a sick leave. Shortly thereafter, thanks to Dr. Genaro Casas, he became a university lecturer, ending his military career (Moreno-Martínez & Martín-Araguz, 2002).

During his military service in Cuba, Cajal nearly died of dysentery. Later, during his Valencia years and his tenure as anatomy chairman there, he witnessed the 1885 cholera outbreak. Owing to his knowledge of microbiology (Ramón y Cajal, 1905; Ramón y Cajal Junquera, 2000), he managed to protect his family by boiling the water (Ramón y Cajal, 1988).

The Claims

Jaraba de Aragón

One of the earliest links of Ramón y Cajal's name with mineral waters dates to 1895 in the *balneario* (spa) of Serón in Jaraba (41°11′36.24″ N, 1°53′0.96″ W, altitude 763 m), 135

[1]University of Macedonia, Thessaloniki, Greece
[2]University of Rochester, NY, USA

Corresponding Author:
Lazaros C. Triarhou, Neuroscience Wing, University of Macedonia, Egnatia 156, 54006 Thessaloniki, Greece.
Email: triarhou@uom.gr

km from Zaragoza (Giménez Herrero, 1994; San Martín Bacaicoa & Valero Castejón, 2004).

Cajal is mentioned as having frequented Jaraba and other resorts in Aragón. In a dedication, dated August 16, 1895, he appears as having written that, after spending a few days in the spa establishment of Serón, he had the opportunity to observe "significant relief and surprising revolutionary cures in diseases such as lithiasis and its common complications of the urinary tract, in gout, in chronic rheumatism, in diabetes mellitus, and in uterine catarrhoea." The beneficial effects at the popular summer resort and *sanatorium* were attributed to the action exerted by the chemical constituents of mineral water on nutrition and secretions (de Gregorio y Guajardo, 1895; Giménez Herrero, 1994; San Martín Bacaicoa & Valero Castejón, 2004).

Cabreiroá de Verín

Verín (41°56′27″ N, 7°26′9″ W) is a town in Galicia (Province of Orense), located 15 km north of the Portuguese city of Chaves, at an altitude of 373 m. The denominated wine region of Monterrey is located in the surrounding area. Three mineral water bottling plants are based in Verín: *Cabreiroá, Fontenova,* and *Sousas*.

The *Cabreiroá* mineral water company was established and began commercial bottling at the source in 1906 (the year that Cajal and Camillo Golgi were awarded the Nobel Prize in Physiology or Medicine). Xosé García Barbón (1831-1909), a Verín native and benefactor, officially started the works after returning from a long and successful stay in Cuba, where he had founded his own bank, as well as the Galician Center of La Habana. Besides founding the Hotel Spa of Cabreiroá, Barbón built in Vigo the theater that bears his name (*Teatro García Barbón*, also housing the *Centro Cultural Caixanova*) and the School of Arts and Crafts (*Escola Municipal de Artes e Oficios*).

The health properties of the Cabreiroá spring water were praised internationally. In 1907, Cajal's post as "director" was printed on labels (Baeza Rodríguez-Caro et al., 2003; Murillo, 1913). Cabreiroá mineral water was imported in Argentina by the Echegaray brothers (Figure 1).

The Cabreiroá company has engaged in the bottling and marketing of its mineral water for over a century. It was advertised that Ramón y Cajal had certified the excellent status of this water and its mineral-medicinal properties. The resort in the vicinity of the spring was in operation through the 1950s (Grupo 2T C.A., 2010).

Ramón y Cajal is reported to have been an ardent supporter of the therapeutic properties of mineral waters (de la Rosa & Mosso, 2004). In September 1909, Cajal spent a few days in Cabreiroá and apparently told a Galician newspaper, "Thanks to the virtues of the Cabreiroá spring I have regained my health that was seriously compromised by the debilitating effects of a chronic intestinal catarrhoea and by the threat of hepatic colic" (Rodríguez Miguez, 1995, p. 107). The words of the man who embodied the national glory would be used to promote the brand.

The company is still in operation (www.magmadecabreiroa.es). The spring is located 100 m under the ground. An octagonal temple stands at the fountain's head. The incandescent magma trapped beneath the Earth's crust releases gas mixing at the spring with the water, which rises naturally at 16°C. It was clinically prescribed for gastroenteropathies, according to the Calpe manual of medical sciences (Doz, Manzaneque, Llord y Gamboa, Rodríguez Pinilla, & Camaleño, 1922) published under Cajal's editorial direction (Figure 2).

In the celebrations that marked the centennial of Aguas de Cabreiroá, S.A., homage was paid to Ramón y Cajal and his "analyses" from the early 1900s. A bronze statue, sculpted by the Galician artist Manuel García Vázquez de Buciños, was erected to honor the Nobel Laureate (Editorial, 2006; Gabinete de Comunicación da Xunta de Galicia, 2006). The base bears an identification. On it, Cajal appears as a gentleman ("caballero") with his frock-coat ("levitón"), walking and holding in his right hand a bottle, whose contents he apparently intends to analyze. The mastery of the sculptor details a face that denotes intelligence and passion, deep intense eyes, and a chin carefully covered by the trimmed thin beard and moustache beneath the protruding nose (Pablos, 2009).

An Argentinian magazine advertisement [ca. 1908] (Figure 1, left) had claimed,

> The greatest bacteriologist of the world, Doctor S. Ramón y Cajal, who won the Nobel Prize by competing with the most eminent scholars of all nations, has affirmed with the unequivocal authority of his signature that the Cabreiroá natural mineral water is bacteriologically pure and of excellent hygienic conditions. The best table water for habitual consumption. Pure, crystalline, fresh, light, of great taste, very absorbable, lightly effervescent. Grand prizes obtained abroad by scientifically proven merits: Paris, May 1908; Genoa, July 1908; Brussels, October 1908. Cabreiroá water is absolutely natural, without chemical manipulations nor artificial additives.

> The salubrious action of Cabreiroá water is perfectly explained by its absolute bacteriological purity and by its remarkable chemical composition. The mineral salts it contains are dosed by nature in a very harmonious and balanced form, such that each, in producing the rightful action, enhances the effect of the others. Thus, the extraordinary proportion of carbonic acid, further makes it eminently digestive, favoring the absorption of alkaline salts, which in turn operate on the blood, removing all of its impurities; the bicarbonates operate on the stomach and the digestive tract, while the lithium oxide exerts its action on the liver and the kidneys.

> Information brochures available. Exclusive dealer for South America: Echegaray Brothers and Co., 1002-1026 Victoria Street [Buenos Aires]. Turn off the faucet. Cholera threatens us, typhoid fever lurks. We must guard against all proper infectious diseases of the season that are acquired through

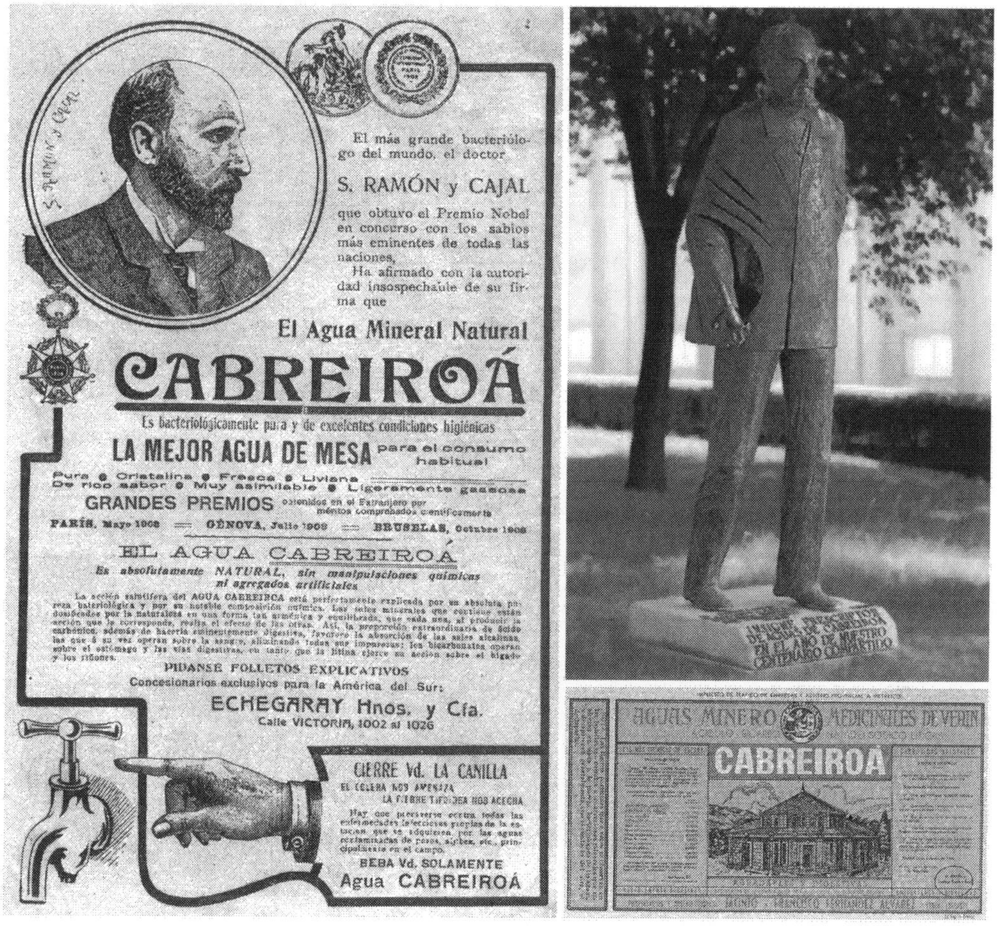

Figure 1. Left: Ramón y Cajal featured in an export advertisement for the Galician bottled water company of *Cabreiroá*, which he directed (from an Argentinian magazine [ca. 1908]; authors' archive). Upper right: Statue of Ramón y Cajal dedicated in 2006 on the occasion of the company's centennial (Pablos, 2009). Lower right: A label from the Cabreiroá water company, with the name of its director, Santiago Ramón y Cajal, appearing at the lower right corner, encircled (Baeza Rodríguez-Caro et al., 2003).

contaminated water from wells, cisterns, etc. mainly in the field. Drink only Cabreiroá water.

The label (Figure 1, lower right) mentions, among other things, "Minero-medicinal water of Verín . . . Pleasant and digestive . . . Naturally carbonated . . . Hygienic analysis . . . The Director, Santiago Ramón y Cajal. Owners and distributors: Jacinto and Francisco Fernandez Álvarez, Verín, Orense." It was advertised as "indispensable for diseases of the stomach, intestine, liver, kidney and diabetes. Ideal table water."

Another figure, mentioned to have praised Cabreiroá was José Casares Gil (1866-1961), the president of the Royal Academy of Pharmacy between January 1940 and June 1958 (Rodríguez Miguez, 2006).

Declared a public utility by Royal Order on December 15, 1906, Cabreiroá achieved reputation for its exceptional qualities, top-ranking not only in Spain but also among famous mineral waters abroad (Figure 3). Its annual exports exceeded 600,000 bottles in 1908; competing against similar national and renowned foreign brands, such as Vichy and Royal of France, and Ems and Fachingen of Germany, Cabreiroá was awarded the *Grand Prix* with special distinction by the Jury of the joint 1908 Spanish–French Exposition of Zaragoza (Editorial, 1908).

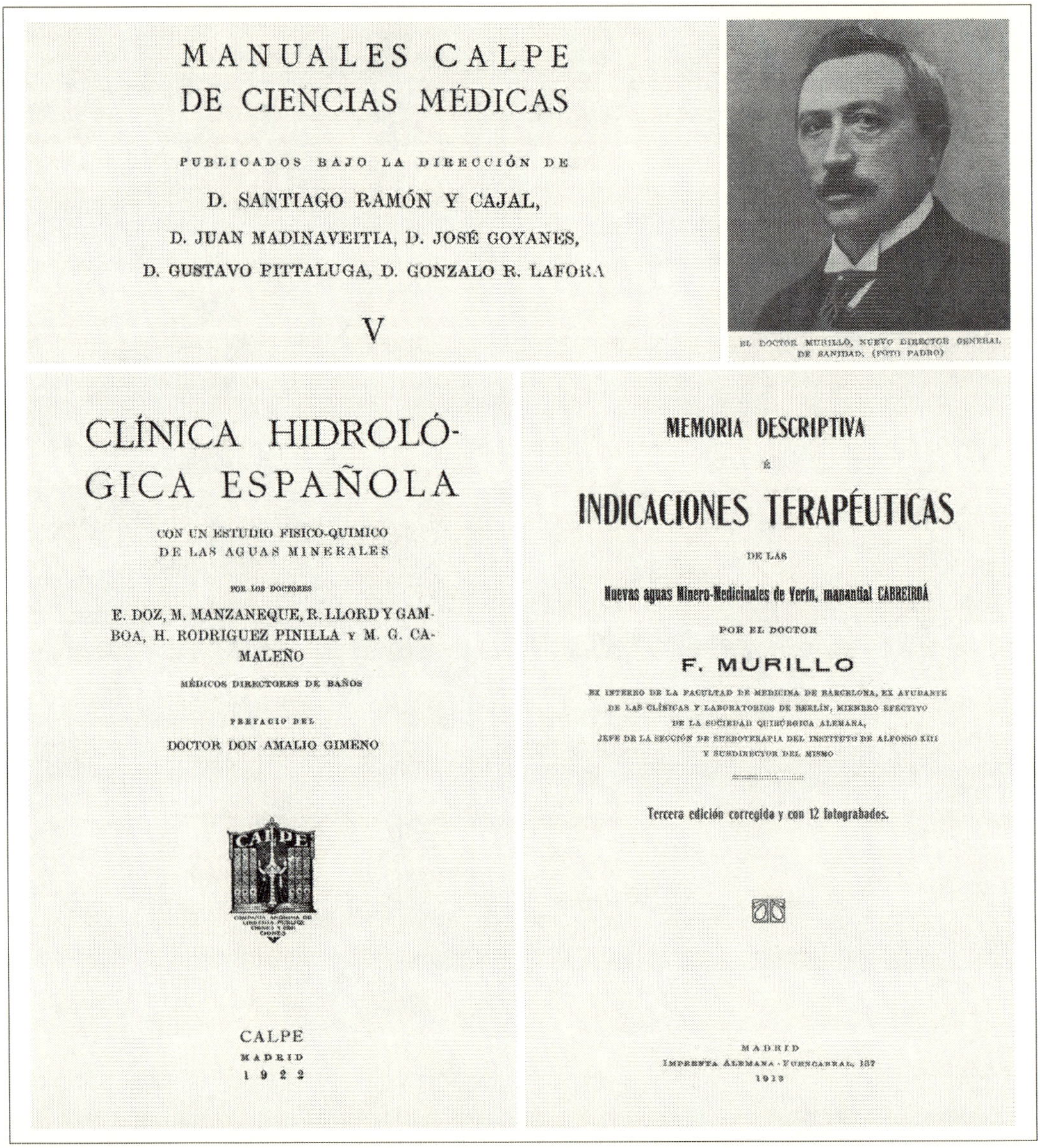
MANUALES CALPE
DE CIENCIAS MÉDICAS

PUBLICADOS BAJO LA DIRECCIÓN DE

D. SANTIAGO RAMÓN Y CAJAL,

D. JUAN MADINAVEITIA, D. JOSÉ GOYANES,

D. GUSTAVO PITTALUGA, D. GONZALO R. LAFORA

V

CLÍNICA HIDROLÓ-
GICA ESPAÑOLA

CON UN ESTUDIO FISICO-QUIMICO
DE LAS AGUAS MINERALES

POR LOS DOCTORES

E. DOZ, M. MANZANEQUE, R. LLORD Y GAM-
BOA, H. RODRIGUEZ PINILLA Y M. G. CA-
MALEÑO

MÉDICOS DIRECTORES DE BAÑOS

PREFACIO DEL

DOCTOR DON AMALIO GIMENO

CALPE
MADRID
1922

MEMORIA DESCRIPTIVA

É

INDICACIONES TERAPÉUTICAS

DE LAS

Nuevas aguas Minero-Medicinales de Verín, manantial CABREIROÁ

POR EL DOCTOR

F. MURILLO

EX INTERNO DE LA FACULTAD DE MEDICINA DE BARCELONA, EX AYUDANTE
DE LAS CLÍNICAS Y LABORATORIOS DE BERLÍN, MIEMBRO EFECTIVO
DE LA SOCIEDAD QUIRÚRGICA ALEMANA,
JEFE DE LA SECCIÓN DE SUEROTERAPIA DEL INSTITUTO DE ALFONSO XIII
Y SUBDIRECTOR DEL MISMO

Tercera edición corregida y con 12 fotograbados.

MADRID
IMPRENTA ALEMANA - FUENCARRAL, 137
1913

Figure 2. Upper left: Editorial committee of Calpe's manuals of medical sciences, headed by Cajal. Upper right: Doctor Murillo, new director general of hygiene (photo by Padro, appearing in *Revista Blanco y Negro [Madrid]*, issue of December 30, 1923, p. 2). Lower left: Monograph titled "Spanish Hydrological Clinic" in the Calpe medical science series (Doz, Manzaneque, Llord y Gamboa, Rodríguez Pinilla, & Camaleño, 1922). Lower right: Murillo's monograph on the Cabreiroá Spring (Murillo, 1913).

Perla del Castellar

Cajal's name was also associated with *La Perla del Castellar* water in Villarrubia de Santiago (39°59′1″ N 3°22′7″ W, altitude 750 m), 65 km from Toledo (Rodríguez Miguez, 1995), which was recommended for its composition of sodium sulfate as a purgative, and promoted for the treatment of scrofula and herpes (Figure 4). The following advertisement had appeared in August 1907 in Barcelona's newspaper *La Vanguardia* (Figure 4, upper right):

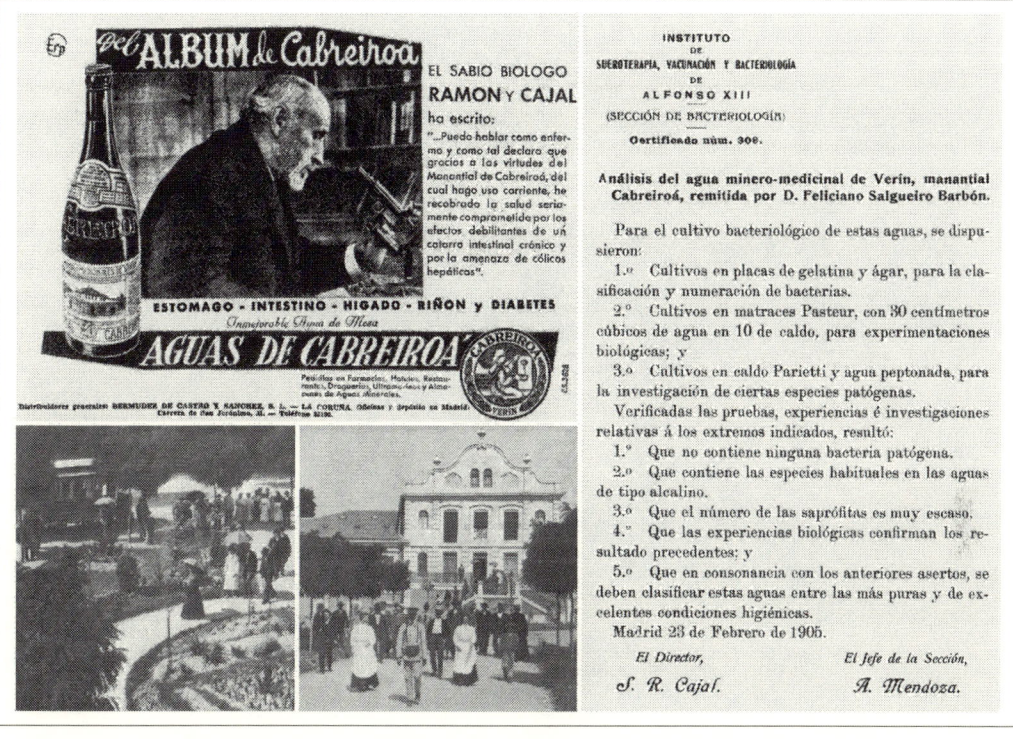

Figure 3. Upper left: An advertisement of *Cabreiroá* mineral water in the Madrid publication *Revista ABC*, citing Ramón y Cajal's comments on its medicinal properties and appearing in print 10 years after his death (issue of November 7, 1944, p. 2). Lower left: The kiosk and garden toward the terrace (far left figure) and the grounds (center figure) of the Cabreiroá spring establishment (Murillo, 1913). Right: Certificate of Cajal's bacteriological analysis on the official letterhead of the "Royal Spanish Institute of Serum Therapy, Vaccination and Bacteriology" (Murillo, 1913).

Natural purgative waters and salts "La Perla del Castellar," analyzed by Dr. S. Ramón y Cajal and other national and foreign eminences, unique in the world, with real medicinal thenardite. Laxative, antibilious, appetizing, diuretic and essentially cleansing. Never irritates or weakens, the most gentle, efficient and economical of all laxatives. Free sampling: Segalá, Rambla Flores, 4. Sold everywhere. Warehouse: Balmes, 83.

"Thenardite" (anhydrous Na_2SO_4) is found in arid evaporite environments, such as dry and volcanic caves. Named after Louis Jacques Thénard (1777-1826)—professor of chemistry at Collège de France, Faculty of Sciences and École Polytechnique of Paris—thenardite forms yellowish, reddish-to-grey-white prismatic crystals and is fluorescent. In humid conditions, it gradually absorbs water and converts to the mineral "mirabilite" ($Na_2SO_4 \cdot 10H_2O$; en.wikipedia.org/wiki/Thenardite).

Agua de Carabaña

In the late 19th century, the mineral water industry of Carabaña *La Favorita* was born when the Chávarri family acquired the property of the spring and surrounding land, and built a spa that became very popular. The Carabaña mineral water was rendered commercially available by Ruperto Jacinto Chávarri on December 11, 1883. It was exported to England, Portugal, Prussia, and Germany. In the early 20th century, Carabaña bottled water was sold in many other countries, including France, Italy, Cuba, and Panama.

Cajal was mentioned as having carried out chemical analyses of Carabaña spring water (Figure 4), along with Gabriel de la Puerta y Ródenas (1839-1908), professor of chemistry at the School of Pharmacy of the University of Madrid. The water was promoted for its curative and medicinal properties. On May 4, 1928, the product became officially qualified as "Highly Recommended for Public Use" (Editorial, 1991, p. 63).

The water contained sodium sulfate (Doz et al., 1922). The town of Carabaña (40°15′25″ N, 3°14′4″ W) at *Cerro de Cabeza Gorda* is 50 km outside Madrid. For centuries, since Roman times, water from the spring had been used for body care with internal and external applications, also known to local countrymen and shepherds. From the mid-1800s, the

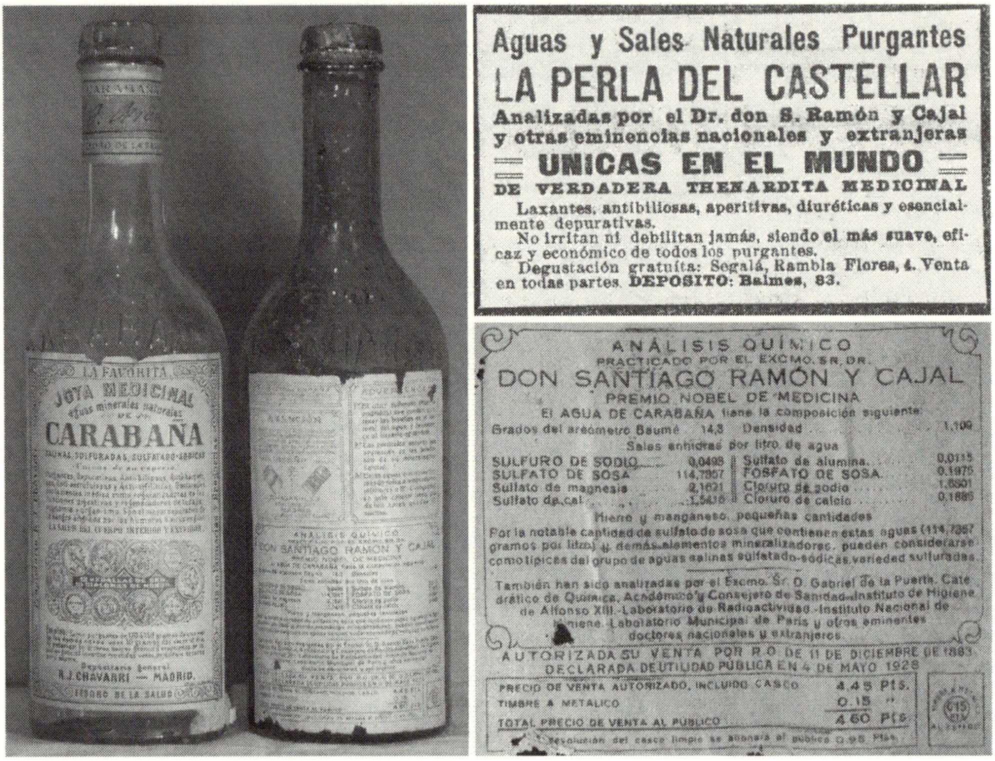

Figure 4. Left: Two bottles of Carabaña company's *La Favorita* mineral water from the outskirts of Madrid. The reverse bottle label on the right shows Cajal's chemical analysis. Salt residue still exists at the bottom of the bottle's inside [ca. 1928]. A detail of the label with Cajal's name can be seen at the lower right figure; the flat image of the label was obtained by rotating the bottle manually on the scanner glass surface, while the light drum was advancing. Upper right: An advertisement for *Perla del Castellar* water approved by Cajal, appearing in Barcelona's newspaper *La Vanguardia* (Thursday, August 22, 1907, p. 9; also appearing on Sunday, August 25, 1907, p. 11; bottles and documents from the authors' private collection).

water was distributed in carafes to nearby places and was used to treat various ailments.

Carabaña's minero-medicinal water gained recognition at Universal Expositions with 12 gold medals and 10 honorary diplomas, including the 1889 Exhibition in Paris. At the beginning of the 20th century, Carabaña water was commercialized in Europe and America, where an estimated figure of four million bottles were being sold in the 1930s.

The water was prescribed for gastrointestinal and hepatic diseases, and externally for skin treatments (Editorial, 1913). The commercial descriptions mentioned "purgative, laxative, antibilious, purifying, anti-herpetic," "medicinal jewel for maintaining health and for curing diseases," and "treasure of health." Beginning in 1904, the company manufactured medicinal soap bars enriched in mineral salts collected from the evaporation of natural spring water. The company remains active today (www.aguadecarabana.com), producing and marketing natural health products.

The following information appears on the label of the bottle shown in Figure 4 (cf. also Editorial, 1913, p. 4):

Chemical analysis carried out by his excellence Dr. Santiago Ramón y Cajal, Nobel Prize in Medicine. The water of Carabaña has the following composition: Baumé aerometer grades 14.3; density 1.109; anhydrous salts per liter of water: Na sulfide 0.0493; Na sulfate 114.7357; Mg sulfate 2.1621; Ca sulfate 1.5416; Al sulfate 0.0115; Na phosphate 0.1975; Na chloride 1.6301; Ca chloride 0.1886; F and Mn small quantities. By its marked quantity of Na sulfate that this water contains (114.7357 g/L) and the other mineral elements it can be considered as typical of the group of Na sulfate mineral waters, the sulfur variety.

Carabaña is one of the best known waters of Madrid, operating since 1883 and being still sold commercially in pharmacies. It comes from the *Charca de la Salina* ("Salty Pond"); the source is known as *La Favorita*. Estimated daily flow is 9,500 dm^3 (Fraguas, 2007; Navarro García, 2010).

In the early 20th century, bottled water was exported by the Carabaña Company to France, Italy, and Portugal, and to the Spanish colonies, including Cuba, Puerto Rico, and the Philippines. The sales, in 1907, were estimated to three million 0.5-L bottles. Shortly after, business was expanded to the production of Epsom salts and soap (el Sáb, 2009).

Agua de Carabaña ranks among the highest in the world regarding the concentration of calcium (505 mg/L) and magnesium (552 mg/L; Vasey, 2006).

La Toja

The "Isla de la Toja" (also "Illa da Toxa" or "Illa de Louxo") is located in the Rías Bajas in the Province of Pontevedra in Galicia, at distances of 30 km from Vilagarcía, 32 km from Pontevedra, and 18 km from Cambados. Famous for its spa, it is covered by green vegetation and surrounded by a sea of crystal clear water. Its thermal mud and medicinal water springs were discovered in the 19th century. Its soaps ("el jabón La Toja") had been a favorite of the Buenos Aires *señoras*.

The 50°C spring with its hypertonic sodium chloride composition, in a granitic terrain of probable volcanic genesis, was indicated for gynecologic conditions (Doz et al., 1922). A liter of "agua de La Toja" in addition contained 20.2 ml anhydrous carbonate, 10.8 ml oxygen, 29.2 ml nitrogen, 0.40 g Mg sulfate, 0.98 g Ca sulfate, 0.18 g Mg carbonate, 0.87 g Ca carbonate, 0.10 g Fe sesquioxide, and 0.12 g silica (Doz et al., 1922).

On the basis of the physicochemical properties of its spring, Cajal is reported to have called the thermal station at La Toja "a true temple of health" (Pérez, 1983, p. 32). He is mentioned to have expressed his views of La Toja as follows:

> Nature created here a salutary and almost unique spring seen as incomparable. The peaceful island is bathed by the most beautiful Galician estuaries, invigorating sea breezes scented by the balmy emanations of the forest, temperature being always spring-like under a clear and bright sky. Art and science, working in concert, have realized the work of nature. By this time, La Toja has fallen into the hands of skilled craftsmen, who have been striving to provide the swimmer with the excellence of a hydrotherapy facility wisely organized, a magnificent residence, a true temple devoted to health, which combines into a happy marriage the refinements of the most demanding comfort with the most scrupulous precautions of hygiene. (Otero Pedrayo, 1954, p. 322)

The Counter-Claim

At first glance, one might surmise that the water analyses in the commercial documents and labels bearing Cajal's name reflected yet another aspect of his diverse scientific avocations.

On one hand, it appears less complicated to explain why Cajal might extol, on several occasions, the medicinal properties of spring waters of the Iberian peninsula. After all, such claims were likely rooted in medical paradigms of his age. The 1800s had seen a widespread enthusiasm for water cures, Darwin being one of thousands of famous patients at water spas. In that aspect of conventional medicine, Cajal might not be doing much different than his contemporaries or anything particularly rigorous by the standards of his work in neuroanatomy.

Furthermore, it is understandable that Cajal, an amateur astronomer and nature lover, felt for the unspoilt corners of his land, such as the tiny town of Verín, one of the many along slow roads from Santiago de Compostela to Salamanca. These are places where the traveler can soak his spirit in the essence of Spain. The night sky is velvet blue, the stars shine as they do not shine in our light-polluted cities. And the silence! It is a silence that "heals the mind."

On the other hand, there is a questionable quality as to how water bottlers were using Cajal's reputation to promote products. Sometimes, a "Great Man" style in industrial advertising can be insufficiently critical, lacking the hard evidence from properly controlled studies for the products being truly efficacious.

The reply comes from a unique, and surprising letter, from Ramón y Cajal himself, hosted in the *Diario Ilustrado ABC* on April 22, 1926 (Figure 5), under an unmistakable title: "How My Modest Name Is Exploited by Certain Unscrupulous Industries" (Ramón y Cajal, 1926). Cajal reiterates that he never practiced any industrial analysis, neither as an individual nor as director of the Alfonso XIII Institute, and clarifies that, if his name appears in some documents, it is only owing to a bureaucratic formality requiring to include the formal approval (B.° V.° or "bueno visto") of the director of the Institute.

The complete text of the letter reads as follows (authors' English translation):

> The most cultivated writer Gómez de Baquero said that the least Spanish virtue is respect. My case eloquently corroborates that sensible observation. I allude to a misuse initiated since I was nominated, at the suggestion of the illustrious doctor Cortezo, director of the Alfonso XIII National Institute of Hygiene. This misuse, committed by quite a lot of industries, consists in gratuitously attributing to me the execution of the analysis of specifics, of medicinal wines, of mineral waters, disinfectants, cigarette paper, toothpaste and other products, of which I have no idea. Such a myth has spread so, that it has even invaded the foreign press (including a current claim in a Swedish newspaper), and has generated within Spain, in magazines of great prestige, commentaries hardly pleasant to me. And yet the tide keeps rising. Today I was informed that the Radio Company has credited me with the analysis of the waters of Venta del Hoyo (waters of which I have not the slightest idea), and that a witted

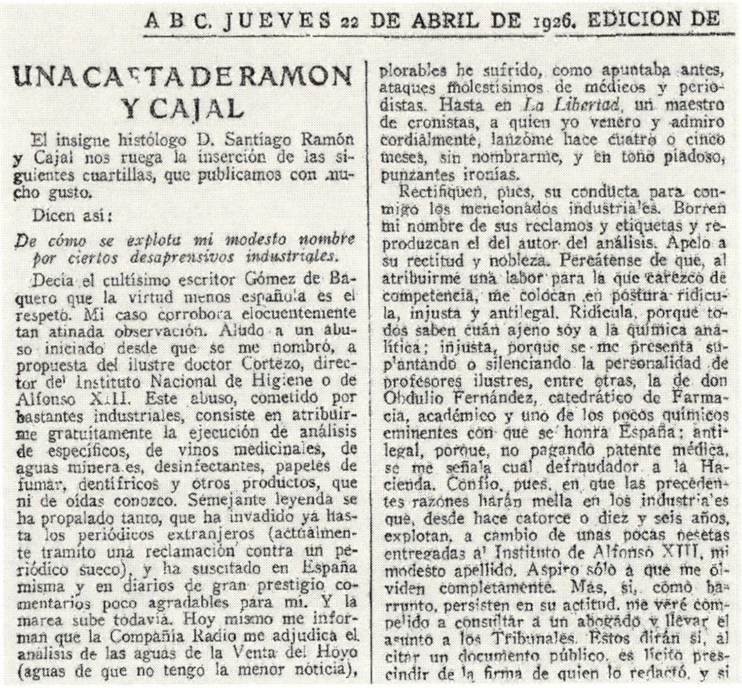

A B C. JUEVES 22 DE ABRIL DE 1926. EDICION DE

UNA CAᵀTA DE RAMON Y CAJAL

El insigne histólogo D. Santiago Ramón y Cajal nos ruega la inserción de las siguientes cuartillas, que publicamos con mucho gusto.

Dicen así:

De cómo se explota mi modesto nombre por ciertos desaprensivos industriales.

Decía el cultísimo escritor Gómez de Baquero que la virtud menos españo'a es el respeto. Mi caso corrobora elocuentemente tan atinada observación. Aludo a un abuso iniciado desde que se me nombró, a propuesta del ilustre doctor Cortezo, director de' Instituto Nacional de Higiene o de Alfonso XIII. Este abuso, cometido por bastantes industriales, consiste en atribuirme gratuitamente la ejecución de análisis de específicos, de vinos medicinales, de aguas minera es, desinfectantes, papeles de fumar, dentífricos y otros productos, que ni de oídas conozco. Semejante leyenda se ha propalado tanto, que ha invadido ya hasta los periódicos extranjeros (actualmente tramito una reclamación contra un periódico sueco), y ha suscitado en España misma y en diarios de gran prestigio comentarios poco agradables para mí. Y la marea sube todavía. Hoy mismo me informan que la Compañía Radio me adjudica el análisis de las aguas de la Venta del Hoyo (aguas de que no tengo la menor noticia), plorables he sufrido, como apuntaba antes, ataques molestísimos de médicos y periodistas. Hasta en *La Libertad*, un maestro de cronistas, a quien yo venero y admiro cordialmente, lanzóme hace cuatro o cinco meses, sin nombrarme, y en tono piadoso, punzantes ironías.

Rectifiquen, pues, su conducta para conmigo los mencionados industria'es. Borren mi nombre de sus reclamos y etiquetas y reproduzcan el del autor del análisis. Apelo a su rectitud y nobleza. Percátense de que, al atribuirme una labor para la que carezco de competencia, me colocan en postura ridícula, injusta y antilegal. Ridícula, porque todos saben cuán ajeno soy a la química analítica; injusta, porque se me presenta suplantando o silenciando la personalidad de profesores ilustres, entre otras, la de don Obdulio Fernández, catedrático de Farmacia, académico y uno de los pocos químicos eminentes con que se honra España; antilegal, porque, no pagando patente médica, se me seña'a cual defraudador a la Hacienda. Confío, pues, en que las precedentes razones harán mella en los industria'es que, desde hace catorce o diez y seis años, explotan, a cambio de unas pocas pesetas entregadas a' Instituto de Alfonso XIII, mi modesto apellido. Aspiro sólo a que me olviden completamente. Más, si, como barrunto, persisten en su actitud, me veré compelido a consultar a un abogado y llevar el asunto a los Tribunales. Estos dirán si, al citar un documento público, es lícito prescindir de la firma de quien lo redactó, y si

Figure 5. A fragment of Cajal's letter published on April 22, 1926, in *Revista ABC* (Vol. 22, no. 7272, p. 21) in Madrid (Ramón y Cajal, 1926).

merchant, in whose house I purchased a spray gun for disinfectants (I paid, naturally), advises his clients to consult me on its efficacy. Finally, as I write these lines, I am informed that in the central theater there appears a sign, which gratuitously attributes to me the analysis of the waters of Hoznayo.

It is urgent, then, to straighten things, by stating that:

First. I have never conducted any industrial analysis, neither as an individual nor as director of the Alfonso XIII Institute, a position that I resigned 6 years ago.

Second. That the experts' certificates handed over to individuals by the said Institute were authorized by the signature of the section chief, the true author of the analysis, with the approval of the director, stamped at the bottom, as required by regulations.

Third. That the tariff of prices, extremely reasonable, were approved by the Directorate of Health, in accordance with a ruling, under which half the amount of the honorarium is destined to bolster the infrastructure and the rest to subsidize the personnel, which, during the initial years of the organization of the Institute, was receiving inadequate stipends.

If the industrial references had pointed on their labels or in their magazine advertisements the official establishment where the expert work was carried out, the name of the authoring professor directly responsible, plus the approval of the director (a bureaucratic imperative, which only expresses the mere sentiment of confidence in the competence and integrity of the analyst), I would be content with all the claims; but the fact is that almost all claims published by the advertisers systematically and maliciously omit the name of the Institute, eliminating that of the illustrious chemistry professor charged with the service, and it is only stated *analyzed, or consulted, by Dr. Cajal, etc.*, even though the report entails bland judgments or formulates restrictions, reservations, and even failures outright unfavorable.

Some will think that all this is suspicions or cogitations of mine. No. Insofar as, even in the minute, the *whole* truth should always shine, for the deplorable tolerances I have suffered, as stated earlier, molestation attacks by doctors and journalists. Even in *La Libertad*, a master of journalists, whom I wholeheartedly revere and admire, expressed 4 or 5 months ago, without naming, and in a pious tone, caustic ironies.

Let the aforementioned industries, then, rectify their conduct toward me. Erase my name from their claims and labels and reproduce that of author of the analysis. I appeal to their rectitude and nobility. Announce that, attributing to me a work for which I am not competent brings me into a ridiculous, unjust, and unlawful position. Ridiculous, because everyone knows how oblivious I am in analytical chemistry; unjust, because I would appear to supplant or silence the personality of the illustrious professors, among others, that of Mr. Obtulio Fernández, Professor and Chairman of Pharmacy, an academic and one of the few eminent chemists honoring Spain; unlawful, because, not paying the medical patent signals that I defraud the Treasury. I trust, therefore, that the preceding reasons will make an impression on the industries, which, for 14 or 16 years, exploit, in exchange for a few pesetas given to the Alfonso XIII Institute, my humble name. I simply aspire to completely forget me. But if, as I suspect, they persist in their attitude, I shall be compelled to consult an attorney and to take the matter to the Courts. These will say whether, in citing a public document, it is permissible to dispense with the signature of the one who authored it, and whether a mere ritualistic approval is equivalent to the paternity of the one who performed in person, and with full competence and responsibility, the meritorious expert work. —*S. Ramón Cajal*

Discussion

This episode is an example of how the exhaustive documentation on a historical topic can prevent us from conceivably passing a message that would not correspond to reality, and from spreading a false legend. By reading Cajal's letter, we see that his view was absolutely contrary to the impression that one might have gathered on the basis of the commercial documents alone.

The story reminds of the Dutch botanist-physician Herman Boerhaave (1668-1738) in 18th-century Leiden, who was often disgruntled by fake publications with incorrect statements and had also sent a letter to the local newspaper warning about claims (mis)using his name (Koehler, 2007). His note appeared in *De Leydsche Courant* on October 9, 1726 (Schulte, 1959; cited by Koehler, 2007). In sharp words, it went as follows:

> Whereas some booksellers of this and other countries, for the sake of lucre only, have highly injured me, and scandalously cheated the public, by printing in my name several books from lectures procured (as they pretended) from my auditors, who were it so, make a very ill requital for my best endeavours to serve them; I find myself obliged to declare that I owe none such for my works, being fraudulently published without my knowledge, contrary to my will. (Lindeboom, 1974, pp. 141-142)

Cajal's medical interests covered a wide spectrum from neuroembryology (de Castro, López-Mascaraque, & de Carlos, 2007; Hamburger, 1980; Lagercrantz, 2006; Puelles, 2009) and neurohistology (Andres-Barquin, 2001, 2002; Berciano & Lafarga, 2001; DeFelipe, 2002; DeFelipe & Jones, 1992; Gibson, 1994; Lafarga, Casafont, Bengoechea, Tapia, & Berciano, 2009; Llinás, 2003; Loewy, 1971; López-Muñoz, Boya, & Alamo, 2006; Sotelo, 2003) to cardiology (de Fuentes Sagaz, 2001) and tumor biology (Martínez, Marín, Junquera, Martínez-Murillo, & Freire, 2005). His first interest in bacteriology and the pathology of inflammation developed early and continued in parallel with his neurohistological work (Iturbe, Pretó, & Lazcano, 2008; Otis, 2001; Ramón y Cajal, 1885a, 1885b, 1905; Ramón y Cajal Junquera, 2000; van Buskirk & Porter-Sánchez, 1961). Cajal's fascination with microbes and the organism's ways of fighting them is also reflected in his early fiction novels (Otis, 2001).

Bottled waters were marketed for their mineral contents, as well as (presumably) for the absence of pathogenic bacteria.

Cholera, another of Cajal's subjects of interest, was a concern in major European cities well into the beginnings of the 20th century. For example, the death of the beloved Ana Cecilia Luisa Dailliez from water-transmitted *fiebre tifoidea* in Madrid in 1912 led Mexican poet Amado Nervo (1870-1919)—also known as Juan Crisóstomo Ruiz de Nervo—to write some of the most sorrowful poetry in the Spanish language. Nervo had spent the first years of the 20th century in Europe, especially Paris, where, in 1901, he met the love of his life and they lived happily for 11 years, until her untimely death. Out of his grief and desperation, Nervo wrote his most important work, *La Amada Inmóvil* ("The Immovable Loved One"), published posthumously in 1922. One can easily imagine don Amado and don Santiago crossing each other in some street of Madrid!

The scientific interests of Ramón y Cajal (1885a, 1885b) had converged with those of Eduardo García Solá (1884, 1885a, 1885b), the Spanish pathologist who became rector of the University of Granada, through simultaneous publications on the virulent bacillus and its treatment during the 1885 cholera outbreak in Spain. The foundations of the promising new science of bacteriology had been laid by the brilliant contributions of Robert Koch (1843-1910) in Berlin, who had recently discovered the *Vibrio cholerae* (Koch, 1884, 1886, 1893).

Cajal introduced for the first time the pioneering concept of a chemical vaccine (Ramón y Cajal Junquera, 2000). For that ground-breaking work on producing a vaccine against cholera, Cajal was presented by the Provincial Government of Zaragoza with a Carl Zeiss microscope. Compared with the new *Statif* and profuse objectives, Cajal's earlier, hard-earned Verick microscope now "seemed like a rickety door bolt" (Andres-Barquin, 2001; Ramón y Cajal, 1988). The Zeiss instrument opened up totally new horizons, enabling Cajal "to attack the delicate problems of the structure of the cells without misgivings and with the requisite efficiency" and eventually to decipher the minute structure of the nervous system. From that work, and that microscope, modern neurobiology was born.

Acknowledgments

The authors express their gratitude to Dr. Peter J. Koehler of Atrium Medical Center, Heerlen, the Netherlands, and to Dr. John Waller of Michigan State University, East Lansing, Michigan, the United States, for invaluable input.

Declaration of Conflicting Interests

The author(s) declared no potential conflicts of interest with respect to the research, authorship, and/or publication of this article.

Funding

The author(s) received no financial support for the research and/or authorship of this article.

References

Andres-Barquin, P. J. (2001). Ramón y Cajal: A century after the publication of his masterpiece. *Endeavour, 25*, 13-17.

Andres-Barquin, P. J. (2002). Santiago Ramón y Cajal and the Spanish school of neurology. *Lancet Neurology, 1*, 445-452.

Baeza Rodríguez-Caro, J., Rubio Campos, J. C., Luque Espinar, J. A., López Geta, J. A., Peinado Parra, T., Reina Laso, J., & Haro Ruiz, M. D. (2003). Las aguas minerales, minero-medicinales y termales de la Provincia de Jaén [Mineral, minero-medicinal, and thermal waters of the Province of Jaén] (Serie "Hidrogeología y Aguas Subterráneas" no. 6). Instituto Geológico y Minero de España, Madrid. Retrieved from http://aguas.igme.es/igme/publica/libro109/pdf/lib109/in_01.pdf

Berciano, J., & Lafarga, M. (2001). Santiago Ramón y Cajal (1852-1934). *Journal of Neurology, 248*, 152-153.

Caullery, M. (1934). Notice sur M. Santiago Ramón y Cajal [Notice on Mr. Santiago Ramón y Cajal]. *Comptes Rendus de l'Académie des Sciences, 199*, 747-748.

de Castro, F., López-Mascaraque, L., & de Carlos, J. A. (2007). Cajal—Lessons on brain development. *Brain Research Reviews, 55*, 481-489.

DeFelipe, J. (2002). Sesquicentenary of the birthday of Santiago Ramón y Cajal, the father of modern neuroscience. *Trends in Neurosciences, 25*, 481-484.

DeFelipe, J., & Jones, E. G. (1992). Santiago Ramón y Cajal and methods in neurohistology. *Trends in Neurosciences, 15*, 237-246.

de Fuentes Sagaz, M. (2001). Santiago Ramón y Cajal y la cardiología: Su descubrimiento poco conocido del sarcolema en el cardiomiocito [Santiago Ramón y Cajal and cardiology: His little known discovery of the sarcolemma of the cardiomyocyte]. *Revista Española de Cardiología, 54*, 933-937.

de Gregorio y Guajardo, A. (1895). *Estudio de las aguas termales cloruradosódicas variedad bicarbonatadas propiedad de don Mariano Serón en Jaraba de Aragón* [Study of the sodium-chloride thermal waters, the bicarbonate variety, property of Don Mariano Serón in Jaraba of Aragón]. Madrid, Spain: C. Apaolaza Impresor.

de la Rosa, M. C., & Mosso, M. Á (2004). Historia de las aguas mineromedicinales en España [History of mineral-medicinal waters in Spain]. *Observatorio Medioambiental, 7*, 117-137.

Doz, E., Manzaneque, M., Llord y Gamboa, R., Rodríguez Pinilla, H., & Camaleño, M. G. (1922). *Clínica hidrológica Española, con un estudio físico-químico de las aguas minerales* [Spanish hydrological clinic, with a physical-chemical study of mineral waters] (Manuales "Calpe" de Ciencias Médicas). Madrid, Spain: Calpe.

Editorial. (1908, November 25). Recompensas obtenidas en la Exposición Hispano-Francesa de Zaragoza: Grandes Premios—Manantial Cabreiroá, Verín (Orense) [Awards obtained at the Spanish-French Exposition of Zaragoza: Grand Prizes—Cabreiroá Spring, Verín (Orense)]. *Revista ABC* (Madrid), p. 13.

Editorial. (1913, December 1). Exposición anexa al IX Congreso Internacional de Hidrología [Exposition annexed to the IXth International Congress of Hydrology]. *Revista ABC* (Madrid), p. 4.

Editorial. (1991, December 11). Chávarri, S.A.—Aguas de Carabaña [Chávarri, S.A.—Waters of Carabaña]. *La Vanguardia* (Barcelona), p. 63.

Editorial. (2006, December 14). Economía—A Xunta destinará 180M€ en 2007 para impulsar a mellora da competitividade [Economy—The Government allocated € 180m in 2007 to promote the improvement of competitiveness]. *Xornal de Galicia*. Retrieved from http://www.xornal.com/artigo/2006/12/14/economia/a-xunta-destinara-180m-en-2007-para-impulsar-a-mellora-da-competitividade/2006121409545800000.html

el Sáb, S. (2009, May 9). Aguas de Carabaña [Waters of Carabaña]. *Tajuña Conecta* (Madrid). Retrieved from http://tajuna.foroactivo.com/carabana-sus-gentes-f8/aguas-de-carabana-t285.htm

Ferrari Billoch, F. (1957). *Ramón y Cajal, un gran sabio Español* [Ramón y Cajal, a great Spanish sage]. Madrid, Spain: Imprenta S. Aguirre Torre.

Fraguas, R. (2007, August 26). Aguas que curan—Recorrido por los manantiales medicinales de la región [Waters that cure—A tour of the medicinal springs of the region]. *El País* (Madrid). Retrieved from http://www.elpais.com/articulo/madrid/Aguas/curan/elpepuespmad/20070826elpmad_9/Tes

Gabinete de Comunicación da Xunta de Galicia. (2006, December 13). Explotación sostible dos recursos naturais [Sustainable exploitation of natural resources]. *Galicia Dixital*. Retrieved from http://www.galiciadixital.org/nota.4282.php

García Solá, E. (1884). La cuestion bactericida y el bacilo colerígeno [The bactericidal question and the cholera-producing bacillus]. *Revista de Medicina y Cirugía Prácticas, 15*, 337-349.

García Solá, E. (1885a). El cólera en Valencia y la vacunación anticolérica [Cholera in Valencia and cholera vaccination]. *Andalusía Médica, 10*, 169-176.

García Solá, E. (1885b). Observaciones sobre el vírgula en la provincia de Valencia [Observations on the cholera bacillus virgula in the Province of Valencia]. *Revista de Medicina y Cirugía Prácticas, 16*, 617-625.

Gibson, W. C. (1994). Ramón y Cajal and his school: Personal recollections. *Journal of the History of Medicine and Allied Sciences, 49*, 546-564.

Giménez Herrero, J. B. (1994). *Perfil socio-sanitario de los agüistas subvencionados del centro de terapia termal Balneario Sicilia-Baños de Serón, en Jaraba, Zaragoza* [Social and health profile of the subsidized curists at the Sicilia Spring–Baths of Serón center of thermal therapy, in Jaraba, Zaragoza] (doctoral thesis). Madrid, Spain: Universidad Complutense de Madrid.

Grupo 2T C.A. (2010, November 30). Magma de Cabreiroá—Un agua que no ha visto luz cientos de años [The magma of Cabreiroá—A water that has not seen the light for hundreds of years]. Retrieved from http://www.tutrago.com/noticia.aspx?cod=1499&;Pagina=8

Hamburger, V. (1980). S. Ramón y Cajal, R.G. Harrison, and the beginnings of neuroembryology. *Perspectives in Biology and Medicine, 23*, 600-616.

Hasselberg, K. B., Pettersson, S. O., Mörner, K. A. H., Wirsén, C. D., & Santesson, M. C. G. (1908). *Les prix Nobel en 1906*

[The Nobel Prizes of 1906]. Stockholm, Sweden: Imprimerie Royale P.A. Norstedt & Söner.

Iturbe, U., Pretó, J., & Lazcano, A. (2008). The young Ramón y Cajal as a cell-theory dissenter. *International Microbiology, 11*, 143-145.

Koch, R. (1884). An address on cholera and its bacillus. *British Medical Journal, 2*, 403-407, 453-459.

Koch, R. (1886). *Die Cholera auf ihrem neuesten Standpunkte* [Cholera from the latest standpoint]. Berlin, Germany: Martin Hampel.

Koch, R. (1893). Wasserfiltration und Cholera [Water filtration and cholera]. *Zeitschrift für Hygiene und Infectionskrankheiten, 14*, 393-426.

Koehler, P. J. (2007). Neuroscience in the work of Boerhaave and Haller. In H. Whitaker, C. U. M. Smith, & S. Finger (Eds.), *Brain, mind and medicine: Neuroscience in the 18th century* (pp. 213-231). New York, NY: Springer Science.

Lafarga, M., Casafont, I., Bengoechea, R., Tapia, O., & Berciano, M. T. (2009). Cajal's contribution to the knowledge of the neuronal cell nucleus. *Chromosoma, 118*, 437-443.

Lagercrantz, H. (2006). Nobel prizes in paediatrics: Santiago Ramón y Cajal (1852-1934) and the founding of neuroembryology. *Acta Paediatrica, 95*, 130-131.

Lindeboom, G. A. (1974). Boerhaave: Author and editor. *Bulletin of the Medical Library Association, 62*, 137-148.

Llinás, R. R. (2003). The contribution of Santiago Ramón y Cajal to functional neuroscience. *Nature Reviews Neuroscience, 4*, 77-80.

Loewy, A. D. (1971). Ramón y Cajal and methods of neuroanatomical research. *Perspectives in Biology and Medicine, 15*, 7-36.

López-Muñoz, F., Boya, J., & Alamo, C. (2006). Neuron theory, the cornerstone of neuroscience, on the centenary of the Nobel Prize award to Santiago Ramón y Cajal. *Brain Research Bulletin, 70*, 391-405.

Martínez, A., Marín, V. G., Junquera, S. R., Martínez-Murillo, R., & Freire, M. (2005). The contributions of Santiago Ramón y Cajal to cancer research—100 years on. *Nature Reviews Cancer, 5*, 904-909.

Moreno-Martínez, J. M., & Martín-Araguz, A. (2002). Santiago Ramón y Cajal: su actividad como médico militar (1873-1875) [Santiago Ramón y Cajal: His activity as a military physician (1873-1875)]. *Revista Neurológica (Barcelona), 35*, 95-97.

Murillo, F. (1913). *Memoria descriptiva é indicaciones terapéuticas de las nuevas aguas minero-medicinales de Verín, Manantial Cabreiroá* [Specifications report and therapeutic indications of the new medicinal waters of Verín, Cabreiroá Spring] (4th ed.). Madrid, Spain: Imprenta Alemana.

Navarro García, C. (2010). Carabaña: Inauguración del primer balneario de la Comunidad de Madrid [Carabaña: Inauguration of the first spa of the Community of Madrid]. *La Voz del Tajuña (Madrid), 75*, 6-7.

Otero Pedrayo, R. (1954). *Guía de Galicia* [Guide of Galicia] (3rd ed.). Vigo, Spain: Editorial Galaxia.

Otis, L. (2001). Ramón y Cajal, a pioneer in science fiction. *International Microbiology, 4*, 175-178.

Pablos, F. (2009). A escultura monumental [A monumental sculpture]. In J. M. Pérez Álvarez, F. Pablos, & M. Moretón (Eds.), *Buciños—Arredor de Si* (pp. 87-130). Ourense, Spain: Centro Cultural Deputación Ourense/Gráficas Rodi.

Pérez, H. (1983, September 3). La existencia relajada de los agüistas en el balneario de la Toja [The relaxed existence of curists in the Springs of Toja]. *Revista ABC* (Madrid), p. 32.

Puelles, L. (2009). Contributions to neuroembryology of Santiago Ramón y Cajal (1852-1934) and Jorge F. Tello (1880-1958). *International Journal of Developmental Biology, 53*, 1145-1160.

Ramón y Cajal, S. (1885a). Contribución al estudio de las formas involutivas y monstruosas del comabacilo de Koch [Contribution to the study of involutive and monstrous forms of the Koch bacillus]. *Crónica Médica, 9*, 197-204.

Ramón y Cajal, S. (1885b). *Estudios sobre el microbio vírgula del cólera y las inoculaciones profilácticas* [Studies on the cholera microbe and prophylactic inoculations]. Zaragoza, Spain: Tipografía del Hospicio Provincial.

Ramón y Cajal, S. (1905). *Manual de anatomía patológica general y fundamentos de bacteriología* [Manual of general anatomic pathology and fundamentals of bacteriology] (4th ed.). Madrid, Spain: Nicolás Moya.

Ramón y Cajal, S. (1926, April 22). De cómo se explota mi modesto nombre por ciertos desaprensivos industriales [How my modest name is exploited by some unscrupulous industries]. *Revista ABC* (Madrid), p. 21.

Ramón y Cajal, S. (1988). *Recollections of my life* (E. H. Craigie & J. Cano, Trans.). Birmingham, AL: The Classics of Neurology and Neurosurgery Library/Gryphon Editions.

Ramón y Cajal Junquera, S. (2000). Ramón y Cajal, microbiologist. *International Microbiology, 3*, 59-61.

Rodríguez Miguez, L. (1995). Estudio histórico bibliográfico del termalismo [Historical-bibliographic study of hydrotherapy]. Orense, Spain: Diputación Provincial.

Rodríguez Miguez, L. (2006). Figuras galaicas del termalismo [Galician figures of hydrotherapy]. *Balnea, 1*, 97-109. Retrieved from http://revistas.ucm.es/med/18870813/articulos/ANHM0606120097A.PDF

San Martín Bacaicoa, J., & Valero Castejón, A. (2004). Acción terapéutica de las aguas de los Balnearios de Jaraba [Therapeutic action of the waters of the Springs of Jaraba]. *Anales de la Real Academia Nacional de Farmacia, 70*, 625-653.

Schulte, B. P. M. (1959). *Hermanni Boerhaave Praelectiones de morbis nervorum. 1730-1735: Een medisch-historische studie van Boerhaave's manuscript over zenuwziekten* [Herman Boerhaave's *Praelectiones de morbis nervorum*, 1730–1735: A medico-historical study of Boerhaave's manuscript on nervous diseases] (Analecta Boerhaaviana, Vol. 2). Leiden, Netherlands: E.J. Brill.

Sotelo, C. (2003). Viewing the brain through the master hand of Ramón y Cajal. *Nature Reviews Neuroscience, 4*, 71-77.

Stefanidou, M., Solà, C., Kouvelas, E., del Cerro, M., & Triarhou, L. C. (2007). Cajal's brief experimentation with hypnotic suggestion. *Journal of the History of the Neurosciences, 16*, 351-361.

Triarhou, L. C, & del Cerro, M. (2008a). Pedro Ramón (Cajal's brother) and his pivotal contributions to evolutionary neuroscience. *Schweizer Archiv für Neurologie und Psychiatrie, 159*, 419-428.

Triarhou, L. C., & del Cerro, M. (2008b). The structure of Lippmann heliochromes: Cajal and the 1908 Nobel Prize in Physics. *Journal of Chemical Neuroanatomy, 35*, 1-11.

Triarhou, L. C., & Vivas, A. B. (2009). Poetry and the brain: Cajal's conjectures on the psychology of writers. *Perspectives in Biology and Medicine, 52*, 80-89.

van Buskirk, C., & Porter-Sánchez, A. (1961). Santiago Ramón y Cajal as a bacteriologist. *Bulletin of the School of Medicine of the University of Maryland, 46*, 38-41.

Vasey, C. (2006). *The water prescription* (J. E. Graham, Trans.). Rochester, VT: Healing Arts Press.

Author Biographies

Lazaros C. Triarhou is professor of neuroscience at the University of Macedonia, Thessaloniki, Greece. His research interests include plasticity and regeneration in the central nervous system, and the evolution of ideas in neurobiology.

Manuel del Cerro is professor emeritus of neurobiology and anatomy, neurology, and ophthalmology at the University of Rochester, New York, USA. His research interests include cerebellar and retinal neurobiology, and the history of the microscope.

THE RENAISSANCE OF THE NEURON DOCTRINE: CAJAL REBUTS THE RECTOR OF GRANADA

Agesilaos M. Partsalis[1],
Pablo M. Blazquez[2],
Lazaros C. Triarhou[3,*]

Abstract

The Spanish histologist Santiago Ramón y Cajal and the Italian anatomist Camillo Golgi, who were jointly awarded the 1906 Nobel Prize in Physiology or Medicine for their discoveries on the structure of the nervous system, are two of the most notable figures in neuroscience. It was the 'Golgi method' that enabled Cajal to gather evidence and defend neuronism (the contiguity of neurons as independent cellular units) against his chief rival's reticularism (the intracellular continuity of the cytoplasm among neurons in a widespread reticulum). Seven months after his Nobel lecture in Stockholm, Cajal wrote a powerful article which he titled 'El renacimiento de la doctrina neuronal' (the rebirth, revival, or renaissance of the neuron doctrine) as a response to an insurrection of reticularist ideas. This new wave of reticularism was instigated in Spain by the pathologist Eduardo García Solá, Rector of the University of Granada at the time, and stemmed from the interpretation of nerve regeneration experiments conducted by the German physiologist Albrecht von Bethe in Strassburg (today Strasbourg, France) and the Hungarian histologist Stephan von Apáthy in Kolozsvár (today Cluj-Napoca, Romania). Cajal's article was hosted by four different journals (three in Spain and one in Argentina). It constitutes an important testimony for the history of the neuron theory that has gone unheeded thus far. Therefore, we provide an English translation of Cajal's Spanish paper, placing it in the context of evolving notions during that first decade of the twentieth century crucial for neurobiology.

Keywords

• History of neuroscience • Neuron theory • Catenary theory • Reticularism
• Santiago Ramón y Cajal (1852–1934) • Eduardo García Solá (1845–1922)

© Versita Sp. z o.o.

[1]*Intensive Care Unit, Hadjikosta General Hospital, 45500 Ioannina, Greece*

[2]*Department of Otolaryngology, Washington University School of Medicine, St. Louis, MO 63110, USA*

[3]*Division of Basic Neuroscience, Department of Educational and Social Policy, University of Macedonia, 54006 Thessaloniki, Greece*

Received 27 November 2012
Accepted 15 December 2012

Introduction

Santiago Ramón y Cajal (Figure 1) gave his Nobel Lecture in Stockholm on December 12, 1906 [1]. Seventh months later, he had to defend the neuron theory again, furnishing cogent arguments after an insurrection of reticularism. That rebuttal (Figure 2) was hosted by three different journals in Spain [2–4], and by the *Archives of Psychiatry and Criminology* in Argentina (the official journal of the Buenos Aires Society of Criminology), founded and edited by the philosopher and psychiatrist José Ingenieros (1877–1925) [5,6]. Cajal forcefully refutes the Rector of Granada, his friend Eduardo García Solá (1845–1922), who had spoken of the "decadence of the neuron" [7].

García Solá (Figure 1), a key figure in Spanish histopathology and microbiology and a proponent of laboratory medicine in the late 19th century, held the Chair of General Pathology in Granada from 1872 until his retirement in 1918 [8]. He published standard works, including a 'Textbook of General Pathology and Pathologic Anatomy' [9], which went through five editions over 30 years, a pioneering 'Manual of Clinical Microchemistry'

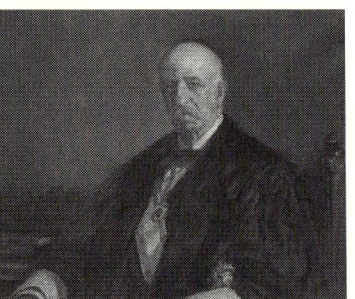

Figure 1. Santiago Ramón y Cajal (1852–1934), left, shortly after the announcement of the Nobel Prize award. Cover portrait in La Ilustración Española y Americana, Madrid, vol. 50, no. 42, November 15, 1906; signature from the Nobel volume [1] digitally etched onto the photograph. Eduardo García Solá (1845–1922), right, Professor at the Faculty of Medicine and Rector of the University of Granada from June 1891 to November 1909. Source: http://rectorado.ugr.es/pages/salon_rojo/rector_1891_egarciasola; signature from La Ilustración Española y Americana, Madrid, vol. 36, no. 38, October 12, 1892, digitally etched onto the painting.

* E-mail: triarhou@uom.gr

[10], and an 'Elementary Textbook of Normal Histology and Histochemistry' [11] based on original material from his tenure at the School of Medicine in Granada.

García Solá [12–14] and Ramón y Cajal [15,16] had earlier converged through their publications on the virulent bacillus and its treatment during the cholera outbreak in Valencia [8]. For his ground-breaking work on producing a vaccine, Cajal was presented with a Zeiss microscope by the provincial government of Zaragoza, which opened up entirely new horizons by enabling him "to attack the delicate problems of the structure of the cells without misgivings and with the requisite efficiency" [17].

Cajal and the neuron theory

Cajal, more than any other single investigator, contributed to our understanding of nervous system organization, laying the foundations of modern neuroanatomy, neuroembryology, and neuropathology [18]. He masterly chartered the microorganization of virtually every region of the central nervous system of vertebrates and compiled his results into the classic *Textura* [19]. He is rightfully recognized internationally as the father of modern neuroscience [20]. Thus, in the history of science and human thought, Cajal is viewed as the conceptualizer and founder, in 1889, of 'neural atomism' [21], *viz.* the Leucippus or the Democritus of the brain. (His groundbreaking discoveries on neural plasticity could also earn him the title of the Heraclitus of the brain [*Panta rhei*, 22].)

Two years later, Waldeyer [23] firmly supported Cajal's *neuronismo* and combined the objective evidence that had been adduced by His, Forel, Gowers, Kölliker, Retzius, van Gehuchten, von Lenhossék, Nansen, Cajal, as well as his brother Pedro Ramón y Cajal [24]. Waldeyer came up with the term *neuron* — a word first appearing in Homer's *Iliad* [25] — to denote what was, until then, called the 'ganglion cell' or 'nerve cell' and systematized the 'neuron doctrine' [1,26–32]. According to the neuron doctrine (Figure 3), or neuron theory today, nerve cells are viewed as polarized structures, contacting each other at specialized synaptic junctions, and forming the developmental,

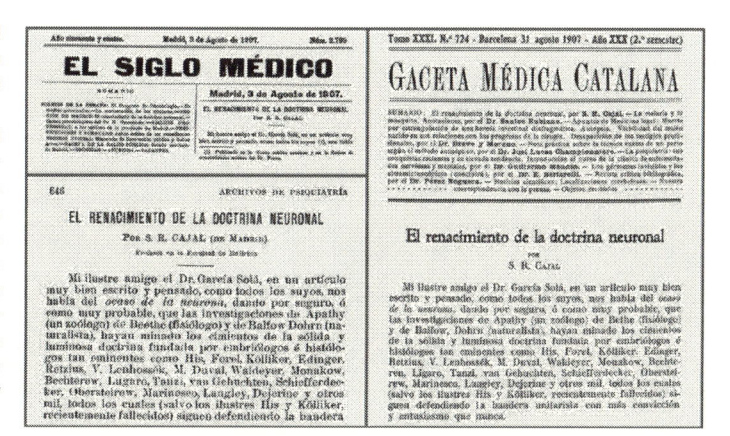

Figure 2. Title page of three variants of Cajal's 1907 'Renaissance' article [2,3,5].

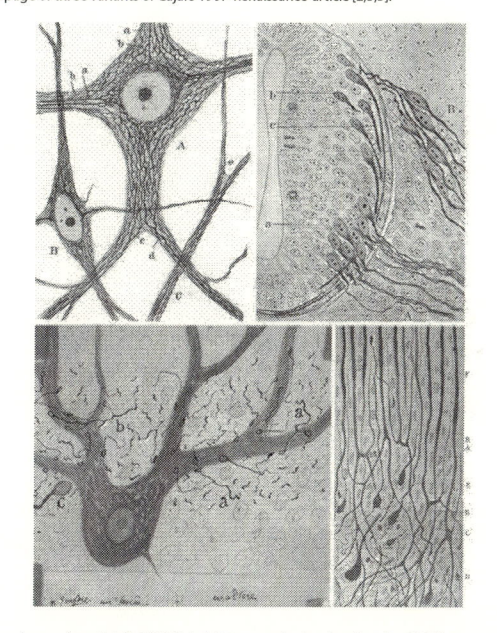

Figure 3. Three schemes from Cajal's 1906 Nobel lecture, and a drawing dated to 1907, in support of the neuron theory. Upper left: Spinal cord cells of a several day-old rabbit. Impregnation by the reduced silver nitrate procedure. A, large funicular corpuscle; B, small corpuscle; a, primary filament; b, secondary filaments; c, d, e, neurofibrillar anastomoses at the level of the dendritic divisions [1]. Upper right: Section from the spinal cord of a chick embryo at day 3 of incubation. Reduced silver method. A, anterior root; B, sensory ganglion and posterior root; a, motor neuroblasts; b, c, commissural neuroblasts whose axon terminates into a growth cone [1]. Lower right: Portion of the central end of the scar in the cut sciatic nerve of a one week-old cat sacrificed 3 days after the operation. A, B, non-myelinated portion of nerve tubes in the process of growth; F, old or myelinated segment of these tubes; C, growth bouton; D, small terminal bouton; G, fiber emitting retrograde branches; a, b, boutons making their way through the cut; c, free neurofibril ending in a ring; e, retrograde bouton; d, bouton from which emanate fine appendages that terminate in small boutons [1]. Lower left: A 1907 drawing by Cajal, depicting a Purkinje cell in the canine cerebellum, with the nerve terminals in a ring. India ink and water-diluted graphite on fine cardboard paper [60].

structural, functional, and trophic units of nervous systems [33].

Definitive proof of the neuron theory was attained half a century later, when the Argentinian cell biologist Eduardo De Robertis (1913–1988), in collaboration with the Uruguayan neurobiologist Clemente Estable (1894–1976), a former pupil of Cajal, put together and described at the ultrastructural level the separation of pre and postsynaptic membranes at the Biological Research Institute in Montevideo, in a Cellular Ultrastructure Department, which housed the first electron microscope in South America [34]. De Robertis carried on his work on synapses and synaptic vesicles with H. Stanley Bennett (1910–1992) in Seattle, studying the sympathetic ganglia of frogs and the nerve cord of earthworms dug from Bennett's own yard [35].

One of the most succinct assessments of the importance of the neuron theory and its implications for neuropsychiatry and biological philosophy, which has received little attention in the English bibliography, is a conference in Buenos Aires given by one of the foremost neuroanatomists of the twentieth century, the ingenious Christofredo Jakob (1866–1956), at a special session of the Society of Neurology and Psychiatry as an homage to Cajal the month after his death, on November 16, 1934. Here is an extract: "The keen eye and deft hand of Ramón y Cajal led us to the *economy of the invisible*, the impenetrability of which was lamented by Schiller. Cajal's powerful brain ousted the *ethereal fluid* of the *channeling systems of the brain* and placed us on the stable pedestal of *facts* in lieu of fancies. The clear mind of the great Spaniard was able to sum up anew a century's preparatory work, from Remak and Deiters to Golgi, Kölliker and Retzius, into the grandiose conception of the neuron theory, the quintessence of which rests on the most brilliant discovery by the astute scholar, i.e., the demonstration and exact interpretation of the function and organization of the axon. Cajal was the first to irrefutably demonstrate the free ending of its terminal ramifications, first in the cerebellum (pericellular baskets, climbing fibers) and subsequently in spinal and cerebral regions. Today this seems trivial, but back then it was the revelation of a new world, freshly leading ever since to our understanding of the principles of conduction, transformation and stabilization of nervous energy. Its philosophical importance rests with the elimination of the supposed immaterial fluids and the demonstration of the natural basis of all neuropsychic functions, whence the elaboration of a psychobiology became possible" [36].

The neuron theory and its repercussions for modern brain research have received a new round of extensive discussions on the occasion of the centennial of the Nobel Prize award to Cajal and Golgi [37–48].

The insurrection and the rebuttal

In his response [2–5], Cajal especially takes aim at the contentions of Albrecht von Bethe (1872–1954) and Stephan (István) von Apáthy (1863–1922), who had attacked the neuron theory [49–51] by insisting that nervous conduction takes place through small fibers passing from one cell into another, a thesis that eventually waned [52]. In particular, Bethe had conducted axonal regeneration experiments, which he interpreted as in line with Viktor Hensen's earlier 'catenary' or 'polygenic' theory of nerve fiber growth and regeneration that defended the fusion of multiple axon segments into a common stump, formed by the coalescence of linear chains of Schwann cells [53]. Cajal showed that this was not the case, and that the new fibers appearing in the distal stump of an experimentally dissected nerve emanated from the axonal sprouting at its proximal stump [20]. Cajal refuted such a resurfacing of reticularism by Bethe and Apáthy on more than one occasion [54,55]. He devised a reduced silver nitrate method, which he used to study the distribution of neurofibrils in the nervous system of vertebrates and invertebrates and their involvement in nerve regeneration [56], and concluded that neurofibrils are linear 'colonies' of particles constituting a dynamic internal skeleton of the neuron [57]. With his comprehensive reply to Apáthy [55], Cajal in effect ended the renewed reticularist campaign against the neuron doctrine [57], and eventually compiled his degeneration and regeneration studies into the classic monograph of 1913/1914 [58].

To our knowledge, this is the first English translation of *El Renacimiento de la Doctrina Neuronal* [2–5]. In brief, Cajal speaks firmly of the adversaries of the neuron doctrine, of the psychology and the vicissitudes of young investigators who, eager for fame and lacking in originality, often succumb to the unhealthy temptation to be negative and to discredit doctrines, even in dominions where science seems to have determined the formulations. Cajal patiently exposes and then rejects the 'arguments' made by anti-neuronists in order to inform those who ignore the actual phase of the problem, based on results from the preceding decade. For Cajal there is no fear: He follows the thinking about the neuron doctrine based on the work of van Gehuchten, Michotte, Donaggio, Tello, Schiefferdecker, Marinesco, Azoulay, Harrison, Neal, Münzer, Mott, Medea, Lugaro, Perroncito, Guido, Room, Krassin, Nageotte, and many others, skilfully refuting the arguments of reticularism and catenarism and arriving at an unmatched degree of solidity [59].

Acknowledgments

The authors are grateful to Dr. Carme Solà of the Consejo Superior de Investigaciones Científicas, Barcelona, and Dr. Manuel del Cerro of the University of Rochester, New York, for their invaluable help, as well as the staff of the libraries of the Instituto Ramón y Cajal, the Universidad Complutense, and the Real Academia de Ciencias Exactas, Físicas y Naturales, Madrid for bibliographic assistance.

References

[1] Ramón y Cajal S., Structure et connexions des neurones (conférence Nobel faite à Stockholm le 12 décembre 1906), In: Hasselberg K.B., Pettersson S.O., Mörner K.A.H., Wirsén C.D., Santesson M.C.G. (Eds.), Les Prix Nobel en 1906, Imprimerie Royale P. A. Norstedt & Söner, Stockholm, 1908, 1–27

[2] Ramón y Cajal S., El renacimiento de la doctrina neuronal, El Siglo Médico (Madrid), 1907, 54, 479-485

[3] Ramón y Cajal S., El renacimiento de la doctrina neuronal, Gaceta Médica Catalana (Barcelona), 1907, 31, 121-133

[4] Ramón y Cajal S., (1907) El renacimiento de la doctrina neuronal, Revista de Especialidades Médicas (Madrid), 1907, 10, 428-441

[5] Ramón y Cajal S., El renacimiento de la doctrina neuronal, Archivos de Psiquiatría y Criminología (Buenos Aires), 1907, 6, 646-662

[6] Ingenieros J., Indice General de Archivos de Psiquiatría y Criminología, Años 1902-1913, Talleres Gráficos de la Penitenciaría Nacional, Buenos Aires, 1914, 3–26

[7] García Solá E., Más sobre el neurona, Gaceta Médica Catalana (Barcelona), 1907, 31, 241-245

[8] Giménez de Azcárate J.C., (2007) Félix Aramendía (1856-1894) y la Patología y Clínica Médicas, ONA Industria Gráfica, Pamplona – Navarra, 2007, 147–151

[9] García Solá E., Tratado de Patología General y de Anatomía Patológica, Moya y Plaza, Madrid, 1874

[10] García Solá E., Manual de Microquimia Clínica, Moya y Plaza, Madrid, 1876

[11] García Solá E., Tratado Elemental de Histología e Histoquimia Normales, Espasa y Compañía, Barcelona, 1888

[12] García Solá E., La cuestion bactericida y el bacilo colerígeno, Revista de Medicina y Cirugía Prácticas (Madrid), 1884, 15, 337-349

[13] García Solá E., Observaciones sobre el vírgula en la provincia de Valencia, Revista de Medicina y Cirugía Prácticas (Madrid), 1885, 16, 617-625

[14] García Solá E., El cólera en Valencia y la vacunación anticolérica, Andalusía Médica (Córdoba), 1885, 10, 169-176

[15] Ramón y Cajal S., Estudios sobre el Microbio Vírgula del Cólera y las Inoculaciones Profilácticas, Tipografía del Hospicio Provincial, Zaragoza, 1885

[16] Ramón y Cajal S., Contribución al estudio de las formas involutivas y monstruosas del comabacilo de Koch, Crónica Médica (Valencia), 1885, 9, 197-204

[17] Ramón y Cajal S., Recollections of my life (translated by E.H. Craigie and J. Cano), The classics of neurology and neurosurgery library – Gryphon editions, Birmingham, AL, 1988

[18] Loewy A.D., Ramón y Cajal and methods of neuroanatomical research, Perspect. Biol. Med., 1971, 15, 7-36

[19] Ramón y Cajal S., Textura del Sistema Nervioso del Hombre y de los Vertebrados, 3 volumes, Nicolás Moya, Madrid, 1897-1904

[20] DeFelipe J., Sesquicentenary of the birthday of Santiago Ramón y Cajal, the father of modern neuroscience, Trends Neurosci., 2002, 25, 481-484

[21] Everdell W.R., The first moderns: profiles in the origins of twentieth-century thought, University of Chicago Press, Chicago, 1997, 100-115

[22] Weiss P.A., "Panta rhei" — And so flow our nerves, Am. Sci., 1969, 57, 287-305

[23] Waldeyer H.W.G., Über einige neuere Forschungen im Gebiete der Anatomie des Centralnervensystems, Deutsche Medizinische Wochenschrift, 1891, 17, 1213-1218, 1244-1246, 1287-1289, 1331-1332, 1352-1356

[24] Triarhou L.C., del Cerro M., Pedro Ramón (Cajal's brother) and his pivotal contributions to evolutionary neuroscience, Schweiz. Arch. Neurol. Psychiatr., 2008, 159, 419-428

[25] Ochs S., A history of nerve functions: from animal spirits to molecular mechanisms, Cambridge University Press, New York, 2004

[26] Ramón y Cajal S., Inducciones fisiológicas de la morfología y conexiones de las neuronas, Archivos de Pedagogía y Ciencias Afines (La Plata), 1906, 1, 216-236

[27] Ramón y Cajal S., Morfología de la célula nerviosa, Archivos de Pedagogía y Ciencias Afines (La Plata), 1906, 1, 92-106

[28] Ramón y Cajal S., Die histogenetischen Beweise der Neuronentheorie von His und Forel, Anatomischer Anzeiger (Jena), 1907, 30, 113-144

[29] Ramón y Cajal S., Die Neuronenlehre (mit 92 Abbildungen), In: Bumke O., Foerster O. (Eds.) Handbuch der Neurologie, erster Band; Allgemeine Neurologie I: Anatomie, Julius Springer, Berlin, 1935, 887– 994

[30] Ramón y Cajal S., Neuron theory or reticular theory? Objective evidence of the anatomical unity of nerve cells (translated by M.U. Purkiss and C.A. Fox), Consejo Superior de Investigaciones Científicas, Madrid, 1954

[31] Ramón y Cajal S., The neuron and the glial cell (translated by J. de la Torre and W.C. Gibson). Charles C Thomas Publisher, Springfield, IL, 1984

[32] Shepherd G.M., Foundations of the neuron doctrine, Oxford University Press, New York, 1991

[33] Guillery R.W., Observations of synaptic structures: origins of the neuron doctrine and its current status, Philos. Trans. Roy. Soc. B., 2005, 360, 1281-1307

[34] Estable C., Reissig M., De Robertis E., Microscopic and submicroscopic structure of the synapsis in the ventral ganglion of the acoustic nerve, 1954, Exp. Cell Res., 6, 255-262

[35] De Robertis E.D., Bennett H.S., Some features of the submicroscopic morphology of synapses in frog and earthworm, J. Biophys. Biochem. Cytol., 1955, 1, 47-58

[36] Jakob C., Santiago Ramón y Cajal — La significación de su obra científica para la Neuropsiquiatría, La Semana Médica (Buenos Aires), 1935, 42, 529-536

[37] Llinás R., The contribution of Santiago Ramón y Cajal to functional neuroscience, Nature Rev. Neurosci., 2003, 4, 77-80

[38] Barbara J.-G., (2006) The physiological construction of the neurone concept (1891–1952), CR Soc. Biol., 2006, 329, 437-449

[39] Glickstein M., Golgi and Cajal: The neuron doctrine and the 100th anniversary of the 1906 Nobel Prize, Curr. Biol., 2006, 16, 147-151

[40] López-Muñoz F., Boya J., Alamo C., Neuron theory, the cornerstone of neuroscience, on the centenary of the Nobel Prize award to Santiago Ramón y Cajal, Brain Res. Bull., 2006, 70, 391-405

[41] Agnati L.F., Genedani S., Leo G., Rivera A., Guidolin D., Fuxe K., One century of progress in neuroscience founded on Golgi and Cajal's outstanding experimental and theoretical contributions, Brain Res. Rev., 2007, 55, 167-189

[42] De Carlos J.A., Borrell J., A historical reflection of the contributions of Cajal and Golgi to the foundations of neuroscience, Brain Res. Rev., 2007, 55, 8-16

[43] Grant G., How the 1906 Nobel Prize in Physiology or Medicine was shared between Golgi and Cajal, Brain Res. Rev., 2007, 55, 490-498

[44] Guillery R.W., Relating the neuron doctrine to the cell theory. Should contemporary knowledge change our view of the neuron doctrine?, Brain Res. Rev., 2007, 55, 411-421

[45] Kruger L., Otis T.S., Whither withered Golgi? A retrospective evaluation of reticularist and synaptic constructs, Brain Res. Bull., 2007, 72, 201-207

[46] Swanson L.W., Grant G., Hökfelt T., Jones E.G., Morrison J.H., A century of neuroscience discovery: Reflecting on the Nobel Prize awarded to Golgi and Cajal in 1906, Brain Res. Rev., 2007, 55, 191-192

[47] Bentivoglio M., Mazzarello P., The anatomical foundations of clinical neurology, In: Handbook of Clinical Neurology, 2010, 95, 149-168

[48] Sotelo C., Camillo Golgi and Santiago Ramón y Cajal: The anatomical organization of the cortex of the cerebellum. Can the neuron doctrine still support our actual knowledge on the cerebellar structural arrangement?, Brain Res. Rev., 2011, 66, 16-34

[49] Bethe A., Über die Regeneration peripherischen Nerven, Archiv für Psychiatrie und Nervenkrankenheiten, 1901, 34, 1066-1073

[50] Bethe A., Zur Frage von der autogenen Nervenregeneration, Neurologisches Centralblatt, 1903, 22, 60-62

[51] Apáthy S., Bemerkungen zu den Ergebnissen Ramón y Cajal hinsichtlich der feineren Beschaffenheit des Nervensystems, Anatomischer Anzeiger, 1907, 31, 481-496, 523-544

[52] Pi-Suñer A., Pi-Suñer J., Ramón y Cajal and the physiology of the nervous system, J. Nerv. Ment. Dis., 1936, 84, 521-537

[53] Jones E.G., Golgi, Cajal and the neuron doctrine, J. Hist. Neurosci., 1999, 8, 170-178

[54] Ramón y Cajal S., Consideraciones críticas sobre la teoría de A. Bethe acerca de la estructura y conexiones de las células nerviosas, Trabajos del Laboratorio de Investigaciones Biológicas de la Universitad de Madrid, 1903, 2, 101-128

[55] Ramón y Cajal S., L'hypothèse de Mr. Apáthy sur la continuité des cellules nerveuses entre ells, Anatomischer Anzeiger (Jena), 1908, 33, 418-448, 468-493

[56] Jakob C., Nuevas teorías de las neurofibrillas (Sociedad Médica Argentina, 8.a Sesión ordinaria del 31 de julio de 1905), Argentina Médica (Buenos Aires), 1905, 3, 347

[57] Frixione E., Cajal's second great battle for the neuron doctrine: the nature and function of neurofibrils, Brain Res. Rev., 2009, 59, 393-409

[58] DeFelipe J., Jones E.G., Cajal's degeneration and regeneration of the nervous system, Oxford University Press, New York, 1991

[59] Rubert A.C., Revista de revistas, Nosotros Publicación Periódica (Buenos Aires), 1908, 2, 92-93

[60] Ramón y Cajal S., Ciencia y Arte, La Casa Encendida, Madrid, 2003

TRANSLATION OF:

Santiago Ramón y Cajal (1907)
Professor in the Faculty of Medicine, Madrid

The renaissance of the neuron doctrine

El Siglo Médico 54: 479–485.
Gaceta Médica Catalana 31: 121–133.
Revista de Especialidades Médicas 10: 428–441.
Archivos de Psiquiatría y Criminología 6: 646–662.

(First English translation by A.M. Partsalis, P.M. Blazquez and L.C. Triarhou from the original Spanish text of *El Renacimiento de la Doctrina Neuronal*, dated by Cajal July 12, 1907).

My distinguished friend, Dr. García Solá, in a very well written and thought out article, as are all of his articles, speaks to us of the "decadence of the neuron" [1907] assuming for certain or quite probable that the research of Apáthy (a zoologist), Bethe (a physiologist) and Balfow, Dohrn (naturalists) have undermined the foundations of the solid and illustrious doctrine founded by embryologists and histologists as eminent as His, Forel, Kölliker, Edinger, Retzius, von Lenhossék, M. Duval, Waldeyer, Monakow, Bechterew, Lugaro, Tanzi, van Gehuchten, Schiefferdecker, Obersteiner, Marinesco, Langley, Déjerine, and a thousand others, all of whom (with the exception of the distinguished His and Kölliker, recently deceased) are today still defending the unitarist flag with more enthusiasm and conviction than ever.

Were I not afraid to offend my dear colleague's sensibilities, I would tell him that, influenced by the noisy flock of young anti-neuronists, he was alarmed too much and, above all, a little too late.

I cannot comprehend, given the mastery of the wise Rector of the University of Granada in the histology literature, why he does not credit in his article the fact that precisely over the past three years we have witnessed a compelling renaissance of the neuron doctrine, thanks to the recent histological works of van Gehuchten, Michotte, von Lenhossék, Donaggio, Tello, Schiefferdecker, Marinesco, Azoulay, Nageotte, Retzius, Athias, and ours; thanks to the histogenetic studies of Kölliker, Harrisson, Neal, Kehr, Gustwisch, Held, and ours; thanks to the histopathological studies (nerve regeneration) of Munzer, Langley, Mott, Halliburton, Medea, Lugaro, Perroncito, Guido, Sala, Marinesco, Krassin, Nageotte, and ours. Not only has the neuron doctrine dismissed the arguments of reticularism and catenarism, but it has also been enriched, thanks to improved tissue staining procedures, with valuable new morphological and histogenetic data, reaching a degree of solidity and prestige never previously attained.

I do not claim that the neuron concept lacks adversaries, and noteworthy adversaries at that. It has had adversaries since it emerged some 18 years ago, it has adversaries today, and will always have them, as long as the psychology of young investigators remains the same, (i.e., their eagerness for reputation). Finding the vein of originality too deep and difficult, they often fall for the unhealthy temptation of doing negative work, discrediting doctrines and tarnishing reputations, even in areas where science seems to have definitely established its principles, such that, with some honorable exceptions, anti-neuronists are not very modest or devoted to scientific truth. A thousand signs show this. Let me just mention one revealing fact of the arrogant egotism and anarchistic rebelliousness concealed in the depths of reticularism. Every anti-neuronist has his structural and dynamic model and defends it as if it were an intangible dogma. Apart from the simple and bright concept brought forth by His and Forel (which is not a theory, as is often said, but a pure and simple expression of facts from observation), there exist six or eight contradictory hypotheses. Thus, the nervous reticulum of Golgi and his disciples bears no resemblance to that of Nissl, Bethe and Apáthy, just as the concept of inter-protoplasmic mesh of Dogiel is not similar to that of Held and Wolff. Favoring imagination and caprice as the norm for their critics, rejecting selective methods for being too clear, and proclaiming the nonselective methods preferable, anti-neuronist schools have regressed to the times of Hence and Leydig, falling into the most deplorable confusion.

However, it is not now appropriate to show the contradiction and emptiness in which the protean phalanges of reticularism revolve and lose authority. I shall deal with such a pleasant and colorful theme in another manuscript. For now I shall examine, as a courtesy, the work of my distinguished friend Dr. García Solá, and I shall also inform those who, disregarding the present state of the subject, stick to the last little celebrity of 10 years ago, the true value and reach of the arguments employed by the most accredited anti-neuronists. These arguments are of three categories: structural, connective (or intercellular relationships), and neurogenetic.

Structural objections by Bethe and Apáthy

The body and expansions of nerve cells contain two factors: neuroplasm, whose sole function is nutritive, and a conductive factor, called the neurofibrils, which are delicate filaments, homogeneous and independent, placed in parallel bundles inside the dendrites and axon, spanning the cell body without ever ramifying or anastomosing. As these wise scientists perceive it, the soma or protoplasmic body is a simple point of crossing of independent nervous conductors; consequently, the neuron is an anatomic feature void of meaning, because the true morphologic and dynamic unit of the nervous system corresponds to the neurofibril.

As can be deduced from the above concept, this theory of Bethe and Apáthy leads to two postulates: the exclusive capability of these elemental filaments, excluding the cellular membrane and neuroplasm, and their perfect insulation inside the cellular body and its expansions.

(a) Independence of the neurofibrils. Leaving aside that the aforementioned wise men have already recognized, in certain cases, the existence of intracellular meshes of neurofibrils, the assertion of perfect and total individuality of the elemental threads loses supporters by the day. Unfortunately for the celebrated discoverers of the neurofibrils technique has advanced with giant steps since 1898. The precarious, difficult, and inconsistent methods used by scientists have been replaced by more perfect and consistent

methods, like those of Simago, Bielschowky, Cajal, Donaggio, DeRossi, Lugaro, etc. Armed with such methods, much more consistent and precise, many researchers have come out to compare their arms with those of the champions of anti-neuronism. And in the fervor created by the new analytical methods, an exuberant literature has sprouted — to which Spain has contributed more than 20 monographs — literature that does not deserve, by the way, the truly surprising silence and disdain of Dr. García Solá. Thanks to the clear and definitive revelations of modern impregnation methods, especially of my laboratory and that of Donnagio, it has been fully demonstrated that the neurofibrils form a complex mesh inside the cell body, instead of a plexus. And it has been clearly shown that the appearance of independent neurofibrils offered in Bethe's preparations were due to his imperfect use of the method, which stains exclusively the thicker filaments of the reticulum, eluding the finer secondary trabecular filaments, which are actually more abundant. This was the judgment, with small variations in interpretation, made by histologists such as van Gehuchten, Donaggio, Lenhossék, Marinesco, Michotte, Athias, Dogiel, Retzius, Azoulay, Nageotte, Legendre, Mahaim, Loudon, etc., the majority, in the end, of those who impartially studied the matter.

(b) *Exclusive conductibility of neurofibrils.* — This is an assertion for which no evidence exists. On the contrary, all we know on the morphology of neurofibrils suggests a conductive ability of the remaining elements of the protoplasm. I shall mention a few facts.

The first is the behavior of the neurofibrils at the level of the nerve terminations. Using the reduced silver nitrate method, I, as well as Dogiel, Loudon, Tello, and others, have provided objective proof that, in the motor plates and sensory endings, the neurofibrillar scaffolding within each branch forms meshes and complicated handles. From this it can be inferred that if, as Bethe and Apáthy maintain, the current flowed only through these threads, a paradoxical situation would occur wherein the motor nerve impulse would return, having reached the motor plate, to the source cell without discharging in the muscle.

In reality, the axon and its branches contain a reticular frame unified in all its parts. This fact, along with the demonstration recently offered by Retzius and Marinesco, that the neuroplasm is continuous at the level of the strangulations (Bethe maintained that the neuroplasm is interrupted at strangulations) have paved the way for the theory of Schiefferdecker, Wolff, and Verworn, for whom the neuroplasm, and not the neurofibrils, is the carrier of the nervous wave. Furthermore, that the neuroplasm and the cell membrane itself have conductive properties is supported by the fact that in the retina, olfactory bulb, cerebellum, etc., interneuronal relations are established by articulations, without it being possible to find any unifying filaments penetrating into the cell body.

Let me add an interesting datum: the dynamic concept of Bethe requires the firmness and stability of the neurofibrillar apparatus. Well, according to my observations, as well as those of Tello and García, confirmed and extended by Marinesco and Donaggio, the neurofibrillar reticulum, far from constituting a stable frame, represents an amoeboid scaffolding susceptible to great quantitative and qualitative transformations, depending on the physiological state (hibernation, effect of cold, fatigue, starvation, poisoning, infection etc.).

Thus, neither are the neurofibrils independent threads, nor do they conduct the nerve pulse individually, nor are they stable; recent structural findings do not contradict, in fact they graciously complete, as van Gehuchten has noted, the neuron doctrine.

Alleged intercellular anastomoses
The second argument derives from studies dealing with intercellular connections, first by Bethe and Apáthy and more recently by Bielschowky. This argument can be formulated thus: Around the nerve cell there exists, apart from the nerve terminations discovered by Cajal and confirmed by many savants, a very fine net of neurofibrils (pericellular net of Golgi — everyone credits Golgi for the discovery of this pericellular reticulated cortex, forgetting that a year earlier [Ramón y Cajal, 1897], I had already mentioned it when I used methylene blue in the nerve centers; the first communication of Golgi on the argument dates to 1898), which receives from an outside anastomosis of the nerve nest, being just a continuation of it, and from inside, bridges of union with the intraneuronal reticulum.

This theory, defended five or six years ago with great tenacity and perseverance by Bethe and his disciples and fervently discussed in schools, has crashed like the previous one against the final revelation of the neurofibrillar methods and the information, no less revealing, learned from the neuroplasm procedures.

I declare, of course, that such a flat pericellular reticulum is not of a nervous nature, nor is it related to the terminal arborizations of the axis cylinders. In fact Golgi, who colored and discovered this net using a modified silver chromate method independently of me, thought of it as a neurokeratin frame, destined to protect the cellular periphery; he never found any indications of communication with the nerve nests. Ehrlich's method, which in some cases stains this pericellular net exclusively and with great precision, according to the studies of Donaggio and ours, presents it as a membrane perforated with round holes and totally separate from both the exterior nerve fibers and the interior reticulum. Also Simarro, who stained this mesh with his method, considers it different from the fibrillar frame. On the other hand, Auerbach and Held share the same opinion. The latter author, who studied this reticulum in detail using a variety of techniques, considers it to be a neuroglial dependency, a view shared by Donaggio and others.

Finally, thanks to Bethe's kindness, we have had the opportunity to study the original specimens of this Strassburg physiologist, ascertaining these two important facts: (a) that the procedure of this author did not color the arborizations of nerve terminals: something which led him to wrongly interpret Golgi's net in his preparations as the pericellular nerve nests, completely invisible or insufficiently stained; (b) that the above specimens, carefully studied with better optics, only show a superposition between the pericellular net and the neurofibrils of the cell body, never the substantial contact predicted by the reticularists. Additionally, the pure neurofibrillar methods (ours and Donaggio's), which lack affinity to non-nervous factors of the grey matter (neuroglia, blood vessels, intercellular cement, interstitial coagulated plasma), never reveal the aforementioned superficial net, while they constantly and admirably stain the intracellular neurofibrils, the nests and the rest of the nerve endings.

From all this it can be logically deduced that the nervous nature of Golgi's net, as well as its purported communications with intra- and extra-cellular neurofibrils, represents an anatomical hypothesis deprived of foundations.

So persuasive are the previous observations that the new reticularists, like Held, Holmgren, and Wolff have definitely abandoned the famous superficial net of Bethe, seeking the desired substantial communications (a true obsession for some spirits), not between this net and the neurofibrillar frame of the cell body, but between the terminal boutons of the pericellular nerve nests (Auerbach's boutons) and the previously mentioned protoplasmic scaffolding, an opinion which, *en passant*, represents another new precarious conjecture based on the misinterpreted results of our staining method (see the critiques by van Gehuchten, Michotte, Mahaisu, Schiefferdecker, Cajal, etc.).

Histogenetic arguments

Faced with the overwhelming headway of the concept of His and Forel, the anti-neuronists, uncertain in the morphological terrain, found refuge in neurogenetic arguments, as if this were an unconquerable bastion.

And this time they defended themselves with such zest and dexterity that, unexpectedly, panic spread among the defenders of the classical doctrine. I must confess that until 1903 most published work dealing with the problem of regeneration and embryonic neurogenesis found inspiration in the principles of polygenism. Dohrn, Büngner, Ballauce, Wieting, Durante, Marchand, Modena, Galeoti and Levi, Marinesco, Grasset, etc. fervently took communion in the new religion which was defined by Alfred Bethe, the most genial and ingenious of all of them.

This new reformatory movement dragged even such a clear and well-oriented spirit as van Gehuchten. Seduced by the ability and experimental genius of the physiologist of Strassburg, the scholar of Louvain, without relinquishing his neuronist faith, abandoned part of his previous convictions. In his opinion, the unity of the nerve cell, indisputable in the morphological terrain, would fail in the histogenetic terrain because axon formation could be the collaborative result of a great number of neuroblasts.

Let me formulate with precision the fundamental objection of anti-neuronists, transcribed by Dr. García Solá. The affirmative mode of this objection constitutes the hypothesis which, for brevity, I shall refer to as the *catenary hypothesis or theory*.

(a) The axis cylinders of the nerves of the embryo are not formed, as supposed by Kupffer, His, Kölliker, Cajal, Lenhossék, etc., by simple continuous growth and ramification of the expansion of a single neuroblast (the embryonic nerve cell of the spinal cord), but they derive, as argued by Dohrn, Balfour, Büngner, Bethe, etc., from the fusion and successive differentiation of several neuroblasts of the periphery, originally arranged in series, or as a chain extending from the cord to the nerve endings. The residual protoplasm of such neuroblasts would remain alongside the axis cylinders, forming the future Schwann cells of the myelin sheath.

(b) In accordance with this concept, when a nerve is cut in a young animal and the immediate reunification of the nerve fragments is prevented, the peripheral end, deprived of its trophic center, auto-regenerates; that is, once the old axons are destroyed, Schwann cells return to their embryonic phase, multiplying actively and forming a solid protoplasmic chain, in which the new nerve fibers sprout by differentiation and in a discontinuous fashion. Ultimately, in some cases, such conductors formed without the aid of trophic centers invade the scar and connect with the persisting central ends.

Such is the new theory that opposes the neurogenetic concept of His and Waller. To obtain experimental anatomopathological support, numerous authors, from Brown-Séquard to Bethe, working with the patience of a Benedictine monk, performed thousands of experiments (nerve transplants, root resection, displacement of the nerve stubs). At the same time, zoologists and histologists like Dohrn, Balfour, Sedgwick, Forel, Bethe, Fragnito, Levi, Capobianco, etc., strived to support it in the domain of neurogenesis.

It is sad to think about the sterility of such efforts and the great experimental ingenuity wasted in defending an error which was avoided by the first observers more than 30 years ago (Waller, Ranvier, Ziegler, Stroebe, etc.). However, I do not imply that the deductions of catenarists totally lack support from observations.

I must admit that there are a few dispositions of dubious interpretation that fertilize catenarism, like the appearance of new fibers in transplanted new segments, the regeneration of the peripheral stub displaced and separated from the central stub, the excitability of the peripheral stub with lack of excitability in the central stub, etc. But in their fervor to rapidly reach the prestige of unanimity, the catenarists committed two serious errors: They based their histological judgment on the results of the imperfect osmic acid method, capable of staining the new fibers only very late in the process when they already have a myelin sheath, and conceded major and almost exclusive importance to experimental physiological fallacies and the wish to resolve an anatomical problem. In vain did wise critics such as Munzer, Sangley, Mott, Haliburton, Purpura, and others, despite working with obsolete and unreliable methods, point attention to interpretation errors by Bethe and his followers. It also proved useless that, from the embryological perspective, Kölliker, Lenhossék, Harrison, Kehr, Gurwits, Neal, etc., actively rejected a doctrine that clashes with the best-demonstrated neurogenetic facts and particularly with the straightforward and unequivocal revelations of Golgi's method. Catenarists, disdainful of criticism, indignantly upheld their assertions, aggravating them with new paradoxes. The conflict would have continued if not for the enrichment of technique with a new procedure: The reduced silver nitrate method, born in Spain, and regularly employed throughout Europe today by histologists and anatomic pathologists.

To elucidate the problem, this method has the ability to perfectly stain, in a transparent coffee-brown color, the neurofibrils of the embryonic or young fibers, in embryos as well as in regenerating fibers, showing with perfect clarity the terminal ending, widened in the shape of a bouton, of the newly-formed, wandering axons of the scar. Provided with this new resource, many observers have joined in anatomic pathological experimentation during the last few years, submitting to sharp and severe criticism all the objective data and physiopathologic deductions that are the foundation and warranty of the catenary theory. In addition to us, Medea, Perroncito, Marinesco, Lugaro, Nageotte, Besta, Tello, Cl. Sala, using the silver nitrate method, and Purpura and Krassin, using the Ehrlich method, have shown beyond doubt that the fiery theory of discontinuity and polygenic development represents (with the exception of a few successes in secondary issues) the sad product of the imperfection of methods and neurogenetic and physiologic prejudices.

Lacking space, I cannot go into the details of the remarkable controversy between neuronists and catenarists over these past three years, nor can I point out the facts and arguments used by the defendants of the classic doctrine of His and Waller. Those wishing to inform themselves on this matter should consult published work by Perroncito, Marinesco, Ramón y Cajal [1905, 1906a, 1906b, 1906c] and Tello y Muñoz [1907].

Here I shall limit myself to recalling the following facts, detrimental to the catenary hypothesis and perfectly in agreement with the observations of Perroncito, Cajal, Lugaro, Marinesco, Medea, Krassin, Purpura, Tello, Mott, etc.

1. From the end of the axis cylinders of the central stub of a sectioned nerve one or more non-myelinated branches sprout early (2nd–4th day), before Schwann cells multiply and form strings,, which cross the scar and exit, ramifying profusely and finally reaching the peripheral stub. Thanks to the bouton or growth rod that crowns the ending of all young axons, and which gets perfectly stained by our method, the as yet impossible task of following the newly-formed axons from their origin to their termination has become easy.

2. Once these fibers reach the peripheral stub, they often ramify at the entrance, seize the old casings or Schwann sheaths, and in their exit towards the periphery they arrive (as was recently demonstrated by Tello) at the matrix plates where they reconstruct the old arborizations. Never in their development are they discontinuous, nor do they have any other relation to the cells of Schwann sheath apart from contiguity.

3. The early and active multiplication of Schwann cells of the peripheral stub is not intended to create new auto-regenerating fibers, but to form guide tubes, which get filled with a chemotactic substance meant to attract and steer the new fibers from the scar.

4. In those cases where, following artificial displacement of nerve fragments, there seemed to be, as catenarists envisioned, no sign of unifying fibers, the new staining method revealed a rich plexus of pale, unmyelinated fibers which establish the continuity between the axons of the central and the peripheral stub.

5. Finally, as my observations in embryos have demonstrated, even during the earliest phases, all the axons of the roots appear denuded and in continuation with the neuroblasts of His and not the slightest sign of the cellular chains described by Balfour, Sedgwick, Bethe, Fraquito, etc. exists. Held recently obtained similar results (with variations that do not apply here), successfully utilizing our procedure in the exploration of salamander and avian embryos.

In summary, the morphological arguments have not been confirmed; the anatomic pathological evidence has been refuted with the aid of methods superior to those used by the catenarists; in the field of embryonic development the recent data strongly support the neuron concept.

Everything announces the imminent and definitive victory. This is also evidenced by the doubts and perplexities of some catenarists, the indicative silence of others and the resolute defection of some of the most authoritative and committed individuals. Because in this scientific controversy a unique event has occurred: During the first skirmishes of the fight, and in view of the arguments made by Perroncito and myself, observers as prestigious as Marinesco, Levi, Medea, and Berta moved to my side. Even the illustrious Dohrn, the most formidable knight of catenarism, the reformer and almost founder of this doctrine, has just recognized his errors and is energetically proclaiming the verity of the neurogenetic doctrine of His. Recent observations of the stingray embryo have allowed him to confirm the centrifugal growth of cranial nerve axons, thereby abandoning opinions which he spiritedly held for a decade. Also ominous for the supporters of polygenism is the fact that Pochariski, a Russian doctor who has worked, with the aid of my method and that of Bielschowky's, in the laboratory of Marchand, one of the centers of catenarism and antineuronism in Germany, is reluctant and unwilling to defend the master's doctrine, but only in part and with great reservations. Finally, even the illustrious Bethe, who defined the school, has been influenced by the new findings. It is clear that the author of a voluminous book written in defense of the theory of discontinuity and reticularism cannot drastically change his opinion; but in his last work, where he tried to refute the serious objections to his theory put forth by Perroncito, Lugaro, Cajal, Marinesco, Mott, etc., he already appears much less exclusive, making the concession, among others, that the fibers of the scar and even those of the peripheral stub might stem from those in the central stub; as a consequence, today he does not even hold as true that the definite re-establishment of the paralyzed member's innervation is provided by Schwann cells of the distal stub.

Finally, before concluding this long and cumbersome article I would like to make some statements of personal character.

Among the colleagues that honor me showing interest in the reach and future of my ideas, there are two kinds: the good friends who, unaware of the majority of my works (unfortunately in Spain there are no more than two or three persons who have read them thoroughly) are afraid that, along with the neuron concept (which has been associated with my name by foreigners) my modest scientific work would sink, too; and those — fortunately very few — who, even more unaware of the value and reaches of my personal scientific contribution, seem to feel ineffable delight and frenetic exaltation as soon as a Mr. Nobody foreign histologist, without prestige or authority, echoing perhaps some error of German origin, is permitted to contradict the neuron concept, or other arguments or deductions of mine. To this latter group of pious and affectionate colleagues undoubtedly belong certain persons who, now and again, and in the event of the alleged failure of the neuron — reported in some weekly French medical journal — send to me, believing it would bother me, anonymous letters full of raw insults and vulgar injustices.

It is not appropriate to answer those who attack with the visor down and hidden in the shadows. Nevertheless, I wish to calm both groups of compatriots. Neither do the former need be afraid, nor the latter rejoice. Understand once and for all that the neuron being a German idea, its possible failure would not affect my work, because my work is based on observations and facts, not theories.

The aforementioned concept (it is necessary to repeat, because as interesting as it might be, when the neuron declines, everybody attributes its paternity to me, and the reverse happens when it is on the rise) was formulated, although without proof, by His and Forel in 1887, as one of many conjectures or possibilities against the theories of Gerlach and Golgi, reigning at the time; however, neither His nor Forel could persuade anyone because in order to gain consent for these new ideas, it would have been necessary to objectively demonstrate the very last terminations of nerve fibers in grey matter. Only in 1888 and 1889 when, with the power of patience and perseverance, I described the true endings of the axis cylinders in embryos and young animals (which occur by gearings, pericellular nests, and climbing branches (i.e., by true articulations established between the soma and dendrites on one side and free nerve endings on the other) did the precarious and disdained hypothesis of His and Forel find scientific foundation, spread rapidly among schools, and, with incontestable impetus, overrun all rival theories. Innumerable morphological studies by Lenhossék, Kölliker, Retzius, van Gehuchten, Edinger, Lugaro, Sala, Harrison, Langley, Held, my brother, etc. confirmed and employed my fortunate findings, and the neuron concept, perfectly harmonizing with conjectures from physiology and pathologic anatomy, was elevated to the range of scientific dogma. Finally, Waldeyer, sheltering the new facts and observations under his high authority, had the merit to condense and popularize them in a brilliant synthesis, baptizing the new morpho-dynamic concept of the nervous system with the name *neuron*, which proved fortunate.

[Dr. García Solá, participating in a very common error in Spain, attributes to Dr. Waldeyer an experimental and observational contribution to the neuron doctrine, which never was. The learned anatomist from Berlin did not carry out any particular research on this point; he merely summarized in a German weekly my work and conclusions (as well as those of His, Kölliker, Lenhossék, Retzius, etc.), reproducing the most compelling figures and giving a name, popular today, to the doctrine. Of the three units implicated in it, the *genetic* was formulated by His, whereas the *morphological* and *physiological* is a logical consequence of my personal investigations.]

The neuron concept is, therefore, not mine; nevertheless, it was nourished by the morphological and neurogenetic facts provided by me; data which, confirmed by numerous wise scientists and various analytic methods, possess their own intrinsic and definitive value, whichever theory with which one interprets them, or whatever new complementary structural data the future may bring.

Let us suppose, as I recently noted in my conference in Stockholm (December 12, 1906), that a new method is discovered, one which reveals that within our nests and climbing nerve plexuses and the cell body, there exists a new system of most subtle unifying threads, hitherto inaccessible to current technique. Thanks to such a valuable discovery, my work would have been completed and perfected; in addition to the contacts I found in vertebrates, and Retzius and von Lenhossék found in invertebrates, we would need to admit that more intimate, heretofore unsuspected, ties between neurons in contact exist. The tenebrous cerebral and cerebellar jungle would become even more entangled. Between the swaying neuronal cups, a system of most delicate threads would entangle branches, creating a tight functional cohesion. But in such a case, would the branches, their roots and foliage cease to exist? And would the scientists who discovered them deserve falling into oblivion? In other words, in the improbable case of the definite abandonment of the notion of neuron individuality, how would this affect my own work and the work of many prominent histologists and embryologists, work essentially consisting of the direction and tracks of nervous pathways, encounters of bifurcations and axon collaterals, differentiation of neuronal populations, study of intercellular connections, determination of contacts, etc.? As far as I am concerned, it would all amount to no more than erasing a couple of paragraphs from some books and 180 monographs.

Only those alien to the morphological sciences and laboratory religion distrust the progress in histology and refer to histology as *celestial anatomy*. Impressed by the changeability of theories, they imagine that nothing is stable in histology, that anything can be overlooked because much is under discussion, when in fact there is discussion because there is advance. When histological images, revealing objects and substances in perfect clarity, present them distinctly and consistently in diverse orders of vertebrates; when, examined with various other complementary techniques, they are found to be well studied and described; when an austere observer with a critical stance eliminates personal bias, similar to what astronomers call *personal equation*, then histological facts represent a definite scientific achievement which should not be affected by the caprices of different schools and the fluctuations of speculation any more than the form or chemical properties of a muscle may be. In histology, as in all the natural sciences, doubts and controversies are not over the facts but over their dynamic interpretation.

This creed of preference for facts, as well as distrust for theories, was always the standard of my conduct. Aware of the fragility and volatility of my synthesis — always premature and based on incomplete and unilateral analysis — theories received only cautious accommodation in my books, and if anyone doubts this, they should read the preface of my book on the histology of nervous centers, written in 1898, when neuronism was in full vogue, where regarding hypotheses and theories I wrote a doctrine that was considered excessively skeptical by more than one author.

Returning to the issue of neuronism, I am afraid that the neuron will be around for a while, and in my opinion the meritorious colleagues I alluded to should calm their nerves. Yes, dear colleagues: *la neurona* or *el neurona* will outlast us, and in its march toward the future the neuron will see new sunrises and sunsets. (Dr. García Solá prefers to say *el neurona*, because the French would write *le neurone*. So be it ... However, with that criterion, the Spanish should say *lo neurona*, because Waldeyer, who created the word, used the neutral gender and wrote *das Neuron*. Foreign usage should not impose on us; since the idea that is conveyed by the term, i.e., the concept of the 'nervous unit' *(la unidad nerviosa)*, is feminine in Spanish, let us use the feminine gender.) And in vain do the anti-neuronists hope for tranquility and unanimity. As I have made clear, new battles are beginning. The reticularist hypothesis of Held and others will replace that of Bethe and Apáthy, and the renewed controversy will only change its theater. It is so easy to destroy without creating! It is so difficult to create without destroying!

On my part, I would not hesitate passing to the reticularist camp, were I to be proven wrong. But it has to be proven with facts.

The good Sancho was willing to proclaim Dulcinea's beauty if only he were to be shown a portrait of hers of the size of a hempseed; I am likewise ready to confess the unmatched beauty of the reticularist doctrine, if only I were shown a constant, clear fact in its favor, not larger than a grain of mustard. But as long as the enthusiastic detractors of neuronism put forth, instead of demonstrations, anatomical hypotheses, and instead of precise and constant images, uncertain and incidental appearances, I shall remain faithful to the old and noble flag of unitarism. Because, although I am much concerned with the peace and tranquility of the spirit (not to be attained by me without renouncing the 'contact' doctrine), and although I sympathize with the ingenuous and romantic champions of reticularism, and although I have confessed that the neuron, as a scientific idea, has not been created by me — despite living persuaded that the positive facts provided by my modest work will sooner win than lose with the new speculative interpretations — there is something in me more powerful and captivating than the fancies and delights of the spirit: the sincere and impartial worship of the truth, wherever it may come from.

And for now ... still, the neuron is the truth, or so it seems.

References cited by Cajal in his article

García Solá E (1907) Más sobre el neurona. *Gaceta Médica Catalana (Barcelona) 31:* 241–245

Ramón y Cajal S (1897) Las células de cilindro-eje corto de la capa molecular del cerebro. *Revista Trimestral Micrográfica 2:* 105–127

Ramón y Cajal S (1905) Mecanismo de la regeneración de los nervios (con 30 grabados). *Trabajos del Laboratorio de Investigaciones Biológicas de la Universidad de Madrid 4:* 192–193

Ramón y Cajal S (1906a) Génesis de las fibras nerviosas del embrión y observaciones contrarias á la teoría catenaria (84 grabados). *Trabajos del Laboratorio de Investigaciones Biológicas de la Universidad de Madrid 4:* 227–294

Ramón y Cajal S (1906b) Notas preventivas sobre la degeneración y regeneración de la vías nerviosas centrales. *Trabajos del Laboratorio de Investigaciones Biológicas de la Universidad de Madrid 4:* 295–301

Ramón y Cajal S (1906c) Les metamorphoses precoces des neurofibrilles dans la régénération et la dégénération des nerfs (con 23 grabados). *Travaux du Laboratoire des Recherches Biologiques de l'Université de Madrid 5:* 47–104

Tello y Muñoz JF (1907) Dégénération et régénération des plaques motrices après la section de nerfs. *Travaux du Laboratoire des Recherches Biologiques de l'Université de Madrid 5:* 117–149

PIONEERS IN NEUROLOGY

Anders Retzius (1796–1860)

Lazaros C. Triarhou

Received: 20 August 2012 / Revised: 30 September 2012 / Accepted: 15 October 2012 / Published online: 31 October 2012
© Springer-Verlag Berlin Heidelberg 2012

Anders Adolf Retzius (Fig. 1) was born on October 13, 1796 in Lund as the son of Anders Jahan Retzius (1742–1821) and Ulrika Beata Prytz (1764–1808), and the younger brother of obstetrician Kristian Retzius (1795–1871); he later became the father of neuroanatomist Gustaf Retzius (1842–1919) [2, 4].

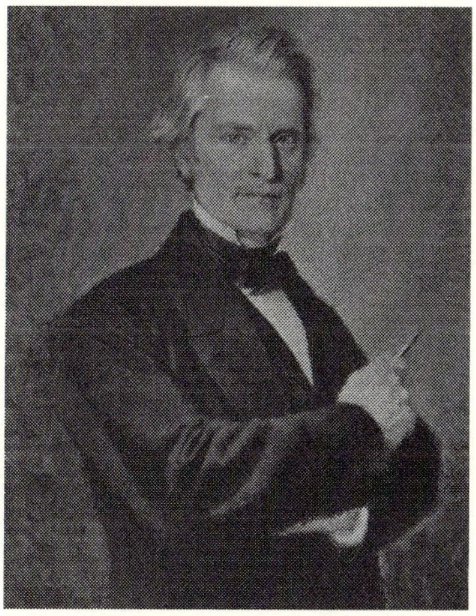

Fig. 1 Oil painting of Anders Retzius by professor Axel Jungstedt (1859–1933), dated 1900; collotype by Chr. Westphal, Stockholm [7]. Copying, redistribution, or retransmission without the author's express written permission is prohibited

L. C. Triarhou (✉)
Economo-Koskinas Wing for Integrative and Evolutionary Neuroscience, University of Macedonia, Thessaloniki, Greece
e-mail: triarhou@uom.gr

Retzius was initiated into zoology by his father, a professor of natural history. He studied anatomy and zoology at the University of Copenhagen and medicine at the University of Lund, graduating from the latter institution in 1819 [4]. His teachers included Arvid Florman (1761–1840), Johannes Reinhardt (1776–1845), Hans Ørsted (1877–1851) and Ludvig Jacobson (1783–1843).

One of his early discoveries was the interrenal organ of elasmobranchs (cartilaginous fish, including sharks), shown later to be homologous to the mammalian adrenal cortex. He published two important morphological studies on the vascular and nervous systems of Myxine glutinosa (hagfish). In collaboration with professor J. S. Billing of Stockholm's Veterinary Institute, Retzius described the ciliary and sphenopalatine ganglia in the horse, and found that the rami communicantes between the cerebrospinal nerves and the sympathetic trunk are connected with the ventral roots as well as with the dorsal roots; he also discovered the peripheral canal of the cornea, later named the 'canal of Schlemm' [4]. In addition Retzius carried out comparative anatomical studies on the avian and reptilian respiratory system, and on the Amphioxus (lancelet).

In 1821 Retzius joined the Veterinary Institute, where he was appointed professor 2 years later. In 1824, endorsed by Jacob Berzelius, Retzius became professor of anatomy at the Karolinska Institute [5]. In 1826, he was elected to the Royal Swedish Academy of Sciences.

His collaborators included Karl von Baer (1792–1876) in Königsberg, Ernst Heinrich Weber (1795–1878) in Leipzig, Johannes Müller (1801–1858) in Berlin, Justus von Liebig (1803–1873) in Giessen and later Munich, Rudolf Wagner (1805–1864) in Erlangen and later Göttingen and Theodor von Bischoff (1807–1882) in Heidelberg. Retzius was introduced to microscopy by Jan Evangelista Purkyně (1787–1869), at the time he attended the Congress of

Naturalists in Breslau in 1833 [4]. Subsequently, he carried out studies on dental histology, describing the brown striae of the tooth enamel or 'contour lines (striae) of Retzius' [6].

Because his eyesight had deteriorated, he devoted his last two decades to gross and topographic anatomy and anthropology. He studied the stomach of rodents, dogs and humans, and defined the divisions of the pyloric antrum and canal, as well as the gastric canal along the inner surface of the lesser curvature. He described the extraperitoneal prevesical space between the symphysis, the bladder, and the anterior abdomen in man, called 'cavum Retzii' or 'retropubic space of Retzius' [1].

The cortical structure with which the name of Anders Retzius is associated by neuroanatomists is a group of gyri he described in 1856 in several mammals (including humans) on the underside of the splenium, in the angle formed by the hippocampus and the dentate gyrus. They appear to be rudimentary in the human brain, but are important in other species, conceivably associated with olfaction. His son Gustaf Retzius named these convolutions 'gyri Andreae Retzii' [8]. Designated as *Balkenwindungen* ('callosal gyri') by Emil Zuckerkandl (1849–1910), and regarded as belonging to the hippocampal formation by Carlo Giacomini (1840–1898) on the basis of their structure, they appear as round or oval eminences on the medial surface of the hippocampus. They are not invariably found in every mammalian species: sometimes they are little more than mere suggestions, whereas when strongly developed they resemble a spirally-wound cord [9]. Cytoarchitectonically, the intralimbic gyri of Anders Retzius belong to the phylogenetically older *allocortex* because they have only three layers of neurons, rather than the six layers of *isocortex*; they are found in a transitional area between the fascia dentata and the fasciolar gyrus [10].

As an anthropologist, Retzius introduced a new classification of humans, based on anatomical cranial characteristics; he coined the term dolichocephalic and brachycephalic [4]. He also pioneered craniometry and is considered one of the founders of physical anthropology.

Influenced by scientific idealism, which viewed perfection as the ultimate goal for history, society and mankind, Retzius favoured an embryological conception of evolution, based on the stages of growth to maturity, as an alternative (spiritual) approach to Darwin's (materialistic) natural selection [3].

A polymath, Retzius also contributed to the history of Scandinavian anatomy, horticulture and to the sanitation and the water supply of Stockholm, and he authored biographical notes on Anders Johan Hagströmer (1753–1830), Arvid Henrik Florman (1761–1840), James Cowles Prichard (1786–1848), Michaël Skjelderup (1769–1852), Georges-Louis Duvernoy (1777–1855), Carl Adolf Agardh (1785–1859), and Jacob Berzelius (1779–1848) [7].

Retzius died on April 18, 1860 in Stockholm. He is among the foremost anatomists and anthropologists of the 19th century, and is credited with introducing the teaching of comparative anatomy and histology into medical curricula in Sweden. In 1896, Gustaf Retzius dedicated his two-volume *Das Menschenhirn* ('The Human Brain'), a classic of macroscopic neuroanatomy, to his late father, in commemoration of the centennial of his birth.

Conflicts of interest None.

References

1. Breimer L (1978) Anders Adolf Retzius (1796–1860). Invest Urol 16:253
2. Grant G (2011) Gustaf Retzius (1842–1919). J Neurol 258: 706–707
3. Gustafsson T (1994) En harmonisk och hierarkisk ordning: synen på utveckling i 1800-talets svenska biologi. Lychnos Lärdomshist Samfundets Årsbok (Uppsala) 1994:87–113
4. Larsell O (1924) Anders A. Retzius (1796–1860). Ann Med Hist 6:16–24
5. Lindblad T (2000) Anders Retzius och Karolinska Institutet. Hagströmer Biblioteket, Stockholm
6. Pindborg JJ (1962) Anders Adolf Retzius and Alexander Nasmyth: a correspondence between two great nineteenth-century dental histologists. J Hist Med Allied Sci 17:388–392
7. Retzius A (1902) Skrifter i Skilda Ämnen jämte Några Bref (Samlade och Utgifna af G. Retzius). Nordiska Bokhandeln, Stockholm
8. Retzius G (1878) Notiz über die Windungen an der unteren Fläche des Splenium corporis callosi beim Menschen und bei Thieren. Arch Anat Physiol Anat Abthlg 1877:474–479
9. Santee HE (1915) Anatomy of the brain and spinal cord with special reference to mechanism and function, 5th edn. Blakiston, Philadelphia
10. von Economo C (2009) Cellular structure of the human cerebral cortex (translated and edited by L.C. Triarhou). Karger, Basel

Cavanna, A.E. (ed.) *Frontal Lobe: Anatomy, Function and Injury*
© 2013 Nova Science Publishers, Hauppauge, New York

Evolution of Christfried Jakob's views on the frontal lobe, 1890–1949

Zoe D. Theodoridou and Lazaros C. Triarhou

Department of Educational and Social Policy, University of Macedonia, Thessaloniki, Greece

Abstract

We review the evolution of the ideas of Christfried Jakob (1866–1956) on the cerebral cortex, with special emphasis on the frontal lobe. For more than five decades, Jakob studied the frontal lobe from the macroscopic to the microscopic level, its function and structure, development, evolution, and pathology. He developed his views on frontal lobe function based chiefly on anatomical works during his 'early' period of the 1890s through the 1910s. In the 1920s, he formulated his psychobiological thought, and in the 1930s and 1940s synthetic neurobiological and neurophilosophical ideas. Arguing that the human cerebral cortex carries within its long natural and social history, he suggested that natural demands have created nervous structures as dictated, at the same time, by the need for cortical specialization and communication. Thus, Jakob attributed a 'humanizing' element to the frontal lobe that lies principally in its praxic character.

Introduction

We track the evolution of the ideas of Christfried Jakob (1866–1956) on the cerebral cortex, particularly on the frontal lobe. Jakob was a German-born neurobiologist, who spent most of his life in Argentina, where he established one of the most important neuropathological laboratories in all of South America. He is considered to be the father of Argentinian neurosciences (Pedace, 1949) and one of the great thinkers of the 20th century. Among his works, the frontal lobe occupied a central part for over five decades (Moyano, 1957).

We have thus divided those works into three 'periods'. During an 'early' period (1890s–1910s), Jakob mostly carried out anatomical works. In his 'middle period' (1920s) he formulated his psychobiological thought. In the 'late' period (1930s–1940s), he developed synthetic neurobiological and neurophilosophical concepts.

Jakob completed his medical studies at the University of Erlangen in 1890. In the early 1890s he worked as an assistant to Adolf von Strümpell at the Erlangen Medical Clinic and privately practised medicine in Bamberg (Orlando, 1995). He published his first book in 1895, an atlas of the normal and pathological anatomy of the nervous system (for details, see Triarhou & del Cerro, 2006a). In 1897, Jakob published an atlas of methods of clinical investigation (an epitome of internal medicine), which was translated into French and English (Triarhou & del Cerro, 2006a).

In 1899, Jakob went to Argentina to direct the Laboratory of the Psychiatric and Neurological Clinic of the Hospicio de Las Mercedes at the National University of Buenos Aires. One of the elements that was crucial in his decision to leave Europe was the prospect of having available 300 brains yearly for pathoanatomical study (López Pasquali, 1965). For a dozen years, Jakob produced works in anatomy, neurology, psychopathology and anthropology (Triarhou & del Cerro, 2007). Then, with his Argentinian contract having ended, he returned to Germany to further his knowledge. At that time, he completed two landmark works on phylogeny, putting forth his original idea on the ubiquity of the sensory-motor dual function of the cerebral cortex (Jakob, 1911; Jakob, 1912a; Jakob, 1912b; Triarhou, 2010a). The works of that 'early' period are mostly centered around the anatomy of the nervous system, reflecting Jakob's German scientific training (López Pasquali, 1965).

The beginning of the 'middle' period of Jakob's work is signalled by his permanent move to Argentina in 1913 (López Pasquali, 1965). At that time, he assumed a triple role consisting of clinical, research and teaching duties. He was appointed Chief of the Neuropathological Institute at the Hospicio Nacional de Alienadas (Mental Asylum for Women) in the Federal Capital, and Professor and Director of the Institute of Biology at the Faculty of Philosophy and Letters of the National University of La Plata. In 1922, Jakob was named Professor of Neurobiology at the Faculty of Humanities and Educational Sciences of the Universidad Nacional de La Plata (Triarhou & del Cerro, 2006b). From 1921 to 1933, he held a joint appointment as Professor of Pathological Anatomy at the School of Medical Sciences of La Plata (Triarhou & del Cerro, 2006b).

A key work from that period is his 1918 article 'From the mechanism to the dynamics of the mind: A critical historical study of organic psychology', in which Jakob pursued his 'dynamic approach'. During that time, Jakob wrote two works which are considered by his biographer and colleague Braulio Moyano (1957) as vital constituents of his psychobiological theorizing: his article 'On he biological bases of memory' (Jakob, 1935b) and his 'Theory on the phylogeny of the kineses' (Jakob, 1935a). However, the emergence of his psychobiological theories becomes obvious in his 1919–1921 work on gnoses and praxes as fundamental factors in cerebral cortical dynamics (Jakob, 1921). Those ideas formed the core for Jakob's future theories (Jakob, 1935a, 1935b).

Gradually, Jakob's thought became more synthetic. He coupled his philosophical background with clinical and research experience. Maintaining that the utmost problem of science and philosophy converges in cerebral function, Jakob studied the brain from the macroscopic to the microscopic level, considered its functional aspects, and pursued its development, evolution, and pathology. He suggested a scientific psychology and a corpus of philosophy (López Pasquali, 1965), in works such as 'The psychogenetic function of the cerebral cortex and its possible localization' (Jakob, 1941), 'The philosophical meaning of the human brain' (Jakob, 1945a), 'The origin of consciousness' (Jakob, 1945b), and 'Common and diverge aspects between biology and philosophy' (Jakob, 1946a) (reviewed in Theodoridou & Triarhou, 2011b, 2011c).

The 'Early' Period (1891–1912)

Between 1906 and 1909 Jakob published eight papers (Jakob, 1906d, 1906f, 1906e; 1906a, 1906b, 1907b, 1907a; 1909), which address biological, anatomo-clinical, pathophysiological and psycholinguistic aspects of the frontal lobe, as well as a series of articles on localization under the title 'Localization of the soul and of intelligence' (Jakob, 1906e). Jakob (1906d) cast doubt on the 'supremacy' previously attributed to the frontal lobe. He argued that "the question concerning superior human functions cannot be answered pointing out their localization in one or another brain lobe but, instead, taking into account issues of another kind" (Barutta, Hodges, Ibañez, Gleichgerrcht, & Manes, 2010).

Jakob's arguments witness a sceptical stance toward strict localization. He highlighted putative historical reasons—from classical Greek philosophy—that might explain the importance attached by various authors to the frontal lobe (Théodoridou & Triarhou, 2011a). In particular, Jakob (1906e) considered the 'Olympian forehead' that is artistically depicted in the sculptures of Zeus as the symbol of 'humanization'.

Having studied preparations with the Weigert method in a series of what are considered as classical contributions, Jakob (1906b) rejected the superiority of frontal myeloarchitectonics by pinpointing at a diminished total density and density of the various layers, a smaller average cell volume and a less developed supraradial layer of the frontal lobe. Campbell (1905) expressed similar views to Jakob regarding the comparatively moderate structural development of the prefrontal cortex, in terms of the low fiber numbers and their delicate nature, as well as the absence of an association system. Regarding Flechsig's proposal of a parallel development of myelination pathways and intellect, Jakob (1906d) remained sceptical.

In regard to the arguments drawn from the clinical literature and placing emphasis on the relation between frontal lobe damage and profound personality changes, Jakob highlighted the rarity of 'pure cases' (1909) in neuropathology. Having studied human brains with frontal lobe tumors, injuries and degeneration, he underlined that (a) the appearance of symptoms does not necessarily coincide with the onset of the disease, and thus, progression may be difficult to determine; (b) tumors compress the brain parenchyma; (c) lesions of vascular origin lead to widespread degeneration; and (d) brain damage may cause either inflammation or concussion that may affect the entire brain (Jakob, 1906b, 1909). Contradictions still exist in the clinical literature that make researchers cautious; case studies may involve either massive lesions extending beyond the frontal lobe or small, unilateral, or asymmetric lesions with correspondingly small and easily compensated effects (Teuber, 2009).

Jakob was fascinated by phylogenetics and viewed it as a means for getting answers about higher human functions, by differentiating between different attributes of the human species and the corresponding evolutionary correlates (Barutta et al., 2010). Jakob's phylogenetic studies on the human brain and over 100 species of the Patagonian fauna (Jakob 1912a, 1912b; Jakob & Onelli, 1913; Triarhou 2010b) provided him with material for formulating original ideas. Jakob (1906d) observed that the evolution of the frontal lobe proceeds from lower to higher mammals in a continual and constant fashion, whereas some other vertebrates do not possess hemispheres with a cortex comparable to that of mammals. Highlighting the similarities between the frontal regions of humans and higher mammals he maintained that productive mentality derives from the frontal lobes. Since the beginnings of the 20th century, human cognitive development was attributed to the large size of the frontal lobes. Modern cytoarchitectonic studies show a very similar organization between human and macaque monkey prefrontal cortex (Petrides, 2005). Moreover, magnetic resonance imaging studies (Semendeferi, Lu, Schenker, & Damasio, 2002) show that the frontal cortex of humans and the great apes occupies a similar proportion of the cortex of the cerebral hemispheres. Accordingly, the enlargement of the human brain has generally preserved the relative proportion of its major lobes (Risberg, 2006).

In the 19th century attempts were made in laboratories where experiments on animals were conducted to show the superiority of the frontal lobe. The experimental confirmation of a motor cortex in the dog brain by Fritsch and Hitzig (1870) was a landmark in the history of functional localization. This tradition continued with new mosaicists and holists. Jakob (1906f) described caveats in such methods, which he considered inappropriate for reaching conclusions about higher human brain functions.

Always considering morphology in a functional context (Tsapkini et al., 2008), Jakob claimed that the elucidation of the anatomical connections of the frontal lobe would decipher its functions (Théodoridou & Triarhou, 2011a). In studying the structure of the frontal lobe, he did not notice any substantial differences from the remaining lobes of the cerebral hemispheres as far as the categories of fibers are concerned, i.e. afferent and efferent projection fibers, association, and commissural fibers (Jakob, 1906f). Emphasizing the importance of studying connections, he anticipated the hodological trend (cf. Catani and ffytche, 2005; ffytche and Catani, 2005). Jakob's writings on cortical connectivity are further attuned to recent theories of frontal systems and neural networks, such as Alexander, de Long and Strick's (1986) concept of parallel but segregated frontal-subcortical circuits, which has been further put into a clinical framework by Chow and Cummings (1999).

According to Jakob (1911), the various centripetal pathways course into all cortical sectors; thus, the cortex has a perceptive activity over its entire extent (Triarhou, 2010b). Based on his anatomical observations, Jakob (1906b) viewed the major part of the frontal lobe as a central station with multiplier and combinatorial characteristics, constantly receiving stimuli from all the motility organs via multiple pathways. He described the sensory-muscular pathways which arrive at the frontal lobe via the cerebellum, the red nucleus and the thalamus, concluding that numerous muscular sensory inputs enter the frontal lobe (Jakob, 1906b).

Based on anatomical and electrophysiological observations, Cappe, Rouiler, & Barone (2009) argued that a connectivity network that includes cortical and thalamocortical pathways as well as the diversity of interactions observed across the thalamus, the cortical sensory or associative areas is involved in multisensory interplay. Thus, most areas in the parietal, temporal, or frontal regions of primates are thought to have connection patterns that relate them to more than one sensory modalities (Cappe, Rouiler, & Barone, 2009).

Jakob's positions apparently antedate some of the modern views on the function of the anterior parts of the human brain, which consider the prefrontal cortex as a locus of synthesis of the outputs of various neuronal systems in providing the basis for the orchestration of complex behavior (Duncan & Miller, 2002). Frontal and prefrontal regions have been linked to visual, auditory and somatosensory inputs (Fogassi et al., 1996; Graziano, Yap, & Gross, 1994; Graziano, Reiss, & Gross, 1999; Wallace, Meredith, M.A., & Stein, 1992). Sensory, mnemonic and response signals that a single neuron displays provide strong evidence that prefrontal neurons behave as sensorimotor integrators (Goldman-Rakic, 2000). Thus, mounting evidence shows that much if not all of the neocortex is involved in multisensory integration (Ghazanfar & Schroeder, 2006). Moreover, the role of the frontal lobe in integrating information from multiple brain areas supports its crucial involvement in learning, comprehension and reasoning (Baddeley, 2002). According to Fuster (2006), actions related to human behavior, reasoning, and language are organized by means of interactions between prefrontal and posterior networks at the top of the 'perception-action cycle'.

The 'Middle' Period (1913-1935)

From 1913 to 1935 Jakob's dynamic approach was gradually refined. He viewed the human brain not as an isolated organ, but as an organ that regulates the internal as well as the external environment (López Pasquali, 1965). In his 1918 paper 'From the mechanism to the dynamics of the mind: A critical historical study of organic psychology' Jakob rejected mechanistic concepts and presented a dynamic approach in explaining cortical function. He argued for an active exchange between the external environment and the adaptive brain (Jakob, 1918).

Jakob incorporated his dynamic views into a phylo-ontogenetic theory of cortical function. He kept moulding his framework (Jakob, 1921; Jakob, 1935a; Jakob, 1946) to include multiple aspects of brain research. According to Jakob's evolutionary postulate (Jakob 1935a; Théodoridou & Triarhou, 2011d; Triarhou & del Cerro, 2006b), phylogeny occurs in two phases. In the first, 'plasmodynamic' phase—or plasmopsychism—elementary biological phenomena such as tropism and pulsatility emerge. The second phase, called 'neurodynamic' and corresponding to 'neuropsychism', is divided into three stages: a phylogenetically older 'archikinetic' stage, where reflex actions emerge; a 'paleokinetic' stage that entails instinctive reactions; and a 'neokinetic' stage, which elaborates conscious motor reactions. 'Neokineses' consist of three kinds of higher neurocognitive processes: (a) 'gnoses', which secure the conscious orientation in one's environment, (b) 'praxes', which underpin active individual intervention and (c) 'symbolisms', which subserve the communication of abstract ideas by means of language, art, etc. Each of these stages corresponds to different levels of organization in the vertebrate C.N.S. The archikinetic stage corresponds to the archineuronal, the paleokinetic to the paleoneuronal, and the neokinetic to the neoneuronal.

Between 1919 and 1921, Jakob presented his theory on gnoses and praxes as fundamental factors in cerebral cortical dynamics (Jakob, 1919, 1921; Théodoridou & Triarhou, 2011d). Gnoses play a key role as the preparatory acts, and praxes as the productive acts, of all psychogenetic processes (Jakob, 1941). For the identification of objects perceived by the senses and the subsequent orientation in the world the integration of the specific features of each object as they are registered in the brain is imperative (López Pasquali, 1965).

Jakob (1921) describes the gnosio-praxic dynamism as follows:

"Through the integration of the sensory information that one normally gets by a certain number of isolated perceptions of distance, color, form, intensity, etc., which characterizes an object one has seen, heard, tasted, etc. normally arrives at a state of 'apperceptive condensation and associative correlation' for the analogous impressions that finally allow the construction of 'the notion of the object', namely its complete gnosis. Thus, gnosis consists in the synthetic condensation of a previous experience with an analogous current situation on the basis of the parallelism of the external and the internal milieu... Gnoses do not result from a special cortical power but from an intricate game of sequential cortical elaborations. Therefore, a gnosis or a sensory perception is not an illusion of the world but a correct approximate representation, proven in practice... Gnoses distribute and organize experience as the securing of orientation in space and time demand it...

All parieto-occipito-temporal cortical zones contribute in the elaboration of gnoses both in animals and in humans. Thus gnoses are represented in the posterior half of the cerebral hemispheres. Nevertheless, gnoses consist in the elaboration and condensation of sensory-motor acts...

Praxis is the cortical process that associates in different combination the series of motor acts during the long learning process in infancy and childhood, to guarantee a determined movement of the limbs, the tongue, the lip, and the trunk or the entire body... The seat of the elaboration of praxes is the whole anterior half of the cerebral hemispheres that is, the anterior Rolandic and the entire frontal lobe with its related associative systems."

Jakob claimed that psychisms are processes of growing complexity (Barutta et al., 2010) and that the human cerebral cortex reflects its long natural and social history (López Pasquali, 1965); the natural demands have created nervous structures in the human brain as they are dictated by the need for cortical specialization and communication at the same time. Based on comparative anatomical studies (Jakob, 1912;

Triarhou, 2010b), Jakob pointed out that the frontal lobe evolved and expanded in a unique way in primates. He wrote (Jakob, 1943, p. 89): "The great development of the frontal lobe is typical of the brain of primates". The evolutionarily older gnosic centers are thought to reside in postcentral 'microdynamics', whereas frontal regions are primarily responsible for praxic processes (Capizzano, 2006).

On the other hand, Jakob considered the strict localization of mental function or dysfunction as misleading. He argued that every gnosic and praxic mechanism comprises localizable elements, such as receptors, assimilators and effectors, but gnosio-praxic dynamics per se are transcortical (Jakob, 1921). By attributing apraxias to the disturbance of transcortical dynamics, Jakob (1921) highlighted the role of cortical communication. Wernicke also opposed the localization of higher functions to specific regions, stressing the importance of association areas (Catani & ffytche, 2005) and claimed that apraxia results from the separation of brain regions (Finger, 1994). Associationist models produced disconnectionist accounts of disorders of higher functions. Liepmann's apraxia model and Déjerine's pure alexia description fall into this tradition, which was revived with Geschwind's neo-associationism. Geschwind (1965a, 1965b) attributed higher function deficits to disconnections that result either from white matter lesions or lesions of association areas, whereas, more recently, Catani and ffytche (2005) updated that model into a hodotopic framework.

Jakob (1921) argued that "gnoses and praxes are neither sensory nor motor, but concomitantly sensory-motor processes" (Jakob, 1911; Jakob, 1912a; Jakob, 1912b; Triarhou, 2010b). Jakob supported the idea of a constant dynamic exchange between the internal and the external milieu, sensation and motion, perception and action.

In his famous book 'Matter and memory' (1896), the French philosopher Henri Bergson (1859–1941) argued that it is impossible to define where perception ends and movement begins (Blumen & Blumen, 2002). The idea of a perception-action cycle has been expressed in various frameworks: in theoretical biology and biosemiotics, by Jakob Johann von Uexküll (1934) to denote perceptual and effector fields that together form a closed unit, the 'Umwelt'; in biocybernetics, by Maturana and Varela (1980; 1987) with the concepts of 'autopoiesis' and 'operational closure'. The German physician and physiologist Viktor Freiherr von Weizsäcker (1950) attempted to represent the unit of perception and movement in a theoretical basis introducing the concept of 'Gestaltkreis', an elaboration of Gestalt psychology. Within ecological psychology, Gibson (1986) saw perception in dynamic terms and emphasized the importance of sensory feedback from movement (Hurley, 2001). Perception and action were thought to be interdependent creating a continuous circle of causes and effects of action (Gibson, 1986). Arbib (1981) put the concept into the framework of computational neuroscience. However, it is Fuster (2006) who is credited with the designation of the perception-action cycle in the cerebral cortex. Therein, the upper stages of the biocybernetic cycle constitute the perception-action cycle where, the sensory information is analyzed in the context of existing perceptual cognits and processed in the context of existing executive cognits.

Although dynamic concepts prevailed in physics in the early part of the 20th century, it took some time for such concepts to be applied to brain theory. Dynamic approaches became popular in many fields after the 1940s confirming the idea that scientific trends reflect an era's broader historical, political and cultural framework (York, 2009). To our knowledge, the first reference to neurodynamics prior to Jakob was made by Trigant Burrow (1943). Wiener's (1948) critical work in cybernetics opened up new vistas (François, 1999). Francisco Varela, a pioneer of modern brain dynamics and cybernetics (cf. Rudrauf, Lutz, Cosmelli, Lachaux, & Le Van Quyen, 2003) supported the view that "consciousness depends crucially on the manner in which brain dynamics are embedded in the somatic and environmental context of an animal's life" (Thompson & Varela, 2001). Thus, influenced by computer science, modern theories use the metaphor of cognition as a dynamic system sustained on spatiotemporal topology (Ibañez & Cosmelli, 2008). Such trends are close to Jakob's views: López Pasquali (1965) emphasizes the fact that certain aspects of Jakob's work such as his studies on the assemblies of circuits seem to anticipate concepts of cybernetics, e.g. autoregulation and feedback.

The 'Late' Period (1935–1949)
Jakob's later years reflect the integration of his thought through the clinical, research and educational experiences, in conjunction with his background in philosophy. Viewing his own self as "a groundworker of a biocentric epistemology", Jakob (1945b) strived to set the foundations of a new interdisciplinary field that would diffuse neurobiological evidence into philosophy. Recognizing the 'humanizing' role of the frontal lobe, Jakob (1943) described the meaning of its dynamics for science and philosophy in a monograph and left that work "rather as a plan for future research and not as an essay with solutions" (Jakob, 1943).

In particular, as far as biology is concerned, he related the progressive perfection that derives from frontal dynamics with the accumulated commemorative function. In neurology, frontal dynamics are thought to be expressed through the evolution from the brutal commands of the generic and irresistible, hereditary and universally obligatory instincts to an elevating liberation that results from an individually orientated intervention in the sphere of consciously caused aims (Jakob, 1943). In psychology, the substitution of the media of communication, conveying exclusively affective information by other, conveying intellectual, was rendered possible by means of the concrete gnosio-praxic experience represented by abstract symbols in language (Jakob, 1943). In sociology, frontal dynamics are related to the possibility of extension and intensification in time and space of the individual and the collective productivity that affects the economic, the cultural and the political spheres in order to progressively become more 'human' (Jakob, 1943). In education, the development of a social intellect that will reinforce individual inclinations and will put emphasis on the active engagement of the student in the formation of concrete knowledge issues from the importance of frontal lobe functions (Jakob, 1943). In neuropsychiatry, it leads to the emergence of objective neuro-psycho-analytical processes for the elaboration of the factors that derive from complex neuropsychological symptoms, reactions and phenomena (Jakob, 1943).

The systematic application of anatomo-clinical methods to study physiological phenomena behind normal and pathological cortical localization and communication leads to the replacement of vague verbal constructions by histo-physio-pathological concrete concepts enabling, thus, the transition from a mechanic to a dynamic phase in neuropsychiatry (Jakob, 1943). Our biopsychism has created unique intellectual, aesthetic and ethical values that enable the explanation of the nature, mental liberty and understanding of the demands and the limits of our mind, thus shedding light onto reality and representation (Jakob, 1943). Praxic (motor) dynamics lead the course of life with the individual and the collective aims; the gnosic intellect, on the other hand, expresses the capability of orientating in one's environment (Jakob, 1943).

Jakob (1943) further proposed that the frontal lobe underpins at the neuronal level the phylogenetic transition from 'blind' desires dictated by impulses to conscious aims planned and executed in order to bring a result. In his late period he revised and updated his phylogenetic postulate in the clinical framework of Pick disease (frontotemporal lobar degeneration). Jakob (1946b) made the supposition that Pick disease represents a model for progressive disintegration of a hierarchical cognitive system (Barutta et al., 2010).

In this revised view, Jakob (1946b) explained that by the Aristotelian concept of 'psyche' he refers to the integrative dynamics issued from sensory-motor regulations. The 'phylopsyche' carries brain activities inherited from phylogenetically older species and is comprised by the 'archipsyche', which contributes to the reflex functions and the 'paleopsyche', which contributes to instinctual functions. The most recent phylogenetic acquisition and typical of the human brain, the 'ontopsyche', is responsible for the elaboration of the individual brain activity mediated by individual experience processes. Ontopsyche or neopsyche, is further divided it into the trophopsyche, an internal milieu regulator whose activity is carried out by the limbic system; the somatopsyche, an external milieu regulator whose activity is performed by the suprasylvian gyri; and the logopsyche, mediator of our symbolization of the world, through the perisylvian gyrus (Barutta et al., 2010). According to Jakob (1946b), Pick disease results in a 'diaschisis', a disruption between the paleopsyche and the neopsyche leading to intellectual and affective disorders. Such a disruption implies the dissociation between the internal and environmental aspects, the subjective and objective world, respectively (Barutta et al., 2010). Therefore, the creation of the most important human ideals is affected because— even though they become realized into the sphere of the intellect—they are rooted in the sphere of the emotions.

Jakob's last publication on the frontal lobe (co-authored with his pupil Eduardo A. Pedace and dated 1949) is entitled 'The task of the frontal lobe in connection with a synthetic quantification of its constitutive elements' (see Triarhou, 2010a). Jakob thought that the frontal lobe reflects the latest acquisitions in the ascending neurophylogeny (Barutta et al., 2010). The fact that the frontal lobe represents 25% of the human brain, i.e. about 350–370 g of cerebral mass, solely considered from a quantitative standpoint, must alone confirm the higher task of their cortical functions. In the frontal lobe, Jakob (1949) recognized the centers of experiential accumulation resulting from personal intervention, progressively elaborated for the elemental and highest human skills, stimulated by the corresponding affective manifestations.

Jakob (1949) viewed the frontal cortex as a locus of interaction between afferent and efferent pathways, the system of transformation of specific stimulations and reactions (endogenous-exogenous frontalization) and with it the final accumulation of its elaborations (frontalized commemorative function). Both areas, in close gnosio-praxic collaboration, execute the conscious activation of human mentality in its creative labor from the concrete to the abstract in an intimate synthesis between their endogenous and exogenous domains, i.e. from their affectivity and intellectuality, reciprocally (Jakob, 1949).

Conclusion

The fact that the human frontal cortex covers about 30% of the total cortical surface has prompted clinicians and basic scientists to hope that unravelling frontal lobe function might eventually explain human behavior (Raichle, 2002). As the riddle of the frontal lobes remains central in modern neurobiology, Jakob's views are still meaningful.

Current theories on the functional localization of cognitive processes in the frontal lobe range from fractionated approaches to central concepts, with concomitant attempts to reconcile contrasting views (Théodoridou & Triarhou, 2010a). The common element in fractionated approaches (cf. Koechlin, Ody, & Kouneiher, 2003; Shallice, 2002; Shallice & Burgess, 1996; Stuss et al., 2002) is the view that there is no unitary frontal lobe process. The anterior part of the brain rather subserves multiple distinct control processes that underpin executive functions (Godefroy, Cabaret, Petit-Chenal, Pruvo, & Rousseaux, 1999). Modularity and fractionation may pertain even to higher human abilities (Baddeley, 1996; Stuss et al., 2002). A more central concept has been put forth by Duncan and Miller (2002) who reject the fixed functional specialization and highlight the adaptability of selected regions of the prefrontal cortex in order to complete a goal-directed activity. Finally, Stuss (2006) argues that the debate between fractionation and adaptability is a false debate and suggested that brain networks may be both locally segregated and functionally integrated. Evidence on the recruitment of the same frontal regions for different cognitive demands (Duncan & Owen, 2000) indicates that in spite of fractionation, frontal processes are applicable to many domain-specific modules; therefore, frontal processes are domain-general (Stuss, 2006).

Jakob used a multilevel approach in studying the frontal lobe in an attempt at being as unbiased as possible. Having understood the limitations and misdirections inherent in any effort to decipher brain-mind relationships, he remained critical of oversimplifying localization explanations (Théodoridou & Triarhou, 2011d) and looked for clues relying on anatomical-clinical correlations. Thus, Jakob's work over 50 years clearly shows a trend that has been discovered anew by modern researchers.

References

Alexander, G. E., DeLong, M. R., & Strick, P. L. (1986). Parallel organization of functionally segregated circuits linking basal ganglia and cortex. *Annual Review of Neuroscience, 9*, 357–381.

Arbib, M. A. (1981). Perceptual structures and distributed motor control. In: V.B. Brooks (Ed.), *Handbook of Physiology; Nervous System, vol. II.* (pp. 1448–1480). Bethesda: American Physiological Society.

Baddeley, A. D. (1996). Exploring the central executive. *Quarterly Journal of Experimental Psychology, 49A*, 5–28.

Baddeley, A. D. (2002). Fractionating the central executive. In: D. T. Stuss, & R. T. Knight (Eds.), *Principles of frontal lobe function* (pp. 246–260). Oxford: Oxford University Press.

Barutta, J., Hodges, J., Ibañez, A., Gleichgerrcht, E., & Manes, F. (2010). Argentina's early contributions to the understanding of the frontotemporal lobar degeneration. *Cortex, 47*, 621–627.

Bergson, H. (1896). *Matière et memoire: essai sur la relation du corps à l'esprit*. Paris: Félix Alcan.

Blumen, S. C., & Blumen, N. (2002). From the philosophy auditorium to the neurophysiology laboratory and back: From Bergson to Damasio. *The Israel Medical Association Journal, 4*, 163–165.

Burrow, T. (1943). The neurodynamics of behavior. A phylobiological foreword. *Philosophy of Science, 10*, 271–288.

Campbell, A.W. (1905). Histological studies on the localisation of cerebral function. Cambridge: University Press.

Cappe, C., Rouiller, E. M., & Barone, P. (2009). Multisensory anatomical pathways. *Hearing Research, 258*, 28–36.

Capizzano, A. (2006). Actualidad del pensamiento de Cristofredo Jakob. *Revista del Hospital Italiano de Buenos Aires, 26*, 71–73.

Catani, M., & ffytche, D.H. (2005). The rises and falls of disconnection syndromes. *Brain, 128*, 2224–2239.

Chow, T. W., & Cummings, J. L. (1999). Frontal subcortical circuits. In: B. L. Miller, & J. L. Cummings (Eds), *The human frontal lobes: Functions and disorders* (pp. 25–43). New York: Guilford Press.

Duncan, J., & Miller, E. K. (2002). Cognitive focus through adaptive neural coding in the primate prefrontal cortex. In: D. T. Stuss, & R. T. Knight (Eds.), *Principles of frontal lobe function* (pp. 278–291). Oxford: Oxford University Press.

Duncan, J. & Owen, A. M. (2000). Common regions of the human frontal lobe recruited by diverse cognitive demands. *Trends in Neurosciences, 23*, 475–483.

ffytche, D. H., & Catani, M. (2005). Beyond localization: From hodology to function. *Philosophical Transactions of the Royal Society of London. Series B, Biological Sciences, 360*, 767–779.

Fogassi, L., Gallese, V., Fadiga, L., Luppino, G., Matelli, M., & Rizzolatti, G. (1996). Coding of peripersonal space in inferior premotor cortex (area F4). *Journal of Neurophysiology, 76*, 141–157.

François, C. (1999). Systemics and cybernetics in a historical perspective. *Systems Research and Behavioral Science, 16*, 203–219.

Fritsch, G. T., & Hitzig, E. (1870). On the electrical excitability of the cerebrum. In: G. Von Bonin (Ed.), *Some Papers on the Cerebral Cortex* (pp. 73–96). Springfield IL: Charles C. Thomas (1960).

Fuster, J. (2006). The cognit: A network model of cortical representation. *International Journal of Psychophysiology, 60*, 125–132.

Geschwind, N. (1965a). Disconnexion syndromes in animals and man. I. *Brain, 88*, 237–294.

Geschwind, N. (1965b). Disconnexion syndromes in animals and man. II. *Brain, 88*, 585–644.

Ghazanfar, A. A., & Schroeder, C. E. (2006). Is neocortex essentially multisensory? *Trends in Cognitive Sciences, 10*, 278-285.

Gibson, J. J. (1986). *The ecological approach to visual perception*. Hillsdale, New Jersey: Lawrence Erlbaum.

Godefroy, O., Cabaret, M., Petit-Chenal, V., Pruvo, J. P., & Rousseaux, M. (1999). Control functions of the frontal lobes. Modularity of the central-supervisory system? *Cortex, 35*, 1-20.

Goldman-Rakic, P. (2000). Localization of function all over again. *NeuroImage, 11*, 451-457.

Graziano, M. S. A., Reiss, L. A., & Gross, C.G. (1999). A neuronal representation of the location of nearby sounds. *Nature, 397*, 428-430.

Graziano, M. S. A., Yap, G.S., & Gross, C. G. (1994). Coding of visual space by premotor neurons. *Science, 266*, 1054-1057.

Hurley, S. (2001). Perception and action: alternative views. *Synthese, 129*, 3-40.

Ibañez, A., & Cosmelli, D. (2008). Moving beyond computational cognitivism: Understanding intentionality, intersubjectivity and ecology of mind. *Integrative Psychological & Behavioral Science, 42*, 129-136.

Jakob, C. (1906a). Consideraciones anátomo-biológicas sobre los centros del lenguaje. *La Semana Médica (Buenos Aires), 13*, 733-737.

Jakob, C. (1906b). Estudios biológicos sobre los lóbulos frontales cerebrales. *La Semana Médica, 13*, 1375-1381.

Jakob, C. (1906c). Existe ó no un centro de Broca? *La Semana Médica (Buenos Aires), 13*, 677-678.

Jakob, C. (1906d). La leyenda de los lóbulos frontales cerebrales como centros supremos psíquicos del hombre. *Arquivos de Psiquiatría, Criminología y Ciencias Afines, 5*, 679-699.

Jakob, C. (1906e). *Localization del alma y de la inteligencia*. Buenos Aires: El libro.

Jakob, C. (1906f). Nueva contribución á la fisio-patología de los lóbulos frontales. *La Semana Médica, 13*, 1325-1329.

Jakob, C. (1907a). Sobre apraxia. *La Semana Médica, 14*, 1344.

Jakob, C. (1907b). Sobre la sintomatología de las afecciones del lóbulo frontal. *La Semana Médica, 14*, 1285.

Jakob, C. (1909). Estudios anátomoclínicos sobre los lóbulos frontales del cerebro humano (Comunicación presentada al IV Congreso Médico Latinoamericano, Rio de Janeiro, 1-8 de agosto de 1909). *Argentina Médica, 7*, 463-472.

Jakob, C. (1911). *Das Menschenhirn: Eine Studie über den Aufbau und die Bedeutung seiner grauen Kerne und Rinde*. J. F. Lehmann, München.

Jakob, C. (1912a). Über die Ubiquität der senso-motorischen Doppelfunktion der Hirnrinde als Grundlage einer neuen, biologischen Auffassung des corticalen Seelenorgans. *Journal für Psychologie und Neurologie (Leipzig), 19*, 379-382.

Jakob, C. (1912b) Ueber die Ubiquität der senso-motorischen Doppelfunktion der Hirnrinde als Grundlage einer neuen biologischen Auffassung des kortikalen Seelenorgans. *Münchener Medizinische Wochenschrift, 59*, 466-468.

Jakob, C. (1918). Del mecanismo al dinamismo del pensamiento: Estudio histórico-crítico de psicología orgánica. *Anales de la Facultad de Derecho y Ciencias Sociales de la Universidad de Buenos Aires, 18*, 195-238.

Jakob, C. (1919). La teoría actual de las gnosias y praxias como factores fundamentales en el dinamismo cortical. *Revista del Círculo Médico Argentino y Centro Estudiantes de Medicina (Buenos Aires), 19*, 1266-1275. Jakob, C. (1921). La teoría actual de las gnosias y praxias como factores fundamentales en el dinamismo de la corteza cerebral. *La Crónica Médica, 38*, 17-24.

Jakob, C. (1935a). La filogenia de las kinesias: Sobre su organización y dinamismo evolutivo. *Anales del Instituto de Psicología de la Facultad de Filosofía y Letras de la Universidad de Buenos Aires, 1*, 109-127.

Jakob, C. (1935b). Sobre las bases orgánicas de la memoria. *Revista de Criminología, Psiquiatría y Medicina Legal, 127*, 84-114.

Jakob, C. (1941). La función psicogenética de la corteza cerebral y su posible localización (Aspectos de la ontopsicogénesis humana. *Anales del Instituto de Psicología de la Facultad de Filosofía y Letras de la Universidad de Buenos Aires, 3*, 63-80.

Jakob, C. (1943). *Folia neurobiológica Argentina, tomo III. El lóbulo frontal: Estudio monográfico anatomoclínico sobre base neurobiológica*. Buenos Aires: Aniceto López-López y Etchegoyen.

Jakob, C. (1945a). El cerebro humano: su significación filosófica. *Revista Neurológica de Buenos Aires, 10*, 89–110.

Jakob, C. (1945b). Sobre el origen de la conciencia: investigaciones neurobiológicas sobre la dinámica cortical en relación con su sectorización conmemorativa. In: E. Mouchet (Ed.), *Temas actuales de psicología normal y patológica, publicados bajo el patrocinio de la Sociedad de Psicología de Buenos Aires* (pp. 345–381). Buenos Aires: Editorial Médico-Quirúrgica/Talleres 'The Standard'.

Jakob, C. (1946a). *Folia Neurobiológica Argentina, tomo V. Documenta Biofilosófica*. Buenos Aires: López & Etchegoyen.

Jakob, C. (1946b). La demencia progresiva: Un analisis neurobiologico de la enfermedad de Pick. *Revista Neurologica de Buenos Aires, 1*, 81-94.

Jakob, C., & Onelli, C. (1913). *Atlas del cerebro de los mamíferos de la República Argentina: estudios anatómicos, histológicos y biológicos comparados sobre la evolución de los hemisferios y de la corteza cerebral*. Buenos Aires: G. Kraft

Jakob, C., & Pedace, E. A. (1949). La misión del lóbulo frontal frente a una cuantificación sintética de sus elementos productores. *Archivos de Neurocirugía, 6*, 467–474.

Koechlin, E., Ody, C., & Kouneiher, F. (2003).The architecture of cognitive control in the human prefrontal cortex. *Science, 302*, 1181–1185.

López Pasquali, L. (1965). *Christfried Jakob. Su obra neurológica, su pensamiento psicológico y filosófico*. Buenos Aires: López.

Maturana, H. R., & Varela, F. J. (1980): *Autopoiesis and cognition. The realization of the living*. Dordrecht: Reidel.

Maturana, H. R., & Varela, F. J. (1987). *The tree of knowledge: The biological roots of human understanding*. Boston, MA, US: New Science Library/Shambhala Publications.

Moyano, B. A. (1957). Christfried Jakob, 25/12/1866–6/5/1956. *Acta Neuropsiquiátrica Argentina, 3*, 109–123.

Orlando, J. C. (1966). *Christofredo Jakob: Su vida y obra*. Buenos Aires: Editorial Mundi.

Pedace, E. A. (1949). Contribución de la escuela neurobiológica Argentina del Prof. Chr. Jakob en el estudio del lóbulo frontal. *Archivos de Neurocirugía, 6*, 464–466.

Petrides, M. (2005). Lateral prefrontal cortex: Architectonic and functional organization. *Philosophical Transactions of the Royal Society of London. Series B, Biological Sciences, 360*, 781–795.

Raichle, M. E. (2002). Foreword. In: D. T. Stuss, & R. T. Knight (Eds.), *Principles of frontal lobe function* (pp. vii–ix). Oxford: Oxford University Press.

Risberg, J. (2006). Evolutionary aspects on the frontal lobes. In: J. Risberg, & J. Grafman (Eds), *The frontal lobes: Development, function, and* pathology (pp. 1–20). Cambridge: Cambridge University Press.

Rudrauf, D., Lutz, A., Cosmelli, D., Lachaux, J.-P., & Le Van Quyen, M. (2003). From autopoiesis to neurophenomenology: Francisco Varela's exploration of the biophysics of being. *Biological Research, 36*, 27–66.

Semendeferi, K., Lu, A., Schenker, N., & Damasio, H. (2002). Humans and great apes share a large frontal cortex. *Nature Neuroscience*, 5, 272–276.

Shallice, T. (2002). Fractionation of the supervisory system. In: D. T. Stuss, & R. T. Knight (Eds.), *Principles of frontal lobe function* (pp. 261–277). Oxford: Oxford University Press.

Shallice, T., &Burgess, P. (1996). The domain of supervisory processes and temporal organization of behaviour [and discussion]. *Philosophical Transactions: Biological Sciences, 351*, 1405–1412.

Stuss, D. T. (2006). Frontal lobes and attention: Processes and networks, fractionation and integration. *Journal of the International Neuropsychological Society, 12*, 261–271.

Stuss, D. T., Alexander, M. P., Floden, D., Binns, M. A., Levine, M., McIntosh, A. R., Rajah, N., & Hevenor, S.J. (2002). Fractionation and localization of distinct frontal lobe processes: Evidence from focal lesions in humans. In: D. T. Stuss, & R. T. Knight (Eds.), *Principles of frontal lobe function* (pp. 392–407). Oxford: Oxford University Press.

Teuber, H. L. (2009). The riddle of frontal lobe function in man. *Neuropsychology Review, 19*, 25–46.

Théodoridou, Z. D., Triarhou L. C. (2011a). Challenging the supremacy of the frontal lobe: Early views (1906–1909) of Christfried Jakob on the human cerebral cortex. *Cortex.* doi:10.1016/j.cortex.2011.01.001.

Théodoridou, Z. D., Triarhou L. C. (2011b). Christfried Jakob's late views on cortical development, localization and neurophilosophy. *Neuroscience Letters* (in press).

Théodoridou, Z. D., Triarhou, L. C. (2011c). Christfried Jakob's late views (1930-1949) on the psychogenetic function of the cerebral cortex and its localization: Culmination of the neurophilosophical thought of a keen brain watcher. *Brain and Cognition* (in press).

Théodoridou, Z. D., Triarhou, L. C. (2011d). Christfried Jakob's 1921 theory of the gnoses and praxes as fundamental factors in cerebral cortical dynamics. *Integrative Psychological and Behavioral Science, 45,* 247–262.

Thompson, E., & Varela, F. J. (2001). Radical embodiment: Neural dynamics and consciousness. *Trends in Cognitive Sciences, 5,* 418–425.

Triarhou, L. C., & del Cerro, M. (2006a). Semicentennial tribute to the ingenious neurobiologist Christfried Jakob (1866–1956). 1. Works from Germany and the first Argentina period, 1891–1913. *European Neurology, 56,* 176–188.

Triarhou, L. C., & del Cerro, M. (2006b). Semicentennial tribute to the ingenious neurobiologist Christfried Jakob (1866–1956). 2. Publications from the second Argentina period, 1913–1949. *European Neurology, 56,* 189–198.

Triarhou, L. C., & del Cerro, M. (2007). Pioneers in Neurology: Christfried Jakob (1866–1956). *Journal of Neurology, 254,* 124–125.

Triarhou, L. C. (2010a). Final publications of Christfried Jakob: On the frontal lobe and the limbic region. In: C. E. Flynn, & B. R. Callaghan, (Eds.), *Neuroanatomy Research Advances* (pp. 165–169). Hauppauge, NY: Nova Science Publishers.

Triarhou, L. C. (2010b). Revisiting Christfried Jakob's concept of the dual onto-phylogenetic origin and ubiquitous function of the cerebral cortex: A century of progress. *Brain Structure and Function, 214,* 319–338.

Tsapkini, K., Vivas, A. B., & Triarhou, L. C. (2008). 'Does Broca's area exist?' Christofredo Jakob's 1906 response to Pierre Marie's holistic stance. *Brain and Language, 105,* 211–219.

von Uexküll, J. (1934). A stroll through the worlds of animals and men. In: C. Schiller (Ed.), *Instinctive behavior* (pp. 5–80). New York: International Universities Press, 1957.

von Weizsäcker, V. (1950). *Der Gestaltkreis.* Stuttgart: Thieme.

Wallace, M. T., Meredith, M. A., & Stein, B. E. (1992). Integration of multiple sensory modalities in cat cortex. *Experimental Brain Research,* 91, 484–488.

Wiener, N. (1948). *Cybernetics or control and communication in the animal and the machine.* Paris: Hermann.

York III, G. K. (2009). Localization of language function in the twentieth century. *Journal of the History of the Neurosciences, 18,* 283–290.

An Avant-Garde Professorship of Neurobiology in Education: Christofredo Jakob (1866–1956) and the 1920s Lead of the National University of La Plata, Argentina

ZOE D. THÉODORIDOU,[1] ATHANASIOS KOUTSOKLENIS,[1] MANUEL DEL CERRO,[2] AND LAZAROS C. TRIARHOU[1]

[1]Neuroscience Wing, Department of Educational and Social Policy, University of Macedonia, Thessaloniki, Greece
[2]Departments of Neurobiology & Anatomy, Ophthalmology, and Neurology, University of Rochester, Rochester, NY, USA

The interdisciplinary trend in "Mind, Brain, and Education" has witnessed dynamic international growth in recent years. Yet, it remains little known that the National University of La Plata in Argentina probably holds the historical precedent as the world's first institution of higher education that formally included neurobiology in the curriculum of an educational department, having done so as early as 1922. The responsibility of teaching neurobiology to educators was assigned to Professor Christofredo Jakob (1866–1956). In the present article, we highlight Jakob's emphasis on interdisciplinarity and, in particular, on the neuroscientific foundations of education, including special education.

Keywords Christfried Jakob, cerebral onto-phylogeny, history of neuroeducation, neurophilosophy

Introduction

Some of the earliest attempts at applying neurobiological findings to education can be traced to the work of the neurologist Henry Herbert Donaldson (1857–1938) and the educator Reuben Post Halleck (1859–1936; Théodoridou & Triarhou, 2009). The new tools of biology and cognitive science have generated vast possibilities for this field, enabling the integration of diverse disciplines that study human learning and development (Fischer et al., 2007). Terms used interchangeably to denote this new branch of knowledge include "neuroeducation" (Battro & Cardinali, 1996), "neurolearning" (Petitto & Dunbar, 2004),

---

The authors gratefully acknowledge Dr. Daniel S. Margulies of the Max Planck Institute for Human Cognitive and Brain Sciences in Leipzig for his invaluable help, the anonymous reviewers for their constructive criticism that led to an improved manuscript, and the courtesy of the staff at Biblioteca de Humanidades de la Universidad Nacional de La Plata, Academia de Medicina de Buenos Aires, Ibero-Amerikanisches Institut Preussischer Kulturbesitz zu Berlin, British Library, Library of Congress, Smithsonian Institution Libraries-National Zoological Park Library, National Library of Medicine of the United States, Ruth Lilly Medical Library of Indiana University, and Bernard Becker Medical Library of Washington University for bibliographic assistance.

Address correspondence to Lazaros C. Triarhou, University of Macedonia, Egnatia 156, Building Z-312, Thessaloniki, GR 54006, Greece. E-mail: triarhou@uom.gr

"nurturing the brain" (Ito, 2004), "developing the brain" (Koizumi, 2004), "mind, brain, and education" (Fisher et al., 2007), "educational neuroscience" (Geake, 2005; Szűks & Goswami, 2007), and "pedagogical neuroscience" (Fawcett & Nicolson, 2007).

The dynamic growth of "neuroeducation" and the opportunities for interdisciplinarity are evidenced by (a) the establishment of academic programs and departments, such as the "Centre for Neuroscience in Education" at the University of Cambridge, the "Mind, Brain, and Education Program" at the Harvard Graduate School of Education, and Dartmouth's "Center for Cognitive and Educational Neuroscience," (b) the emergence of the "International Mind, Brain and Education Society" and the launch of its official journal in 2007, as well as the launch of another new journal in 2012, the *Trends in Neuroscience and Education*, (c) the organization of congresses, meetings, and seminars at both the international (European Association for Research on Learning and Instruction, Zürich, 2010; International Mind, Brain and Education Society, Philadelphia, 2009, San Diego, 2011) and local levels (Collaborative Frameworks for Neuroscience and Education, UK, 2005–2006), and (d) the attention received in the mainstream press and by the lay public (see also Beauchamp & Beauchamp, 2012).

There are additional examples of the worldwide impact of the neuroeducation movement. In the United Kingdom, the Teaching and Learning Research Programme administered by the Economic and Social Research Council (TLRP-ESRC) organized a seminar series on Neuroscience and Education which brought together national and international education and science experts to discuss how these two areas may collaborate. At its conclusion, in June 2006, over 400 teachers, educational researchers, psychologists, and neuroscientists had participated in the series. In Germany, the Federal Ministry of Education and Research found it reasonable to concentrate on the latest line of research in educational neuroscience to improve education (Stern, 2006). In Finland, a national network on neuroscience and education hosted its activities in the University of Helsinki, beginning in 2009, under the theme "The Brain, Learning and Education Network."

Still, it remains a little known fact that the National University of La Plata in Argentina holds a historical precedent as most likely the world's first institution of higher education that formally introduced and included neurobiology in the curriculum of an education department. It was Christfried Jakob (1866–1956; Figure 1), a Bavarian-born neuropathologist, who promoted the initiative to teach brain structure and function to students of the Faculty of Philosophy and Letters as early as 1922.

Prior to 2006, a literature search in the PubMed database would yield no returns on Jakob, save an article by Meyer in Spanish (Théodoridou, 2011). Since 2005, a systematic effort began by one of us (LCT) and his colleagues to retrieve and revive Jakob's writings; this ongoing project has aimed at placing Jakob's ideas in a modern neuroscientific perspective (Théodoridou & Triarhou, 2011, 2012a, 2012b; Triarhou, 2008a, 2008b, 2009, 2010a, 2010b; Triarhou & del Cerro, 2006b, 2006c, 2007; Tsapkini, Vivas, & Triarhou, 2008; Vivas, Tsapkini, & Triarhou, 2007). In the present study, we review Jakob's contributions to education, an endeavor that he pursued throughout his career.

Jakob's Professional Life

Jakob (his forename castillianized to "Christofredo"), the founder of neuropathology in Argentina, adopted that country as his home and lived there from 1899 until his death in 1956, with only a brief visit to Europe from 1910 to 1912 (Moyano, 1957; Fumagalli & Saredo, 2005). He was recognized for his neuroanatomical work, particularly for the systematization of brain sectioning and the application of the Weigert method to the study of

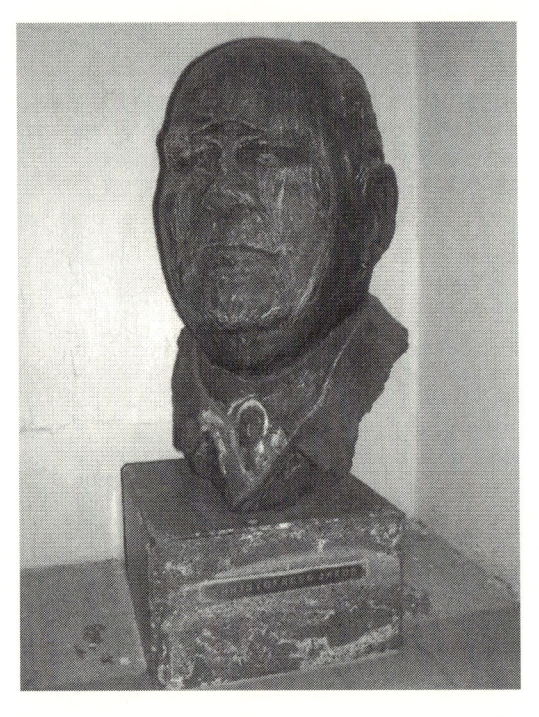

Figure 1. Bust of Christofredo Jakob at the Pathology Laboratory, Moyano Psychiatric Hospital, Buenos Aires. Credit: http://www.flickr.com/photos/theodor_meynert/4695367482.

myelinated fiber tracts (Allegri, 2008). He authored 30 books and 200 articles on developmental, evolutionary, anatomical and pathological neurobiology (Figure 2; Triarhou & del Cerro, 2006c). His approach was largely based on studying species of Argentinian fauna (Papini, 1978, 1988). For example, his theory on the phylogenetic origin of the neocortex (Jakob, 1945) issued from his histological studies on *Amphisbaena*, a small apod reptile (Papini, 1988). Jakob is credited with combining phylogenetic, embryological, and functional approaches in a quest to explain the role of the cerebral cortex in cognition and behavior (Triarhou, 2008b). From such an attempt ensued his theory of a dual developmental-evolutionary origin and ubiquitous sensory-motor function of the cerebral cortex (Jakob, 1911, 1912a, 1912b; Triarhou, 2010b). He further studied and highlighted the fields of neurophilosophy, affective neuroscience, and educational neuroscience (Triarhou, 2008a; Théodoridou, 2011). He did so based on his collective academic, clinical, and research experience from multiple vocational frameworks, including universities (National University of Buenos Aires and National University of La Plata), hospitals (Las Mercedes Hospital in Buenos Aires and National Psychiatric Hospital for Women in the Federal Capital), and research laboratories (Laboratory of the Psychiatric and Neurological Clinic of Las Mercedes Hospital, Neuropathological Institute at the National Psychiatric Hospital for Women in the Federal Capital, and Institute of Biology at the Faculty of Philosophy and Letters of the National University of La Plata; Triarhou & del Cerro, 2006b, 2007).

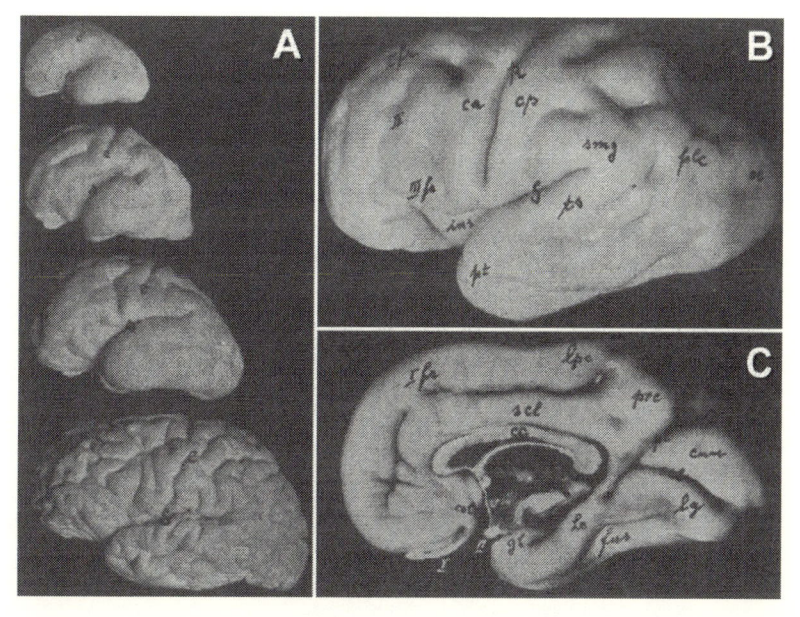

Figure 2. One of Jakob's main interests was developmental neurobiology, human and comparative. (a) Lateral view of left cerebral hemisphere in human embryos at 4, 5, 6, and 8 months of gestation, showing the progressive gyration (Jakob, 1941, p. 428). (b) Lateral view of left cerebral hemisphere in a fetus at a gestation age of 5½ months (Jakob, 1941, p. 433). (c) Midsagittal facies of right cerebral hemisphere in a human fetus at 5 months of gestation (Jakob, 1941, p. 433). From the private archive of L. C. Triarhou. Copying, redistribution, or retransmission without the author's express written permission is prohibited.

His work can be roughly divided into three periods, each having a slightly different focus. Jakob shared the "early period" of his work (1890–1912) between Germany and Argentina, carrying out anatomical studies (Théodoridou & Triarhou, 2012a). During his "middle period" (1913–1935), he developed his psychobiological ideas (Théodoridou & Triarhou, 2011). In the "late period" (1936–1949), he formulated a neurobiophilosophical synthesis (Théodoridou & Triarhou, 2012b).

Overall, Jakob realized the essence of the current definition of the mind, brain, and education convergence, that is, "the integration of disciplines that investigate human learning and development bringing together education, biology, and cognitive science" (Fischer et al., 2007, p. 1) as his life's paradigm. In 1899, at 33 years of age, Jakob had already attained renown after publishing a handbook of neuroanatomy and neuropathology that was translated in multiple languages (Triarhou & del Cerro, 2006b). In that year, he accepted an offer by Domingo Cabred (1859–1929), the Argentinian Professor of Psychiatry, to take over the organization of the Laboratory of the Psychiatric and Neurological Clinic of the Hospital of Las Mercedes at the National University of Buenos Aires (Orlando, 1966). The prospect of having 300 brains available for pathological study on an annual basis was a key factor that influenced his decision to leave Germany for South America (López Pasquali, 1965). Thus, he moved to Argentina, having signed a three-year contract.

During that time, he struggled to transform his innovative ideas into action. Already in 1906, encouraged by the visionary Minister of Public Education, Joaquín V. González

(1863–1923),[1] Jakob asked for permission from the University of Buenos Aires to introduce a new course under the title "The Nervous System and its Relationship to Education" (Orlando, 1966). However, he met with resistance, and it took several years for such an initiative to be effected. (It is not surprising that even in the past, the idea that neuroscience is or should be an important aspect of educating educators often sounded foreign to pedagogues or psychologists, who, not knowing a neuron from a glial cell, had little interest in neurobiology and avoided any serious study of the brain like the plague. The attitude that neuroscience was irrelevant for educators, other than as a subject matter to be taught by someone else, and the predilection exclusively for behavioral and psychological theories and practices are fortunately waning.)

The "Universidad Provincial de La Plata" was inaugurated on April 18, 1897 under the Administration of Dr. Guillermo A. Udaondo (1859–1922), Governor of Buenos Aires, with Dr. Dardo Rocha (1838–1921) serving as Rector.[2] The University of La Plata became nationalized by Act 4609 of Congress and by Provincial Law on September 29, 1905. When González was appointed its President the following year, he integrated several municipal scientific institutions into the university and brought substantial change by placing an emphasis on experimental and natural science methods (González, 1905). For example, he introduced modern academic physics to the country (Glick, 1996).

Jakob held faculty positions at the University of Buenos Aires from 1913 to 1944 and at the University of La Plata from 1922 to 1933 (Papini, 1988). In 1912, the Faculty of Philosophy and Letters of the University of Buenos Aires created a Professorship of Biology in an attempt to enhance the scientific status of the School (Nazar Anchorena et al., 1927; Orlando, 1966).[3] Jakob was then appointed Professor and assumed the task of building a solid biological basis for psychological and philosophical studies (Talak, 2008). The reverberation of the success of Ramón y Cajal in the Hispanic world and his Nobel Prize award must have played a part in the emphasis placed by the University of La Plata on the brain sciences. For instance, in 1906, the *Archives of Pedagogy* (official journal of the Faculty of Education) published in the inaugural volume two papers by Cajal on the

---

[1] González was admitted into the *Real Academia Española*, the Royal authority on the Spanish language, in 1906, and was elected to the Argentine Senate in 1916 (while still President of the University). Retiring from the latter in 1918, he returned to the University of Buenos Aires, where he taught Constitutional Law, Public Law, and a course in the History of Foreign Relations of Argentina. He contributed regularly to *La Nación* as a columnist and translated Rabindranath Tagore's *One Hundred Poems of Kabir*. He joined the International Law Association in 1919, and advocated on behalf of the League of Nations, as well as U.S. President Woodrow Wilson's efforts towards its ratification by a recalcitrant Senate. His most controversial work, *Patria y Democracia* (Fatherland and Democracy), was published in 1920 and delved into regional and political tensions in Argentina. González's efforts on behalf of the League of Nations helped lead to his nomination to the International Court of Justice at The Hague, becoming a member in 1921. González died in Buenos Aires in 1923; he was 60. *Fábulas Nativas*, a work of cultural anthropology, was published posthumously in 1924, and González left a bibliography of over a thousand works, including 50 books on a variety of academic subjects.

[2] Rocha was an Argentine naval officer, lawyer, and politician best known as the founder of the city of La Plata and of the University of La Plata. La Plata was planned by the architect Pedro Benoit in a regular pattern of diagonals and precisely placed squares. His success in La Plata led the Governor to seek his party's nomination for the presidency in 1886. Rocha was a well-known, well-connected, and persuasive candidate who had secured his place among Argentina's paramount "Generation of 1880" but lost the nomination to Miguel Juárez Celman, the Governor of the Province of Córdoba and President Roca's son-in-law.

[3] The Anchorenas were one of the most traditional, socially prominent, and richest families of Argentina. There was a saying: "Rich as the Anchorenas."

morphology and connections of nerve cells (Ramón y Cajal, 1906a, 1906b). The inclusion of highly technical neuroanatomical papers in a purely pedagogical journal is in itself a remarkable act. The following year, on December 14, 1907, the Science Museum of the University of La Plata bestowed Cajal the title of "Honorary Academician" (Ramón y Cajal, 1988, p. 628).

In 1913, Jakob published the "Atlas of the Brain of Mammals of Argentina" in collaboration with Clemente Onelli (1864–1924), the director of the Buenos Aires Zoo. Jakob and Onelli (1913) intended to establish the biological basis of mental phenomena, underscoring that psychology would either use the comparative method in studying nervous function and structure, in order to shed light on psychological phenomena, or it would be limited to the descriptive method (Papini, 1988). Eventually, in 1922, the National University of La Plata appointed Jakob as Professor of Neurobiology at the Faculty of Humanities and Educational Sciences (Triarhou & del Cerro, 2006c), rendering him one of the first academic teachers of neurosciences in a department of education (Figures 3 and 4). In fact, his course "Anatomy and Physiology of the Nervous System" (Figure 5) was taught in freshman year to the future teaching workforce of the country (Gotthelf, 1969).

Jakob's insight into the evolutionary basis of behavior, founded on his research in comparative developmental neuroanatomy, became known and cited. In one of the early textbooks of biological psychology (translated in French and German and prefaced by Wilhelm Ostwald, Nobel laureate in chemistry), the philosopher-psychiatrist José Ingenieros (1877–1925) credits Jakob and the palaeontologist Florentino Ameghino, along with Ramón y Cajal, van Gehuchten, Golgi, and von Lenhossék, for their fundamental discoveries in the anatomy and phylogeny of the nervous system (Ingenieros, 1922; Triarhou & del Cerro, 2006a). In the postscript to his autobiography, the great Ramón y Cajal (1988, p. 602) acknowledges Jakob (1922) among the foreign scientists of prestige who contributed to the two-volume *Festschrift* on the occasion of his retirement at the age of 70, including the Vogts, Loeb, Herrick, Sherrington, von Monakow, Marie, Houssay, and numerous others. Finally, in their monumental *Cytoarchitectonics*, von Economo and Koskinas (1925) argue that future research on the human cerebral cortex will have to be based on the work of three of the most important cortical neuroanatomists, that is, Theodor Kaes, Ramón y Cajal, and Christfried Jakob, whose ideas on cortical phylo-ontogeny they call ingenious.

In the capacity of Professor of Neurobiology in the School of Humanities and Educational Sciences, Jakob epitomized the neuroeducational idea through his teaching and research activities, discussed next.

Teaching Neurobiology to Educators

In considering the fervent growth of Educational Neuroscience, we note that the attempt to bridge neuroscience with the humanities goes back more than a century. The books of Donaldson (1895) and Halleck (1896) were published at the same time as Jakob's first atlas of the normal and pathological nervous system (1895). We do not have any evidence that Jakob was aware of Halleck's or Donaldson's books. Nevertheless, some years later he laid a new stone in the formation of Educational Neuroscience.

Throughout his career, Jakob defended the dissemination of neuroscientific knowledge into the humanities. He dealt with that topic in his *Documenta Biofilosófica* (Biophilosophical Documents; Jakob, 1946). He developed his rationale as follows (Théodoridou & Triarhou, 2012a): First of all, life sciences form a justified basis for an

FACULTAD DE HUMANIDADES Y CIENCIAS DE LA EDUCACIÓN

Decano

Doctor Ricardo Levene.

Vicedecano

Doctor Juan José Nájera.

Consejeros académicos titulares

Señor Rafael Alberto Arrieta.
Doctor Alfredo D. Calcagno.
Señor Rómulo D. Carbia.
Doctor Juan Chiabra.
Profesor Pascual Guaglianone.
Doctor Enrique Mouchet.

Consejeros académicos suplentes

Doctor Tomás D. Casares.
Profesor Mateo Heras.
Profesor Francisco Legarra.
Doctor Enrique Loedel Palumbo.
Doctor Juan Millé Giménez.
Abogado Alberto Palcos.

Representantes de los estudiantes al Consejo académico

Señor José Armando Seco.
Señorita Araceli Saborido Gómez.

Secretario

Profesor Carlos Heras.

Profesores titulares

Historia de la filosofía: Doctor Alejandro Korn.
Lógica: Doctor Alfredo Franceschi.
Psicología: Doctor Enrique Mouchet.
Biología y anatomía y fisiología del sistema nervioso: Doctor Christofredo Jakob.
Higiene escolar: Ingeniero Antonio Restagnio.
Psicopedagogía: Doctor Alfredo D. Calcagno.
Legislación escolar argentina y comparada: Doctor Juan E. Cassani.
Ética: Doctor Coriolano Alberini
Didáctica general: Profesor José Rezzano.
Introducción a la filosofía: Doctor Coriolano Alberini.
Prehistoria argentina y americana: Doctor Luis María Torres.
Historia argentina: Doctor Ricardo Levene.
Historia de la civilización antigua: Profesor Pascual Guaglianone.
Historia de la civilización moderna: Profesor José A. Oría.
Introducción a los estudios históricos argentinos y americanos: Señor Rómulo D. Carbia.
Sociología: Doctor Ricardo Levene.
Composición y gramática: Señor Arturo Marasso.
Literatura castellana: Señor Arturo Marasso.
Literatura de la Europa meridional: Señor Rafael Alberto Arrieta.
Literatura de la Europa septentrional: Señor Rafael Alberto Arrieta.
Literatura argentina y de la América española: Doctor Arturo Capdevila.
Literatura griega y latina: Doctor Leopoldo Longhi.
Latín, primer curso: Doctor Juan Chiabra.
Latín, segundo curso: Doctor Juan Chiabra.
Griego, primer curso: Doctor Leopoldo Longhi.

Figure 3. Roster of administrative officers and members of the Faculty of Humanities and Educational Sciences, National University of La Plata (Nazar Anchorena et al., 1927, pp. 20–21). The faculty roster includes some remarkable names. The Dean, Doctor (probably Law Doctor) Ricardo Levene, professor of Argentinian History and Sociology, was the author of the most respected and widely read *Historia de la República Argentina* available in the midtwentieth century. Alejandro Korn (1860–1936) was an Argentine physician, psychiatrist, philosopher, reformist, and politician. For 18 years, he was the director of the psychiatry hospital in Melchor Romero (a locality of La Plata in the province of Buenos Aires), named for the city. He was the first university official in Latin America to be elected, thanks to the students' vote. He is considered the pioneer of Argentine philosophy. Along with Florentino Ameghino, Juan Vucentich, Almafuerte, and Carlos Spegazzini, he is considered to be one of the five wise men of La Plata. He was still remembered with respect in the university days of one of the authors (MdC) as a man of extraordinary culture and liberal ideals. Rafael Alberto Arrieta was one of the best known and respected writers around 1945–1964 (MdC). Leopoldo Lugones: If Arrieta was the man of letters that saw the present and dreamed the future, Lugones was the man that saw the present and wanted to live in the past. A respected poet, we reluctantly have to admit. His son Leopoldito, as he was sarcastically called, became the chief torturer of the Argentinian police, or so it was said. Apparently he wanted to restore "la Argentina de la Cruz y de la Espada." From the private archive of L. C. Triarhou. Copying, redistribution, or retransmission without the author's express written permission is prohibited.

objective, rational, and scientific development of philosophical orientations (Jakob, 1946). Thus, the scientific field that studies nervous structure and function is indispensable for psychology and its related sciences. Further, knowledge of the evolution of the human brain in correlation with cognitive development, as well as brain alterations and their sequelae on memory, behavior, language, and other abstract processes, forms the natural foundation of a conscious learning science, as the creation and preservation of higher cognitive functions (intellect, volition, and emotions), instincts and reflexes depend on human cerebral organization. Thus, Jakob called for a learning science aware of the biological mechanisms that underpin learning.

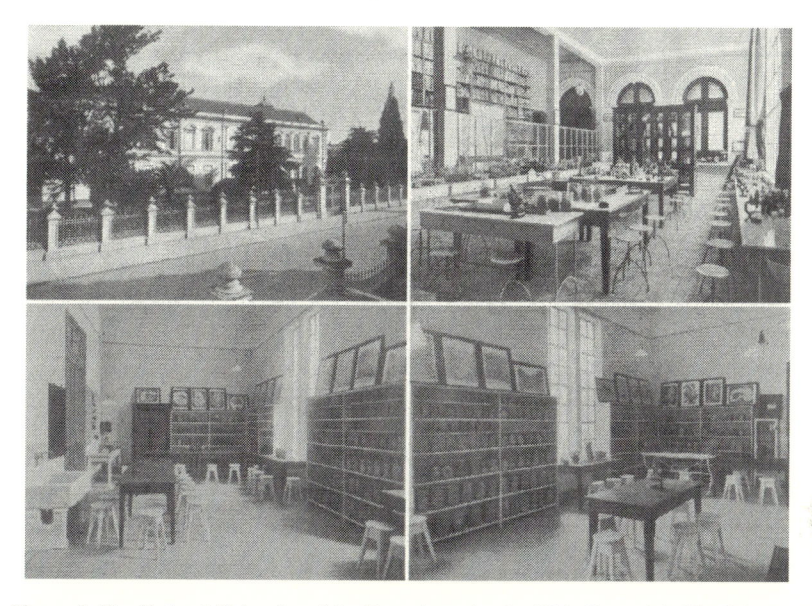

Figure 4. The National University of La Plata, Argentina in 1926. *Upper left:* The School of Humanities and Educational Sciences. Central building of the University. *Upper right:* Jakob's Laboratory of the Nervous System at the School of Humanities and Educational Sciences. *Lower:* Jakob's Laboratory of Pathological Anatomy and Physiology at the School of Medical Sciences viewed from two different angles (Nazar Anchorena et al., 1927, pp. 297, 309, 350). From the private archive of L. C. Triarhou. Copying, redistribution, or retransmission without the author's express written permission is prohibited.

In a commentary on "The Function of Biology in a Faculty of Philosophy and Letters," Jakob (1942) argued that future teachers and professors, aware of their highest mission, ought to know the fundamental facts of brain development as well as the physiological capacity of its mentality and disorders, because development and its dynamics form the anatomical-physiological substrate of their instructional efforts.

Jakob presented these ideas in a monograph on the frontal lobe, which he characterized "rather as a plan for future research and not as an essay with solutions" (Jakob, 1943b, p. 9). Recognizing the "humanizing" role of the frontal lobe, he described the meaning of its dynamics for science and philosophy (Théodoridou & Triarhou, 2012b).

The fact that the human frontal cortex covers about 30% of the total cortical surface generated the hope that unravelling its function might eventually explain human behavior (Raichle, 2002). Jakob (1906) viewed the major part of the frontal lobe as a central station with multiplier and combinatorial characteristics, constantly receiving stimuli from all the motility organs via multiple pathways. The role of the frontal lobe in integrating information from multiple brain areas supports its crucial involvement in learning, comprehension, and reasoning (Baddeley, 2002). According to Fuster (2006), actions related to human behavior, reasoning, and language are organized by means of interactions between prefrontal and posterior networks at the top of the "perception-action cycle." Jakob placed in the frontal lobe the centers of experiential accumulation that results from personal intervention, elaborated progressively for elemental and higher human skills and stimulated by affective states.

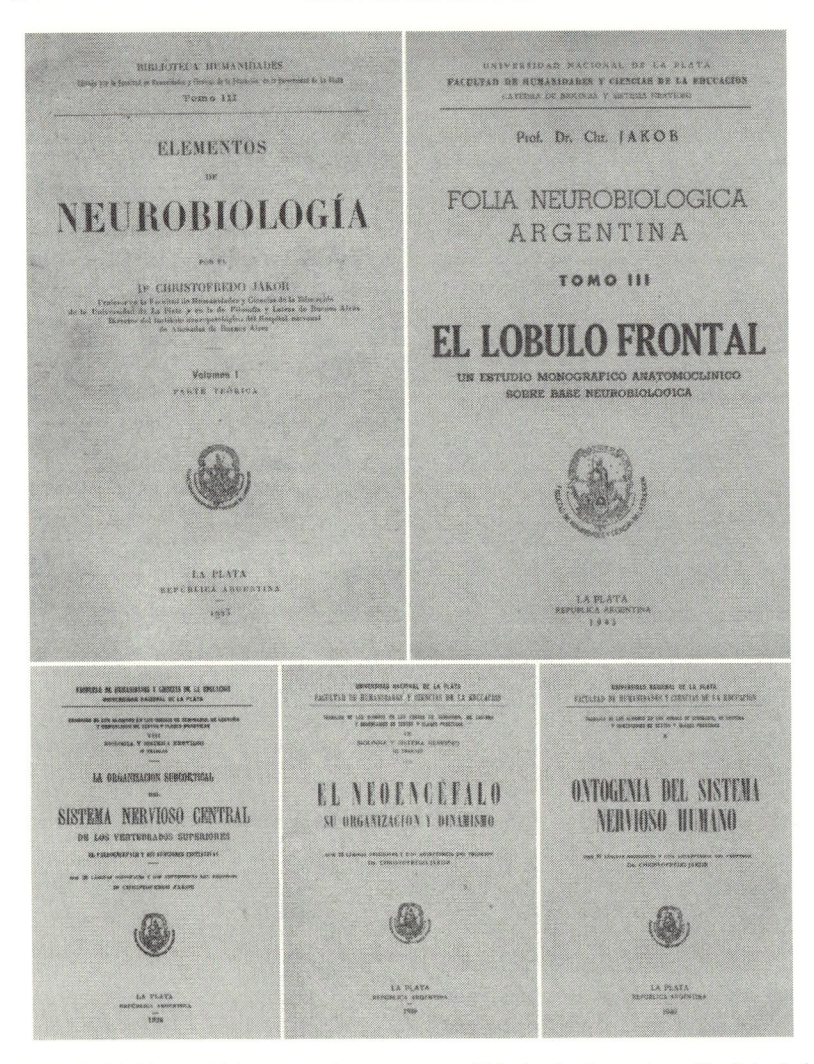

Figure 5. Jakob's neurobiology textbooks, *upper row*, published under the auspices of the School of Education at La Plata: the "Elements of Neurobiology," *left*, and "The Frontal Lobe," *right* (Jakob, 1923, 1943b). Jakob's booklets on the nervous system, lower row, based on his lectures at the School of Education in La Plata: "The Subcortical Organization of the Central Nervous System," "The Neoencephalon, its Organization and Dynamics," and "Ontogeny of the Human Nervous System" (Jakob, 1936, 1939, 1940). From the private archive of L. C. Triarhou. Copying, redistribution, or retransmission without the author's express written permission is prohibited.

In particular, Jakob explained the relation of the frontal lobe to education as follows: "The development of a social intelligence that will reinforce individual inclinations and will put emphasis on the active engagement of the student in the formation of concrete knowledge issues from the importance of frontal lobe functions" (Jakob, 1943b, p. 140).

As a result of the progress in the brain sciences in recent decades, traditional philosophical questions have been steered in new directions (Churchland, 2008), inviting a broad and divergent body of scientists to work together. Following philosophy, education has been enriched with new information stemming from the neurosciences.

For example, imaging studies pinpoint to neural systems that are responsible for the acquisition of reading skills and further support the idea that we can remedy inefficiencies in those systems through intervention; behavioral outcomes are accompanied by neural changes in the expected areas (Goswami, 2006). Concerning arithmetic, the finding that the brain has a preferred mode of representation bears directly on the teaching of mathematics: It suggests that teachers should build on this spatial system when teaching ordinality and place value. Other aspects of education that have been informed by neuroscience include second language learning, lifelong learning, and early learning (Blakemore & Frith, 2005).

However, a fair and fruitful dialogue among the sciences presupposes a minimum amount of knowledge and familiarity. The current demand for educators' literacy in neuroscience seems very attuned with Jakob's arguments (Ansari & Coch, 2006).

In a survey of teachers, almost 90% thought that knowledge of the brain was important, or very important, in designing educational programs (Pickering & Howard-Jones, 2007). In 1999, the Teaching and Learning Research Programme (TLRP) commissioned Blakemore and Frith to review neuroscientific findings that might be of relevance to educators. At the same time, a project on "Learning Sciences and Brain Research" was launched by the Centre for Educational Research and Innovation (CERI) at the Organisation for Economic Cooperation and Development (OECD). Major research and funding institutions from all over the world took part in that attempt: the Sackler Institute (United States), the University of Granada (Spain), and the RIKEN Brain Science Institute (Japan); the National Science Foundation (United States), the Lifelong Learning Foundation (United Kingdom), and the City of Granada (Spain); and INSERM (France) (OECD, 2001). The first phase of the project (1999–2002) brought together international scientists to review the potential implications of brain research for policy makers. The second phase (2002–2006) focused its activities on three areas: literacy, numeracy, and lifelong learning (Howard-Jones & Economic and Social Research Council, 2007).

Brain Topics, Psychological Theories, and Educational Implications

The potential cross-fertilization of neuroscience and education and its inherent limitations are one of the main points of discussion in the educational neuroscience literature (Beauchamp & Beauchamp, 2012). The production of "usable knowledge" (Christodoulou, Daley, & Katzir, 2009, p. 65) has proven a demanding task for researchers, as it entails an innate danger of misapplication, that is, oversimplification, misunderstanding, or generalization of scientific data (Beauchamp & Beauchamp, 2012).

Jakob's elaborations form a justified basis for educational implications, given that they cover multiple aspects of learning, both horizontally (evo-devo processes, normal and pathological conditions, structure, and function) and vertically (in-depth analyses and formulation of original theories). In addition, one of the most influential schools of educational thought, that is, the Piagetian, is based on a cognitive theory with biological roots.

Piaget (1964) argued that learning is subordinated to development. In a similar line of thinking, Jakob held the firm belief that cognitive and socioemotional development go hand in hand with cerebral development in a course he termed "psychogenesis" (Jakob, 1913,

1919, 1921, 1935). Thus, he explored its evolution and development in his neurodynamic postulate (for reviews see Théodoridou & Triarhou, 2011, 2012b).

Jakob's theory on cognitive development could have impact on the formulation of learning theories and practices, as the quest for a mutual understanding among cognitive scientists, neuroscientists, and educators is at the epicenter of current research.

In Jakob's neurodynamic theory, every system is an arc or circuit, composed of long ramifications or afferent and efferent pathways, "macrodynamics" of charge and discharge, and of a center or an inserted formation of increasing complexity, comprising cells and short fibers that constitute the "microdynamics" or "associative and commissural systems" (López Pasquali, 1965). The first macrodynamic circuit (reflexes) is only capable of responding in an instant and invariable form. The second macrodynamic circuit (instincts) preserves the information and mounts it up through discharges. In the third macrodynamic circuit, any entering or exiting element becomes registered and furthermore interacts interfocally. Such a system subserves the emergence of "psychism," that is, "the neurobiophylactic complex of neuroenergetic reception, assimilation and reaction, which regulates the organism's vital necessities against variable factors in the external and internal milieu" (Jakob, 1939, p. 8). Psychogenesis crescents in the "neopsychic" stage. Then, three kinds of neurocognitive processes occur: (a) *gnoses*, which secure the conscious orientation in one's environment; (b) *praxes*, which underlie active individual intervention; and (c) *symbolisms*, which subserve the communication of abstract ideas by means of human language (Jakob, 1919, 1921, 1935).

Treating Developmental Disorders

One of the most important of Jakob's contributions to education is his effort to establish a biological treatment theory for developmental disorders (Théodoridou, 2011). Jakob (1913) viewed mental retardation as the result of a degenerative psychogenetic process that necessitates a biological treatment. Thereby, the introduction of principles for a biological classification with practical and functional value would be meaningful. Jakob condemned the existing classifications as insufficient and ineffective for the formulation of both psychological and educational intervention.

Still, he acknowledged the contribution of existing classifications (clinical, anatomo-pathological, and educational) to psychology, medicine, and education, respectively. However, he stressed the importance of a functional connection between these aspects on the grounds of the dynamic nature of mental retardation. He noticed that each of those aspects and their interactions may influence prognosis in a child with mental retardation, for example, the time of onset of a disease, the extent of a lesion, individual differences, and the amount and quality of educational opportunities.

On that basis, Jakob (1913) divided normal cognitive and socioemotional development into the following psychogenetic stages (see also, Théodoridou, 2011):

1. "Psychobiomolecular stage," characterized by the irritability of the protoplasm.
2. "Psychoneuromolecular stage," when elementary nervous organization is not differentiated, although there is a nervous irritability.
3. "Elementary psychoreflexive stage," signalled by the differentiation of the reflexive, the nuclear, the spinal, and the bulbar systems.
4. "Complex psychoreflexive stage," when the successive maturation of instincts, impulses, and subcortical arcs is realized, along with the differentiation of afferent and efferent arcs.

5. "Crepuscular stage," when the reflexes and functions such as respiration, sucking, some movements, and mimicry dominate as primary, diffuse, and preconscious cortical perceptions.
6. "Stage of provisory psychological fixations":
   a. "Stage of elementary temporary fixations," when the superior instincts, affects, active mimicry and combined voluntary perceptions and actions first appear;
   b. "Stage of complex temporary fixations," when elements of articulate language, concrete ideas, orientation in the environment in terms of space and time as well as affective and voluntary actions emerge.
7. "Stage of definitive psychoenergetic associations":
   a. "Stage of permanent concrete associations," when an egocentric realism, the formation of personality, actions of affective inhibition, elementary consciousness, as well as the perception of time, space, and causality are observed.
   b. "Stage of elementary abstract associations," when the conscious personality is formed with elements of self-critisism and egoism; judgment, reasoning, and acts of intellectual inhibition are also evident in this stage of infantile analytic empiricism.
8. "Puberty," when the synthesis of ideas is possible, and aesthetic and ethic tendencies are evident.
9. And finally, "second puberty," when thought becomes rational and speculative.

Jakob's designation of egocentric realism precedes once again a Piagetian concept (see also, Théodoridou & Triarhou, 2011, 2012b). Piaget (1926, 1932) introduced the concept of egocentrism in his early writings (Light, 1983). The roots of the concept of egocentrism can be traced back to Freud's influence on Piaget, in particular on Freud's concepts of the "primary process" (i.e., the mode of functioning in service of the immediate gratification of needs) and the "secondary process" (i.e., the regulation and control of needs to attend to the demands of reality; Kesserling & Müller, 2011). Piaget (1920) initially distinguished between autistic (i.e., symbolic) and logical, scientific thought. Piaget's (1920) notion of autistic thought is derived from Bleuler and is much different from the contemporary use of this term as a designator of a particular developmental disorder (Kesserling & Müller, 2011). The pleasure principle dictates autistic thinking that is "personal, incommunicable, confused, undirected, indifferent to truth, rich in visual and symbolic schemas, and above all, unconscious of itself and by the affective factors by which it was guided" (Piaget, 1928, pp. 204–205). Later, Piaget introduced the concept of egocentrism as an intermediate level between these modes of thought. However, Piaget's study of his own infants led to a revision of the concept of egocentrism, which from the mid-1930s was conceptualized as a phenomenon that recurs at the beginning of different developmental stages.

Jakob (1913) viewed developmental disorders as energetic and dynamic conditions defined by multiple components. Thus, he stressed the importance of elucidating the internal and external causes of developmental cognitive arrest and their complex consequences on cerebral growth. He maintained that such knowledge would help scientists to contain the extent and severity of the factors that compromise the learning powers of the brain.

Apart from their biological characteristics, in his 1913 article, Jakob further provided the psychological profile that corresponds to each stage. He maintained that "degenerative psychogenesis" runs through the same stages as normal psychogenesis. He further made suggestions for suitable interventions, according to the stage that the child with disabilities falls into. Finally, Jakob discussed the concept of *patopedagogía* ("pathopedagogy") long before the fields of special and remedial education were formally introduced (Théodoridou, 2011).

In 1940, Jakob, in collaboration with Antonio Scaravelli, published a study of eight siblings from Tupungato with familial mental retardation, deafness, and spastic quadriplegia (Jakob & Scaravelli, 1940). Maintaining his interest in disability, Jakob dealt with heredity factors that cause pathological characteristics both from a neurological and from a socio-anthropological viewpoint.

Until the end of the eighteenth century, charity rather than education served as the underlying guidance for any special provisions for disabled children (Winzer, 1993). Afterwards, some sparse attempts were made for a methodologically sound, science-informed special education by pioneers such as the French physician-educator Jean Marc Gaspard Itard (1774–1838), the French psychologist Eduard Seguin (1812–1880), the Italian physician-educator Maria Montessori (1870–1952), the Belgian teacher and psychologist Jean-Ovide Decroly (1871–1932), and the Soviet defectologists Aleksandr M. Shcherbina (1874–1934), Lev S. Vygotsky (1896–1934), and Ivan A. Sokolyanskii (1898–1960).

The demand for a neuroscience-informed special education (Goswami, 2004) ensued from the unification of the mind, brain, and education sciences under modern attempts defined as neuroeducation (Battro, Fischer, & Léna, 2008) and educational neuroscience (Petitto & Dunbar, 2004; Szűks & Goswami, 2007). Learning and education can be viewed as a new field of the natural sciences with the entire human lifespan as its subject, including various problems such as fetal environment, childcare, language acquisition, general and special education, as well as rehabilitation (Koizumi, 2004). In this line of thought, Ito (2004) suggested that research should aim at providing new knowledge about the pathogenesis of developmental disorders on the solid basis of neuroscience. New knowledge should aid the appropriate assessment and treatment of patients, based on an accurate identification of individual-specific deficiencies, and environmental factors that might prevent children from behaving appropriately. Therefore, it would be helpful in solving problems rooted in antisocial behaviors of students. Further advantages of the adoption of a biological perspective include the timely diagnosis of special educational needs, the monitoring and comparison of the effects of different kinds of educational input on learning, and an increased understanding of individual differences in learning, and the best ways to customize input to the learner (Goswami, 2004).

Conclusion

A polymath, Jakob contributed original ideas to diverse aspects of education and pedagogy. Jakob's organizational skills have been considered exceptional (Papini, 1978). Throughout his career, Jakob became heavily involved in the organization of services, laboratories, clinics, and academic departments (Jakob, 1916, 1937, 1943a) and is credited as the father of Argentinian neurobiology and neurology (Orlando, 1966; Triarhou & del Cerro, 2007), having established an intellectual lineage of distinguished researchers and clinicians that included José Ingenieros, Braulio Moyano, and many others.

With his deep understanding of human brain function, he shed light on cognitive development and consciously aimed at the enhancement of learning theories and practices. Jakob further promoted the right of handicapped children to an appropriate education, paving the path for the grounding of special education on a scientific basis (Jakob, 1913). Impressively, he put forth the idea of teaching a course on "The Nervous System and Its Relationship to Education" as early as 1906. Although such a ground-breaking idea did not find fertile soil right away, eventually, in 1922, he became one of the first academics to formally teach neurobiology in a School of Education, at the National University of La Plata in Argentina.

Thus, Jakob introduced fundamentals of neuroeducation many decades before the discipline was formalized. At the same time, the National University of La Plata should be credited for its pioneering administrative decisions on educational and research policies that rendered such a neuroeducational connection possible. Ninety years later, Jakob's innovative thinking may still open up new horizons for a neuroscience-informed learning science and interdisciplinarity.

References

Allegri RF (2008): The pioneers of clinical neurology in South America. *Journal of the Neurological Sciences* 271: 29–33.

Ansari D, Coch D (2006): Bridges over troubled waters: Education and cognitive neuroscience. *Trends in Cognitive Sciences* 10: 146–151.

Baddeley AD (2002): Fractionating the central executive. In: Stuss DT, Knight RT, eds., *Principles of Frontal Lobe Function*. Oxford, Oxford University Press, pp. 246–260.

Battro AM, Cardinali DP (1996): Más cerebro en la educación. *La Nación*. [Online]. Retrieved from http://www.byd.com.ar/cereln.pdf

Battro AM, Fischer KW, Léna P (2008): *The Educated Brain: Essays in Neuroeducation*. Cambridge, Cambridge University Press.

Beauchamp M, Beauchamp C (2012): Understanding the neuroscience and education connection: Themes emerging from a review of the literature. In: Della Sala S, Anderson M, eds., *Neuroscience in Education: The Good, the Bad, and the Ugly*. Oxford, Oxford University Press, pp. 13–30.

Blakemore S-J, Frith U (2005): *The Learning Brain: Lessons for Education*. Malden, Massachusetts, Blackwell.

Christodoulou JA, Daley SG, Katzir T (2009): Researching the practice, practicing the research, and promoting responsible policy: Usable knowledge in mind, brain, and education. *Mind, Brain, and Education* 3: 65–67.

Churchland P (2008): The impact of neuroscience on philosophy. *Neuron* 60: 409–411.

Donaldson HH (1895): *The Growth of the Brain: A Study of the Nervous System in Relation to Education*. London, Walter Scott, Ltd.

Fawcett AJ, Nicolson RI (2007): Dyslexia, learning, and pedagogical neuroscience. *Developmental Medicine and Child Neurology* 49: 306–311.

Fischer KW, Daniel DB, Immordino-Yang MH, Stern E, Battro A, Koizumi H (2007): Why mind, brain, and education? Why now? *Mind, Brain, and Education* 1: 1–2.

Fumagalli A, Saredo G (2005): Christofredo Jakob (1866–1956) and the birth of neurology in Argentina. *Journal of the Neurological Sciences* 238(Suppl. 1): 160–161.

Fuster J (2006): The cognit: A network model of cortical representation. *International Journal of Psychophysiology* 60: 125–132.

Geake J (2005): Educational neuroscience and neuroscientific education: In search of a mutual middle-way. *Research Intelligence (Warborough)* 92: 10–13.

Glick TF (1996): Science in twentieth century Latin America. In: Betthel L, ed., *Ideas and Ideologies in Twentieth Century Latin America*. New York, Cambridge University Press, pp. 287–359.

González JV (1905): *La Universidad Nacional de La Plata: Memoria sobre su Fundación*. Buenos Aires, Talleres Gráficos de la Penitenciaría Nacional.

Goswami U (2004): Neuroscience, education and special education. *British Journal of Special Education* 31: 175–183.

Goswami U (2006): Neuroscience and education: From research to practice? *Nature Reviews Neuroscience* 7: 406–411.

Gotthelf R (1969): Historia de la psicología en la Argentina, segunda parte. *Revista Latinoamericana de Psicología (Bogotá)* 1: 183–198.

Halleck RP (1896): *The Education of the Central Nervous System: A Study of Foundations, Especially of Sensory and Motor Training*. New York, Macmillan Company.

Howard-Jones P, Economic and Social Research Council (2007): *Neuroscience and Education: Issues and Opportunities*. London, TLRP.

Ingenieros J (1922): *Prinzipien der biologischen Psychologie*. Leipzig, F. Meiner.

Ito M (2004): "Nurturing the brain" as an emerging research field involving child neurology. *Brain and Development* 26: 429–433.

Jakob C (1895): *Atlas des gesunden und kranken Nervensystems nebst Grundriss der Anatomie, Pathologie und Therapie desselben*. München, J. F. Lehmann.

Jakob C (1906): Estudios biológicos sobre los lóbulos frontales cerebrales. *La Semana Médica* 13: 1375–1381.

Jakob C (1911): *Das Menschenhirn: Eine Studie über den Aufbau und die Bedeutung seiner grauen Kerne und Rinde*. München, J. F. Lehmann.

Jakob C (1912a): Über die Ubiquität der senso-motorischen Doppelfunktion der Hirnrinde als Grundlage einer neuen, biologischen Auffassung des corticalen Seelenorgans. *Journal für Psychologie und Neurologie (Leipzig)* 19: 379–382.

Jakob C (1912b): Ueber die Ubiquität der senso-motorischen Doppelfunktion der Hirnrinde als Grundlage einer neuen biologischen Auffassung des kortikalen Seelenorgans. *Münchener Medizinische Wochenschrift* 59: 466–468.

Jakob C (1913): La psicopatogenia de los niños retardados: Psicogenesis degenerativa y su tratamiento biológico. *Revista de la Asociación Médica Argentina* 21: 1003–1016.

Jakob C (1916): Encuesta sobre en plan de estudios de medicina y la formación del profesorado universitario. *Revista del Círculo Médico Argentino y Centro de Estudiantes de Medicina* 16: 1–2.

Jakob C (1919): La teoría actual de las 'Gnósias y Práxias' como factores fundamentales en el dinamismo cortical. *Revista del Círculo Médico Argentino y Centro de Estudiantes de Medicina (Buenos Aires)* 19: 1266–1275.

Jakob C (1921): La teoría actual de las gnosias y praxias como factores fundamentales en el dinamismo de la corteza cerebral. *La Crónica Médica (Lima)* 38: 17–24.

Jakob C (1922): Sobre tumores teratogénicos del cerebro (A propósito de un teratoma del conducto de Sylvio). In: Junta para el homenaje a Cajal, eds., *Libro en honor de D. S. Ramón y Cajal—Trabajos Originales de Sus Admiradores y Discípulos, Extranjeros y Nacionales*, tomo II. Madrid, Jiménez y Molina Impresores, pp. 415–431.

Jakob C (1935): La filogenia de las kinesias: Sobre su organización y dinamismo evolutivo. *Anales del Instituto de Psicología de la Facultad de Filosofía y Letras de la Universidad de Buenos Aires* 1: 109–127.

Jakob C (1937): La enseñanza universitaria de la anatomía cerebral. *Revista de la Asociación Médica Argentina* 51: 799–803.

Jakob C (1939): *El Neoencéfalo: Su Organización y Dinamismo*. Buenos Aires, Universidad Nacional de La Plata–Imprenta López.

Jakob C (1941): La función psicogenética de la corteza cerebral y su posible localización (Aspectos de la ontopsicogénesis humana). *Anales del Instituto de Psicología de la Facultad de Filosofía y Letras de la Universidad de Buenos Aires* 3: 63–80.

Jakob C (1942): La función de la Biología en la Facultad de Filosofía y Letras. *Logos (Buenos Aires)* 1: 159–161.

Jakob C (1943a): Clinica–Laboratorio. *Revista de la Asociación Bioquímica Argentina* 9: 42–44.

Jakob C (1943b): *Folia Neurobiológica Argentina, III. El Lóbulo Frontal: Estudio Monográfico Anatomoclínico sobre Base Neurobiológica*. Buenos Aires, Aniceto López-López y Etchegoyen.

Jakob C (1945): *Folia Neurobiológica Argentina, IV. El Yacaré (Caimán latirostris) y el Origen del Neocortex: Estudios Neurobiológicos y Folklóricos del Reptil más Grande de la Argentina*. Buenos Aires, Aniceto López Editor.

Jakob C (1946): *Folia Neurobiológica Argentina, V. Documenta Biofilosófica*. Buenos Aires, López y Etchegoyen.

Jakob C, Onelli C (1913): *Atlas del Cerebro de los Mamíferos de la Republica Argentina: Estudios Anatómicos, Histológicos y Biológicos Comparados sobre la Evolución de los Hemisferios y de la Corteza cerebral*. Buenos Aires, Guillermo Kraft.

Jakob C, Scaravelli A (1940): A propósito de un caso de ocho hermanos con idiocia, sordomudez y cuadriplejía espasmódica familiar. *Revista Neurológica de Buenos Aires* 5: 283–299.

Koizumi H (2004): The concept of "developing the brain": A new natural science for learning and education. *Brain and Development* 26: 434–441.

Kesserling T, Müller U (2011): The concept of egocentrism in the context of Piaget's theory. *New Ideas in Psychology* 29: 327–345.

Light P (1983): Piaget and egocentrism: A perspective on recent developmental research. *Early Child Development and Care* 12: 7–18.

López Pasquali L (1965): Christfried Jakob. *Su Obra Neurológica, Su Pensamiento Psicológico y Filosófico*. Buenos Aires, López.

Moyano BA (1957): Christfried Jakob, 25/12/1866–6/5/1956. *Acta Neuropsiquiátrica Argentina* 3: 109–123.

Nazar Anchorena BA, Amaral SM, Alegre PJ (1927): *La Universidad Nacional de La Plata en el Año 1926: Publicación Oficial*. La Plata & Buenos Aires, Casa J. Peuser, Ltda.

OECD (Organisation for Economic Co-operation and Development) (2001): *Preliminary Synthesis of the Third High Level Forum on Learning and Sciences and Brain Research: Potential Implications for Education Policies and Practices*. Retrieved from http://www.oecd.org/edu/ceri/15302896.pdf.

Orlando JC (1966): *Christofredo Jakob: Su Vida y Obra*. Buenos Aires, Editorial Mundi.

Papini MR (1978): La psicología experimental argentina durante el período 1930–1955. *Revista Latinoamericana de Psicología (Bogotá)* 10: 227–258.

Papini MR (1988): Influence of evolutionary biology in the early development of experimental psychology in Argentina (1891–1930). *International Journal of Experimental Psychology* 2: 131–138.

Petitto LA, Dunbar K (2004): New findings from educational neuroscience on bilingual brains, scientific brains, and the educated mind. *Conference on Building Usable Knowledge in Mind, Brain, and Education*, 6–8 October 2004, Cambridge, MA.

Piaget J (1920): La psychanalyse dans ses rapports avec la psychologie de l'enfant. *Bulletin Mensuel de la Société Alfred Binet* 20: 18–34 & 41–58.

Piaget J (1926): *The Language and Thought of the Child*. London, Routledge & Kegan Paul.

Piaget J (1928): *Judgment and Reasoning in the Child*. New York, Harcourt, Brace and Company.

Piaget J (1932): *The Moral Judgment of the Child*. London, Routledge & Kegan Paul.

Piaget J (1964): Cognitive development in children: Development and learning. *Journal of Research in Science Teaching* 2: 176–186.

Pickering SJ, Howard-Jones P (2007): Educators' views on the role of neuroscience in education: Findings from a study of UK and international perspectives. *Mind, Brain, and Education* 1: 109–113.

Raichle ME (2002): Foreword. In: Stuss DT, Knight RT, eds., *Principles of Frontal Lobe Function*. Oxford, Oxford University Press, pp. vii–ix.

Ramón y Cajal S (1906a): Inducciones fisiológicas de la morfología y conexiones de las neuronas. *Archivos de Pedagogía y Ciencias Afines (La Plata)* 1: 216–236.

Ramón y Cajal S (1906b): Morfología de la célula nerviosa. *Archivos de Pedagogía y Ciencias Afines (La Plata)* 1: 92–106.

Ramón y Cajal S (1988): *Recollections of My Life* (translated by E. H. Craigie and J. Cano). Birmingham, Alabama, The Classics of Neurology and Neurosurgery Library–Gryphon Editions.

Stern E (2006): *Educational Research and Neurosciences—Expectations, Evidence and Research Prospects*. Berlin, Bundesministerium für Bildung und Forschung.

Szűcs D, Goswami U (2007): Educational neuroscience: Defining a new discipline for the study of mental representations. *Mind, Brain, and Education* 1: 114–127.

Talak AM (2008): Christofredo Jakob: La tradición neurobiológica en la primera psicología en Argentina. *VI Encuentro de Filosofía e Historia de la Ciencia del Cono Sur Montevideo*, 27–30 May 2008, Montevideo, Uruguay.

Théodoridou ZD (2011): *Christfried Jakob on the Cerebral Cortex: Neurobiological, Neurophilosophical and Neuroeducational Concepts* (Unpublished Doctoral Dissertation). Thessaloniki, Greece, University of Macedonia.

Théodoridou ZD, Triarhou LC (2009): Fin-de-siècle advances in neuroeducation: Henry Herbert Donaldson and Reuben Post Halleck. *Mind, Brain, and Education* 3: 117–127.

Théodoridou ZD, Triarhou LC (2011): Christfried Jakob's 1921 theory of the gnoses and praxes as fundamental factors in cerebral cortical dynamics. *Integrative Psychological and Behavioral Science* 45: 247–262.

Théodoridou ZD, Triarhou LC (2012a): Challenging the supremacy of the frontal lobe: Early views (1906–1909) of Christfried Jakob on the human cerebral cortex. *Cortex* 48: 15–25.

Théodoridou ZD, Triarhou LC (2012b): Christfried Jakob's late views (1930–1949) on the psychogenetic function of the cerebral cortex and its localization: Culmination of the neurophilosophical thought of a keen brain observer. *Brain and Cognition* 78: 179–188.

Triarhou LC (2008a): Centenary of Christfried Jakob's discovery of the visceral brain: An unheeded precedence in affective neuroscience. *Neuroscience and Biobehavioral Reviews* 32: 984–1000.

Triarhou LC (2008b): The books of Christofredo Jakob: Lasting treasures of evolutionary neuroscience. *Society for Neuroscience Abstracts* 38: 221.16.

Triarhou LC (2009): Tripartite concepts of mind and brain, with special emphasis on the neuroevolutionary postulates of Christfried Jakob and Paul MacLean. In: Weingarten SP, Penat HO, eds., *Cognitive Psychology Research Developments*. Hauppauge, New York, Nova Science Publishers, pp. 183–208.

Triarhou LC (2010a): Final publications of Christfried Jakob: On the frontal lobe and the limbic region. In: Flynn CE, Callaghan BR, eds., *Neuroanatomy Research Advances*. Hauppauge, New York, Nova Science Publishers, pp. 165–169.

Triarhou LC (2010b): Revisiting Christfried Jakob's concept of the dual onto-phylogenetic origin and ubiquitous function of the cerebral cortex: A century of progress. *Brain Structure and Function* 214: 319–338.

Triarhou LC, del Cerro M (2006a): An early work [1910–1913] in *Biological Psychology* by pioneer psychiatrist, criminologist and philosopher José Ingenieros, M.D. (1877–1925) of Buenos Aries. *Biological Psychology* 72: 1–14.

Triarhou LC, del Cerro M (2006b): Semicentennial tribute to the ingenious neurobiologist Christfried Jakob (1866–1956): 1. Works from Germany and the first Argentina period, 1891–1913. *European Neurology* 56: 176–188.

Triarhou LC, del Cerro M (2006c): Semicentennial tribute to the ingenious neurobiologist Christfried Jakob (1866–1956): 2. Publications from the second Argentina period, 1913–1949. *European Neurology* 56: 189–198.

Triarhou LC, del Cerro M (2007): Christfried Jakob (1866–1956). *Journal of Neurology* 254: 124–125.

Tsapkini K, Vivas AB, Triarhou LC (2008): "Does Broca's area exist?"—Christofredo Jakob's 1906 response to Pierre Marie's holistic stance. *Brain and Language* 105: 211–219.

Vivas AB, Tsapkini K, Triarhou LC (2007): Anatomo-biological considerations on the centers of language: An Argentinian contribution to the 1906 Paris debate on aphasia. *Brain and Development* 29: 455–461.

von Economo C, Koskinas GN (1925): *Die Cytoarchitektonik der Hirnrinde des erwachsenen Menschen: Textband und Atlas*. Wien, J. Springer.

Winzer MA (1993): *The History of Special Education: From Isolation to Integration*. Washington, DC, Gallaudet University Press.

Chapter 2
The Cytoarchitectonic Map of Constantin von Economo and Georg N. Koskinas

Lazaros C. Triarhou

Abstract In 1925 Constantin von Economo (1876–1931) and Georg N. Koskinas (1885–1975), working in the Psychiatric Clinic of Julius Wagner-Jauregg (1857–1940) at the University of Vienna, published their monumental *Atlas and Textbook of Cytoarchitectonics of the Adult Human Cerebral Cortex*, following in the footsteps of Theodor Meynert (1833–1892) and Korbinian Brodmann (1868–1918). Von Economo and Koskinas provided a much more detailed verbal and pictorial description of the variations in cellular structure (cytoarchitecture) of cerebral cortical layers, compared to Brodmann. By dissecting each gyrus and sulcus perpendicularly to its axis, von Economo and Koskinas successfully addressed the core problem of flattening out the convoluted polyhedral surface of the human cerebral mantle. They defined five structural cortical *types* (agranular, frontal, parietal, polar, and granulous) and 107 cytoarchitectonic area *modifications* (35 frontal, 13 limbic, 6 insular, 18 parietal, 7 occipital, 14 temporal, and 14 hippocampal). Their numerous discoveries include the *koniocortex*, i.e. the dusty appearance of sensory areas, and the identification, at the boundaries of koniocortex with ordinary isocortex in parietal, temporal and occipital areas, of thin bands with giant pyramidal cells, the so-called *parasensory zones*. Von Economo and Koskinas also provided the first comprehensive description of the distinct rod and corkscrew cells in cingulate and frontoinsular areas known today as "von Economo neurons" that are putatively involved in social behavior and the pathophysiology of neurodevelopmental and mental diseases. The cortical cytoarchitectonics system of von Economo and Koskinas may be especially meaningful in conjunction with modern studies on functional imaging in the human brain.

L.C. Triarhou (✉)
Economo-Koskinas Wing for Integrative and Evolutionary Neuroscience, University of Macedonia, Egnatia 156, Bldg. Z-312, 54006 Thessaloniki, Greece
e-mail: triarhou@uom.gr

S. Geyer and R. Turner (eds.), *Microstructural Parcellation of the Human Cerebral Cortex*, DOI 10.1007/978-3-642-37824-9_2, © Springer-Verlag Berlin Heidelberg 2013

2.1 Introduction

"The cortex is both chaos and order, and therein lies its strength." With these words the neuroanatomist Gerhardt von Bonin (1890–1979) summarized in his classical essay on the cerebral cortex (von Bonin 1950) the quintessence of the cerebral hemispheric mantle.

The inextricability of cerebral morphology and function was exemplified in the writings of the neurobiologist Christfried Jakob (1866–1956): "Form is stabilized function and function is change of form; the organism is a single entity that presents itself as form in the latent state and as function in the kinetic state... Form, structure and function are inseparable, if not identical, and only scholastic science has managed to separate them... Only a basis that is fundamentally biological, morphostructural and histophysiological at the same time, unified in an ample ontogenetic and phylogenetic context, can let us address in legitimate ways the fundamental questions of modern neuro- and psychobiopathology" (Jakob 1939, 1941; Triarhou 2010; Triarhou and del Cerro 2006).

One of the overarching grand challenges of neuroscience for the twenty-first century is how does the brain work and produce mental activity and how does physical activity in the brain give rise to behavior (Hougan and Altevogt 2008). It is argued that the field of understanding how the mind works may move forward to its full potential only when we gain a better insight into the physical instantiation of nervous systems by constructing connectional maps that integrate anatomy, neuronal activity and function.

In the early twentieth century, the holding tenet among neuroanatomists was that deciphering cortical cell architecture is a preamble to understanding the mind. Essential contributions to cortical histology by Félix Vicq d'Azyr (1748–1794), Theodor Meynert (1833–1892), Vladimir A. Betz (1834–1894), W. Bevan Lewis (1847–1929), Santiago Ramón y Cajal (1852–1934), Theodor Kaes (1852–1913), Christfried Jakob (1866–1956), Alfred Walter Campbell (1868–1937), Korbinian Brodmann (1868–1918), Oskar Vogt (1870–1959), Sir Grafton Elliot Smith (1871–1937), and Cécile Mugnier-Vogt (1875–1962) formed the basis upon which Baron Constantin von Economo (1876–1931) and Georg N. Koskinas (1885–1975), from patrician Greek families rooted in the Hellenic regions of Macedonia and Lacedaemonia, respectively (Fig. 2.1), produced their *magnum opus* on the adult human cerebral cortex (von Economo and Koskinas 1925). The historical merit and its modern perspective are discussed elsewhere (von Economo 2009; von Economo and Koskinas 2008; Zilles 2004; Zilles and Amunts 2012).

With his landmark monograph, Brodmann (1909) defined 44 cortical cytoarchitectonic areas in the human brain (and a total of 52 areas in the primate brain overall). He studied cortical cytoarchitecture in numerous mammals, from the hedgehog, with its unusually large archipallium, to primates and humans, and introduced the terms *homogenetic* and *heterogenetic formations* to denote two different basic cortical patterns with either the typical six layers or lacking the six-layer stage, respectively (Garey 2006; Zilles and Amunts 2010).

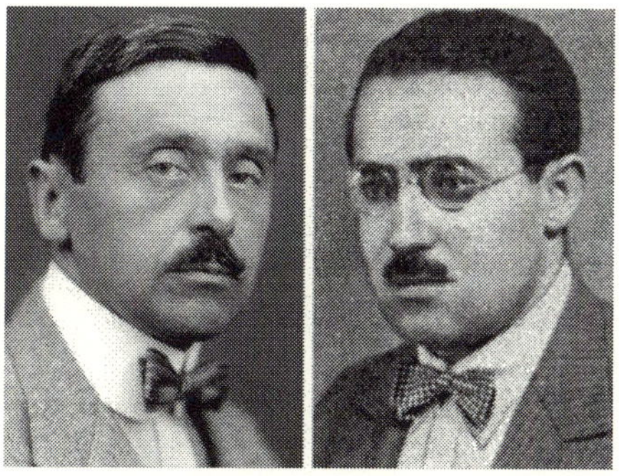

2 The Cytoarchitectonic Map of Constantin von Economo and Georg N. Koskinas

Fig. 2.1 Constantin von Economo (1876–1931), Professor of Psychiatry and Neurology at the University of Vienna, *left*, and Georg N. Koskinas (1885–1975), former Assistant at the Psychiatric and Neurological Clinic of the University of Athens, *right*. For his discovery of encephalitis lethargica, von Economo was nominated three times for the Nobel Prize in Physiology or Medicine between 1926 and 1932. Koskinas returned to Greece in 1927; after an unsuccessful application for the chair of Neurology at the University of Athens, he devoted himself to private practice in the suburb of Kifisia (Triarhou 2005) (Photo credits: Bildarchiv und Grafiksammlung der Österreichischen Nationalbibliothek, Vienna (Economo); Helios Encyclopedic Lexicon, Athens (Koskinas). Used by permission and protected by copyright law. Copying, redistribution or retransmission without the author's express written permission is prohibited)

Vogt and Vogt (1919) laid the foundations of myeloarchitectonics (the architecture of fiber pathways) and defined the structural features of *allocortex*, *proisocortex* and *isocortex*; they also analyzed the differences between *paleocortical*, *archicortical*, and *neocortical* regions (Vogt and Vogt 1919; Vogt 1927; Zilles 2004; Zilles and Amunts 2012).

Von Economo commenced his work on cortical cytoarchitectonics in 1912, and Koskinas joined him in 1919. Their Atlas and Text Volume were published in 1925, and included 150 new discoveries (Koskinas 1931). Von Economo and Koskinas (1925, 2008) defined 107 area *modifications*, and more than 60 area *transitions* (von Economo 2009), virtually raising the "resolution" of our cortical cytoarchitectonic register, compared to Brodmann's data, by a factor of four.

In subsequent decades, by combining cytoarchitectonics with myeloarchitectonics, Sanides (1962, 1964) placed emphasis on transitions or gradations that accompany "streams" of neocortical regions coming from paleocortical and archicortical sources (Pandya and Sanides 1973), while Vogt and Vogt (1919) had already spoken of "areal gradations".

Comprehensive tables correlating the 107 cortical areas defined by von Economo and Koskinas with the Brodmann areas can be found in a previous review article (Triarhou 2007b) and in the English edition of the Atlas (von Economo and Koskinas 2008).

The work of von Economo and Koskinas represents a gigantic intellectual and technical effort (van Bogaert and Théodoridès 1979). Their attempt to bring the existing knowledge into a more orderly pattern was emphatically acknowledged by von Bonin (1950) and Bailey and von Bonin (1951).

Spyridon Dontas (1878–1958), Professor of Physiology and Pharmacology at the University of Athens and President of the Academy of Athens, had remarked in 1926 upon meeting Koskinas: "The work of von Economo and Koskinas is monumental and constitutes a milestone of science, charting new paths for understanding the brain from an anatomical, physiological and pathological viewpoint. It stands as the first comprehensive reference on the architecture of the adult human cerebrum and will persevere as a perpetual scientific testimony" (Triarhou 2012).

The brain map and the systematic area naming by von Economo and Koskinas have regrettably not passed into widespread general use. However, it is clear that they brought together concepts and ideas of cortical organization and structure that had been developing over the preceding 30 years and which remain with us in the present era of cortical research; moreover, they introduced original terms and, by applying in a systematic manner nomenclatures derived from other authors and themselves, they codified the language that we use to describe the cortex to this day, essentially providing the first "ontology" of the cerebral cortex (Jones 2010).

2.2 Method

At the outset of their studies, von Economo and Koskinas devised an entire system of new methods to overcome the existing obstacles and difficulties, from the autopsy to the photographic documentation (Koskinas 1926, 1931; von Economo 2009; von Economo and Koskinas 2008). The following are some of the introduced innovations.

2.2.1 Sectioning

Instead of the widely adopted method of sectioning the whole brain serially, perpendicular to its fronto-occipital axis, von Economo and Koskinas obtained tissue sections always perpendicular to the axis of each gyrus or sulcus and in directions corresponding to their convoluted pattern (Figs. 2.2 and 2.3). They arrived at that idea by considering that, in order to be able to compare the various brain areas cytoarchitectonically, sections had to have a consistent orientation relative to the gyral surface, insofar as only then could the breadth of the entire cerebral cortex and of each cortical layer as well be represented in the sections in a precise way.

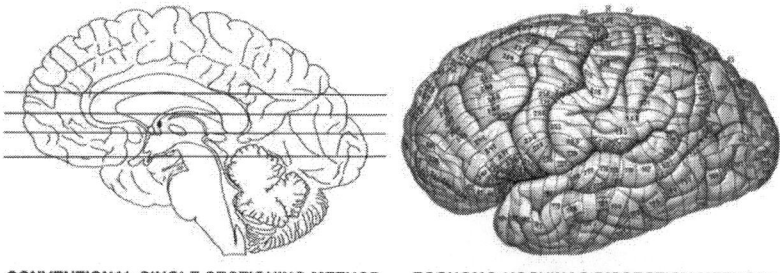

CONVENTIONAL SINGLE SECTIONING METHOD OF ENTIRE CEREBRAL HEMISPHERE   **ECONOMO-KOSKINAS DISSECTION METHOD FOR PERPENDICULAR GYRAL SEGMENTS**

Fig. 2.2 The difference between the widely used method of obtaining whole single sections of the cerebral hemispheres, *left*, and the method devised by von Economo and Koskinas (1925, 2008) for dissecting each hemisphere into 250–350 tissue blocks, 4 mm in thickness, always perpendicular to the axis of each gyral or sulcal segment, *right*; hatched areas indicate "cancelled" tissue

2.2.2 Staining

The staining of the preparations was perfected such that a uniform tone was achieved not only of the single sections, but of all the series of sections into which each brain had been divided. That was mandated by the need, firstly, to define gradual differences of histological elements in neighboring areas of the cerebral cortex, and secondly, to achieve consistent photographic registrations.

2.2.3 Specimen Depiction

Most of the previous histological studies on cortical cytoarhitecture depicted their results schematically, and therefore subjectively. Instead of schematic drawings, and aiming at an exact documentation of the specimens, with all the relationships of the diverse neurons, von Economo and Koskinas used photography, which is the most objective testimony regarding form, size and arrangement, and turned to branches of science such as advanced optics and photochemistry.

The stained cortical sections were photographed using Carl Zeiss Planar lenses, which are special macro objectives with a considerably larger field than the common microscopy objectives, especially valuable for large area objects under relatively large magnifications. Planar lenses are used without an eyepiece. Additional details on technique can be found in my historical notes on Koskinas (Triarhou 2005) and von Economo (Triarhou 2006).

The depth of field that von Economo and Koskinas achieved in their photomicrographs, as well as the clarity and detail with which individual neurons can be visualized is remarkable. Their plates probably still represent the most comprehensive set of high resolution images of cortical histology ever assembled (Jones 2008).

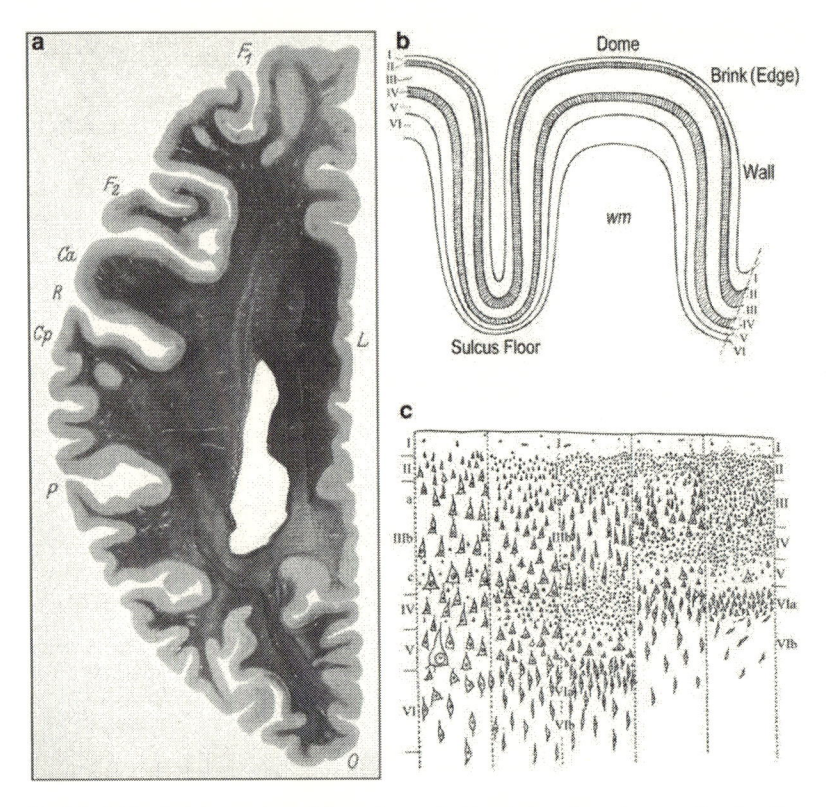

Fig. 2.3 (a) In obtaining sections of the entire cerebral hemisphere through conventional sectioning techniques, the real variations in layer thickness and cellular architecture cannot be studied consistently. The horizontal section through the left human cerebral hemisphere depicts such sizeable regional differences in cortical thickness and the random orientation of the gyri (von Economo and Koskinas 1925). Weigert method. F_1 and F_2, superior and middle frontal gyrus; *Ca*, precentral gyrus; *R*, central sulcus; *Cp*, postcentral gyrus, *P*, parietal lobe; *O*, occipital lobe; *L*, limbic gyrus. (b) A schematic drawing that depicts the varying thickness of the six cortical layers (I through VI) at the level of the *dome, brink (edge), wall* and *valley (sulcus floor)* in a cortical gyrus. The two granular layers (external and internal) are hatched; *wm*, subcortical white matter (von Economo 2009). (c) The five fundamental structural types of isocortex: 1, agranular; 2, frontal; 3, parietal; 4, polar; 5, granulous or *koniocortex* (von Economo 1925, 1929, 2009; von Economo and Koskinas 1925, 2008)

2.3 General Part

The "General Part" of the Text Volume (von Economo and Koskinas 1925) covers introductory concepts on the cerebral cortex and its nerve cells, the structure and the development of the cortical layers, the composition and the meaning of the cortical laminar structure, the definition of cortical areas, and methodological issues (Fig. 2.4).

Brodmann (1909) grouped his 44 human cortical areas as 4 postcentral, 2 precentral, 8 frontal, 4 parietal, 3 occipital, 10 temporal, 6 cingulate, 3 retrosplenial, and 4 hippocampal.

Von Economo and Koskinas (1925, 2008) divided the cortex into seven lobes, which they denoted by their initials. The lobes were further subdivided into regions: the frontal lobe (F) into prerolandic, anterior (prefrontal) and orbitomedial (orbitomedial) regions; the superior limbic lobe (L) into anterior, posterior and retrosplenial regions; the parietal lobe (P) into postcentral (anterior parietal), superior, inferior and basal regions; and the temporal lobe (T) into supratemporal, temporal proper, fusiform and temporopolar regions. The insular (I) and occipital (O) lobes were not subdivided. The inferior limbic lobe consists of the hippocampus (H). For cytoarchitectonic area designations, they did not continue Brodmann's system of random numbers, but instead used letter codes, consisting of a Roman capital letter (the initial of the lobe), followed by a calligraphic capital to note the sequence of a gyrus within a lobe (e.g. F*B* means the second gyrus of the frontal lobe), and a Latin or Greek subscript for characteristic microscopic features (e.g. m = magnocellular, p = parvicellular, γ = gigantopyramidal).

Von Economo and Koskinas (1925, 2008) defined five fundamental "supercategories" of structural cortical types (agranular, frontal, parietal, polar and granulous) (Fig. 2.3c), further arranged into 54 *ground*, 76 *variant* and 107 cytoarchitectonic *modification* areas, plus more than 60 *transition* areas (von Economo 1925, 2009; von Economo and Horn 1930). Topographically, the 107 modification areas of von Economo and Koskinas are grouped into 35 frontal, 13 superior limbic, 6 insular, 18 parietal, 7 occipital, 14 temporal, and 14 inferior limbic or hippocampal (Figs. 2.5 and 2.6). Of the 107 modifications, 22 are allocortical, 22 heterotypic isocortical, and 63 homotypic isocortical. Von Economo and Koskinas (1925, 2008) separately analyzed the *dome, edge, wall* and *floor* of each cortical gyrus (Fig. 2.3b).

For certain cortical areas with a granular appearance of their cells in most layers, especially of gyral walls, associated primarily with sensory functions, von Economo and Koskinas (1923, 1925) introduced the term *koniocortex* to denote their dusty appearance.

Von Economo and Koskinas (1925, 2008) regularly saw a special type in a small band in sublayer IIIc at the boundary between any koniocortex (or sensory isocortex) and the ordinary surrounding isocortex in sensory parietal, occipital and temporal areas. Such zones contain giant pyramidal cells. They called these margin regions with magnocellular characteristics *parasensory zones*.

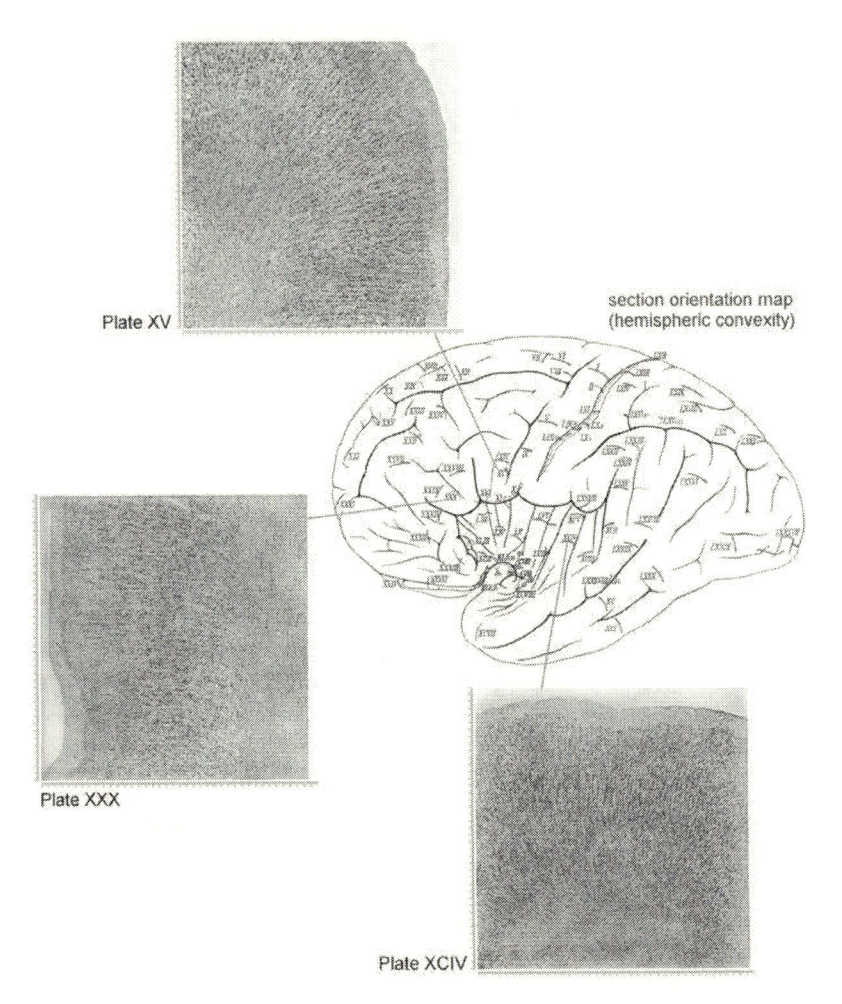

Fig. 2.4 Schematic map of the lateral (*convex*) facies of the hemispheric surface and three microphotographic plates from the Atlas of von Economo and Koskinas (2008), shown as examples: *Plate XV* – Magnocellular intermedio-agranular frontal area FCB$_m$ (*Broca's area*) at the *foot* of the inferior frontal gyrus, anterior wall. *Plate XXX* – Triangular granular frontal area FD$_\gamma$ in the inferior frontal gyrus, wall of the notch of pars triangularis *(incisura capi)*. *Plate XCIV* – Supratemporal area granulosa TC in first gyrus of Heschl (primary auditory cortex), middle, dome, with the typical "rain shower formation" *(Regenschauerformation)*. The detailed descriptions of the normal histological structure of the cerebral cortex depicted in the 112 microphotographic plates of the Atlas were explained in the accompanying Text Volume (von Economo and Koskinas 1925). The printing size of the original plates was 40 × 40 cm at a magnification of × 100, therefore covering a 4.0 × 4.0 mm true cortical area

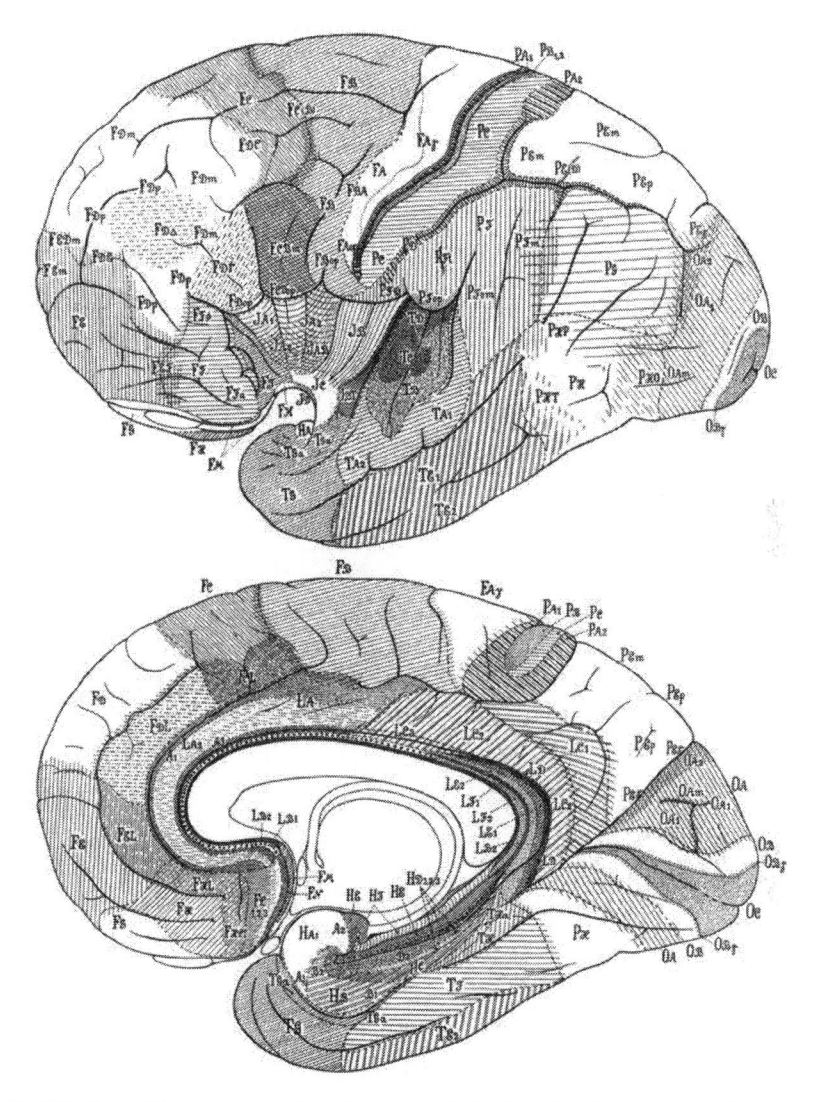

2 The Cytoarchitectonic Map of Constantin von Economo and Georg N. Koskinas 41

Fig. 2.5 Cytoarchitectonic maps of von Economo and Koskinas, showing cortical modification areas in the convex and median hemispheric facies of the human brain

Another crucial discovery was that of the large, spindle-shaped bipolar projection neurons in the inferior ganglionic layer (Vb) of the dome of the transverse insular gyrus, which are now called "von Economo neurons" (Watson et al. 2006) – although a more succinct term might be "von Economo-Koskinas neurons". The

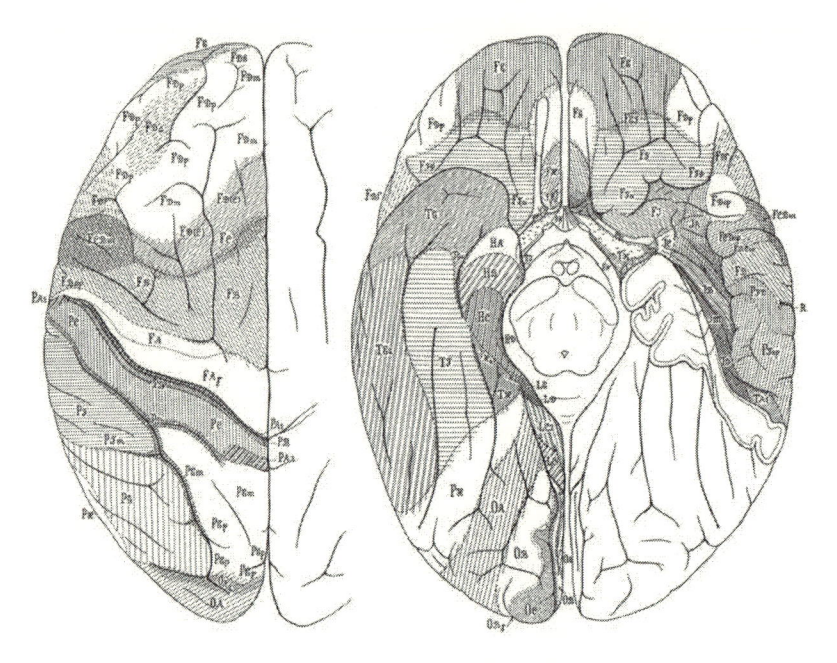

Fig. 2.6 Cytoarchitectonic maps of von Economo and Koskinas for the dorsal and ventral hemispheric surface

detailed morphology of these rod cells *(Stäbchenzellen)* and corkscrew cells *(Korkzieherzellen)* was documented by von Economo and Koskinas (1925) in cingulate (anterior) limbic and frontoinsular areas.

2.4 Special Part

The following text is a selection of some ideas discoursed in previous reviews (Triarhou 2007a, b) and in the new English editions of the Atlas (von Economo and Koskinas 2008) and of von Economo's shorter textbook of cortical cytoarchitectonics (von Economo 2009).

2.4.1 Frontal Lobe

Broca's motor speech area FCB_m in the inferior frontal gyrus was considered as a particular human characteristic by von Economo and Koskinas (1925), as well as by Brodmann (1909). The surface area of the pars opercularis of the inferior frontal gyrus is characterized by a distinct type of cortex, distinguishable from the posteriorly lying premotor cortex in area FB in the precentral gyrus; it continues rostrally as area FD_γ (Fig. 2.4).

Anteriorly one finds portions of areas FD and FE, which are rich in granule cells. Lesions in the prefrontal region result in disturbances of attention, psychomotor activity, will and emotivity. Von Economo (2009) termed such higher mental functions, localized in the frontal regions of the brain, "the active part of the psychic personality". Area FA_γ resembles the frontal core area more closely, with the consequence that a large part of area FA belongs to nonprimary motor cortex.

Area FF partly corresponds to the orbitofrontal proisocortex of the monkey that lies intercalated between the caudal orbitofrontal isocortex rostrally, and the orbitofrontal peripaleocortex caudally. Area FF_a in the human brain probably corresponds to the granular isocortex in the anterior part of the orbital surface of the frontal lobe in the macaque. Areas FH and FHL correspond to the paralimbic dysgranular isocortex on the ventromedial surface of the prefrontal cortex in the macaque, which lies intercalated between the frontopolar granular isocortex rostrally and the orbitomesial archicortical proisocortex of the straight gyrus caudally. Area FJ appears to correspond to peripaleocortex in the inferior part of the transverse gyrus of the insula, and to the orbitofrontal peripaleocortex in the monkey (de Olmos 1990). The area FF lies rostrally and ventrally to area FD_γ.

Von Economo and Koskinas (1925) mark transitional types of cortex in their maps, beyond the 107 "standard" modifications; such transitions comprise the areas FBA, F$C(B)$, FCD_{op}, FDC, FDE, FED_m, FEF and FE_m. Areas FBA, FDC, FDE and FEF denote transition forms (e.g. FBA marks the transition of area FB into FA, FDC the transition of FD into FC, and so on). The designation F$C(B)$ implies a part of area FC with an admixture of the type of the neighboring area FB, whereas the subscript m in the areas FED_m and FE_m signifies cellular variations with magnocellular features. Area FCD_{op} is a transitional opercular variant between areas FC_{op} and FD_{op}.

2.4.2 Parietal Lobe

Brodmann (1909) defined four areas (1, 2, 3, 43) in the postcentral region, whereas von Economo and Koskinas six (PA_1, PA_2, PB_1, PB_2, PC and PD). In the parietal region, Brodmann defined four areas (5, 7, 39, 40), and von Economo and Koskinas nine (PED, PE_m, PE_p, PE_γ, PF, PF_t, PF_{op}, PF_{cm} and PG). The basal parietal region PH most likely belongs to the visual cortex and includes the functionally defined areas V4 and V5 (Zilles and Palomero-Gallagher 2001). The proposed subdivisions of the anterior parietal cortex by von Economo and Koskinas are still in use.

Area PA is located in the depths of the central sulcus. Area PB is "sensory koniocortex", located on the caudal bank of the central sulcus. Concerning the primary somatosensory cortical areas and the subdivision of the posterior parietal lobe into a superior and an inferior lobule, the accepted terminology of von

Economo and Koskinas forms the basis for modern cytoarchitectonic analyses and experiments in primates (Zilles 2004). Brodmann did not delineate any transition zones in the posterior parietal lobe, whereas von Economo and Koskinas marked such transition zones between the areas P*E*, P*F*, P*G*, P*H* and O*A*, in agreement with the observations of Eidelberg and Galaburda (1984).

Beyond the standard modifications, transition parietal areas are PC_γ, P*E(D)*, P*FD* and PF_m. Areas PC_γ and PF_m denote cellular variations containing giant pyramidal and magnocellular neurons, respectively. Area P*E(D)* is a variant of area P*E* with an admixture of the neighboring cortical type P*D*. The functionally defined secondary somatosensory cortex (SII) is located in the parietal operculum, hidden within the Sylvian fissure. Brodmann areas 40 and 43 extend into the parietal operculum and are candidates for SII on topographic grounds; they partially correspond to the opercular modification PF_{op} and to the subcentral area P*FD*, respectively. In the supramarginal gyrus of the rostral inferior parietal cortex, von Economo and Koskinas subdivide Brodmann area 40 into the five areas P*F*, PF_{cm}, PF_m, PF_{op} and PF_t, confirmed in general lines by Caspers et al. (2006). In the caudal inferior parietal cortex, Caspers et al. (2006) distinguish a caudal region termed P*G*p and a rostral region termed P*G*a, this latter fitting to area P*G* in the angular gyrus (roughly Brodmann area 39).

2.4.3 Temporal Lobe and Insula

Based on pathological and physiological considerations, von Economo (1927, 2009) localized the understanding of word *speech* in area TA_1 of the left hemisphere, the understanding of word *sense* in the caudal transitional region of area TA_1 towards area P*F*, and the understanding of *music* in area TA_2 and the temporal pole; the appreciation of higher tones in parts in the bottom of the Sylvian fissure, while that of lower tones more towards outer portions. Area T*C* is koniocortex, i.e. sensory cortex representing *primary audition*, and receiving fibers from the medial geniculate body.

Von Economo and Horn (1930) investigated the cytoarchitectonics of the auditory cortex further in the adult and juvenile human brain. They found the superior temporal surface and the length of the Sylvian fissure larger on the left side. Initial attempts at investigating the cytoarchitectonics of the auditory cortex by Campbell (1905), Rosenberg (1907) and Brodmann (1909), who had identified it with Brodmann area 41, had missed the most characteristic feature that this area shares with all other "sensory" cortices, i.e. the "granularity" (Meyer 1977); that was first described by von Economo and Koskinas (1925). Von Economo and Horn (1930) attribute the striking variations in size among individuals and between the two hemispheres possibly to handedness or differences in musicality.

The koniocortex of the human temporal lobe encompasses areas T*C* and T*D* and is located on Heschl's gyrus (transverse temporal gyrus); area T*A* contains Wernicke's speech area, while the cerebral "belt" areas most likely correspond to areas T*A* and T*B* (Chiry et al. 2003; Webster and Garey 1990). Within the area T*C*, which closely corresponds to the "core" region of Hackett et al. (2001), von Economo and Horn (1930) describe 11 distinct types of granular cortex. The "belt" field of the human auditory cortex, on the other hand, seems to correspond to the medial portion of the koniocortical T*D* sector of von Economo and Koskinas (1925).

In sections cut perpendicularly to the radial orientation of layer III apical dendrites, the small pyramidal cells are arranged in short radial columns that partially extend into layers II and IV (Hackett et al. 2001); such a feature seems to correspond to what von Economo and Koskinas called the "rain shower formation" (Fig. 2.4). With regard to the columnar organization of the belt region, layer III pyramidal cells are arranged in organized vertical columns, which von Economo and Koskinas called the "organ pipe formation".

Von Economo and Koskinas (1925) and von Economo and Horn (1930) were among the first investigators to notice individual differences of the auditory fields and marked asymmetries between the two hemispheres: Heschl's gyrus is generally single and longer on the left side and double and shorter on the right side; the *planum temporale* (located caudally to Heschl's gyrus, in area T*B*) is larger on the left side (Webster and Garey 1990). Such asymmetries may underscore the modern idea of a functional differentiation of the two cerebral hemispheres and the predilection of the left hemisphere (right ear) for verbal tests, and that of the right hemisphere (left ear) for music recognition (Brodal 1981).

In contrast to Brodmann, von Economo and Koskinas divide the medial temporal lobe into a rostral area T*G* and two caudal areas, T*H* and T*F*, with area T*G* further subdivided into a medial area TG_a and a larger lateral area T*G* (Suzuki and Amaral 2003). Like Elliot Smith (1907), von Economo and Koskinas also illustrate the temporal polar cortex as being continuous with the anteroventral portion of the medial temporal lobe. The nomenclature and cortical demarcations of Brodmann (1909) regarding the medial temporal lobe in primates is somewhat vague and varying across species, whereas the analyses of von Economo and Koskinas are more detailed (Suzuki and Amaral 2003). Areas T*F* and T*H* belong to the posterior part of the parahippocampal gyrus; the anterior part of the parahippocampal gyrus comprises mainly the entorhinal cortex and the associated perirhinal cortex (Amaral and Insausti 1990). Area T*J* seems to be homologous to the hyperchromic, coarse-cell temporopolar peripaleocortex in the macaque (de Olmos 1990). Besides area T*J* the peripaleocortical agranular claustral region (Brodmann area 16 in the *Cercopithecus*) is also homologous to a certain extent to the human area I*D* (Zilles 2004).

The insula includes areas IA_1, IA_2, I*B*, I*C* and I*D*. The gradual transition of area I*A* backwards over the central sulcus of the insula to area I*B* is denoted by von Economo and Koskinas as area I*AB*, which is characterized by a condensation of the granular layers and a reduction of pyramidal cell size.

2.4.4 Occipital Lobe

The primary visual area or striate cortex is area O*C*, the parastriate cortex is area O*B*, and the peristriate cortex is area O*A*. A borderzone at the boundaries of Brodmann areas 17 and 18, containing giant pyramidal cells in the lower part of layer III, is area O*B*$_\gamma$ *(limes parastriatus gigantopyramidalis)*. The total surface of koniocortex in the visual sensory sphere (area O*C*) in both hemispheres was estimated at about 50 cm^2 and the total number of cells at about 1.4×10^9, i.e. 10 % of the total number of neurons of the entire cerebral cortex. Thus, the area striata appears four times richer in cells than any other cortical region (Koskinas 1969; von Economo 1927; von Economo and Koskinas 2008).

2.4.5 Superior Limbic and Inferior Limbic (Hippocampal) Gyrus

One concern in the localization of functions in the human cerebral hemispheres is the boundary between the retrosplenial/cingulate and the parahippocampal cortices. Brodmann (1909) depicted the retrosplenial cortex as fully surrounding the posterior and ventral edge of the splenium of the corpus callosum. Von Economo (1927, 2009) provided the first subregional map of the posterior cingulate gyrus and showed a termination of the retrosplenial areas L*E* and L*D* at a plane caudal but not ventral to the splenium (Vogt et al. 2001).

Every section through the retrosplenial cortex includes a segment of allocortical hippocampus and ectosplenial area L*F*. At allocortical-isocortical transition points in the primate telencephalon, modern anatomists recognize the concept of a "dysgranular" cytoarchitecture (a weakly defined layer IV); such points are found in orbitofrontal, insular, and anterior and posterior cingulate cortices (Vogt et al. 2001). Ngowyang (1934) had described a "dysgranular region" in the frontal lobe, associated with areas F*C* and F*CL*. Going forward, the granular layer appears sporadically, making this area "hypogranular" or "dysgranular"; forward of Brodmann area 6, the prefrontal cortex, and continuing through the frontal pole, the cortex is "eugranular" (DeMyer 1988).

The area L*D* is dysgranular rather than agranular, as it was originally thought (Vogt et al. 2001); its layer IV has a variable thickness, interrupted by large SMI-32 immunopositive neurons in the sublayers IIIc and Va. Brodmann (1909) referred to area 30 as agranular. Von Economo (1927, 2009) was quite explicit that area L*D* is not merely agranular, but that the "granulous" layer of area L*E* is not continuous with the isocortical layer of area L*C*$_2$. Von Economo vacillated on the presence of a layer IV in area L*D* and showed a layer III(IV) below layer III. A dysgranular layer IV has a variable thickness and may even disappear as the neurons of the sublayers IIIc and Va intermingle. The dysgranular concept for a cortical architecture was obviously not defined during the early years of cortical cytoarchitectonics in terms of the chemical signature of neurons, since histochemical methods were not available. In a series of studies spanning over 30 years, Vogt et al. (2001) have described in the primate brain the dysgranular nature of area LD and its profound differences with the cytoarchitecture of the granular Brodmann area 23a.

The inferior limbic lobe comprises the hippocampal gyrus from the isthmus until near the temporal pole and contains the entire uncinate gyrus, the subiculum, the dentate gyrus and Ammon's horn. Above the splenium, the hippocampal rudiment, the indusium griseum, or areas LB_2 and HF, there is a single layer of densely packed SMI-32 (nonphosphorylated neurofilament) immunopositive neurons. Adjacent to the indusium griseum is the subicular rudiment or area HE, which has fewer and more dispersed neurons. These two areas together form the fasciolate gyrus on the dorsal surface of the corpus callosum (Vogt et al. 2001).

2.5 Discussion

Brodmann maps are commonly used to either designate cytoarchitectonic areas as such, or as a "shorthand system" to designate some region on the cerebral *surface* (DeMyer 1988). Macroscopic extrapolation of Brodmann projection maps are effected on the atlas of Talairach and Tournoux (1988), rather than being based on real microscopic cytoarchitectonics. Such specifications of Brodmann areas may lead to erroneous results in delineating cortical regions, something that may in turn lead to erroneous hypotheses regarding the involvement of specific brain systems in normal or pathological situations (Uylings et al. 2005).

Von Economo (1927, 2009) was the first to use subregional maps, which are invaluable in resolving difficult topological problems (Fig. 2.7). Talairach and Tournoux (1988) emphasize the shortcoming of Brodmann's reconstruction technique in not distinguishing areas on the gyral surfaces from areas in the sulcal depths, something may lead to miscalculations of the depth of the callosal sulcus and related areas, and placing e.g. Brodmann areas 29 and 30 on gyral surfaces. Because the architecture of each cortical area cannot yet be determined by the current imaging modalities, it is imperative that standardized atlases seeking to localize specific areas rely heavily on neuroanatomical observations, rather than Brodmann's reconstructions onto the convoluted human brain surface (Vogt et al. 2001).

On the other hand, the *perpendicular* sectioning method of von Economo and Koskinas (1925, 2008), which was consistently used to analyze the dome, wall and floor of each cortical gyrus, practically solves the generalized mapmaker's problem of flattening nonconvex polyhedral surfaces (Schwartz et al. 1989), which also constitutes a core problem in cortical research.

Microscopically-defined borders usually differ from gross anatomical landmarks; cytoarchitectonics reflect the inner organization of cortical areas and their morphofunctional correlates (Zilles 2004). Despite the integration of multifactorial descriptors such as chemoarchitecture, angioarchitecture, neurotransmitter,

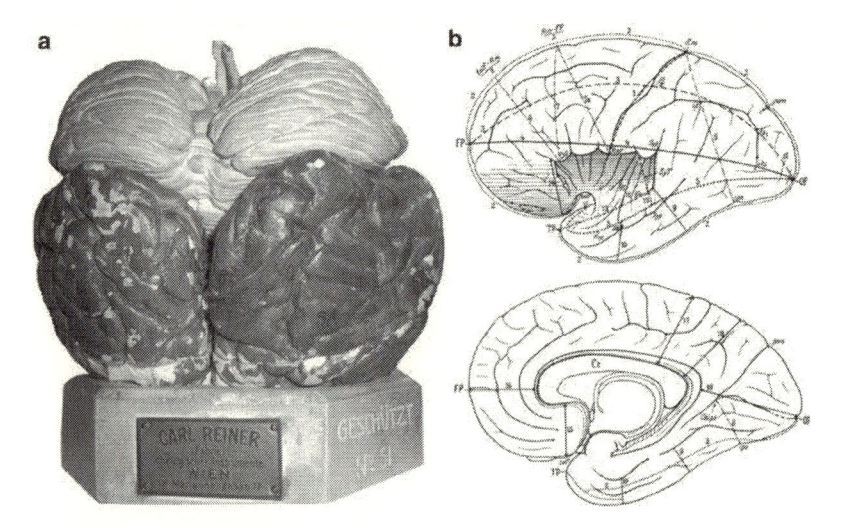

Fig. 2.7 (a) A plaster model of the human brain made in the 1920s, with cytoarchitectonics marked according to the system of von Economo and Koskinas (1925, 2008), used by von Economo (2009) for his lectures (courtesy of Fabrikation Chirurgischer Instrumente Carl Reiner GmbH, Vienna). (b) Schematic drawing of 26 encephalometric constants in the lateral and medial cerebral hemispheric facies, suggested by von Economo (1929) on the basis of macroscopic and cytoarchitectonic criteria as reference points, for future studies to determined variations among individuals, gender and talent differences, and alterations associated with nervous and mental diseases

receptor and gene expression patterns, as well as white matter tracts, it is clear that the knowledge of the classical anatomy remains fundamental (Toga and Thompson 2007). The structure of the cerebral cortical layers incorporates, and reflects, the form of their constitutive cells and functional connections; the underpinnings of neuronal connectivity at the microscopic level are paramount to interpreting any macroscopic clue yielded by neuroimaging studies.

The century-long endurance of the cytoarchitectonic analyses of Brodmann (1909) and of von Economo and Koskinas (1925) is in part due to the fact that these brain scientists did not hypothesize much about function; their only supposition was that anatomical subdivisions reflect functional variations, and that future functional and clinical studies would validate their anatomical subdivisions. In fact, there are examples of such cytoarchitectonic subdivisions in the motor, parietal and striate cortex that reflect functional differentiation to an unexpected degree (Bartels and Zeki 2005).

In a similar line of reasing, Koskinas (1926) argued: "The mind has its organic locus, its seat, its altar in the cerebral cortex. That is why one may be justified in claiming that the anatomical and the physiological exploration of that noblest of the organs deserves the utmost attention of science." And later wrote: "Provided that, as a general principle, each physiological function presupposes a corresponding anatomical basis, one understands how important the study of brain structure becomes. From a precise knowledge of the structure of the cerebral cortex, we may expect to shed light upon issues of the utmost importance, such as the anatomical basis of mental phenomena and the relationship between certain attributes and brain structure. But can we not hypothesize that the limitations of anatomically tracing deficits of the mind is simply a matter of the sophistication of our methods and the acuity of our foresight?" (Koskinas 1931).

The underlying concept is that cytoarchitectonic differences indicate functional differences (the "neural hardware" that includes cell types, connectivity, synaptic interactions and molecular events) and that functional differences necessitate cytoarchitectonic differences; by being "blind" with respect to function, the cytoarchitectonics approach ensures a degree of objectivity and data longevity, since observers document mere facts (Bartels and Zeki 2005).

Modern "probabilistic" atlases of the human brain bridge high-resolution in vivo data with neurocytology, and spatially normalize them to a common reference space; thus, they provide the means for moving from a descriptive to a hypothesis-driven science (Mazziotta et al. 1995). Nonetheless, in hypothesis-driven neuroimaging research, the interpretation of findings may vary depending on the specific paradigm, and attributing a function to a given area rarely goes unchallenged (Bartels and Zeki 2005).

In the fad of "cognitive brain mapping" and its purported representations in the human brain, color images generated by software can be adjusted to denote so-called "activations" with much ambiguity, and occasionally lead to fallacious findings unworthy of attempted replication. "Functional segregation", i.e. the common notion that mental functions are localized in cell clusters at specific cortical sites, is based on the old, hard-dying conception that a particular conscious process must have a delineated seat in the brain (Smith 2010), as "modern phrenologists, equipped with the powerful tools of functional MRI, seek to relate tiny pseudo-colored patches of slightly enhanced cortical activity associated with some limited cognitive function to an underlying structural correlate" (Jones 2008).

Functional MRI, as one technique that allows a correlation between structure and function, has limitations insofar as the measurements are not in real time and the spatial resolution only recently reached the mm level. Even the hypothetical development of a technique, which would noninvasively image neural activity at a spatial resolution of 1 mm and a temporal resolution of 1 msec, would still appear coarse relative to the size of the neuronal soma (5–100 μm) or the synaptic gap (20–40 nm) (Hougan and Altevogt 2008).

A key element in defining cortical areas is connectivity, and the guiding principle of neurohistologists that cortical areas form parts of connectional networks is now being adopted by the neuroimaging community; besides the streams of intrinsic cortico-cortical connections, no cortical area is without re-entrant projections from the thalamus, while each cortical area is undoubtedly governed, like the thalamocortical connections, by ontogenetic mechanisms (Jones 2008).

Particular emphasis on the U-shaped fibers of the frontal lobe and its connections with subcortical nuclei of the thalamus and the medial temporal lobe was placed by Christfried Jakob in his hodological approach of the early 1900s (Théodoridou and Triarhou 2012). Those pathways are currently emphasized in imaging studies (Catani et al. 2012). Jakob had identified all the major tracts of the limbic circuitry early on, preceding James W. Papez (1883–1958) by almost three decades (Triarhou 2008, 2009). Bearing a direct relevance to the clinic, Jakob's network approach provided a prescient anatomical framework for the concept of "diaschisis" – as elaborated by Constantin von Monakow (1853–1930) in 1914 to highlight the possible recovery of dysfunctional distant regions connected to destroyed areas – and for what would eventually become an intense area of research on the neural underpinnings of memory, emotion and behavioral disorders associated with frontal lobe damage (Catani and Stuss 2012).

As the necessity emerges to move from brain localization to connectivity imaging, methods such as high-resolution two-photon imaging are used to visualize functionally-defined afferent inputs on cortical dendritic spines in vivo with single-synapse resolution (Chen et al. 2011), and the relationship between structure and function in cortical synaptic circuits is studied by combining in vivo physiology with network anatomy. For example, a functional property of specific cortical neurons can be characterized by two-photon calcium imaging and a portion of these neurons' local interconnections can be traced with large-scale electron microscopy of serial thin sections (Bock et al. 2011). Thus, it is becoming possible to address hitherto intractable neurobiological questions through the technological advances that permit the combination of functional imaging and neuronal wiring (Briggman et al. 2011) through a high-speed reconstruction of neurite connectivity while performing reliable analyses of large neuroanatomical datasets (Helmstaedter et al. 2011).

The novel approaches for analyzing brain imaging data aim at providing levels of specificity with narrower confidence intervals in determining the dynamics of local neural population responses to their native temporal resolution (Tyler and Likova 2011). Furthermore, to better understand the anatomical organization of structures that form the basis of cognitive information processing, morphological data may be distilled and synthesized into a single interactive visualization that represents a fundamental blueprint upon which cognitive functions must be implemented (Solari and Stoner 2011). In such a framework, functional circuits corresponding to memory, cognition and cortical information flow are described in terms of distinguishable neuronal groups and cortical systems in order to elucidate the basis of distinct homotypical cognitive architecture in multiple independent visualizations that constitute an annotated view of "neuroanatomical consilience" (Solari and Stoner 2011).

Acknowledgments The author gratefully acknowledges the support of Karger Publishers, the Bodossakis Foundation, the Academy of Athens, the Hellenic Ministry of National Education, the Hellenic Neurological Society, and the University of Macedonia in his effort to revive the neuroanatomical works of von Economo and Koskinas, as well as the invaluable encouragement by the family members of the two eminent scientists.

References

Amaral DG, Insausti R (1990) Hippocampal formation. In: Paxinos G (ed) The human nervous system. Academic, San Diego, pp 711–755

Bailey P, von Bonin G (1951) The isocortex of man. University of Illinois Press, Urbana

Bartels A, Zeki S (2005) The chronoarchitecture of the cerebral cortex. Philos Trans R Soc Lond [Biol Sci] 360:733–750

Bock DD, Allen Lee W-C, Kerlin AM, Andermann ML, Hood G, Wetzel AW, Yurgenson S, Soucy ER, Kim HS, Reid RC (2011) Network anatomy and in vivo physiology of visual cortical neurons. Nature 471:177–182

Briggman KL, Helmstaedter M, Denk W (2011) Wiring specificity in the direction-selectivity circuit of the retina. Nature 471:183–188

Brodal A (1981) Neurological anatomy in relation to clinical medicine. Oxford University Press, Oxford

Brodmann K (1909) Vergleichende Lokalisationslehre der Großhirnrinde. J.A. Barth, Leipzig

Campbell AW (1905) Histological studies on the localization of cerebral function. Cambridge University Press, Cambridge

Caspers S, Geyer S, Schleicher A, Mohlberg H, Amunts K, Zilles K (2006) The human inferior parietal cortex: cytoarchitectonic parcellation and interindividual variability. Neuroimage 33:430–448

Catani M, Stuss DR (2012) At the forefront of clinical neuroscience. Cortex 48:1–6

Catani M, Dell'Acqua F, Vergani F, Malik F, Hodge H, Roy P, Valabregue R, Thiebaut de Schotten M (2012) Short frontal lobe connections of the human brain. Cortex 48:273–291

Chen X, Leischner U, Rochefort NL, Nelken I, Konnerth A (2011) Functional mapping of single spines in cortical neurons in vivo. Nature 475:501–505

Chiry O, Tardif E, Magistretti PJ, Clarke S (2003) Patterns of calcium-binding proteins support parallel and hierarchical organization of human auditory areas. Eur J Neurosci 17:397–410

de Olmos J (1990) Amygdaloid nuclear gray complex. In: Paxinos G (ed) The human nervous system. Academic, San Diego, pp 583–710

DeMyer W (1988) Neuroanatomy. Harwal Publishing, Malvern

Eidelberg D, Galaburda AM (1984) Inferior parietal lobule: divergent architectonic asymmetries in the human brain. Arch Neurol 41:843–852

Elliot Smith G (1907) A new topographical survey of the human cerebral cortex, being an account of the distribution of the anatomically distinct cortical areas and their relationship to the cerebral sulci. J Anat Physiol (Lond) 41:237–254

Garey LJ (2006) Brodmann's localisation in the cerebral cortex. Springer, New York

Hackett TA, Preuss TM, Kaas JH (2001) Architectonic identification of the core region in auditory cortex of macaques, chimpanzees, and humans. J Comp Neurol 441:197–222

Helmstaedter M, Briggman KL, Denk W (2011) High-accuracy neurite reconstruction for high-throughput neuroanatomy. Nat Neurosci 14:1081–1088

Hougan M, Altevogt B (2008) From molecules to minds—challenges for the 21st century: workshop summary. National Academies, Washington, DC

Jakob C (1939) Folia neurobiológica Argentina, Atlas I: El cerebro humano—su anatomía sistemática y topográfica. Aniceto López Editor, Buenos Aires

Jakob C (1941) Folia neurobiológica Argentina, Tomo I: neurobiología general. Aniceto López Editor, Buenos Aires

Jones EG (2008) Cortical maps and modern phrenology. Brain 131:2227–2233

Jones EG (2010) Cellular structure of the human cerebral cortex. Brain 133:945–946

Koskinas GN (1926) Cytoarchitectonics of the human cerebral cortex. Proc Athens Med Soc 92:44–48

Koskinas GN (1931) Scientific works published in German. Pyrsus, Athens

Koskinas GN (1969) Lobus occipitalis: makroskopische und mikroskopische Beschreibung. Privately Published, Athens

Mazziotta JC, Toga AW, Evans AC, Fox PT, Lancaster JL (1995) Digital brain atlases. Trends Neurosci 18:210–211

Meyer A (1977) The search for a morphological substrate in the brains of eminent persons including musicians: a historical review. In: Critchley M, Henson RA (eds) Music and the brain: studies in the neurology of music. William Heinemann, London, pp 255–281

Ngowyang G (1934) Die Cytoarchitektonik des menschlichen Stirnhirns I. Cytoarchitektonische Felderung der Regio granularis und Regio dysgranularis. Monogr Natl Res Inst Psychol Acad Sin (Shanghai) 7:1–68

Pandya DN, Sanides F (1973) Architectonic parcellation of the temporal operculum in rhesus monkey and its projection pattern. Z Anat Entwickl-Geschichte 139:127–161

Rosenberg L (1907) Histologische Untersuchung über die Cytoarchitektonik der Heschl'schen Windungen. Neurol Cbl 14:685–686

Sanides F (1962) Die Architektonik des menschlichen Stirnhirns. Springer, Berlin/Göttingen/Heidelberg

Sanides F (1964) The cyto-myeloarchitecture of the human frontal lobe and its relation to phylogenetic differentiation of the cerebral cortex. J Hirnforsch 47:269–282

Schwartz EL, Shaw A, Wolfson E (1989) A numerical solution to the generalized mapmaker's problem: flattening nonconvex polyhedral surfaces. IEEE Trans Pattern Anal Mach Intell 11:1005–1008

Smith DF (2010) Cognitive brain mapping for better or worse. Perspect Biol Med 53:321–329

Solari SVH, Stoner R (2011) Cognitive consilience: primate non-primary neuroanatomical circuits underlying cognition. Front Neuroanat 5:1–23. doi:10.3389/fnana.2011.00065 (article 65)

Suzuki WA, Amaral DG (2003) Where are the perirhinal and parahippocampal cortices? A historical overview of the nomenclature and boundaries applied to the primate medial temporal lobe. Neuroscience 120:893–906

Talairach J, Tournoux P (1988) Co-planar stereotaxic atlas of the human brain. 3-dimensional proportional system: an approach to cerebral imaging (trans: Rayport M). G. Thieme Verlag, Stuttgart

Théodoridou ZD, Triarhou LC (2012) Challenging the supremacy of the frontal lobe: early views (1906–1909) of Christfried Jakob on the human cerebral cortex. Cortex 48:15–25

Toga AW, Thompson PM (2007) What is where and why it is important. Neuroimage 37:1045–1049

Triarhou LC (2005) Georg N. Koskinas (1885–1975) and his scientific contributions to the normal and pathological anatomy of the human brain. Brain Res Bull 68:121–139

Triarhou LC (2006) The signalling contributions of Constantin von Economo to basic, clinical and evolutionary neuroscience. Brain Res Bull 69:223–243

Triarhou LC (2007a) The Economo-Koskinas atlas revisited: cytoarchitectonics and functional context. Stereotact Funct Neurosurg 85:195–203

Triarhou LC (2007b) A proposed number system for the 107 cortical areas of Economo and Koskinas, and Brodmann area correlations. Stereot Funct Neurosurg 85:204–215

Triarhou LC (2008) Centenary of Christfried Jakob's discovery of the visceral brain: an unheeded precedence in affective neuroscience. Neurosci Biobehav Rev 32:984–1000

Triarhou LC (2009) Tripartite concepts of mind and brain, with special emphasis on the neuroevolutionary postulates of Christfried Jakob and Paul MacLean. In: Weingarten SP, Penat HO (eds) Cognitive psychology research developments. Nova, Hauppauge, pp 183–208

Triarhou LC (2010) Revisiting Christfried Jakob's concept of the dual onto-phylogenetic origin and ubiquitous function of the cerebral cortex: a century of progress. Brain Struct Funct 214:319–338

Triarhou LC (2012) Cytoarchitectonics of the human cerebral cortex: the 1926 presentation by Georg N. Koskinas (1885–1975) to the Athens Medical Society. In: Bright P (ed) Neuroimaging—cognitive and clinical neuroscience. InTech Publishers, Rijeka/Vienna, pp 1–16

Triarhou LC, del Cerro M (2006) Semicentennial tribute to the ingenious neurobiologist Christfried Jakob (1866–1956)—2. Publications from the second Argentina period, 1913–1949. Eur Neurol 56:189–198

Tyler CW, Likova LT (2011) Estimating neural signal dynamics in the human brain. Front Syst Neurosci 5:1–17. doi:10.3389/fnsys.2011.00033 (article 33)

Uylings HBM, Rajkowska G, Sanz-Arigita E, Amunts K, Zilles K (2005) Consequences of large interindividual variability for human brain atlases: converging macroscopical imaging and microscopical neuroanatomy. Anat Embryol 210:423–431

van Bogaert L, Théodoridès J (1979) Constantin von Economo: the man and the scientist. Verlag der Österreichischen Akademie der Wissenschaften, Vienna

Vogt O (1927) Architektonik der menschlichen Hirnrinde. Zbl Gesamte Neurol Psychiatrie 45:510–512

Vogt C, Vogt O (1919) Allgemeinere Ergebnisse unserer Hirnforschung. J Psychol Neurol (Leipz) 25:279–461

Vogt BA, Vogt LJ, Perl DP, Hof PR (2001) Cytology of human caudomedial cingulate, retrosplenial, and caudal parahippocampal cortices. J Comp Neurol 438:353–376

von Bonin G (1950) Essay on the cerebral cortex. Charles C. Thomas, Springfield

von Economo C (1925) Die fünf Bautypen der Grosshirnrinde. Schweiz Arch Neurol Psychiatrie 16:260–269

von Economo C (1927) Zellaufbau der Grosshirnrinde des Menschen: Zehn Vorlesungen. Julius Springer, Berlin

von Economo C (1929) Wie sollen wir Elitegehirne verarbeiten? Z Gesamte Neurol Psychiatrie 121:323–409

von Economo C (2009) Cellular structure of the human cerebral cortex (trans, ed: Triarhou LC). Karger, Basel

von Economo C, Horn L (1930) Über Windungsrelief, Maße und Rindenarchitektonik der Supratemporalfläche, ihre individuellen und ihre Seitenunterschiede. Z Gesamte Neurol Psychiatrie 130:678–757

von Economo C, Koskinas GN (1923) Die sensiblen Zonen des Großhirns. Klin Wochenschr 2:905

von Economo C, Koskinas GN (1925) Die Cytoarchitektonik der Hirnrinde des Erwachsenen Menschen: Textband und Atlas mit 112 Mikrophotographischen Tafeln. Springer, Vienna

von Economo C, Koskinas GN (2008) Atlas of cytoarchitectonics of the adult human cerebral cortex (trans, rev, ed: Triarhou LC). Karger, Basel

Watson KK, Jones TK, Allman JM (2006) Dendritic architecture of the von Economo neurons. Neuroscience 141:1107–1112

Webster WR, Garey LJ (1990) Auditory system. In: Paxinos G (ed) The human nervous system. Academic, San Diego, pp 889–944

Zilles K (2004) Architecture of the human cerebral cortex: regional and laminar organization. In: Paxinos G, Mai JK (eds) The human nervous system, 2nd edn. Elsevier/Academic, Amsterdam/London, pp 997–1055

Zilles K, Amunts K (2010) Centenary of Brodmann's map: conception and fate. Nat Rev Neurosci 11:139–145

Zilles K, Amunts K (2012) Architecture of the cerebral cortex. In: Mai JK, Paxinos G (eds) The human nervous system, 3rd edn. Elsevier/Academic, Amsterdam/London, pp 836–895

Zilles K, Palomero-Gallagher N (2001) Cyto-, myelo-, and receptor architectonics of the human parietal cortex. Neuroimage 14:S8–S20

Made in the USA
Columbia, SC
01 December 2023

52461e31-f828-4ab9-8443-f450b75eb2cfR01